D1597041

Strategic Practice Management

Second Edition

Strategic Practice Management

Business and Procedural Considerations

Second Edition

Robert G. Glaser, PhD
Robert M. Traynor, EdD, MBA

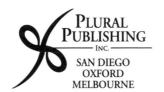

PLURAL
PUBLISHING
— INC. —
SAN DIEGO
OXFORD
MELBOURNE

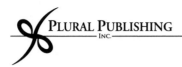

PLURAL PUBLISHING
INC.

5521 Ruffin Road
San Diego, CA 92123

e-mail: info@pluralpublishing.com
Web site: http://www.pluralpublishing.com

Library of Congress Cataloging-in-Publication Data

Glaser, Robert (Robert G.)
  Strategic practice management : business and procedural considerations / Robert G.
Glaser, Robert M. Traynor.—2nd ed.
      p. ; cm.
  Includes bibliographical references and index.
  ISBN-13: 978-1-59756-522-6 (alk. paper)
  ISBN-10: 1-59756-522-9 (alk. paper)
  I. Traynor, Robert M. II. Title.
  [DNLM: 1. Practice Management, Medical—organization & administration.
2. Audiology—organization & administration. WV 270]

  617.80068—dc23
                                                      2012049153

Contents

Foreword by Brad A. Stach   vii

Acknowledgments   ix

Contributors   xii

Prologue: Leadership and Successful Practice Management   xiii
by Robert G. Glaser, PhD

1   **The Economic Realities and Competitive Landscape of Audiology Private Practice**   1
Robert M. Traynor, EdD, MBA

2   **Strategic Business Planning**   39
Robert M. Traynor, EdD, MBA

3   **Legal Considerations in Practice Management**   75
Glenn L. Bower, JD, and Michael G. Leesman, JD

4   **Ethical Considerations in Private Practice**   97
Jane M. Kukula, AuD

5   **Fundamentals of Marketing the Audiology Practice**   119
Robert M. Traynor, EdD, MBA

6   **Effective Marketing: Developing and Growing the Practice**   161
Kevin D. St. Clergy, MS

7   **Optimizing Pricing Strategies for the Practice**   195
Robert M. Traynor, EdD, MBA

8   **Fiscal Monitoring: Cash Flow Analysis**   243
Robert M. Traynor, EdD, MBA

9   **Coding, Reimbursement, and Practice Management**   289
Debra Abel, AuD

10   **Policy and Procedures Manual**   335
Robert G. Glaser, PhD

11   **Patient Management**   357
Robert G. Glaser, PhD

12 **Supporting Practice Success: Counseling Considerations**   **389**
for Patient and Employee Management
John Greer Clark, PhD

13 **Referral Source Management**   **403**
Robert G. Glaser, PhD

14 **Personnel Management**   **415**
Robert G. Glaser, PhD

15 **Career Management: What It Takes to Make It**   **429**
Patrick N. Mangino, AuD

16 **Compensation Strategies**   **443**
Robert M. Traynor, EdD, MBA

17 **Hearing Instrument Manufacturers and Suppliers**   **469**
Robert G. Glaser, PhD

18 **Practice Management Considerations in a University**   **491**
Audiology Clinic
Gail M. Whitelaw, PhD, MHA

19 **Transitions: Optimizing Entry and Exit Strategies**   **513**
Gail M. Whitelaw, PhD, MHA

Index   539

Foreword

The founder of Plural Publishing, Dr. Sadanand Singh, began his career as an academician. He was a professor of speech science who took his love for knowledge and turned it into the business of selling books. And by creating this business, he helped us all to gain and share that knowledge. Dr. Singh knew well that the only way he could be successful in sharing knowledge was to run a successful business.

The provision of health care is no different, of course. Those of us who practice the profession of audiology do so to help people. Traditionally, we were brought up to think of ourselves as being part of a "helping" profession. The idea of profiting while providing this help was made to seem almost crass; so much so, in fact, that as students we were traditionally not exposed to the business side of health care. But we eventually came to the realization that we cannot help anyone if we do not make money. The businesses we work in need to be financially successful in order for us to take care of our patients.

The business of audiology has changed as dramatically as the profession itself over the last seven decades. The profession of audiology in the United States owes much of its heritage to the aural rehabilitation programs that were developed in the military hospitals during World War II. Early practices developed in the newly formed Veteran's Admin-istration hospitals, in rehabilitation and hospital settings, and in educational institutions. Training programs developed alongside the profession of speech pathology, largely in colleges of education or arts and sciences. The prospect of understanding the nuance of the business side of a health care private practice was years away.

When we fast-forward a half-century, the landscape of the profession is vastly changed. Audiologists are now recognized by the federal government as "health diagnosing and treating practitioners." Audiologists hold state licenses to practice and are credentialed by third-party payers. They are doctoral-level practitioners in diverse health care, private practice, and group practice settings. The business model has been transformed. It is now not only not crass to talk about making money, but also essential to talk about making money.

The second edition of Glaser and Traynor's *Strategic Practice Management* is about the business of audiology. Together, Glaser and Traynor bring decades of practical experience in their own very successful private practices. They have rearranged the content of this second edition and assembled additional contributors to expand their coverage of practice ethics, economic influences, marketing, compliance, counseling, and career management.

Whether you are a student, an independent practitioner, a clinician employed in an audiology/ENT practice or hospital, educational audiologist, or manager of a university-based clinic, this second edition contains information that is essential to the operation and business management of your practice setting. This excellent text is an informative resource for any health care practitioner considering a start-up venture, purchasing an ongoing practice, reinventing their current practice, or interested in sharpening their clinical service delivery model in today's competitive and dynamic health care marketplace.

For the practice of audiology to thrive in the current tumult that is health care, sound business practice is essential. If we are going to continue to help people with their hearing care needs, we will to need to run our businesses successfully. This book lays the foundation for that success.

Brad A. Stach, PhD
Director, Division of Audiology
Department of
    Otolaryngology—Head
    and Neck Surgery
Henry Ford Hospital
Editor-in-Chief
Plural Audiology

Acknowledgments

I am fortunate to have a satisfying career rich in the interest, support, and guidance of personal and professional role models and mentors. Thank you for all that you have provided over many years: Kenneth W. Berger, PhD, Joseph P. Millin, PhD, John R. Alway, DO, A. Lee Fisher, RPh, Floyd E. Billette, OD, Michael J. Setty, MHA, Michael Kincaid, CPA, and William Forsthoefel, CPA. My goal was to exceed your expectations in all that I was to do both clinically and in the business and financial management of my practice.

If you can find a hard-working, dedicated friend to partner with you in your professional career, I hope you are as fortunate as I have been over many years of professional collaboration in writings, presentations, and other practice management ventures to work with a respected colleague like Dr. Robert Traynor. His talent is seen in these pages and in his love for our profession.

Grateful thanks is extended to my associates at Audiology & Speech Associates of Dayton—they tolerated my inattention and covered the practice in their usual, excellent fashion.

Special thanks must go to each contributor to this second edition. Each is at the top of their respective game and their participation ensures an important range of critical information set forth with tremendous depth and focus.

I thank my immediate and extended family: my parents Helen and Robert, Sr.; my sister Gayle; M. J. Willhelm and Rosella Randolph; my daughter Erin and husband Mark and their children Oscar, Milo, Mary Jane, and Leo; and my sons Matthew and Graham.

Last, but certainly not least, special gratitude and appreciation goes to my wonderful wife, Annie. She goes through each day with such effortless style and grace, confirming that "all that is done for love's sake is not wasted and will never fade." She remains my inspiration and the light of my life, the shadow sewn to my soul. She is as well a tremendous editor and reviewer.

Robert G. Glaser, PhD

Acknowledgments

I have been blessed with tremendous opportunity in the field of audiology and a unique vantage point by which to observe the growth of our scope of practice and emergence of audiologists into the business world, not only in the United States but around the world. In addition to the "school of hard knocks," I have many friends, relatives, and colleagues to thank for my contribution as coauthor of the second edition of *Strategic Practice Management*. Initially a university professor, I began my private practice to pay for children to go to college and to augment a very meager income. I have not only built the practice but have had the experience of being a consulting audiologist for hearing aid and equipment manufacturers, serving as a member of research and development teams, as well as the opportunity to lecture on most aspects of audiology in over 40 countries. I learned much about the business of audiology and the hearing industry from good friends, Erich Spahr, Bruno Keller, Nicolai Krarup, Gustav Nussle, Patrick Perler, Stefan Schafroth, Christina Krauchi, Hoover Blessing, Arthur Schaub, and a number of other colleagues within the hearing industry. I have also learned much about international business operations from distributors within the industry, especially Brito Lousandro (Brazil), Barry Lin (China and Taiwan), Esam Khalil (United

Arab Emirates), Carlos Valdivia (Chile), and Mohammad Shabana (Egypt).

I want to recognize my friends and colleagues at the University of Florida, especially Alice Holmes, who in 1998 asked me to teach a business course for the UFL Doctor of Audiology Program; from which much of my material in this volume was generated.

I will never forget lifelong otolaryngology colleagues James H. Peterson, MD, Keith E. Peterson, MD, and Thomas T. Peterson, MD., who gave me my initial taste of audiology practice as a technician in 1972 performing audiograms for ENT exams and drug testing, which evolved into a 40-year audiology practice.

As most clinicians know, successful audiology practices are not organized and maintained by only one person. Without Karen S. Swope, AuD, audiology colleague for 20 years, and Barbara Jones, my office manager with the practice now for 28 years, the clinic may not have survived through some of those tough times. When distracted by international travel, manuscript preparation, teaching, and other activities, I can always depend on Barbara and Karen to insure that all the patients are seen, the bills are paid, and the practice continues.

I would also like to thank Col. Calvin Zen, MD, former State Surgeon Colorado Army National Guard, who gave me the chance to be his executive officer for a few years that ultimately was instrumental in allowing for retirement from the United States Army.

I cannot, of course, forget to mention Robert G. Glaser, PhD, a personal and professional friend for over 35 years and my partner in both editions of *Strategic Practice Management.* Dr. Glaser's taste for Italian cuisine and fine wine is only superseded by his passion for the field of audiology and its advancement into the medical private practice community. There are few true partners in book projects, but Bob is an exception. I sincerely thank Bob for his true partnership in completing both editions of this book and contributing his expertise in practice management, his steadfastness on task, his editorial skills, and, most of all, his friendship and counsel.

Certainly this work would have never been completed without the support from my family. I thank my daughter Alison and husband Michael Sarantakos, little Emma and their new child that will be with us soon, and my daughter Andrea J. Fuller, MD, Brian, and Henry, for their encouragement and love over the past year. I also want to remember my father, (the late) Robert M. Traynor, and my mother, Peggy L. Traynor, now 87, who taught me that with the right education and lots of hard work I could do anything.

And lastly I give special thanks to my wife, Krista; without her academic, moral, and inspirational support and unwavering love, my portion of this book would have never come to fruition. The person that knows you the best, of course, also knows your advantages, limitations, shortfalls, mistakes, anxieties, and aspirations. A supporter of Audiology Associates of Greeley, Inc., during its highs and lows, she is my partner in life and involved in virtually all of my successful projects. In the words of Ghandi, "Where there is love there is life." Krista gives so much life.

Robert M. Traynor, EdD, MBA

Contributors

Debra Abel, AuD
Arch Health Partners
Adjunct Instructor
A.T. Still University
Salus University
Poway, California
Chapter 9

Glenn L. Bower, JD
Attorney
Coolidge Wall Co., LPA
Dayton, Ohio
Chapter 3

John Greer Clark, PhD
Clark Audiology, LLC
Middletown, Ohio
Department of Communication
    Disorders
University of Cincinnati
Cincinnati, Ohio
Adjunct, Division of Communication
    Disorders
Louisville, Kentucky
Chapter 12

Kevin D. St. Clergy, MS
Audiologist, Chief Practice Building
    Expert, and CEO
EducatedPatients.com, LLC
Chapter 6

Jane M. Kukula, AUD, AAAF
Board certified in Audiology
Co-owner, Clinical Audiologist

Advanced Audiology Concepts
Mentor, Ohio
Chapter 4

Robert G. Glaser, PhD
President and CEO
Audiology Associates of Dayton, Inc.
(dba) Audiology and Speech Associates
Dayton, Ohio
Chapters 10, 11, 13, 14, and 17

Michael G. Leesman, JD
Attorney
Coolidge Wall Co., LPA
Dayton, Ohio
Chapter 3

Patrick N. Mangino, AuD
Member of the American Academy of
    Audiology
Westerville, Ohio
Chapter 15

Robert M. Traynor, EdD, MBA
President and CEO
Audiology Associates of Greeley
Greeley, Colorado
Chapters 1, 2, 5, 7, 8, and 16

Gail M. Whitelaw, PhD, MHA
Department of Speech and Hearing
    Science
Ohio State University
Columbus, Ohio
Chapters 18 and 19

Prologue

Leadership and Successful Practice Management

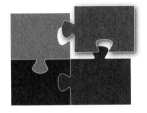

ROBERT G. GLASER, PhD

"Management is doing things right; leadership is doing the right thing."

— Peter Drucker, Founder of Modern Management

Introduction

Unquestionably, leadership skills permeate all that we do as clinicians. Patients rely on our professional skills as audiologists for the leadership needed to appropriately manage their hearing loss. Leadership skills are equally important in both matching their auditory needs with advanced technologies and managing the critical counseling interface with their family members and significant others in their lives. Leadership is critical to the success of our profession.

There are as many definitions of leadership as there are leaders. In a simple amalgamation, leadership can be defined as a process set into motion by an individual or a team of people to create a meaningful collaboration of focused thinking resulting in action(s) for a common purpose. Agreeing on a definition helps to focus on the topic; however, it is the varied critical elements, the components, that create the opportunities for leadership to work its particular magic.

Leadership is complicated, and the process of developing these skills does not evolve overnight. Leaders demonstrate many, distinct characteristics: competence, commitment, positive attitude, emotional strength, vision, focus, discipline, relationship building, responsibility, initiative, people skills; the list goes on. Many of these intermingled factors are intangible, and that is why leaders require so much seasoning to be effective in the venues of their influence.

Clinical Training and Leadership Skills

Talent is never enough (Maxwell, 2007). No person reaches his or her potential unless they are willing to practice their way there. Preparation positions talent and practice sharpens it. Practice enables development in the clinical domain. Clinicians get better at what they do when they have opportunities to see more patients. That is true, but there must be an important proviso: practice creates a better clinician as long as there is a guide, a mentor, a coach straightening the wrinkles and providing feedback on the functional characteristics of their interactions with patients and their families and significant others. Change is never easy but seemingly always essential to success. Guided change is essential to improving clinical skills and, in the long haul, improving patient outcomes. The difficult changes must be done in concert with direction and feedback from another source skilled at evaluation and promotion of better tactical use of whatever talent you bring to the mix. Max DePree, a preeminent leadership expert, recognized that people, in general and no matter the situation, are resistant to change: "We cannot become what we need to be remaining what we are" (DePree, 2004). His directives were clear; to sharpen your talent through guided practice, you need to do more than just be *open* to change; you have to *pursue* change. And that pursuit must be consistent and vigorous and never ending because your competitors are on the same track to improve their talents. Those who sit and wait for change to happen will be covered in dust as those determined to excel on a diet of change and improvement roar pass them in a thunderous stampede.

Selected Characteristics of Leaders

Positive Attitude

"A successful man is one who can lay a firm foundation with the bricks others have thrown at him."
—David Brinkley, Television Journalist (Maxwell, 1999, p. 88)

Every profession enjoys a cadre of successful people, whether teaching students, managing a productive research laboratory, or creating opportunities in the many and varied venues where we practice. There will always be those who accelerate the profession by example. Of the individuals who have achieved lasting success in our discipline, there seems to be a singular thread; their positive outlook on life and their profession. Each has overcome difficulties in some fashion, yet each has excelled despite the "bricks others have thrown" in the course of their path to contribution. Maxwell (1999) made two important points about attitude: it is a matter of personal choice and it unequivocally determines your actions. No matter what happened yesterday, your attitude is your choice today. Attitude becomes the decisive factor for success, because it determines how you act.

Competence

Competence can be defined in a word as "capability" or "expertise." Competence goes beyond words: it is the leader's ability to say it, plan it, and do it in such a way that others know that you know how, and know that they want to follow you (Maxwell, 2007). Leaders are admired for both inherent competence and perceived capabilities. There are several key elements that must be a part of a leader's armament for success. They are simple elements, easy to accomplish on a consistent basis.

Show Up Every Day

Responsible people show up when they are expected. Highly competent people come ready to play every day, no matter how they feel, what kind of circumstances they are facing in their personal or professional life, nor how difficult they expect the game to be.

Keep Improving

Highly competent people are constantly engaged in learning, growing, and improving. They do that by asking *why*. After all, the person who knows *how* will always have a job, but the person who knows *why* will always be the boss.

Follow Through with Excellence

Performing at a high level of excellence is a choice, an act of will. As leaders, we expect our people to follow through when we hand them the ball. They expect that and much more from us as their leaders.

Accomplish More Than Expected

Highly competent people always go the extra mile. For them good enough is never good enough; they need to do the job, and then some, day in and day out.

Inspire Others

Motivating others to perform at high levels is not a skill that develops overnight, nor can it be taught in a classroom. It is a talent commonly learned by watching effective leaders succeed. Excellent leadership has no stops and starts, no clear edges, nothing but smooth transition from concept and plan to effective action completing a well-defined goal.

Engage

Skilled leaders spend their time advancing conversations, not avoiding or ending them. The more you engage others, the better leader you will become both in your clinical efforts and in managing your practice. It is difficult to bring about the type of confidence, trust, and loyalty a leader must possess without being *fully engaged* in person, over the telephone, via email, through social media or even by sending personal, handwritten notes—likely the most surprising and, therefore, perhaps the most effective example of engagement in this age of rapid, often impersonal informational exchanges.

Communication Skills

"Developing excellent communication skills is absolutely essential to effective leadership. The leader must be able to share knowledge and ideas to

transmit a sense of urgency and enthusiasm to others. If a leader can't get a message across clearly and motivate others to act on it, then having a message doesn't even matter."
—Gilbert Amelio, President and CEO National Semiconductor Corp. (Maxwell, 1999, p. 23)

Your communication skills will make you the kind of leader that people will want to follow—or not. Your message must be clear and well articulated. People will not follow you if they cannot see clearly where you are going and how you intend to get there. Keep your message simple. Before you can convince others to follow, you have to believe in what you are promoting, what it is that is so important to you that it can readily become important to others. The goal of all communication is action. Simply providing information is not enough. Leaders must provide an incentive to listen, an incentive to remember the importance of the tasks ahead, and, most importantly, a plan of action and involvement to reach the desired outcome(s). At the root of effectiveness is the ability to communicate meaningful information in a clear and concise manner such that all involved in the processes leading to accomplishing the goals know the path, even when blindfolded.

If you want to become an effective leader, it is best to stop talking and start listening. There is far more to gain by surrendering the floor than by trying to dominate it. As mentioned earlier there is a seeming rush to communicate what is on one's mind without considering the value of everything that can be gleaned from the minds of others: as my father used to say so effortlessly and consistently—*you can't learn anything with your mouth open.*

Commitment

"Followers expect a leader to face up to tough decisions. When conflict must be resolved, when justice must be defined and carried out, when promises need to be kept, when the organization needs to hear who counts—these are the times when leaders act with ruthless honesty and live up to their covenant with the people they lead."
(DePree, 2008)

The obligation inherent in assuming positions of leadership requires personal sacrifice. Consider the many audiologists who have made the commitment to advance their professional acumen by completing their AuD. They have done so not only at financial expense but also in terms of valuable time spent away from family and friends. Consider as well the incalculable hours spent volunteering for professional organizations: our colleagues sacrifice their time, talent, and personal assets to take on various roles of leadership in our professional organizations. They are involved because they are committed to their profession, what it stands for, what it does for others, and because it is needed to secure our future as important and significant contributors to the health of our nation.

Pursuit

Pursuit is an often overlooked quality of leadership. Exceptional leaders are never satisfied with traditional practice, static thinking, conventional wisdom, or common performance; they are simply uncomfortable with anything that embraces the status quo. You cannot attain that which you do not pursue.

Myatt (2011) states explicitly: "Leadership is pursuit—pursuit of excellence, of elegance, of truth, of what's next, of what if, of change, of value, of results of relationships, of service, of knowledge and of something bigger than themselves. Smart leaders understand it is not just enough to pursue, but pursuit must be intentional, focused, consistent, aggressive and unyielding. You must pursue the right things, for the right reasons, and at the right times."

Teamwork

"Teamwork makes the dream work."
(Maxwell, 2007)

Teamwork divides the effort and multiplies the effect. It is working toward a common goal that joins people in an effort that they might never engage in as an individual. It is an opportunity for growth for all involved, leaders and members of the group as well. Teamwork is not always as easy as getting a few folks together to solve a problem or change a direction. Teams do not usually come together and develop on their own; they require ardent leadership and cooperation within the group. Teamwork, however, is superior to individual effort.

■ Teams involve more people, thus affording more resources, ideas, and energy than an individual possesses.
■ Teams maximize a leader's potential and minimize weaknesses.
■ Teams provide multiple perspectives on how to meet a need or reach a goal, thus devising alternatives for each situation. Individual insight is seldom as broad and deep as a group's when it takes on a problem.

■ Teams share the credit for victories and the blame for losses, fostering genuine humility and authentic community. Individuals take credit and blame alone.
■ Teams keep leaders accountable for the goal. Individuals connected to no one can change the goal without accountability.
■ Teams can simply do more than an individual.

Ability to Empower

"People under the influence of an empowering person are like paper in the hands of a talented artist."
(Maxwell, 2002)

If you are in a leadership role in an organization, your ability to empower others is not an option unless, of course, you plan on running the entire show alone. Empowering others is as critical to the success of the organization as it is critical to the success and effectiveness of the leader. Empowerment has an incredibly high return. When you empower a person to take on a task, to lead a team or research a topic important to organizational advancement, it not only helps the individuals you raise up by making them more confident, more at ease in making decisions, and more productive, it also frees you to actively promote the growth and health of your organization or practice.

Achievement comes to someone who is able to do great things for himself. Success comes when he empowers followers to do great things *with* him. Significance comes when he develops leaders to do great things *for* him. But a legacy is created only when a person puts his organization into the position to do things *without* him (DePree, 2004).

A Final Note on the Responsibility for Your Profession

Respect for the future, regard for the present, understanding the past. Leaders must forever move between the present and the future. Our perception of each becomes clear and valid if we understand the past. The future requires our humility in the face of all we cannot control. The present requires attention to all the people to whom we are accountable. The past gives us the opportunity to build on the work of our elders (DePree, 2008).

Although it seems like yesterday, a long time ago, as young students, budding practitioners and teachers and researchers-in-the-making, we accepted the torch of leadership willingly. We recognized early on that there was no substitution for clear communication and effective collaboration within our ranks and across the boundaries of our organizations. We were eager to not only perpetuate our profession but to improve upon the efforts of those who had come before us. Strong challenges remain today and each must be met head on and without fear. Our profession requires vigilant stewards willing to accept the torch and make it burn brighter than ever before. Without your eagerness to accept the responsibility of leadership, our profession will

have a restricted future dictated by others seeking to minimize our impact and lessen our rightful place in today's health care market place. Take the torch and continue the journey. Make us proud.

References

DePree, M. (2004). *Leadership is an art.* New York, NY: Random House.

DePree, M. (2008). *Leadership jazz: The essential elements of a great leader.* New York, NY: Random House.

Drucker, P. (n.d.). BrainyQuote.com. Retrieved May 27, 2012, from BrainyQuote.com, http://www.brainyquote.com/quotes/quotes/p/peterdruck131069.html

Glaser, R. G. (2011). *If not you then who?* Keynote presentation, Ohio Academy of Audiology Fifth Biennial Audiology Conference, Columbus, OH.

Maxwell, J. C. (2002). *Leadership 101: What every leader needs to know.* Nashville, TN: Thomas Nelson.

Maxwell, J. C. (2007). *Talent is never enough.* Nashville, TN: Thomas Nelson.

Maxwell, J. C. (1999). *The 21 indispensable qualities of a leader.* Nashville, TN: Thomas Nelson.

Myatt, M. Forbes. Retrieved May 28, 2012, from www.forbes.com/sites/mikemyatt/2011/12/19/this-one-leadership-quality-will-make-or-break-you/

Myatt, M. Forbes. Retrieved May 28, 2012, from www.forbes.com/sites/mikemyatt/2011/12/27/leadership-and-the-power-of-yes/

Traynor, R. M, & Glaser, R. G. (2010). *Positive emergence: Optimization strategies for a difficult economy.* American Academy of Audiology Annual Meeting, San Diego, CA.

Sadanand Singh, PhD

The late CEO and founder of Plural Publishing, Inc.

Beyond his favorite proverb below, nothing more can be said about this brilliant star of a man who helped so very many in so many ways. And through the strife and turmoil that visited his life, his bright light shined through to the happiness he created for his beloved Angie and all his children, friends, and colleagues around the world:

"He does not live in vain who employs his wealth, his thought and his speech to advance the good of others."

Ancient Hindu proverb

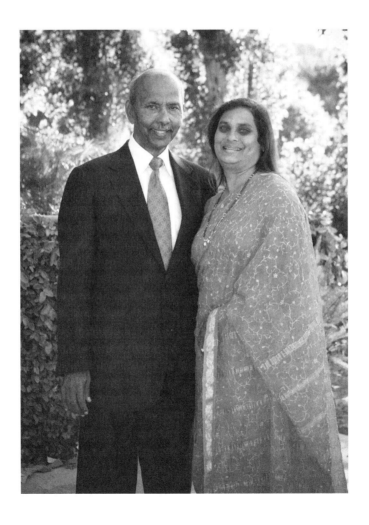

1

The Economic Realities and Competitive Landscape of Audiology Private Practice

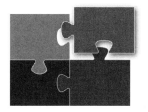

ROBERT M. TRAYNOR, EdD, MBA

When audiologists get together at meetings or socially it is rare that the economic and business issues of our profession will come up in the conversation. We often discuss the latency of waveforms, new amplification and/or evaluation technology, surgically implantable hearing instruments, cochlear implants, research, certification requirements, and other topics. Furthermore, we might also discuss ethical considerations to keep our professional standards at the highest possible level to insure that our patients obtain the best hearing healthcare possible. It is not in our nature to be concerned with economic statistics, the value of a dollar or the boom/bust of economic cycles. The decade of 2010 is an interesting time to be in the private practice of audiology. There are many unseen forces threatening quality patient care and the very existence of audiology as a profession: companies are consolidating; insurance companies, hearing aid manufacturers, buying groups, and others that would like to increase their profits by dealing directly with consumers.

Drucker (2008) stated that a practice manager's concern and their responsibility is everything that effects the performance of the practice and its success. No matter, offered Drucker, if it is a variable controlled internally by the manager or an external variable that creates a situation for strategic adjustments. Most audiology practice managers are quite capable of adjusting to internal variables as they manage their practices. It is the adjustments to the external variables, such as general economic climate, industry consolidation actions, and the competitive landscape in their communities that can be the most baffling. It is these sorts of variables that require the most vigilance and strategic modification in the process of management. Porter (2008a) feels that industry changes bring the opportunity to spot and claim promising new strategic positions if the strategist has a sophisticated understanding of the competitive forces and their underpinnings.

Economic Realities of Audiology Private Practice

Although we would like to think that our services are so important to our patients that we are immune from the economic realities of difficult economic circumstances. Recently, patients, third-party payers, suppliers, and subsequently audiology businesses have been affected by the worst economic downturn since the 1930s Great Depression. These difficulties have been amplified by governmental intervention with new banking and finan-cial regulations, controversial healthcare legislation, and an unsuccessful economic stimulation that results in significant uncertainty within the business community at large. Difficult economic issues are not solely in the United States or North America but are the result of changes in the world economy. The situation is compounded by European economic difficulties in Greece, Italy, Spain, and Portugal that have greatly affected the US stock market and other economic indicators.

These issues suggest to practice managers that, in this new century, the economies of the various countries of the world are intertwined and difficulties in one country can cause major problems in other parts of the world. This tenuous situation creates instability in banks and other financial institutions that loan funds to other nations and world financial stability can teeter on their ability to repay the loans. A classic example of world financial influence was the Lehman Brothers debacle. Considered by many "too big to fail," the company was bankrupt overnight with bad loans and investments, not only in the United States but abroad as well. The uncertain world economy combined with an ambiguous, yet unknown health care system, impending higher taxation, increased governmental spending, and an unprecedented national debt growing for many years has significant implications for our profession and our practices. These economic uncertainties trigger a realization that our practices are fragile and vulnerable in periods of overall economic downturn for a variety of reasons. Therefore, an understanding of basic economic concepts is essential to making sound strategic business decisions. Although this discussion is not a comprehensive presentation of economics, it is an important primer of terms and situations that have a direct effect on audiology practices.

Fundamentally, there are two general divisions of economics. Microeconomics refers to the economic behavior of a specific person, a household, a particular business, or an industry, while the behavior of the aggregate or overall economy is macroeconomics. Although microeconomics involves important concepts relative to individual units, such as an audiology practice within a local economy, macroeconomics presents industry and marketplace trends that may require strategic adjustments. Flynn (2011) says that macroeconomics studies the economy as a whole. Seen from on high, either businesses or the government do the production of goods and services. Businesses produce the bulk of what people consume, but government also provides many goods and services, including public safety, national defense, and public goods such as roads and bridges. Additionally, the government provides the legal structure in which businesses operate and also intervenes in the economy to regulate pollution, mandate safety equipment, and redistribute income from the rich to the poor.

Macroeconomics is part of the 24-hour news cycle and bombards viewers each day with a myriad of incomprehensible terms and economic rationales from around the world. As Audiologists, we do not typically attend to these terms and, subsequently, clues to necessary strategic adjustments in our practices become lost the background noise of evening news. Calculations and terms that describe the direction and/or health of the economy are known as *Economic Indicators*. While the economic calculations used and manipulated by the news pundits might well be background noise to most

of us, these indicators can provide valuable information regarding the strength or weakness of the economy leading to knowledge of an expansion or contraction of the economy in advance.

Market Economies and Economic Cycles

The first of many concepts essential to the comprehension of how the economy works in general is that of the *Market Economy* and *Economic Cycles*. The United States is thought to be a market economy where prices are set by supply and demand. In a market economy the amount of a product that is demanded by consumers usually indicates to managers within a particular industry how much of that product is manufactured and distributed to the marketplace.

The assumption is made that market forces, such as supply and demand, are the best determinants of what is right for a nation's well-being. In contrast, the opposite is a *Command Economy*, such as North Korea or the former Soviet Union, countries where all markets, from hearing aids to toilet paper, are controlled by a committee within the communist party. In command economies there are often shortages of various products creating huge black markets that meet the product demands by the consumers. In reality, the US economy and most other "free" markets are mixed economies and, to some degree, controlled by the government. For example, if you were in the business of marketing alcoholic beverages, the market would demand alcohol for minors but the government does not allow the sale of this product to minors, thus limiting the free market. The same limitation is for harmful drugs the drug company would like to (and probably would) sell their drug to anyone, the government only allows the sale of certain drugs when prescribed by a licensed physician and dispensed by a licensed pharmacist. The US free market is then limited for sales of many products to certain governments, specific age groups, those with specific diseases and other situations. These markets, such as the US market and other western economies are generally free markets, but there is some government intervention that regulates certain products and services, so they are technically referred to as *Hybrid Markets*.

Market economies are subject to natural economic cycles or periods of expansion and contraction, sometimes called *boom* or *recession*. These expansions and contractions in the economy (Figure 1–1) are part of a continuous economic fluctuation that creates periods of prosperity and austerity. In a boom economy businesses flourish, there is high employment, home values increase, and capital is readily available. The opposite cycle, a recession creates situations where austerity prevails and business is difficult, people lose jobs, mortgages are foreclosed, and business capital is scarce. A recession has many different definitions, depending upon the orientation of those offering the definition. Generally, a recession occurs when an economic indicator, the Gross Domestic Product (GDP) has declined for two consecutive quarters, whereas a *depression* is a serious recession that lasts longer than 18 months, such as the economic slowdown that occurred in the 1930s and, possibly, as recently as 2008 to 2012.

Defining Economic Indicators and their Implications for Audiologists

To fully appreciate some of these terms associated with a market economy and the economic business cycle, it is fun-

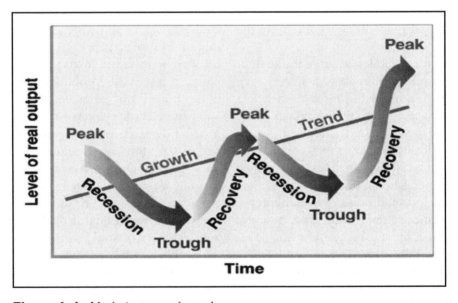

Figure 1–1. Market economic cycles.

damental to interpret terms known as *economic indicators*. There are many economic indicators including (but not limited to), gross domestic product, national debt, deficit, interest rates, inflation, deflation, tax increases/decreases, currency value, retail sales, pending home sales, petroleum prices, unemployment, and others available on the news and from various Web sites. Unlike the precise audiologic data necessary to discuss new procedures and evaluations essential to ensure that a procedure is beneficial and a true measure of what it purports to be, economic data sometimes depends upon the analysis and the particular point of view or political position.

Gross Domestic Product (GDP)

Gross Domestic Product (GDP), according to Investor Words (2012), is a calculation of the total market value of all final goods and services produced in a country in a given year (Figure 1–2). These values are usually published quarterly and offer some idea of the performance of the economy during the period. The GDP report is released on the last day of each quarter and reflects the growth in the value of goods and services over the past quarter. Growth in GDP is what is important and the US GDP growth historically has averaged about 2.5 to 3% per year but with substantial deviations. Recently, during the current recession, GDP has had some huge swings been between −5% (negative) to 3.5% (positive) growth and is currently only at about 1.8%.

For example, if the GDP calculation is up by 4% the suggestion is that the economy grew by 4%. Conversely, if the economy is down by 4% then the economy shrunk by 4% and the value of goods and services has become less in the period. GDP can be figured on the expenditures of companies but is more commonly considered on the income as income figures are used for tax reporting in most countries. Companies report and pay their taxes quarterly allowing for the quarterly measurement of the GDP. In the United States and other countries, reductions or increases in the GDP typically affect the stock market

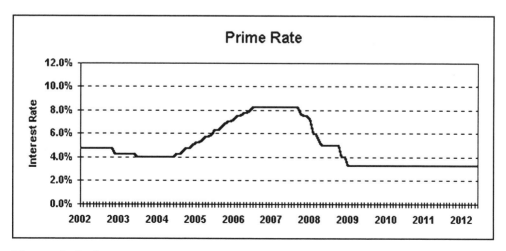

Figure 1–2. Growth in GDP 2007–2012.

either positively or negatively. The market is affected due to the suggestion of the productivity of companies and, as the GDP falls, there is less demand for goods and services company profits are affected. Reduced corporate profit is an indication that there is less demand for the company's goods and services causing a reduction of production which, if the trend continues, causes companies to lay off or discharge employees, creating unemployment. GDP is an indication of the performance of the economy but politicians, government agencies, and other measurers of GDP manipulate the data by including some things and leaving out others that can change the GDP calculation either up or down to suit their needs. For example, in the current calculation of the GDP, leaving out the housing market makes the figure look much better than if it is figured into the GDP. Particularly during this latest recession, exclusion of housing market causes the GDP to go up, whereas the inclusion causes a downward trend. These manipulations have caused difficulties in reviewing the health of economies around the world, such as Greece, Spain, and, of course, the United States. Although the GDP is a major indicator of the health of an economy, interpretation of these figures can be difficult as it requires knowledge of the figures used in its calculation.

It also is important to differentiate Gross Domestic Product (GDP) from Gross National Product (GNP). GDP includes only goods and services produced within the geographic boundaries of the United States, regardless of the producer's nationality, whereas GNP doesn't include goods and services produced by foreign producers, but does include goods and services produced by US firms operating in foreign countries.

Interest Rates

The Federal Reserve is a major institution in the United States directly responsible for maintaining economic stability. According to Kennon (2012) it is primarily responsible for maintaining full employment by keeping unemployment at 4 to 5% and simultaneously maintaining a low inflation. The most powerful weapon at the disposal of the Federal Reserve to maintain this economic balance is the capability to influence the direction of interest rates either higher or lower. *Interest rates* are amounts charged for borrowing money from a bank or other funding source. Basically, the Federal Reserve sets interest rates that they charge banks for funds that they lend to the general public. Banks and other financial institutions review the current Federal Reserve rate then decide how much to charge their customers for funds so that they make a profit on loans. The interest rate at which eligible banks may borrow funds directly from a Federal Reserve bank is called the *prime rate*. When these prime interest rates are low, capital is usually easier to acquire and when these rates are higher funds are difficult obtain. The interest rates that banks and other lenders charge their customers for the use of their funds are a "retail" interest rate. The difference between the basic rate charged by the Federal Reserve to the banks to acquire the funds to loan and the interest rate charged by banks to their customers is the bank's profit. Currently, Money Café (2012) reports that the Federal Reserve prime rate is 3.25% for funds they receive through the system (Figure 1–3).

So, if the bank charges 6% to borrow funds, their profit is 2.75% on the loan. Typically, when the economy is in recession and requires stimulation inter-

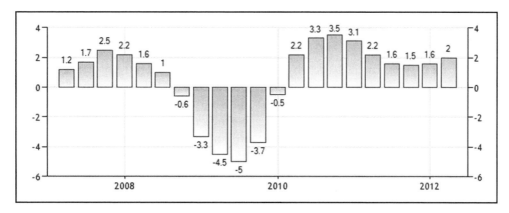

Figure 1–3. Prime interest rates 2002–2012.

est rates are lowered so that funds are more available. When the economy is in a boom the economy is kept in check by raising interest rates. Typically, this controls the flow of capital, which subsequently controls economic growth. Although that seems like a rather simple concept, new and restrictive banking regulations imposed by the government have made the process extremely complex. Since the economy is in recession, the current strategy is to keep interest rates low to stimulate and grow the economy. Although interest rates are currently at their lowest in 50 to 60 years, funds are still difficult to obtain, application processes are lengthy, and capital is still scarce due to all of these new regulations. As a result, audiologists will find it difficult to obtain funds to purchase practices, finance expansion and obtain working capital loans from banks and other financial institutions. Currently, funds are available and interest rates are low, but the financial markets are still insecure with new regulations and borrowing requirements. This lender insecurity insures difficulty in the application process and raises the bar for creditworthiness facilitating a very slow and frustrating process.

Inflation/Deflation

Flynn (2011) defines *inflation* as the word that economists use to describe a situation in which the general level of prices in the economy is rising. Whereas inflation refers to prices rising, *deflation* is a term that denotes prices lowering.

The Federal Reserve causes interest rates to rise and fall to reduce the possibility of inflation or deflation. When the economy is in a boom, funds are easy to obtain and interest rates are favorable and, but when not controlled, inflation occurs. If the economic stability is out of balance, there can be an increase or decrease in the cost of goods and services suggesting that the value of money becomes less, *Inflation,* or the value of money is greater, *Deflation.* The Federal Reserve uses their prime rate to control the supply of available funds and the overall (or retail) interest rate. Traditionally, the more funds are available at lower interest rates, the more likely inflation will occur. By raising the prime rate the Federal Reserve makes it more expensive for banks to borrow at the prime rate and the "retail" interest rate becomes higher. Subsequently, the higher cost of funds causes money to become scarce and slows the economy down reducing the possibility of inflation.

Inflation is typically measured by the *Consumer Price Index (CPI)*. Investopedia (2012) defines the Consumer Price Index (CPI) as a measure that examines the weighted average of the price of a basket of consumer goods and services within various economic sectors, such as transportation, food, medical care, and other areas. The CPI is calculated by taking price changes for each item in the predetermined basket of goods, averaging them, and comparing to the previous period. While changes in the CPI are used to assess and discuss price changes associated with the cost of living, weighted according to the relative importance of various sectors; changes CPI or the costs of living are measured by the higher (inflation) or lower (deflation) cost calculations of these baskets of goods and services.

Figure 1–4 presents the annual inflation rate over the past 10 years in the United States.

National Debt

National Debt is the total amount of debt that the federal government owes on funds that it has borrowed to keep the country solvent (Figure 1–5). At this writing, the US national debt is over 16 trillion dollars and can be easily checked anytime for the exact amount owed by the government at National Debt Clock (2012) (http://www.brillig.com/debt_clock). This site not only presents the amount that is owed overall but how much is owed by each individual citizen, currently hovering at over $50,000. Although simply owing money is critical in itself, the public policy problems that created the debt must be adjusted or the country will go bankrupt. The adjustments involve one of three modifications, Print more money, raise taxes, or reduce spending by cutting entitlement and other expensive programs. Entitlement programs are those that offer benefits to specific groups of individuals. Programs such as Medicare, Medicaid, Social Security, Welfare, and many others

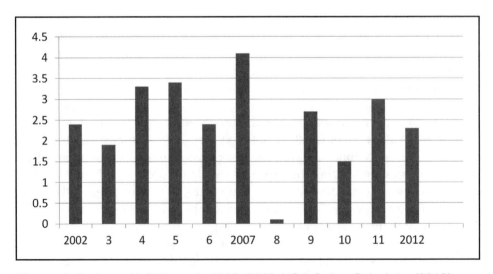

Figure 1–4. Annual inflation rate 2002–2012. US Inflation Calculator (2012).

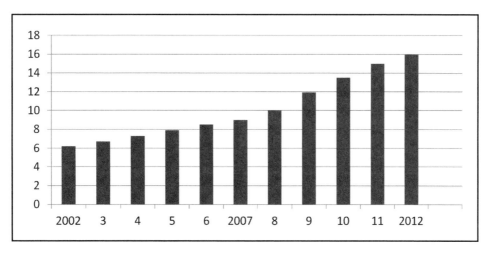

Figure 1–5. National debt 2002–2012.

can be considered entitlement programs. In many cases, these are programs that citizens have paid into most of their lives, and the government has used those funds to do other things, thus, there is no funding for the benefit when it comes their turn to receive it, such as Social Security. The choices are for the government to print more money so it has funds to meet its obligations, to make citizens pay more in taxes, or reduce the benefits available to the citizens to a lower, more affordable level. The likelihood of more money being printed to pay the government's obligations is minimal since this process leads to rampant inflation and within a short period of time the the the currency becomes worthless. Therefore, the options of either a tax increase or reducing benefits become realistic options. No matter which of these solutions is chosen, neither solution is good for Audiology.

■ *Raising Taxes*
Although raising revenue seems to be a logical solution for a lack of funding, as patients are taxed at a higher rate there is less disposable

income available for other necessities. Since most audiology patients are in the last one-third of their life, the greater tax reduces a patient's capability to pay their co-payments for services, amplification, and/or other clinical products. Basically, patients have less cash to make purchases or to service existing products that they use every day. Additionally, revenue would also be raised by taxing businesses at a higher level, causing the practice manager to cut expenses, personnel, and other expensive fixed expenses.

■ *Reducing Government Spending*
By the reduction of costs for programs the debt can be reduced with existing funds taken in through taxes. The question then becomes which programs should be cut, how much, and the effects of cutting these programs that are difficult to fund. The reduction or elimination of programs such as Medicare, Medicaid, Social Security, and others would have significant effect on the country in general and certainly

on the practice of audiology. Reimbursement is already minimal for most procedures and cuts could be disastrous to some practices. Although the new Affordable Care Act promises audiology direct access to their patients, there is (at this writing) so much that is unknown about the new healthcare system that leaves all health care providers asking serious questions about how they will be paid for their services.

A high national debt creates other issues, such as reduced value of the dollar, interest rate increases, inflation, and other problems.

Deficit Spending

Deficit spending simply refers to the amount that has been borrowed in a specific period of time. If the federal government has spent a dollar of their funds and they had to borrow 40 cents of that dollar, then 40 cents of each dollar is the deficit between available revenue, 60 cents and the borrowed funds, 40 cents to make up the total dollar required for the obligation. Since the government does not have that 40 cents and must borrow it, for each dollar there is a 40 cent deficit.

Currency Values are usually the result of a high or low national debt. The US dollar has been known as one of the world's most stable and reliable currencies for well over 100 years and is even used in many countries as their currency as well. As the US national debt has increased, the value of the US dollar has decreased. In most countries, however, they use their own currency which reflects their national identity, the value of the specific country's goods and services according to *their* national debt, and the country's political policies. When residing in another country most people that reside in that country prefer that you pay your bills and other financial obligations in their currency. It is a system that they understand and use daily as preferred method of payment. As the national debt has increased over the past 10 years, the value of the US dollar has decreased significantly. For example, in 1999 when changing US dollars into Swiss francs (the currency of Switzerland) the dollar was worth $1.80 in Swiss francs (CHF), in June 2012, the same US dollar is only worth .96 Swiss francs (CHF). This substantial decrease is a direct result of the high national debt brought about by the substantial deficit spending during the past 10 years. In another example, in 1999 the US dollar was on par with the euro (1 US dollar = 1 euro) the currency used by most of the countries in Europe. In June 2012 the same US dollar that was on par with the euro in 1999 is now worth about .79€. Although many audiologists might wonder why the concern over the value of the dollar, consider that when the dollar is low against European currencies, it costs more to travel in places where the dollar has less value and costs more for products from these countries. Then consider where audiologists purchase most amplification products and many other products, Europe. If your costs have gone up for equipment and amplification products, it is likely due to the fact that the value of the dollar is down significantly relative to the euro, Swiss franc, and other currencies.

Sidebar 1–1
FUNDING IN A DIFFICULT ECONOMY

In difficult times when banks and other business funding sources are over regulated with better opportunities to grow their assets than to loan money, where does a practitioner go to obtain working capital, equipment, and/ or expansion funds. When times are good, everyone wants to loan money to a business operator as there is ample cash to repay the loan easily at a rate of return that offers the cash to the borrower and a good rate of return for the lender. In tough times, however, particularly at a time when there is more opportunity for banks to invest their money with less risk, how does the practitioner obtain the funds to operate. Community banks, usually a good source of capital for small businesses, have been especially hard hit by the recent economic downturn. These local banks often know the practitioners, their practices and may even be patients. While the large banks were bailed out by the government, stringent new regulations were imposed upon community banks. As of January 1, 2011 new banking regulations increase the amount of assets that these local banks must have to loan funds and to keep existing loans to existing customers (FDIC, 2012a). As a result, community banks must have 5% more assets put aside for each new loan that they fund or have outstanding. For example, if a practice has a $20,000 loan at a community bank. In the past, the bank was required to have $2,000 (or about 10%) in assets to fund the loan. The new regulations require that they must now have $3,000 (or about 15%) in assets to make the same loan or to continue a loan already in force. Although an increase of $1,000 (or 5%) in assets is not that much in this case, when the total loans that a community bank might have outstanding is considered, it might be impossible the bank to meet the government's demand to cover the required increase in assets to cover all the outstanding loans. This and other new banking regulations have caused problems with the distribution of the money supply and contributed to the failure of 389 banks in the past three years (FDIC, 2012b). These and other issues have created a situation where most audiologists will have difficulty when applying for a loan for any purpose. Lenders are currently not in a mood to lend funds and, consequently, make the application process impossible by requiring unrealistic down payments, extreme amounts of collateral, impeccable credit, and other unrealistic standards, impeding business. So where does the enterprising practitioner obtain working capital, equipment, or expansion, funds for their practice?

Business Defense Assets

The best place to obtain funds for working capital or other uses is the practices own Defensive Assets. Another name for the business's defense assets is the practice's savings account. These accounts are the very best place to borrow funds as they belong to the clinic and, although the funds will not be gaining interest, they can be paid back when it is comfortable for the practice and no interest is charged for the funds borrowed. There are no qualifications necessary to obtain the funds and they are available immediately.

Personal Savings Account

Probably the second best source of funds is a personal savings account. Since these funds are owned by the practitioner, who likely owns the practice and may even be the only stockholder in the practice's corporation; these funds can be immediately available with no application process and provide the capital necessary to facilitate a down period. Borrowing from personal funds should be conducted properly to avoid "co-mingling" by simple loan documents indicating that the practice has borrowed so much from the personal assets. No matter the business structure, sole proprietorship, partnership, corporation, professional corporation, limited partnership, or others; borrowing from a personal account needs to be done formally. This should be conducted in close consultation with an accountant to insure that there is no appearance of mingling personal and corporation's assets. Care should be taken not to take funds from the children's college money, a 401(k), or other retirement account. Funds taken from retirement accounts by those under age 59½ will be subject to a 10% penalty and ordinary income tax as it was not paid when the funds were earned.

Ten Strategies for Positive Emergence from an Economic Downturn

Successful emergence from an economic downturn involves learning as much about how the practice interacts with the economy as possible. Over the years Audiology has been thought to be rather immune from economic ups and downs as the products and services were required for communication. With all of the Medicare and insurance cuts to providers, additional competent competition, and the new government Affordable Health Care Act, the landscape has changed and it is necessary for clinicians to be aware that their practice can be vulnerable to economic, governmental, and other pressures. Positive emergence from a economic downturn or over regulation by the government is based upon how prepared the practice is for these difficulties. Is your practice prepared for the new government health insurance? What if the economic downturn lasts another five years? What the manager knows about the economy and the practices' operation prepares them to manage a myriad of situations. Once prepared, the manager will need to strategically plan for the necessary adjustments to the economic and competitive concerns that are created by the situation. Strategic planning involves an analysis of the difficulties encountered and the development of methods to cope in a difficult business environment. Economic downturns will be with the practice as long as it is in existence; thus, it is fundamental to success to figure out how to deal with them. Preparing for these economic highs and lows, obtaining the skills to analyze each situation rationally, and strategizing how to insure that the business will survive are essential to positive emergence. Ten general strategies that can facilitate positive emergence from difficult times are as follows:

1. Improve Your Business Skills
   - Study economics—know what's coming
   - Study business—know the basics
   - Study marketing—innovative and conservative
   - Do a budget and follow it
2. Learn New Audiology Skills
   - The more skills you have the more opportunities arise.
   - Tinnitus, APD, vestibular, operative monitoring, and so forth.
3. Local Networking
   - Physicians
   - Nontraditional medical professionals
   - Chamber of Commerce
   - Service Clubs—Rotary, Kiwanis, Sertoma
   - Others
4. Modify Fees and Product Prices
   - Less unit sales. . . higher prices
   - Lower/higher according to market and image
   - Careful in price modification as it may not be necessary
5. Increase Marketing Activities
   - Not easy in down economy
   - Presentations
     - Service clubs
     - Health care facilities
   - Internet/social media
   - Modify USP
6. Review Policies and Procedures
   - Customer service
   - Follow up
   - Other procedures
7. Watch the Economic Indicators
   - Down times are normal
   - Watch for the economic cycles
   - In down times, thieves appear, beware of the embezzlers they abound in clinical practices and disguise themselves as practice managers.
8. Watch Out for Your Referral Sources
   - Others will want to steal them
   - Cater to their needs and wishes
9. Offer Patient Financing Programs
   - 90 days same as cash
   - 6 to 12 months—no interest
10. Stay Motivated
    - Down times are normal
    - Patient centrism

■ Take care of your patients and they will take care of you!

Many of these survival strategies are offered in more detail in subsequent chapters. It is essential for the practice manager to prepare the practices' own outline of changes necessary to survive in an economic downturn. A further step to the goal of preparing for practice survival is knowledge of the competitive landscape in which all practices operate.

The Competitive Landscape of the Hearing Industry 2012

The hearing industry is a highly competitive environment and various product manufacturers fiercely compete for our business. When walking the halls of major audiology conventions, such as the American Academy of Audiology, the exhibit hall is full of 2- and 3-story exhibition booths purveying amplification, assessment equipment, buying groups, marketing programs, and ancillary products and programs that are of great benefit to our practices and the hearing impaired. We are lured to one booth or another by product innovations, modifications, special financial incentives, a particular representative, or often just to go to their party at the end of the week. Although these manufacturers compete fiercely with each other, their competitive nature has taken on a new complexion in the past few years. Fueled by the static nature of the hearing industry, adoption rates for amplification, and the economic promise of a baby boomer generation that will require more of our products and services, there is intense rivalry among manufacturers for our business as manufacturers attempt to steal market share each other. When profits begin to shrink the natural industry consolidation process becomes the place to secure profits from acquisitions, mergers, and entering into unchartered channels.

Bofah (2012) describes Industry consolidation as a process that occurs among businesses that serve a particular market by merging together, rather than competing for profits. Industry consolidation is categorized into either horizontal or vertical integration. *Horizontal integration* combines similar firms and products within the market segment. *Vertical integration* consolidates companies along the same supply chain. Kocic (2012) reports that the US Federal Trade Commission (FTC) supports industrial consolidation as benefiting competition and consumers by allowing firms to operate more efficiently. Kocic (2012) presents that industry consolidation improves investment returns, cuts costs, creates new products, and leads to production gains. These consolidations can be voluntary, or hostile by the management of one firm resisting the advances of the other, Conversely, Kocic (2010) also offers that mergers and consolidation can lead to monopolistic positions, which may lead to higher prices, decreased innovation and/or a drop in the quality or availability of goods or services. Industry consolidation has been going on for quite some time in Audiology and the Hearing Industry. This process is considered a normal part of a maturing industry and happens in all infant professions and industries as they develop.

Industry consolidation is not a new phenomenon, but a natural part of the industrial business cycle. In the early part of the 20th century, there were literally hundreds of small automobile companies in the United States. For a few years, they all flourished as companies struggled to manufacture enough cars to meet the consumer demand. Initially, the need for vehicles was so great that consumers did not care too much about brand, only that it was available, affordable, and reliable transportation. After a few years, the excessive demand for vehicles diminished and these small automobile companies struggled against each other and larger competitors for component parts, metal, and other essential manufacturing materials; many went out of business or were purchased by larger, better managed companies. Eventually, smaller automobile manufacturers banded together to buy their materials in bulk and in return they were given very favorable prices, whereas those that did not "band together" were charged at the going rate, compromising their profits and their competitive capabilities. Although those that banded together, had to deal with buying group politics, the nonbuying group participants, paid a higher price for component parts, metals, and other essential materials and, subsequently had less funds for marketing, and other operating expenses. By the 1950s, due to industry consolidation there were only three major automobile competitors, General Motors, Ford, and Chrysler. Having horizontally consolidated as much as possible, vertical consolidation moved forward as the automobile manufacturers began purchasing dealerships to offer their products directly to the consumers without sharing the profit with a dealership owner, thus increasing their profits.

In the hearing industry, competitors have been horizontally consolidating for quite some time. Major hearing aid manufacturers have created holding companies (such as William Demant Holding (WDH), Sonova, etc.), others are owned by corporate conglomerates such as Great Nordic (GN Resound) and still others, such as Siemens, own huge controlling portions of other companies that are influential in the product distribution system. Holding companies (WDH and Sonova) have become publically traded, big business enterprises involved in horizontal industry consolidation by purchasing smaller hearing aid companies, equipment companies, and in vertical consolidation by purchasing other ancillary companies such as buying groups, retail outlet companies, and others that will assist them in dominating distribution channels as well. Their ultimate goal is not to simply own the manufacturing of products, but the distribution channels as well; controlling the whole market by manufacturing and directly distributing their products to the consumer. For example, WDH owns not only Oticon, but also Bernafon, Sonic (formerly Sonic Innovations), Maico Audiometers, Interacoustics, Grason-Stadler, Amplivox, Phonic Ear, and has interests in Sennheiser. They also own the Avada Network and are controlling stockholders in the American Hearing Aid Associates (AHAA), among others. Sonova not only owns Phonak, but Unitron, Hansaton, Lyric, Advanced Bionics, and retail distribution chains in various countries, including the United States. Sonova is also involved in Internet hearing aid sales through their recently acquired company, Hearing Planet. Additionally, in 2012, Sonova is rapidly purchasing practices across the United States that, as a corporate owned entity, will directly compete with independent private practitioners. Siemens has also been involved in the consolidation process for a number of years owning Rexton, Electone, and other product brands and controlling shareholders in many operations that are part of the industry distribution channel, such as and HEARx, HEARPO, and other holdings solidifying their horizontal and vertical acquisitions. Others that are involved in the industrial consolidation process include, Resound, Starkey, and others all with their respective horizontal and vertical consolidations.

Vertical consolidations assist in bringing hearing aid products into nontraditional distribution channels, such as Costco and Walmart. For example, the major manufacturers offer their flagship technology to audiologists and dispensers but use their second brands, Bernafon (WDH), Interton (GN Resound), Rexton (Siemens), offered through discount warehouse stores such as COSTCO, Wal-Mart to expand their profits. As part of the industrial consolidation of sales channels, many of these companies own buying groups such as AHAA and Audigy (WDH), HEAR PO (Siemens) and others. Audiologists participating in these groups need to evaluate that their business with these groups and the control that they exercise on their practice and the profession.

Commoditization of Amplification Devices

Another issue that is a current threat to audiology private practice and part of our current landscape is the commoditization of amplification products. Commoditization, according to Business Dictionary (2012), is the result of a lack of differentiation of products within an industry. Without differentiation, products become a commodity and can be perceived as the same no matter the vendor or the place of purchase. Commoditized products have thin margins and are sold on the basis of price and not brand. This situation is characterized by standardized, ever cheaper, and common technology that invites more suppliers who lower the prices even further. Patients do not realize the performance differences among amplification products and most instruments physically look very similar. The commoditization process is not to be confused with the movement toward "starter hearing aids," as these products are meant to begin patients toward the use of better products over time. The threat of commoditization is a part of our practice as it is in front of us at all times. For example, Internet hearing aid sales, magazine ads (Rotary Club magazine, Elks Club magazine, AARP, and other publications), late night television ads, offer products such as the Bionic Hearing Aid and others claiming provide the same benefit as products from reliable, flagship manufacturers for thousands less in cost. Basically, the suggestion is that it makes no difference in who makes the product or where you obtain it, performance will be the essentially the same. This commoditization process has recently been reinforced by insurance companies. For example, United Healthcare's (UHC) program to sell hearing aids directly to their subscribers through their "front" company, Hearing Innovators (HI), via the Internet with only an audiogram typifies the move toward commoditization. Although initially, UHC was to have their subscribers take a totally invalid, and unreliable online hearing evaluation, the Food and Drug Administration (FDA) has disallowed their online hearing evaluation. Subscribers using this program must now obtain an audiogram from a reliable source, such as an audiologist, for entry into the system. Once the audiogram is received, Hearing Innovators will program the device, and mail it to the patient, no counseling, fine tuning or other aural rehabilitation services. Of course, this is not the way to provide high quality instrumentation or aural rehabilitation, but if UHC can bypass audiologists, there is more profit for the provision of this insurance benefit. After all, in their opinion, it makes no difference as to the device or how you obtain the device as audiologists are superfluous and all products will provide the same benefit.

Buying Groups

As briefly suggested earlier in this chapter buying groups have changed the landscape of how our practices are managed. Over the years many successful practices have developed and prospered by providing patient centric services, offering experience, hard work, and expertise. In the early 1990s, buying groups began to offer clinicians large discounts, bill consolidation, business advice, marketing assistance, insurance referrals, trips, continuing education, and/or other benefits. To the casual observer, these "benefits" do not appear to compromise ethical standards as, on the surface, the financial incentives were not offered by a specific product manufacturer. Unknown to many audiologists, however, is that most buying groups are owned partially or wholly by the hearing instrument manufacturers. There is probably more ethical compromise than is obvious as the buying groups have their favorite manufactures, and present better "deals" on some products over others. Buying groups make their money by selling audiologists product at

a lower discount better rate than could be obtained by the audiologist from the manufacturer directly. For example, if an audiologist was to obtain product X from a manufacturer and purchase 10 or more per month, they would probably obtain a 25 to 30% discount on the devices. If they only purchased 2 to 3 instruments per month, they may not obtain more than 10% discount when purchasing direct from the manufacturer. Buying groups obtain huge discounts by agreeing to sell a large number of hearing instruments. Their discounts can be as much as 45% or more on selected products. The audiologist joins the buying group and then obtains the very same 2 to 3 hearing instruments a month, but through the buying group they obtain a 30% discount. The buying group obtained the devices for 45% discount and offers the audiologist member a 30% discount on all products. Thus, the buying group that purchased the instrument at 45% off single unit price, sells the product to the audiologist for 30% off and pockets the 15% as profit. They did not even see the instruments and as long as the buying group pays their bill and meets the minimum number of sales they are in business. The buying group makes money, the audiologists save money, and keeps their business healthy so what is the problem? These groups often "hook" young audiologists with loans, business or financial advice, marketing assistance, and/or insurance referrals (which may or may not actually exist) these audiologists often end up strung out and thus obligated to the buying group for loans, marketing, discounts, or other incentives. This is not simply a phenomenon of Audiology or hearing aid dispensers, it is happening in all types of health care practices including, optometry, dentistry, chiropractic, and other professions. From the 1970s until recently, Audiologists have felt that they were in control of their destiny, particularly after the advent of the Doctor of Audiology, but it is now product manufacturers, those that build the hearing instruments and our equipment that have the power in the hearing industry. This whole process is very reminiscent of the industry consolidation of automobiles early in the previous century.

Sidebar 1–2
TYPICAL STEPS IN INDUSTRY ANALYSIS

Define the relevant industry:

- What products are in it? Which ones are part of another distinct industry?
- What is the geographic scope of the competition?

Identify the participants and segment them into groups, if appropriate:

Who are . . .

- The buyers and buying groups?
- The suppliers and the supplier groups?
- The competitors?
- The substitutes?
- The potential entrants?

Assess the underlying drivers of each competitive force to determine which forces are strong and which are weak and why.

Determine overall industry structure, and test the analysis for consistency:

- Why is the level of profitability what it is?
- Which are the controlling forces for profitability?
- Is the industry analysis consistent with actual long run profitability?
- Are more profitable players better positioned in relation to the five forces?

Analyze recent and likely future changes in each force, both positive and negative.

Identify aspects of industry structure that might be influenced by competitors, new entrants, or by your company.

Porter (2008)

Generic Competitive Strategies

The objective of a strategy should be to modify competitive forces in a way that improves the position of the organization relative to the competition. Porter (1980) suggested that there were three potentially successful generic approaches to outperforming other firms within an industry:

- Overall Cost Leadership
- Differentiation
- Focus

Although these strategies can be implemented at the same time, they rarely are executed together as successful implementation requires total commitment from the firm, its executives, and support mechanism.

Overall Cost Leadership Strategy

In an attempt to be the cost leader, there must be a great deal of managerial attention to cost control. Low cost relative to the competitors becomes the theme running through the entire strategy, though quality, service and other areas cannot be ignored (Porter, 1980). Alagse (2012) indicates that a low cost strategy is centered on the capability of the company to produce and deliver a product or products of competitive quality at lower costs. Cost leadership strategy is much more than cost reduction initiatives that get prominence in strategic planning and review of any company as a means to improve the bottom line by improving its efficiency. Some companies use their efficient cost structures to protect their markets from the competitors by responding to competitors' in the market by reducing prices. Lash (2007) states that customers are price sensitive, and if you can deliver a product for less than the competition, you will be successful at generating more sales. Even if your product isn't as good as the competition, if it's cheaper, more people will buy it. One of the advantages of low pricing is that it often leads to a more consistent or predictable demand. Suppliers or retailers are able to more effectively control and forecast production, inventory costs, and shipping costs thus stabilizing demand. Hurwich (2012) cautions that, although his strategy works in some markets, it doesn't make sense where demand is so high that price increases are warranted, or when demand declines to the point that price discounts are needed to reduce inventories. In the hearing industry it is obvious that Costco and Walmart are leaders in the cost leadership strategy. Depending upon the market, products offered through these outlets are usually about one-third less in cost than through a typical audiology clinic.

Differentiation Strategy

The second of Porter's generic strategies is one of differentiating the product or service offering into something that is perceived as truly unique and different. In a product differentiation strategy the firm still looks to control costs, but costs are not the focus nor the primary target. Differentiation provides insulation against competition by generating brand loyalty resulting in low sensitivity to price. This is usually coupled with a lower market share as it requires a perception of exclusivity but yields higher margins with which to deal with suppliers. Buyers perceive that there is no other place to obtain the product or service with the same differentiation; thus, they are less price sensitive. Most product manufacturers are differentiation; strategy companies. One has only to watch the marketing materials, presentations, and journals to see that the major effort in the hearing industry is that of differentiation.

Focus Strategy

The final generic strategy is focusing on a particular buying group, segment of a product line, or geographic market and, as with differentiation can take many forms. Although the other two strategies are aimed at the total industry, focusing does just that, focuses on a specific target. Functional policies are tuned for a specific audience and to the benefit of a specific group or groups. A hearing industry example of focusing is Bernafon's deliberate strategy to focus their business in the United States on Costco and the Veteran's Administration, not seeking nor turning away the business of private clinics.

As strategies go a firm or a practice should pick one and move in that direction as the worst place to find themselves in "stuck in the middle" with no direction. Firms stuck in the middle must make a fundamental strategic decision. Porter (1980) indicates it is critical for these firms to take the steps necessary to achieve cost leadership or least parity, which usually involves aggressive investments to modernize and perhaps the necessity to buy market share, or it must orient itself to a particular target (focusing) or achieve some uniqueness (differentiation). A hearing industry firm that

is an example for "stuck in the middle" was Sonic Innovations. Although a rather profitable, unique group for a number of years, their products lacked cost leadership, differentiation, or focus creating lackluster business performance. The result of this nonstrategic performance was that the company was floundering and finally acquired William Demant Holding in 2011.

Porter's Five Forces— Assessing the Balance of Power in Business

So, what are the powers that trigger strategies, competitive spirit, consolidation, and commoditizing? Although horizontal and vertical industrial consolidation, commoditization, buying groups, and other natural modifications of our industry situations are confusing to most audiologists, the best method of understanding the balance of power in a competitive situation and the reasons why these processes are a natural result of the maturation of an industry is to consider Porter's Five Forces (Manktelow & Carlson, 2012). Porter (1980, 1998, 2008) developed a model that is used routinely by business professionals to evaluate competition and how it affects their industry. An industry is defined as a group of firms that produce products that are close substitutes for each other. Industry, of course, is not a closed system; as competitors exit/enter the market, suppliers and buyers exert significant influence on their profitability as well as the overall outlook for the industry in question. Porter's model is a simple, but powerful, business tool that provides an understanding of where the power lies among competitors within a specific industry. Understanding the structure of the industry is fundamental to the formulation of a competitive strategy (Porter 1980, 1998, 2008). Changes in industrial structure are usually slow but nevertheless can create social or cultural change within an industry. These changes are usually due to political, labor, or economic issues. Slow structural change is not typically effected by the general economic climate or short-term fluctuations in the market demand which makes the industry structure somewhat easier to predict using the model.

Recklies (2001) states that the basis of Porter's classic model is that strategy should meet the opportunities and threats to the organizations external environment and a thorough understanding of industry structures can and will change over time. Porter (1980, 1998) identified five specific competitive forces that shape virtually every industry and market no matter how large or small. These forces determine the intensity of competition and, hence, the profitability and attractiveness of a particular business.

Porter's model (1980, 1998, 2008a,b) analyzes competitive driving forces in a particular industry and, based on the information derived, a manager can decide how to influence or exploit particular characteristics and situations within their industry. The five forces analysis assumes that there are five important forces that determine competitive power within a specific business situation. The model shown in Figure 1–6 presents these five forces: (1) *Threat of New Entrants*, (2) *Bargaining Power of Buyers*, (3) *Bargaining Power of Suppliers*, (4) *Threat of Substitutes*, and (5) *Rivalry Within the Industry.*

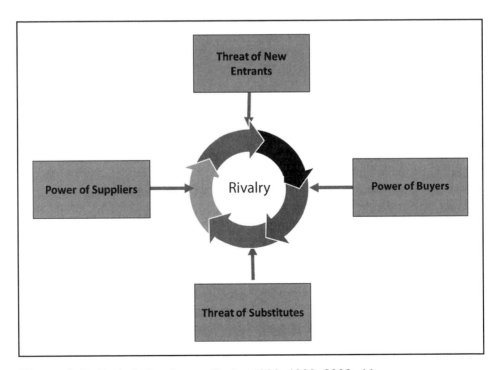

Figure 1–6. Porter's five forces (Porter 1980, 1998, 2008a,b).

Threats of New Entrants into the Market

Porter's first concern is for *new entrants* into the industry. New entrants into an industry add capacity. If the capacity added is greater than the growth in demand the added capacity reduces the profitability of whole the industry. Essentially, the easier it is for new companies to enter the industry the greater the chance for more competition. New entrants can emerge at any time changing an industry's character for market share, price, and customer loyalty disrupting other critical balances within the business environment. There is always a latent pressure for reaction and adjustment among the existing businesses (or incumbents) within the industry. The threat of new entries into the industry will depend on the extent to which there are *barriers to entry*. Significant barriers to entry in most industries include:

■ If *significant capital* is required to start a company. Some industries require huge amounts of capital to begin operations and follow up with marketing efforts to facilitate entry. Especially in times when capital is scarce, and significant amounts are required, funding can be a major barrier to entry into a particular industry. In the hearing industry the manufacturer of most products requires high capital investment and this provides a major barrier for entry into the marketplace.

■ If *economies of scale* or producing enough product volume efficiently is difficult. Firms that have been in the marketplace have learned manufacturing techniques, component suppliers, and other skills that allow them to manufacture enough products at costs that allow them to stay profitable. If not capable of manufacturing enough of the product, volume will suffer and subsequently profitability. Similarly, if the cost of manufacturing is more than other existing products within the industry, the cost of each of the new entry products will be priced too high for the market to absorb.

■ If *access to resources*, such as trained staff or patents, is limited. Often access to valuable resources can be controlled by the competition. These may be product components, capabilities, or some other essential feature valuable to production. If the new entrant is not able to access some of the essential resources standard to service delivery or product manufacture, the entrant product or service will be seen as substandard and, without significant compromise in price, sales will lag other industry products, reducing profitability for the entrant.

■ If *access to distribution channels* is limited. New entrants to the market need access to the traditional distribution channels or to create new ones to be successful. If the distribution channels are controlled by another entity within the industry, entrance can be difficult and, thus, a barrier to entry to the industry. Furthermore, if the major industry manufacturers have long-term contracts with large key customers these can tie up the market and act as a barrier. Many of the product brands are owned by the major manufacturers, holding companies and/or buying groups in the hearing industry, this creates a significant barrier to entry into the market.

- If *buyer's switching costs* are high. Some customers are brand loyal and prefer not to switch to a new entrant into the industry. Additionally, if the costs involved in training for the entrant product, obtaining spare parts, or other costs of switching are too expensive, the new product will not be adopted by the industry and profitability lost. Usually the costs of switching hearing aid suppliers is not much, the software, cords, and peripherals are usually complementary and the education required to switch is minimal; thus, this is not much of a barrier to entry. For equipment, however, there is a tendency to go with proven manufactures as these providers will offer an ease of repair, servicing, and other reliability factors.

- If there is *government intervention* within the industry. Governments often make rules as to who may be sold certain products. For example, a US company cannot sell war planes to communist countries. If the industry was selling war planes to Iran, selling them to Iran would be illegal. There are certain Medicare and Medicaid rules relative to service and product provisions that can be prohibitive to a new entrant into the hearing industry.

Power balance is affected by the ability of *new entrants* to enter the industry. If it costs little in time, energy, effort or funds to enter the industry and compete effectively, if it is easy to manufacture enough of the product (easily obtain economies of scale), and if there is little protection for product technology then the new competitor can and will enter the industry and the added capacity weakens the market position of all incumbent companies. The object of competitive strategy should be for incumbent companies to have strong and durable barriers for entry into the industry.

Bargaining Power of Buyers

In general, the prices that can be obtained for products and services have the most contribution to the profitability of a business. The *bargaining power of buyers* determines how customers can impose pressure on product or service margins and volumes. In most cases, a buyer of a particular product will shop around for the best deal causing downward pressure on prices. Buyers bargaining power is likely to be high in the following situations:

- If *switching costs are low*. When buyers can easily switch to another brand with relatively low cost and frustration, they are empowered to purchase from the lower cost provider. In the hearing industry switching costs are relatively low exerting pressure on suppliers to offer existing customers deals that keep them purchasing and mounting efforts to cause audiologists to switch to their product by incentives.

- If *buyers purchase in large volume* within a particular industry. In the hearing industry these can be large key customers, such as insurance companies, the Veteran's Administration, or buying groups that purchase huge lots of product. Suppliers are under major pressure to keep these buyers satisfied as they can disrupt cash flow if they were to not purchase, disrupting the balance within the industry.

- If buyers *manufacture the products in-house.* If, for example, the Veteran's Administration began manufacturing hearing instruments within their system, this would pose a significant threat to suppliers.
- If the supplying industry *comprises a large number of small operators.* The greater number of suppliers insures more price competition among the suppliers. If most buyers need to deal with a small number of suppliers, then the margins will be high for each product sold.
- If the supplying industry operates with *high fixed costs.*
- If the *product is undifferentiated* and can be easily replaced by substitutes. Products or services that are essentially the same can be purchased from any supplier for the lowest possible price. Manufacturers go to great lengths to differentiate their products and services even if they are similar so that buyers will not realize the similarities. Is not an audiometer an audiometer? Are there really differences among hearing instruments? Are these realities or simply our perceptions created by the differentiation process?
- If *switching to an alternative product is relatively simple* and is not related to high costs. As suggested earlier, it is a minor issue to switch hearing instrument suppliers.
- If buyers have *low margins* and are price-sensitive. Although most audiologists are price sensitive, for most clinics margins are large enough that minor adjustments in price can be tolerated.

- The product is *not strategically important* for the buyer.
- The *customer knows production costs* of the product.
- There is the possibility for the *buyer to integrate backward* or go into the business of supplying.

Essentially the concern with *Buyer Power* is the ease with which buyers can drive the prices down. Of course, this is driven by the number of buyers, the importance of each individual buyer, and the cost of switching products and services to those of another offering within the industry. If a supplier deals with a few powerful buyers, these buyers are then able to dictate their terms to the supplier.

Bargaining Power of Suppliers

Appreciating the *power of suppliers* can assist in understanding interactions within an industry and the strength of a particular business's current or future competitive position. The term "suppliers" comprises all sources for inputs or products that that are required for the business to provide goods or services to their customers (buyers). Assessing where the competitive power exists allows a new or expanding enterprise to take fair advantage of their strength, improve upon their weaknesses, and, possibly, avoid taking the wrong steps in a competitive business situation. Supplier bargaining power is likely to be high when:

- If the market is *dominated by a few large suppliers* rather than a fragmented source of supply. The hearing industry with its vertical and horizontal consolidation is now reduced in the number of suppliers each exercising much influence over their buyers.

- If there are *no substitutes for certain products*. It is well known that with a specific amplification manufacturer audiologists can fit 85% of their patients. For some patients, however, there are no substitutes for the products that they require. Phonak's Lyric is an example where they are the only manufacturer of a specific product that is required by the patients and providers that use them. For these instruments the supplier dictates price, availability and terms of use and there are no alternatives giving the supplier great power over the buyers.

- If the *supplier's customers are fragmented*, so their bargaining power is low. In independent audiology practices, not involved in a buying group, are at the mercy of the supplier for pricing. For most, independent practices their volume is minimal to the supplier so they are unable to negotiate a better price.

- If the *switching costs from one supplier to another are high*. Switching costs are not high and in the buyers favor within our industry, except where there is only one supplier of a specific product.

There is always the possibility of a supplier integrating forward or moving into supplying the consumer directly in order to obtain higher prices and/or margins.

This threat of forward integrations is especially high when:

- If the *buyers have higher profitability* than the supplying industry. Most audiology private practices have a greater profit margin than the manufacturer supplying the

products. Our industry is ripe for suppliers to forward integrate and this is occurring daily at this writing.

- If *forward integration, owning practices,* or *buying groups provides economies of scale* (or more sales) for the supplier. When a manufacturer purchases a practice, they expect the clinic to do 95% of their product. This substantially increases the suppliers economy of scale as they sell more product for a higher margin than if an audiologist purchased the product from them and then sold it to the consumer.

- If the *buying industry is hindering the supplying industry in their development* (e.g., reluctance to accept new releases of products). In the days of analog hearing instruments, there was a movement that felt that digital amplification was not necessarily better. This hindered the manufacturers in obtaining acceptance for their products by many buyers. Buyer acceptance of new products is essential for suppliers to obtain adoption of new technology. Sometimes it is seen as an opportunity to integrate forward and use the new product or technology.

- If the *buying industry has low barriers to entry*. In the hearing industry it does not take much of an investment for a manufacturer to enter the consumer market by either the purchase of a practice or simply stealing market share from the incumbents by heavy marketing, thus the tendency for forward integration from suppliers is ever present to the independent practitioner.

Basically, *Supplier Power* is how easy it is for suppliers to drive up prices. This is usually driven by the number of suppliers of each key input, the uniqueness of their product or service, their strength and control over the buyers within the industry, the cost of switching from one supplier to another. The fewer the supplier choices, the more supplier help is necessary to continue in practice, and the more powerful the suppliers become. When forward integration occurs, the buying industry often faces high pressure on margins from their suppliers that have become competitors. The relationship to powerful suppliers can potentially reduce strategic options for a business.

Threat of Substitutes

A *threat of substitutes* exists if there are alternative products used for the same purpose with lower prices that have better performance parameters than incumbent products already in the industry. These products could potentially attract a significant proportion of market volume and, hence, reduce the potential sales volume for incumbent companies. Similar to the threat of new entrants, the threat of substitutes is determined by factors such as:

- *Brand loyalty of customers.* Many audiologists are brand loyal as they have their philosophical reasons for using particular brands of equipment and/or amplification. There is a faction of professionals that are early adopters looking for a better product each day. These professionals are constantly looking for new products that will provide more benefit for patients. Substitutes for traditional amplification are instruments such as Lyric or middle ear implantable devices such as Esteem, modifications of cochlear implants, and others. Although these devices pose no real threat in 2012, there are possibilities that these instruments can become substitutes over time.

- *Close customer relationships.* Suppliers need to keep their customers happy as this will determine how easily they will switch to substitute products when they become available.

- *Switching costs for customers.* The switching costs to an implantable product are probably high in training and relationships with surgeons that will implant the device as well as follow-up support. These costs notwithstanding, there is a threat from these products on the horizon.

- *The relative price for performance of substitutes.* Why do I need a high end product for a patient with a limited lifestyle? Why should an implantable device be used when a traditional hearing instrument costs much less and provide the same benefit?

- *Current trends.* The trend at this point is to integrate amplification products into other devices and manufacturers that do not have this capability will not be considered by many buyers. Additionally, audiometer manufacturers have successfully used the PC as a format for their products, those that do not have a PC format will likely not be seriously considered for audiometric and special testing equipment.

The *Threat of Substitution* generally refers to the threat that buyers may find a new way to do what the incumbent companies have traditionally provided. There are often new inventions created that may, as they develop, significantly threaten the market for a product that is the standard of the industry or even replace these products. For example, a product such as Voice Over Internet Providers (VOIP) of telephone service. VOIP products are significant threat to substitute existing telephone companies and, subsequently, the incumbents within the industry are in the process of adjusting to this new technology by offering this VOIP telephone service bundled with cable TV, Internet service. In the hearing industry this would parallel advancements in technology that make implantable devices the method of choice for amplification, or research finding a cure for sensorineural hearing loss.

Rivalry Among the Incumbents

Rivalry refers to the intensity of competition between existing players (incumbents) within an industry. A highly competitive climate results in severe pressure on prices, margins, and, therefore on profitability for every company in the industry. Competition among existing players is likely to be high when:

- There are *many incumbents about the same size*. The hearing industry market has a few major incumbents and the number is being reduced due to horizontal and vertical consolidation.

- The *incumbent companies have similar strategies*. Competition is high from most of these companies as their have similar strategies. Basically, they have taken the differentiation strategy by attempting to present their product as different from others in the industry for one feature or another. Competition for differentiation among amplification, assessment, and other audiologic products is fierce.

- There is *not much differentiation among incumbents* and/or their products, thus the price competition is intense. On one side there is fierce competition for differentiation of products but simultaneously there is the commoditization of amplification that attempts to undifferentiate products. For some products where differentiation is minimal, there is intense price competition, while for those products that are successfully differentiated, price is not a major issue.

- *Low market growth rates* indicating that the growth of a particular company is possible only at the expense of a competitor. For quite some time, the market for amplification has been static. This static market suggests that growth of a company that supplies amplification products will only grow at the expense of another incumbent. As there is much market share stealing going on among the major incumbents, intense rivalry exists in the hearing industry.

- *Barriers for exit are highly expensive* as the companies have specialized equipment and procedures that cost dearly if they exited the manufacturing process.

Sidebar 1–3
PORTER'S FIVE FORCES (1980, 1998, 2008a)

Reducing the Bargaining Power of Suppliers

Partnering

Supply chain management

Supply chain training

Increase dependency

Build knowledge of supplier costs and methods

Take over a supplier

Reducing the Bargaining Power of Customers

Partnering

Supply chain management

Increase loyalty

Increase incentives and value added

Move purchase decision away from price

Cut powerful intermediaries (go directly to customer)

Reducing the Threat of New Entrants

Increase minimum efficient scales of operations

Create a marketing / brand image (loyalty as a barrier)

Patents, protection of intellectual property

Alliances with linked products / services

Tie up suppliers

Tie up distributors

Retaliation tactics

Reducing the Threat of Substitutes

Legal actions

Increase switching costs

Alliances

Customer *surveys* to learn about their preferences

Enter substitute market and influence from within

Accentuate differences (real or perceived)

Reducing the Competitive Rivalry Between Existing Players

Avoid price competition

Differentiate products

Buy out competition

Reduce industry overcapacity

Focus on different market segments

Communicate with competitors

Porter's Five Forces— How Does This Concept Apply To My Practice?

How does this apply to the management of a small independent practice? I am just a small clinic, why do I need to know this? As was presented earlier in the chapter, there are significant consolidations occurring each day in the overall hearing industry. Our suppliers are constantly reviewing these forces and their impact upon them so it behooves audiologists to at least understand these forces since we are vulnerable to them on the local level. Let's examine each of the five forces and how they apply to a small independent audiology practice. For our purposes, we define the industry as patients with a hearing impairment in a particular part of the country and the business as providing general audiological services and amplification products.

The Threat of New Entrants Into *My* Market

Porter's first competitive concern is new entrants into the industry. In the old days, before clinical doctorates, manufacturer's assistance, and other new concepts, barriers to entry were high. The start-up fixed and variable costs relative to the benefits were enormous, not to mention the expertise of running a business. Over the past 10 years this has drastically changed as the barrier to entry is significantly reduced. New entrants into the industry in your community may be another audiology private practitioner, an ENT physician, a new dispenser, or very likely a buying group or manufacturer disguised to look like another clinic. New entrants into your market are not necessarily a negative, unless the demand stays the same for services and products. Recall that new entrants to an industry add capacity to the available services and products and if the demand is not greater than the growth in availability it reduces the profitability for each individual practice within the whole industry. It is obvious that these new entrants into the small industry of practices within a particular community can change major components of the market environment, such as market shares, prices, patient loyalty, and other balanced factors. This situation may occur at any time and will create pressure for reaction and adjustment among the incumbents or existing practices within the industry (your particular small town). Since we know that the threat of new practices entering into our industry will depend on the extent to which there are *barriers to their entry*. A review of these barriers and how they apply to this small practice is germane to this discussion:

- *Significant capital.* Significant capital means different amounts to various people as it is relative to their resources. A new Audiology graduate is has a significant debt from school and the 75,000 to 100,000 in start-up costs seems like a major barrier to entry into practice in this small town. To a chain of practices with financial support, or a manufacturer owned clinic, this is often pocket change compared to the amount of products that can be sold. Profits in our industry are rather high, but with more competitors within the small town the margins will be compromised, marketing expenses will be greater and the patient population will be split into a lower market share for the incumbent practice. Although young competitors will have difficulties obtaining capital, especially in times when it is scarce; they may be funded by a buying group anxious to increase their buying power to suppliers. Chain practices usually funded by buying groups or manufacturers will still be able to secure the funding even if difficult times by purchasing the required increase in the number of products necessary to open a competitive clinic. Manufacturer owned clinics have the necessary cash to sustain themselves until they take over your market, demand becomes higher, or they have decided to buy out the competition.

■ *Economies of scale.* This refers to how well a new practice can compete with an existing practice. For example, if they are only open 3 days per week, they may not be able to provide enough service, follow-up, or product volume to become competitive. Conversely, if the competitors are open on weekends and the existing practice is not, this can be a concern. Building a new operation from scratch is difficult and either takes a very long time, lots of advertising or both, while the small practice has been in the marketplace, learned the culture of the community (industry), and specific procedures and products necessary to sustain the patient population. They have further

decided on product and equipment suppliers, reviewed the profitable services, and secured reliable referral sources that allow them to conduct enough business to stay profitable. Since they know the specific methods of conducting business within this particular community, this knowledge is the economy of scale serves as another significant, though not insurmountable, barrier to entry.

■ *Access to resources*, such as trained staff is limited to the number of trained professional staff and clerical support available. Often, access to these valuable resources can be controlled by the competition. Resources may be equipment, office space, referral sources, or some other essential feature valuable to attracting perspective patients. If the new entrant is not able to access some the essential capability standard to a practice within the community, the practice will be seen as substandard and, without significant compromise in price, sales will lag competitive practices, reducing profitability.

■ *Access to distribution channels* is limited. A significant barrier to entry for a new practice is obtaining patients or accessing the distribution of their services and products. New entrants to the market begin with no referral sources, no patients and need to either access to the traditional distribution channels such as referral sources or to create a new channel, usually from intense marketing to be successful. If the distribution channels are controlled by another entity (such as the incumbent or existing practices), entrance into the market may be difficult and, thus, serve as a barrier to entry. Furthermore, if the existing businesses have long term contracts with insurance companies or others, these may tie up the market and create yet another barrier to entry.

■ *Buyer's switching costs* are high. Some patients are simply brand loyal; they are thoroughly convinced that the existing practice is the best and prefer not to switch to the new entrant into the community. Additionally, they may have a warranty or after care program that offers discounts on products, repairs, and follow-up visits that serve as a barrier for them to switch to the new practice. If switching costs of learning the new practice, obtaining repairs, cleanings, developing new relationships, and other products/services seem too expensive, the new practice will not be adopted by the patient population and profitability for the new practice will be lost. Clinicians should be aware that the newest group of patients, baby boomers, are not very loyal and extra effort is necessary to keep them with the incumbent.

■ *Government intervention* within the industry. Although this is not usually a barrier for another practice to enter a particular market. It could be that licensure, continuing education, tax collection licenses, and other governmental issues maybe a barrier to entry.

Competitive power is affected by the ability of new practice to enter the industry. If it costs little in time, energy, effort, or capital to enter the market and compete effectively; if it is easy to provide enough appointment times, appropriate services, and other economies of scale, and if there is little protection for the technology surrounding the methods and model in which the products and services are provided; new competition can enter the industry and weaken the market position of all incumbent practices. The object of a competitive strategy should be to have strong and durable barriers to entry into the community deterring new entrants by preserving a favorable position for the practice and taking fair advantage of this position.

Bargaining Power of Buyers— What Is *My* Power?

As a purchaser of products for your practice there may be significant power or very little power. Since the prices you can obtain for your products and services have the most contribution to the profitability of the business, it is essential to obtain the best possible price for products and keep costs low for the provision of services. It makes good sense to shop around for the best deal on employees, products, equipment, and other items essential to the practice. If the practice is large enough this can have some effect on reducing costs for these items, but most of practices are small enough that our efforts will not obtain much supplier negotiation. In this situation, buying groups are another choice to keep costs down by purchasing products as part of a much larger group. Often, there are other buying group benefits, such as marketing, loans, or business support. Buying groups, though beneficial in lowering costs to a practice, can also be a source of frustration if the buying group changes their policies, or if they gain too much power over the practice. Your power as a buyer is likely to be high in the following situations:

■ When *switching costs are low*. If the buyer (the practice) can easily switch to another brand with the same results and relatively low cost, minimize frustration, and relearning, then they are empowered to purchase from the lower cost provider.
■ *Buyers purchase in large volume* within a buying group, keeping their costs reasonable, but service support high.
■ Buyers *manufacturing the products in-house*. Not usually possible in an average audiology practice. At times it is possible to obtain components and manufacture in house, but it is usually impractical, thus, not part of the buyers power in our industry.
■ The supplying industry *comprises a large number of small operators*.
■ The supplying industry operates with *high fixed costs*.
■ The *product is undifferentiated* and can be replaced by substitutes.
■ *Switching to an alternative product is relatively simple* and is not related to high costs.
■ The product is *not strategically important* for the *buyer*.
■ The *buyer knows production costs* of the product.

Essentially, the concern with buyer power is how easy it is to for the buyers to drive the prices for product down. Of course this is driven by the number of buyers, the supplier importance of each individual buyer, and the cost of switching products and services to those of another offering in the industry. If a supplier deals with a few, powerful buyers these buyers are then able to dictate their terms to the supplier, while the small independent audiology practice will struggle.

The Power of Suppliers— How Am I Being Managed by Suppliers?

As audiologists we are concerned with the ethics of various situations but none is more tedious than that of manufacturer relationships. Although we are concerned about great technology, support, and other benefits for our patients, manufacturers compete very hard for our business. Foster's forces suggest that supplier power begins with having some control over the Industry. There is much competition for our business among the major manufacturers, all offering state of the art technology, customer service, support, and special features. Since there are a number of major suppliers of amplification products, supplier control is not as much of an issue unless the practice has given control of product supply to a particular manufacturer with some sort of an agreement. Phonak's Lyric is a classic example supplier power. As the only purveyor of this product, they have substantial supplier power over the small audiology practice. If they cut off supply, charge a higher price, modify the product, decide only to sell to high volume customers, there is no recourse or buyer control over their decisions. The small practice is totally at the mercy of the supplier's power in this example. Conversely, if a small practice is dealing a major manufacturer, such as Siemens, and there are unfavorable modifications in price, competition, terms, product technology, or other issues; simply switch to Phonak, Resound, Oticon, Widex, or others. In this situation the small audiology practice has significant buyer power.

Appreciating the power of suppliers can assist in a knowledge of what is happening in the industry and an understanding of the strength of a practice's current or future competitive position using their products. Supplier bargaining power is likely to be high when:

- The market is dominated by a few large suppliers rather than a fragmented source of supply. For our small audiology practice the supplier power is rather low as the clinic has the opportunity to obtain product from others that are also of high quality and performance.
- There are no substitutes for the particular for certain products for specific patients, as in the Phonak Lyric example.
- The supplier's customers are fragmented, so their bargaining power is low, as with independent practices. Many audiologists are independent practices and purchasing power is fragmented. If involved in a buying group, the buyer power is much greater and the power is the large number of sales from the buying group. Thus, members of a buying group are not subjected to supplier power from the manufacturers, but there is supplier power from the buying group. The "member" of the buying group must follow the rules

and regulations of the buying group to continue involvement.
- The switching costs from one supplier to another are high. As presented earlier, in audiology practices there is not much cost in switching to another manufacturer as suppliers are eager to offer the software for no cost, and demonstration units at minimal cost. They also offer training at no cost on their products so costs are minimal to switch; reducing supplier power.

As suggested earlier in this chapter there is significant move by suppliers toward owning audiology practices. This is an effort to control the manufacturer and distribution of the products to increase margins and profits. The threat of suppliers "moving forward" or purchasing direct outlets for their products is especially high when:

- The buying industry has a higher profitability than the supplying industry. It is well known that retail outlets, such as audiology clinics, have significant margins that have been coveted by product manufacturers for generations. This is the reason that manufacturers are purchasing audiology clinics and will continue to do so for some time.
- Forward integration, owning practices or buying groups provides economies of scale (or more sales) for the supplier. When the supplier owns or has a significant interest in a buying group they can feature their own products, selling a greater volume of them then if offered to fragmented audiology clinics. The purchase of a practice by a

manufacturer not only insures sales of their products but also generates good margins with profit once on the product sale to the practice and a second profit opportunity for the retail margin as well.

■ The buying industry hinders the supplying industry in their development. Often, audiology has not rapidly accepted new product styles or new generation technology. In the 90s, it took digital hearing aids some time to become standard of care. It took some time for thin tube instruments, receiver in the canal (RIC) instruments, and Bluetooth technology to be used in big volumes.

■ The buying industry has low barriers to entry. To a manufacturer or a buying group (suppliers), it takes a minimal amount to begin a new audiology or hearing aid dispensing operation.

Supplier power can be a huge consideration if the small Audiology practice:

■ Has supplier loans and is committed to the purchase of a certain number of products over a particular period of time.

■ If the supplier is the sole provider of products with a unique technology, such as Phonak's Lyric or if the practice is a franchise, such as Beltone or Audibel, where only one brand of product is used exclusively.

■ If the supplier is a buying group and the practice has only one bill for all products obtained. These statements from one supplier (the buying group) can be very convenient, but if the payables get behind the buying group will cut off the supply.

As in most industries, the fewer the supplier choices, the more supplier help is necessary, and the more powerful the suppliers become. In our industry there are a number of options to obtain traditional products and services, unless the practice has relinquished their power as buyers by entering into contracts or use a product for which there is only one supplier. In such situations, the buying industry often faces a high pressure on margins from their suppliers that can potentially reduce strategic options.

Threat of Substitutes—Will Audiologists Become Obsolete?

A threat from substitutes exists if there are alternative products used for the same purpose with lower prices that have better performance parameters than those incumbent products already in the industry. In a small audiology practice most of its income from the dispensing of amplification products the treat of substitutes always exists. New research that cures sensorineural hearing loss, development of affordable implantable hearing devices, Internet hearing aid sales, and insurance programs that exclude some clinics all threaten as substitutes to the independent small audiology practice. These cures, concepts, and philosophies could potentially attract a significant proportion of market volume and, hence, reduce the potential sales volume for the clinic and threaten its very existence. Although many of these possible substitutes are impossible, some are improbable, and others remain, at this time the threat of substitutes is rather low in audiology. The threat of substitutes is determined by factors such as:

- *Brand loyalty of customers.* "Take good care of patients and they will take good care of you," goes the proverb. Brand loyalty in this this sense refers to how loyal your patients and referral sources are to the practice. The higher the loyalty, the less the threat from substitutes to the practice.
- *Close customer relationships.* Related to brand loyalty, it is necessary to communicate and build close relationships with the patients so that they will not want to go to another provider.
- *Switching costs for customers.* Although it may not cost much for the patient to switch, you want to instill the perception that if they do switch they will not get much value, less product, less warranty, less expertise, less care, and so forth. Basically, it is up to the practitioner to convince the patient or referral source that they are settling for less when they substitute another practice for yours.
- *The relative price for performance of substitutes.* The substitutes may have a better price, but is the product the same, does it have a better warranty, or is it "good value for money"? Is the substitute really a substitute or just a different place where services and products will be at a lower level?
- *Current trends.* There are a number of current trends that can have an effect on the small audiology practice.
  - Manufacturers purchasing practices.
  - Development of implantable middle ear devices, that is, Esteem, Otologics, Symphonics, and others.

- Buying groups.
- Insurance programs unfriendly to audiologists
- Internet hearing aid sales.

The *Threat of Substitution* refers to the possibility that the patients may not need the products and services or find a new way obtain what the practice has always offered. There are often new inventions created that may, as they develop in technology, significantly threaten to cut into the market for a product that is the standard of the industry or even replace these products, that is, middle ear and cochlear implants replacing hearing aids. Although these substitute technologies for amplification or cures for sensorineural hearing loss are unlikely, they are nevertheless possibilities for the future.

Rivalry Among the Incumbents—Competitive Spirit Among Audiologists

Rivalry refers to the intensity of competition between existing practices within a particular market. In most markets there is a highly competitive climate that results in severe pressure on prices, margins, and, therefore on profitability in all of the practices within the market. Competition among existing practices within a particular market is likely to be high when:

- There are many practices about the same size.
- Various existing practices within the market that have similar strategies. Many practices use preprepared marketing programs offered by manufacturers. The more similar these programs, the higher the

competition will be and the more it makes sense to use a strategy than the different from the competition.

- There is not much differentiation among incumbents and/or their products, thus the price competition is intense. The more differentiation among the practices within the market, the less competition will be a factor.
- Low market growth rates indicating that the growth of a particular company is possible only at the expense of a competitor. It is well known that the market for amplification is a stagnated yet only a fraction of those that could use our services and products actually seek them. Thus, with a market that is not growing, competition is high for each patient that is seeking treatment.
- Barriers for exit are highly expensive as practices have invested in equipment, facilities, and education; hence, it is not easy to exit practice once the clinic is opened.

To apply Porter's five forces to an individual problem, such as your practice, a product manufacturer, or other industry endeavors, explore the Internet. Consider sites such as Mind Tools (2012) offering worksheets and other tools that can be extremely helpful to assessing the competition.

References

Alagse. (2012). Customer focused low cost strategy. Alagse.com. Retrieved June 2, 2012, from http://www.alagse.com/strategy/s10.php

Bofah, K. (2012). What is industry consolidation. eHow Money. Retrieved May 20, 2012, from http://www.ehow.com/facts_5965961_industry-consolidation_html

Business dictionary.com. (2012). Commoditization of products. Retrieved June 2, 2012, from http://www.businessdictionary.com/definition/commoditization.html#ixzz1weZHLrWO

Drucker, P. (2008). *The Essential Drucker: The Best Sixty Years of Drucker's Essential Writing on Management.* New York, NY: Harper Collins Publishing.

Federal Deposit Insurance Corporation (FDIC). (2012a). New federal banking regulations. Retrieved May 30, 2012, from http://www.fdic.gov/regulations/laws/rules/index.html

Federal Deposit Insurance Corporation (FDIC). (2012b). Failed bank list. Federal Deposit Insurance Corporation. Retrieved June 7, 2012, from http://www.fdic.gov/bank/individual/failed/banklist.html

Flynn, S. (2011). *Economics for dummies.* Indianapolis, IN: Wiley.

Hurwich, M. (2012). Everyday low pricing. Strategic Pricing Management Group. Retrieved June 2, 2012, from http://www.spmgpricing.com/Every%20day%20low%20pricing.pdf

Investor Words. (2012). Definition of Gross Domestic Product (GDP). Investorwords.com. Retrieved June 7, 2012, from http://www.investorwords.com/2153/GDP.html

Investopedia. (2012). Definition of Consumer Price Index. Investopedia.com. Retrieved May 30, 2012, from http://www.investopedia.com/terms/c/consumerpriceindex.asp

Kennon, J. (2012). The Federal Reserve and interest rates. About.com: Investing for beginners. Retrieved June 6, 2012, from http://beginnersinvest.about.com/od/banking/a/aa062405.htm

Kocic, A. (2012). Definition of industry consolidation. eHow.com. Retrieved May 16, 2012, from http://www.ehow.com/about_6555139_definition-industry-consolidation.html

Lash, J. (2007). Low cost is not a strategy. Goodproductmanager.com. Retrieved June 2, 2012, from http://www.goodproduct manager.com/2007/06/25/low-cost-is-not-a-strategy/

Manktelow, J., & Carlson, A. (2012). Assessing the balance of power in a business situation. *Mind tools video.* Retrieved May 30, 2012, from http://www.youtube .com/watch?v=KlNlYeS0JTI&feature= player_embedded

Mind Tools. (2012). Porter's five forces: Assessing the balance of power in a business situation. Retrieved May 30, 2012, from http://www.mindtools.com/pages/ article/newTMC_08.htm

Money Café. (2012). Prime interest rates. Moneycafe.com. Retrieved June 7, 2012, from http://www.moneycafe.com/library/ primerate.htm

Porter, M. (1980). *Competitive strategy.* New York, NY: Free Press.

Porter, M. (1998). *Competitive strategy* (2nd ed.). New York, NY: Free Press.

Porter, M. (2008a). Five competitive forces that shape strategy. In M. Porter (Ed.), *On competition* (p. 9), Cambridge, MA: Harvard Business Press.

Porter, M. (2008b). *On competition.* Cambridge, MA: Harvard Business Press.

Recklies, D. (2001). Porter's five forces. The Manager.org. Retrieved May 21, 2012, from http://www.themanager.org/Models/p5f. htm

Trading Economics. (2012). United States annual GDP growth rate. Retrieved June 7, 2012, from http://www.tradingeconom-ics.com/united-states/gdp-growth-annual

US Inflation Calculator. (2012). Annual inflation rates 2002–2012. Retrieved June 7, 2012, from http://www.usinflationcalc ulator.com/inflation/current-inflation-r ates/

US National Debt Clock. (2012). Outstanding debt by date and time. Retrieved May 30, 2012, from http://brillig.com/debt_clock/

2

Strategic Business Planning

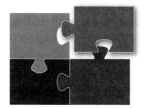

ROBERT M. TRAYNOR, EdD, MBA

Introduction

Independent private practice is a rapidly expanding sector of the audiology profession. Practitioners are choosing not to practice in hospitals, government clinics, and ENT practices as these settings are increasingly viewed as restrictive to professional autonomy and/or financial opportunity. With the advent of the Doctor of Audiology (AuD) degree over the past few years, private practice has become the "new frontier" for entrepreneurial, business oriented, audiologists. These independently practicing audiologists are truly fostering the successful transition of audiology into an entrepre-

neurial doctoring profession, taking its rightful place with optometry, dentistry, chiropractic, and other doctoring professions. In a new century, armed with a doctorate that uniquely designates the profession, independently practicing audiologists have become a stand-alone professional business enterprise poised to treat the huge baby boomer hearing-impaired population. Baby boomers are more likely to go directly to allied health professionals and are not necessarily dependent upon their physician to direct them to the correct professional to treat specific disorders. Due to their education, the Internet, and a changing medical community this new generation of patients is more apt to seek treatment by audiologists, chiropractors, nurse practitioners, and other emerging allied professions without visiting their physician for a formal referral. Fueled by legislation that may offer patients direct access to audiology services, the possibility of government sponsored health care, and hearing aid tax credits; those with hearing impairment will seek care direct from independently practicing audiologists.

Although the profession of audiology is recognized by individuals seeking resolution of their hearing difficulties more than ever before, it remains much less prominent to bankers and other perspective lenders. These business professionals loan money to unfamiliar businesses every day but there are specific rules by which they evaluate each of these investment opportunities. One of the "rules of the road" for the evaluation of an unfamiliar enterprise is to review a business plan offered by the perspective business. Since the business of audiology is an unfamiliar model to most funding sources, practitioners must develop a sound business plan that clearly establishes their fundamental business strategy and a realistic plan, not for just taking good care of patients, but the generation of revenue. Even in the best of times, the prevailing attitude among lenders is that of skepticism and to raise capital for an existing or new audiology practice, the owner must present an extremely convincing business plan (Tracy, 2005). In these challenging economic times, where new government regulations prevail and when perspective funders are extremely reluctant to loan funds to anyone; the challenge is to construct a conservative, straightforward, concise, yet detailed business plan that will demonstrate the lucrativeness of the investment opportunity. A well-thought-out business plan has become an essential component of the rules of engagement and the basic link between perspective lenders and investors and the entrepreneurial practitioner.

As audiology expands as a profession, offering clinicians a variety of practice opportunities across a number of venues, each type of audiology practice begins with a conceptual framework. This framework is a general concept of how the products and services are provided, the populations to be served, an assessment of the competition within the market area, projected costs to provide these products and services, and a detailed analysis of the projected income versus these projected costs. Once the concept, needs, and other infrastructural components begin to solidify, a detailed business plan is then developed from the framework to describe the operational and economic realities of the practice concept. Built upon a sound conceptual framework, the formal business plan provides a clear and complete picture of resources required to turn the practice concept into a profitable business reality over a specific time period. For a new or expanding audiology practice, the business plan includes the important business and clinical parameters to be evaluated by investors at beginning of the venture as well a review of the assets required to nourish the business through its three-year start-up phase and beyond. For the plan to serve as an effective roadmap to success, it must be exhaustive in its clarity of concept and present an accurate, yet conservative, depiction of the anticipated costs and the revenues to be generated. Additionally, the plan must include necessary milestones for the measurement of success or failure with known instruments and have individuals assigned to monitor and conduct the measurements.

Business plans are not simply for the private practice venue. Other practice settings use business planning, but often call them by another name, such as, a "New Program Proposal" or "Departmental Prospectus." These alternative plans may be labeled with other titles specific to the practice venue and the business concept under consideration but are nonetheless a business plan. In an educational setting a new program proposal may be used to present the clinical and financial benefits of offering a new service to students. In a hospital setting a departmental prospectus might be used to conceptually present a new service, the costs of providing that service and the financial benefits to the department for the provision of the new service. Regardless of the venue or the name of the document, these business plans are utilized to establish the need, set forth operational and fiscal requirements necessary to establish and maintain the new or expanded enterprise and, most importantly, the financial benefit to the enterprise.

The purpose of this chapter is to present the rationale for the framework or business preplanning and formal business planning for start-up and existing audiology practices. Additionally, it offers the mechanics of how to go about planning for an audiology practice, tips for success, and checklists to ensure that all the planning has been accomplished. It is, however, highly recommended that those preparing a business plan consider the use of a myriad of computer programs to facilitate the components of the planning process. Recently, Web sites such as http://www.liveplan.com have surfaced offering business planning expertise for a reasonable cost and work very much like the business planning programs and, for either Mac or PC computers. These relatively inexpensive, yet very sophisticated Web sites or business planning programs bring the expertise of seasoned business professionals to the table as they take the preparer from the most basic business planning concept to the completion with shear professionalism.

Is the Business World Really for Me?

Before beginning the planning process, the first question that must be considered is, "Is running a business really for me"? Some audiologists have dreamed of owning their own clinic since they began in the field, whereas others may not be interested in running a business and are best served working for a company or a practice as an employee. Those without the entrepreneurial spirit are better off not beginning a business that, due to interest or aptitude, may be ill managed and ultimately fail.

For those that share the dream of owning their own business, they will never be satisfied as an employee and will work for others only until they can begin their own practice. These audiologists yearn to work for themselves and be their own boss, have the freedom to take days off at will, paying themselves a higher salary, set the policies and procedures of the practice, while obtaining earned benefits or perks from manufacturers for conducting business. If these are the motivations for beginning a practice caution should be observed as these and other benefits may or may not be immediately available, and some may never be achieved. As an employee, the benefits of owning the business may be observed, but often it is difficult for employees to experience the hard, nonclinical work necessary (usually in addition to a full clinic schedule) that goes into management of an audiology clinic. The real truths and myths of owning a practice are often not obvious until the employee becomes responsible for toiling in the clinic every day seeing patients, simultaneously ensuring employees are paid, payroll and other taxes are paid, as well as meeting fixed costs such as rent, leases, lights, telephone, payables, and other expenses each month. Before progressing much further in business planning process, it is necessary to review a few of the truths or myths of running a business such as a private audiology practice.

Being Your Own Boss

While working for others as employees, many audiologists may have felt that it would be better to "work for themselves" or "be their own boss." On the surface, the idea of "being your own boss" in a business seems reasonable. There is no one to tell you what to do, when to do it, how to do it, or if you should do it. Therefore, the idea of "being your own boss" has some face validity to the uninitiated. In reality "being your own boss" is a myth as a business owner has many bosses and an audiology practice owner is no exception. In an audiology clinic, there are many bosses and foremost among them are the patients, to whom the practitioner is ultimately responsible to provide services, products, and follow up the products with warranty service. Practice owners are also responsible to the patients for all other administrative issues, such as keeping malpractice insurance, timely return of product deposits, maintaining

the competence and certification of not only themselves, but their employees, and virtually everything else that goes with the provisions of high quality services and products.

The practice's valuable referral sources are another "boss" that requires constant maintenance as the competition will always be going after them in an attempt to win them for their practice. Competition for referral sources in the marketplace makes it just that much more important to turn reports around promptly, keep communications constant, and reinforce the referral sources expertise routinely (see Chapter 13). A private practice proverb is that, "If you take good care of your patients and referral sources, they will take good care of you."

If the practice has a bank loan, it must be paid no matter if there is business or not, so another "boss" are bankers or the investors in the practice. Because they have put up funding for the clinic, bankers and those to whom long-term or short- term loans are owed have a vested interest in the success or failure of the business. Their main goal is to receive a good return on their investment and their interests may not be the same as your goals. Although your goals are to provide the highest quality audiological services and products, these people simply want to be paid and make a profit.

Often, the first to observe success or failure of the business, the practice accountant is still another "boss." As those that monitor the books and the success or failure of the methods, procedures, dispensing products, and other routine business practices, it is a wise practice owner that listens carefully to their accountant. Their recommendations may involve changes in the provision of specific products and services, pricing, tax issues, or other business modifications that are essential to the financial stability of the practice, all of which makes the accountant another "boss" to whom the wise practice owner listens carefully.

Even the most ethical and conscientious Audiology practices are plagued with legal issues from time to time which makes their attorney another "boss." Legal issues such as business structure, leasing space, equipment, employee issues, collections, difficult patients, taxes, and other legal issues can create situations where the practitioner must conduct business as indicated by their attorney (see Chapter 3). As we discuss later in this text, generally, in patient-centric practice we work with our patients first and foremost; if we do a good job with our patients, then usually the other bosses will be served as well. Thus, concept of "being your own boss" is not really true in that the audiology practice owner has many bosses, all of whom are extremely important to keep satisfied for a practice to succeed. Being your own boss is a myth.

Take Time Off

It is good (and necessary) to have time off to relax, forget those problem patients, the employee's problems, or the frustrations of paying the months expenses but if the practice is successful, there may not be very much time or funds for days off or personal vacations. Especially in a solo practice, when the clinician is away and the clinic is closed there is no income into the clinic. Unless the practitioner has responsible employees that can keep the doors open and see patients in their absence, time off must be scheduled around the clinic schedule and other low pressure times, such as holiday periods or when business is usually slow. For example, if the practice is in a very

hot climate, such as Arizona or Florida, summertime is probably the best time to close and, similarly, if in Minnesota it might make sense to close in a difficult period in the wintertime. Even in a practice that has good clerical employees and colleague clinicians it is difficult to get away for much longer than a week without frustrating situations arising during the absence or upon return. These difficulties can sometimes be devastating to the practice so it is best to err on the side of caution and be careful about absences whether they be elected vacations, or necessary emergencies. As in other businesses, an audiology practice requires that the owner be available most of the time for business and clinical decisions that are required each day. Often, well-meaning employees may make decisions that they feel are in the best interest of the clinic, but these could be inaccurate based upon the full knowledge of clinic operations and plans for the future. The business world is unforgiving and a proprietor or CEO who is absent will be punished severely by the marketplace. Getting more time off is a myth.

Getting a Higher Salary

Clerical and professional employees observe the income into the practice as they are involved in its generation and collection. It is a normal reaction, given the costs of services and products, to perceive that these gigantic sums coming into the practice should generate enough income to the practice to increase their compensation (see Chapter 14). The issue is that while an employee observes the income they typically do not have much information regarding the expenses that must be paid by that income. The practice owner's salary is determined by many things, but mostly by the amount of business conducted and the control of costs. When business is good, cash flow is created and it is the cash flow as well as the control of fixed and avoidable costs that facilitate the level of the practice owner's salary. In a new practice, it could very well be that the generation of income will be significant and, accordingly, the salary and benefits will be very high. Realistically, however, a new audiology practice will typically not generate much initial cash flow and, subsequently, not much income for the practitioner until the business is established in the marketplace. In a new clinic, cash flow is limited and as expenses such as rent, utilities, telephone, employees, and payroll taxes need to be paid first, it is not unusual that the owner's salary begins at a lower level than they experienced when working as an employee elsewhere. Another old private practice proverb is, "The owner is always paid last." After a period of time, it may be possible for the clinic to generate a greater cash flow, meeting all the expenses; then (and only then) can salary and benefit increases can be considered for the owner. Just the entry into private practice does not insure a higher salary and/or benefits, the survival of the business is foremost and takes priority over how much the practice owner will be compensated. Obtaining a higher salary is usually a myth in the beginning and may become a reality as the practice matures.

Setting the Rules of the Practice

Clinicians who have worked for others have often found themselves feeling that they could manage the clinic better than their boss. In their opinion, the clinic should have different hours of operation, better/newer equipment, more or less procedures, less paperwork, better (or different) products, more precise evaluative protocols, higher or lower prices, better credit terms, higher or lower attire standards, better benefit packages, better policies, and/or various other issues that, in their opinion, should be managed differently. Although these management modifications in policies and procedures seem perfectly reasonable to the employees from their perspective, once they realize the rationales for the positions taken by their employer, they often arrive at the same or similar decisions they criticized as employees. Thus, owning a practice to be able to change the management technique, policies, and procedures is often a myth.

Obtaining Earned Benefits from Manufacturers

Obtaining "benefits" from manufacturers of hearing instruments have become a very controversial issue in the second decade of the 21st century. In the past, these benefits included trips, equipment, loans, and many other perks offered from hearing instrument manufacturers that could be earned as part of simply conducting business with a particular supplier. These benefits could be earned by selling a specific number of units of a manufacturer's product and thus, trips to exotic places, new equipment, low interest loans, special cash accounts, and other benefits were provided to practice owners. These perks and special benefits were provided to the practice owner with no out of pocket expense. Although these benefits are often considered a normal part of conducting business by manufacturers of most products, audiological recommendations for hearing devices are involve a special fiduciary trust relationship. Over the years, ethical practice boards for both national and state audiology organizations have found on numerous occasions that obtaining these benefits are unethical, ruling that these "gifts or benefits" could (and do) influence the clinician's choice of hearing instruments chosen for their patients. The ethical concern is that a practice manager in need of a few more units to pay for the trip to Europe, that ABR unit, or this month's payment on the loan, might possibly compromise patient care recommending instruments that count toward the trip when the patient would be better served by another manufacturer's product. Of course, most audiologists are ethical and would not let these product choices be influenced by trip qualification or units for equipment, etc; it is, however, considered unethical practice nonetheless by the American Academy of Audiology, American Speech-Language Association, the Academy of Doctors of Audiology, and many state licensure boards. If the practitioner does not care about ethics or keeping their certification, then these perks are possible (see Chapter 4). Owning a practice for the "benefits" offered by manufacturers is most likely a myth unless you are willing to compromise your ethical standards.

Is Owning a Business Right for You?

Even those that contemplate owning a practice need to ask themselves serious questions that can shed light on if they *really* should be the person responsible for the clinical and financial success of a practice. SBA (2011) offers 20 questions that should be considered before arriving at the final decision to own any business. These questions have been modified to reflect the audiology private practice rather than a generic business. The answers to these questions assist a clinician in the determination if they have a general aptitude toward becoming a small business owner.

1. Am I prepared to expend the time, money, and precious resources required to generate my new audiology practice?
2. What kind of a practice do I want?
3. What products/services will my practice provide to the public?
4. Why am I starting a new practice?
5. What/who is my target market?
6. Who is the competition in the chosen market?
7. What is unique about this particular idea and the products/services provided that distinguish this clinic from the competition?
8. How much time will pass before my products/services are available?
9. How much funding will be required to get this new practice up and running?
10. How long will the practice need funding before it begins to make a profit?
11. Will the company require outside funding?
12. How will prices be computed compared to the competition?
13. How will the practice be marketed?
14. What legal business structure should be used for the practice?
15. How will the practice be managed?
16. Where will the practice be located?
17. How many employees will practice require at start up?
18. Who will be the suppliers for the practice?

19. What kind of insurance policies are necessary for my practice?
20. What is necessary to insure that taxes are paid correctly?

These are essential questions that must be answered to accurately assess if the world of practice management is an good fit or if it is best to let others manage the clinic and simply take good care of someone else's patients.

What Is a Strategy?

Organizations that succeed and organizations that fail have one link, strategy. A strategy that succeeds and one that does not offer success are still strategies nonetheless. But what goes into a strategy? Probably one of the world's authorities on strategy was Dr. Paul Drucker (1909–2005), a professor of management and, even today, is still considered one of the world authorities in management, ethics, and planning. Cohen (2010) discusses Drucker's concept of strategic development as the continuous process of making entrepreneurial (risk taking) decisions systematically in the present with the greatest knowledge of their futurity while organizing systematically the efforts needed to carry out these decisions through organized systematic feedback.

Drucker is basically presenting that strategizing or strategic development is a continuous process that involves risk-taking decisions that must be made in the present for things that will happen in the future and, of course, only thing we know about the future is that it will be different from the present. Since we must develop a concept of how we will progress in the future while in the "here and now,"

decisions of how to proceed should be made with the greatest knowledge available of what could happen in the future and the probable implications of these decisions. Thus, when taking decisions as to how to approach the situations created by a new business, Drucker felt that an organized and detailed plan (i.e., a business plan) must be generated to insure that all future variables are covered at least to the extent that they can be predicted in the present. Finally, he felt that all this planning and strategizing was a moot point without systematic feedback to make modifications if the future did not actually turn out as predicted. The directors of a clinic, a private practice owner, or others in charge of the clinic are the leaders, and leaders are responsible for pointing out the general direction, directing the implementation of the strategy, obtaining and analyzing feedback and adjusting the actions and movement toward the desired results. The leaders should consider the statistics, and other valuable data points, but paramount in development of a strategy is the leader's judgment, leadership, and vision.

What then is a strategy? Cohen (2010) describes it as more than a combination of objectives, resources, and well thought out approaches to where the plan hopes to go, but rather it is a roadmap that guides the organization forward to the future that is being created.

Arrival at a strategy involves asking some questions (Cohen, 2010):

- What opportunities does it want to pursue and what risks is it willing to take?
- What is the scope and structure of the plan including the right balance among such aspects as specialization, diversification, and integration?

■ What is the acceptable tradeoff between time and money and between in-house execution as opposed to merger, acquisition, joint venture or other external means to reach the desired objectives?

■ What organizational structure is appropriate to economic realities, opportunities, and performance expectations?

Why Plan?

Another old business proverb states that, "If you do not plan, you are planning to fail." This is true for any new business, especially an audiology business. Although the increase in the number and quality of private practices is good for the profession, the increase in quality competition makes it even more necessary to exert the effort to plan a new practice or a practice expansion. Furthermore, it is impossible to predict economic future and other variables that can affect a business. Planning the business allows the owner to bring, as much as is possible, the future into the present so that issues relating to the success or failure of the business can be strategized in the present. SBA (2011), Berry (2006), and many others suggest that a business plan should be a *work in progress* since businesses evolve over

---

Sidebar 2–1
TEN PRINCIPLES ESSENTIAL TO THE DEVELOPMENT OF A STRATEGY

In the development of specific strategies it is necessary to consider the following elements that Cohen (2010) has derived from his readings and interactions with Peter Drucker. These have been interpreted into language that should be easily understood by audiologists as they develop their strategies on how to attack the marketplace.

1. Commit fully to a definite objective. Another old planning proverb is, "You cannot get to where you are going until you know where that is." A full commitment to the goals and objectives of your project. This will be your very soul until the project is outlined, planned, executed, meets success, or is revised or abandoned.

2. Seize the initiative and keep it. If you have a good idea for a practice or a new twist on the marketplace or other opportunity that makes your brand of audiology different from the competition, seize the moment. Take the initiative and keep it until the goal is achieved. There are many stories of those that delayed entrance or never entered the marketplace and others use your idea and enter the market with success.

3. Economize to mass your resources. You cannot do everything as there are only so many hours in a day and resources are always limited. You must choose your most profitable, beneficial products and services. Economize where efforts and resources are not critical and concentrate them to areas of importance. This involves the economic concept of opportunity costs described in Chapter 8.

4. Use strategic positioning. This involves flexibility by moving to the unexpected changes that will most likely occur when a business concept moves toward reality. The environment, competition, economy, insurance discounts, governmental regulations, government sponsored health care and other unforeseen issues create the need to change plans, modify direction and other strategic maneuvers as the plan is exercised.

5. Do the unexpected. Surprise the competition by doing something that truly makes you and your new entry into the audiology marketplace unique. Set your brand of audiology apart for the competition by daring to do something different.

6. Keep things simple. An old acronym, *KISS* or *"keep it simple stupid"* applies here. The more complex your plans, the more that can go wrong when it hits the reality of the marketplace. Keep the strategy simple and one that all in your organization can understand easily.

7. Prepare multiple alternatives. Always have a backup plan as things will be different and it is necessary to anticipate as many as possible of the difficulties that could arise, preparing a backup strategy to deal each of the issues identified.

8. Take the indirect route to your objective. Sometimes the direct route is a tough road to the eventual goal. Employees and others are resistant to change and movement against the grain does not usually win friends nor elicit cooperation with a new strategy. Sometimes the best way to obtain cooperation with the employees or others is to involve them in the conversation as the strategy develops, bringing them into the decisions creating cooperation.

9. Practice timing and sequencing. Cohen (2010) indicates that implementing the right strategy at the wrong time is as ineffective as implementing the wrong strategy. The new practice idea needs to be one that the marketplace is ready to receive as well as offering leading edge technology or assessment techniques that others, particularly the market or referral sources do not understand.

10. Exploit your success. Once successful, continue to lead the market, as if you let up, even for a second, the competition will be simply given another chance to outperform the practice that you have built.

time and are influenced by many outside factors such as the economy, local conditions, competition and other unforeseen events. Even if a practice is successful, a current business plan should be maintained to ensure fresh knowledge of the elements affecting continued success. Many factors critical to business success depend upon the planning process, such as obtaining outside funding, credit from suppliers, management of your operation's finances, promotion, and marketing of your business.

Some perspective business owners assume that if they are not going to seek financial support from lenders or investors to open their practice that it is not necessary to prepare a business plan, but *every* business should have a plan or as Cohen (2010) calls it, a *roadmap,* no matter if it funded by third parties or with personal funds.

Berry (2006) indicates that perspective business owners should know the obvious reasons for planning, but there are a number of other issues that must be considered as establishing or expanding a business is considered. These planning considerations, modified from Berry (2006), are 15 answers to the question, "Why plan?"

1. Grow your existing business. Establish strategy and allocate resources according to strategic priority. Reviewing the benefits of the expansion, the costs involved, competition in the expansion area, and the perspective revenues required.

2. Back up a business loan application. As presented previously, lenders want to see a plan as to how *their* funding will be spent and review how long it will take

for the business to make a profit. They will expect the business plan to cover their main points of interest which usually varies from reviewer to reviewer and institution to institution.

3. Seek investment for a business. Whether it's a start-up or not, investors need to see a business plan before they decide whether or not to invest. Even if the investor is "Rich Uncle Harry" who is investing in your practice there will be an expectation for your business plan to cover the main points of the practice and present how long it will take to pay the investors the return on their investment.

4. Create a new business. Use a plan to establish the correct steps to establishing a new business, including what you need to do, what resources will be required, and what you expect to happen.

5. Valuation of the practice. Another reason for a business plan is to determine the value the business for formal transactions related to divorce, inheritance, estate planning and/or tax issues. A valid valuation usually incorporates a business plan, as well as a professional with experience. The plan tells the valuation expert what the business is doing, when, why, and how much that will cost as well as how much income it will produce.

6. Selling your practice. If selling the practice a business plan can be a very important part of sale. A good business plan will assist the buyers in understanding what you have, what it's worth, and why they want it.

7. Information for professionals that deal with the practice. Share selected highlights or your plans with the attorney, accountant, financial people, and others who have a need to know your operation. This facilitates better advice from these professionals as they know your goals and objectives for the clinic.

8. Develop new business alliances. The business plan can be used to set targets for new alliances, such as joint marketing programs, product suppliers, and insurance provider programs.

9. Share and explain business objectives with the management team, current and new employees. Make selected portions of the business plan part of new employee training. This will instill knowledge of the goals and objectives of the practice by everyone involved and present a vision to those that assist in making the practice a success.

10. Decisions on the necessity new or expanded assets. Considerations as to if these assets are actually required, how many needed, and if to purchase or lease these assets. Among the first decisions the new practice owner must make is regarding equipment. Leasing is usually a good choice (see Chapter 8) for assets that depreciate, but if cash flow could be a problem, it can make sense to purchase equipment, furniture, and computers outright and not have the monthly expense.

11. Hiring new or more employees. This is another new obligation or fixed cost that increases the risk of success. Difficult decisions must be made as to maintaining enough personnel to operate the business yet poise it for growth over time. Serious thought as to how many employees will be necessary to get up and running in the new practice or the expansion? In an existing practice how will new people help the business grow and prosper? What exactly are they supposed to be doing? What are some milestones that must happen before new people are hired?

12. Decide whether or not to rent new or expanded space. Rent is an obligation, usually considered a fixed cost that must be paid each month. Of course, in a new practice space is a necessary expense and in an expansion more space may be required, it is necessary to consider both the immediate needs and those for the future. This is a delicate balance as too much space can be an extra obligation that reduces cash flow and not enough can cause lost business if the practice is successful. Do your growth prospects and plans justify taking on this amount of fixed cost? The business plan can assist in the evaluation of space and allow for revisions of the requirement according to projected costs and benefits.

13. Deal with displacement. Displacement is similar to the economic concept of opportunity costs (see Chapter 8) where, if you do something that uses valuable clinic time, then you cannot do something else during that time. Displacement lives at the heart of all small business strategies and business planning assists in prioritizing various projects necessary to getting the business up and

running as well as allowing for a semblance of a personal life.

14. Share your strategy, priorities, and specific action points with your spouse, partner or significant others. Starting a new business is a hectic endeavor and requires a lot of extra time, energy, and effort. In addition to seeing patients, the practice owner will spend an inordinate amount of time in the rush of answering phone calls, "putting out fires," insuring that milestones are met, etc. The other people in involved in the practice owner's life need to know what's supposed to be happening as well, if they know the plan for the practice they are more likely to understand if you miss the soccer game, get home late, need to work on the weekends, and so forth.

15. Set specific objectives for managers. Good management requires setting specific objectives and then tracking and following up. A business plan communicates the objectives and necessities for success to all of those concerned and assists them in making adjustments to the plan when necessary.

In addition to the general reasons for planning, a good business plan can assist in filtering through many of the other essential business thought processes as the strategy develops:

■ What you will need to do to get started and what resources (time, money, etc.) you will need to expend?
■ What are the variables necessary for this business to be profitable?
■ How long it will take to make this business profitable?

■ What information on potential customers is available to justify this practice in this location conducting these perspective procedures and selling these products?
■ What information and financial data is necessary to demonstrate to vendors and investors that your practice will be profitable?

Writing a business plan also forces objective thinking and an opportunity to stand back and review the business as an outsider critically considering the positives and negatives. At the end of the planning process there is usually a more realistic perspective *of the effort* this practice will require and if it is a venture that will be worth the time, energy, and funds to be invested when compared with the generated profit. The planning task is intimidating but can foster creativity as well as lead to new business strategies and concepts that may not have been previously considered. Written business objectives enable continuous focus on the practice so that the vision is not lost once the practice is up and running.

Strategic Conceptual Planning for an Audiology Practice

Before a formal business plan is generated for an audiology practice a strategic preplanning planning exercise is conducted. This preliminary planning allows the practitioner to consider their resources and the general economic climate to design the type of audiology practice that will be viable within the community. The preplanning exercise is similar to a discussion that might be conducted with friends over a beer written on a cocktail napkin outlining a conceptual overview of the business. An organizational concept that greatly assists in preliminary planning is offered by Harrison and St. John (2004) and updated by Traynor (2008) in the first edition as a preplanning model for an audiology practice. The model, presented in Figure 2–1, describes a simple preliminary planning exercise that, in this example, has been applied to an audiology practice. The model describes preplanning as a process where the perspective practice owner analyzes and learns from external and internal environments to formulate goals, establishes a direction for the practice by creating strategies that are intended to assist in the achievement of those formulated goals, and then safely execute those strategies.

Internal and External Analysis

The internal preliminary planning process begins with an analysis of the internal resources available, such as personnel,

office policies, equipment, physical location, space, and capital. Reviewing these internally controllable resources allows for the development of a *realistic* conceptual plan that transfers easily into the formal business plan. Similarly, there are external limitations to the business that require analysis including the economic climate, competition, suppliers, referral sources, insurance companies, and other factors that have an effect on the preliminary plan but out of the control of the perspective practitioner. Although there is usually no control over these factors, it is essential to the overall success of the business to formulate solid strategies to face these critical issues.

Strategic Direction

Another component of the preliminary planning exercise is to strategize the practice's direction. This exercise ponders the type of a practice offered to the marketplace and involves asking the question, "What type of an audiology

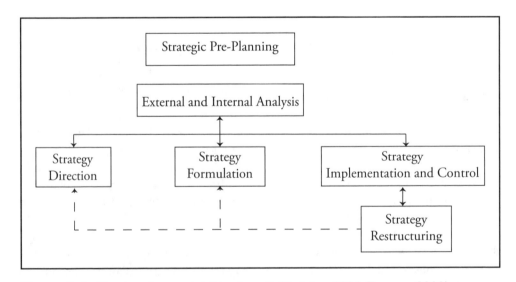

Figure 2–1. Preplanning model (Harrison & St. John, 2004; Traynor, 2008).

practice do I want?" Part of that discussion should be other questions including, "Should the practice be general audiology?" "Should the practice only sell hearing instruments"? "Specialize in pediatric patients or adults or both?" "Should the new clinic offer balance services, ABR, middle ear implantable hearing instruments, cochlear implant follow up and fine tuning?" "Should the practice offer operative monitoring?" Cohen (2010) indicates that Drucker called this exercise "looking out the window." Drucker suggested that his would involve finding and assessing the target market, considering cultural, ethnic, religious, racial, and social variables. Other issues considered would be demographics, buying group participation, competitors, technology, economics, politics, and legal issues. Strategy formulation is just that: how will my practice or project take on the market and, in general, what brand of audiology should be offered to fill the void or improve the available services in the marketplace?

Strategic Formulation

Once the overall strategy for the direction of the practice is outlined, it is necessary to consider the methods incorporated to interface with the market. Preplanning decisions necessary at this point are if the practice will utilize heavy or light marketing techniques, referrals only, or some combination of both. The perspective practitioner will also need to develop a pricing strategy to price products and services appropriately so as to position their brand of audiology within the marketplace. Decisions as to patient centrism, risk management, ethics, and other conceptual factors must also be decided

to further refine the type of practice that will be presented into the market.

Strategy Implementation and Control and Restructuring

As the market and practice patterns change, it may be necessary to revisit this preliminary planning process to restructure or fine tune the concept before the development of the formal business plan or a formal update of an existing business plan. Even before the formal business plan is ever considered, a preliminary strategic plan must be formulated and sometimes reformulated to fine tune unique, well-developed arguments for the proposed success of the practice.

Preliminary Considerations in Developing the Formal Business Plan

A formal business plan is a complete and detailed description of exactly how you intend to operate your proposed practice, as well as a communications tool for investors and others interested in understanding the operations and goals. Berry (2011) indicates that a business plan is any plan that works for a business to look ahead, allocate resources, focus on key points, and prepare for problems and opportunities. A normal or customary business plan includes a standard set of elements, but formats and outlines vary somewhat according to the type of business that is to be planned. Generally, a formal business plan will include components such as descriptions of the company, product or service, market, forecasts, management team, and financial analysis.

The formal business plan is a succinct document that addresses how you are going to build and maintain your practice by specifying the specific components of a longitudinal business strategy developed in the preplanning exercise. Specifically, the plan describes to *stakeholders* (those concerned with the long-term success of the venture) how the practice will function within the marketplace. These formal plans also present what is being sold, by whom, the background and qualifications of those involved in the company, prospective customers, where they can be found, what is needed to build the business, and how the practice plans to promote and determine the viability of the venture in a designated market. Not only is formal business planning a clarification of the practitioner's goals but it establishes a plan of action for reaching those goals with general concepts and specific ideas.

A good formal business plan is also an operational tool that spells out the specific goals to optimize the success of the practice. It determines how much money will be needed for start-up costs and includes financial projections over a 3- to 5-year period. It must reassure lenders and other financial stakeholders that the analysis of the current market and the projections for the market in the future are based on sound statistics and logical projections about the needs of the hearing and balance impaired populations as well as a detailed response strategy to competitive encroachment, expansion into new markets and the opportunities that may come available by advancing technology. Formal business plans should establish the specific goals of the practice for the projected

3- to 5-year period with objectives and anticipated milestones stated for each year. For example, hearing instrument sales should be *realistically, even conservatively,* projected on a monthly basis for at least the first 3 years of the projected period. Milestones to consider include hiring additional audiologists to assist in the practice, as specific milestones are met. Each decision to add personnel, expand to a second or third office must be tied to definitive and measurable evidence before the action is put into motion.

Since the practice business plan is so important, there are components of bad business plans must be avoided. Berry (2004) offers some general do's and don'ts in business planning. They are adapted here for an audiology practice:

Formal Business Plan Do's

- A mission statement must be crafted to reflect the purpose and long-term vision and goals of the practice.
- As part of your strategy, formulate concrete goals, responsibilities, and deadlines to guide the practice from start-up through 3 to 5 years.
- Milestones must be established and, once achieved, describe other actions that can develop, such as obtaining more or updated equipment or hiring another audiologist contingent on attaining specific revenue milestones.
- Assign action to achieve goals and milestones to a specific individual in the practice for implementation and monitoring progress.
- The competition must be exhaustively researched and accurately characterized.

■ Describe why this business is unique and differentiate it from the other practices in the area. Why this clinic going to get the business and not the competition?

■ As part of the implementation of a business plan, scheduled times for evaluation and assessment of the plan—at least quarterly in the first three years, semiannually thereafter.

■ Good business plans provide a practical *roadmap* with clear metrics for achieving goals and objectives relative to the mission of the practice.

Formal Business Plan Don'ts

■ Don't use a business plan to show how much you know about your business.

■ Don't have an executive summary more than 1 page.

■ Nobody reads a long-winded business plan: not bankers or other sources of capital, keep it to no more than 25 pages.

■ Don't overhype the opportunities; keep your enthusiasm visible in the document but avoid the temptation of overselling the product.

■ Don't set forth unattainable goals; be realistic relative to the demographics: the patients and referral sources to be served.

■ Don't underestimate the need for the services to be provided.

■ Don't underestimate nor lose sight of the competition;

■ Don't develop unrealistic or unattainable financial projections; be conservative in estimates and projections.

■ Don't underestimate the effects of reducing margins on hearing instru-

ments and the necessary strategy to counteract the trend.

■ Don't make the assumption that hearing instrument manufacturers would rather deal with you than directly with the consumer of their products.

Formal Business Planning: The Advantages and Utility of a Business Plan

There were audiologists, though few in numbers in the 1970s, 1980s, and 1990s, who had both entrepreneurial spirit and the capacity to develop an appropriate business plan. They knew that the bankers and lenders of the day would not consider funding a venture that was not well conceived and carefully delineated in the context of a business plan. They understood that the business plan was (and remains) a highly stylized document involving a logical progression of information in a commonly accepted format. The content requirements may have changed over the years, largely as a function of changing technologies and advancing clinical protocols; however, these changes have resulted in additional opportunities to generate revenue. Furthermore, there is improved accessibility to information important to defining the patient base, potential sources of patient referral, insurance information and general demographic data including information about services provided by competitive practices.

One thing has not changed: the lenders of today expect an exhaustive market analyses. They will expect to know how the patients will get to your office, what the marketing and promotional plans will be at start-up and over at least a 3-year period. They will want to understand the metrics for the practice over that period and if they are providing serialized financial support, those metrics must be validated before each note is reissued and funds are transferred to the practice. The plan must contain a complete forensic on the competition, how your venture exceeds the competition and how your practice will provide that information to referral sources and potential patients so that they have the opportunity to choose your practice for the hearing and balance segment of their patient's care.

Staffing projections and equipment costs including clinical and business equipment, office furnishings, Informational technologies to be instituted at start-up, Web site development, and planning for a consistent Internet and social media presence will need to be addressed in the plan. Anything less will constitute a lack of due diligence in the eyes of potential lenders. In short, the comprehensive business plan develops all the components of a successful practice based on the vision of the person seeking financial support. The audiologist seeking funding must be able to answer a single question about the business plan. If the business plan contains the appropriate balance of information, realistic projections, well-developed demographics, and information about services available within the market, the answer to the question will be simple. The question: "If you were a venture capitalist or a banker with money to invest, would you invest in this practice?" To put it another way, did your business plan develop an opportunity for a lender to become a partner in your venture with limited risk relative to the due diligence set forth in the business plan?

Brassil (2007) calls the business plan a management and financial blueprint of the practice that clearly identifies and defines the goals of the practice while precisely outlining the methods of achieving these goals. The business plan is a document that may be critical to the start-up of the practice but it is also critical to the ongoing good health of the practice. Some believe the business plan should be placed in the circular file after start-up funding has been obtained. Instead, it should be considered a live and growing document to be renewed and updated from time-to-time as the practice grows and flourishes. The business plan should be in close-to-current form at all times so that when the need for expansion capital arises, the plan will be ready to submit with minimal intervention and revisions. Keep it handy and review it occasionally if for nothing else but to remind yourself where the venture began, how it is evolving, and whether or not the practice is on its planned schedule.

Business Plans Change with Market Changes

The start-up business plan represents concept and vision couched in operational actions coupled with financial forecasting. It is the early roadmap for the practice. The business plan at 3 years post start-up will likely be considerably different from the original. As roadmaps change with the addition of new highways, so too does the business plan as the venture flourishes, hits bumps in the road, encounters market changes, relocation or considerations, the addition of a second or third office location. Time changes everything and that is particularly true in health care. What was a good direction and a meaningful path for the practice at start-up may not be the best direction three or five years down the road. In a matter of a few years an office location once considered the best spot in the target demographic can change abruptly for a number of reasons:

- A hospital can internalize a large family practice group immediately dictating their referral patterns to providers participating in the hospital's network or provider panel.
- Older patients move to assisted living facilities or move in with their children outside a reasonable drive time to the practice.
- Competitive practices move into the area and begin to impact what was once an exclusive referring relationship with several primary care practices.

Other market changes are driven by factors well outside the realm of health care. For example, if the practice is dependent on a large, single employer and the plant closes or moves to another state, the impact on the entire community and the health care market in particular will be felt across the board and perhaps especially so in the practice. In the case of an impending plant closing, the business plan should be revisited to consider adjustments such as marketing to those workers and retirees who will remain in the area following the closing or issuing information about the need to take advantage of their hearing care benefits while they remain in full force. Adapting to changing market parameters is vital to the long-term survival of many

practices today—not just audiology, but in primary care and other medical specialties as well.

Formal Business Plan Format for an Audiology Practice

Business plans, as mentioned earlier, are stylized reports describing elemental information about start-up needs and projections, milestones, objectives, and actions needed to meet the goals established throughout the course of the practice. Business plans conform to generally accepted guidelines of form and content. The format may vary depending on the nature of the business. Health care business plans require specificity of the patient population to be served, the referral sources as pathways to the market, equipment and personnel necessary to provide the services and in-depth analyses across each market segment of care to be provided by the practice. A business plan specifically adapted for audiology practices is proposed below:

- Executive Summary
- Mission Statement
- Practice Overview
- Market Assessment
- Competition Analysis
- Personnel/Human Resources
- Operational Plan
- Financial Components.

Executive Summary

The executive summary is the single most important segment of any business plan. It is the section that is read first and creates the first impression. If it is well crafted, it may become the basis for the decision to fund or not to fund a venture. The executive summary must not exceed two pages; preferably it should be completed on one page. It needs to be precisely written and generate a wide enough snapshot of the practice to provide the reader with the most important facts and concepts that are or will become the practice. Ward (2012) presents that the purpose of an executive summary is to provide the reader with an overview of the business plan. The Executive Summary can be thought of as an introduction to your business. It is suggested that the best format for constructing the executive summary is to put the issue (problem) and purpose in the first paragraph to formulate interest in the reader. The scope and limitations as well as the alternatives (procedures) will go in the next paragraphs, while the significant considerations, analysis,

and decisions will comprise the final paragraphs. Care must be taken to only include significant considerations, analysis, and decisions as extra information in these sections is not appropriate. Since each segment of the executive summary should contain key facts and information gleaned from the other sections of the business plan, experts agree that the executive summary should be written last. Each paragraph should mirror the sections of the business plan.

Mission Statement

The mission statement should be considered the starting point of the business plan. It must be a concise statement that depicts both the purpose and the long-term vision of the practice. Hamilton (2011) indicates that some companies list both their vision and their mission statements on their sites. The difference between a mission statement

---

Sidebar 2–2
EXECUTIVE SUMMARY QUESTIONS

Abrams (2005) suggests that when completed, the executive summary should answer the following questions for your readers:

- Does your basic concept make sense?
- Has your business been thoroughly planned?
- Is the management team capable?
- Is there a clear-cut market need for your product/service?
- What advantages do you have over your competition?
- Are your financial projections realistic?
- Is the business likely to succeed?
- Will investors be able to make money?
- Will lenders be able to get their money back?

and a vision statement is that a mission statement focuses on a company's present state while a vision statement focuses on a company's future. However, some companies tend to blend these statements. Most practice business plans, however, use the mission statement to present what the practice does, for whom they do it, and how well they do it. The mission statement is a proclamation of the general nature and direction of the practice—it is an assertion of what the practice will do and what it potentially can be. Its value is twofold:

- To serve as an internal guidance statement for all working together in the practice.
- To inform those who come to the practice about the practice philosophy and commitment to excellence in all aspects of the services to be provided: *Audiology Associates will work honestly and diligently every day to exceed the expectations of our patients and referral sources by providing the best hearing and balance care in our community.*

Practice Overview

Following an opening section describing the profession of audiology and its important contributions to contemporary hearing and balance care, the practice overview should delineate basic information about the practice including office locations, Internet presence (Web site, Facebook, Twitter, LinkedIn), legal business structure (sole proprietorship, corporation, LLC, etc.), and a list of principals participating in the practice and what they will bring to the business. It should contain the history and developmental stages of the practice to date. An expan-

sive narrative describing diagnostic and treatment procedures, hearing instrument assessment and assistive device selection, and fitting and follow-up care must be set forth so that the reader readily understands the operational core of the practice and clinical opportunities available to patients and referring practitioners.

The path a patient takes from referral source to the office and through a comprehensive hearing examination, interpretation and counseling should be portrayed to illustrate the many interactions between the patient, clerical and clinical staff members, specialized environments and equipment used in the clinical process. Pathways can be developed for each clinical presentation; those patients referred for hearing assessment and management, evaluation of equilibrium, and for specialized protocols such as tinnitus management and central auditory processing assessment as well as treatment recommendations. No matter the clinical pathways to be described, this section must be written with the nonaudiologist reader in mind.

The practice overview should characterize contemporary service and treatment trends in audiology and relate them to the needs of patients in the relevant market area. It should also describe specific business and clinical parameters that will make the practice profitable and an effective yet competitive force in the existing market. It must establish the practice's competitive edge whether based on personnel with advanced degrees and licenses, specific assessment, or therapeutic protocols not offered by others in the market (e.g., tinnitus assessment, preventative noise control, and rehabilitation), or a unique marketing approach to primary care physicians that has not been considered in the particular market of interest. The reader of this section should develop a clear picture of the services to be provided, understand what the practice will bring to the existing provider mix in the area, and an appreciation of what differentiates the practice competitively.

Market Assessment

The market is defined by individuals who will seek services directly and by other health care providers with whom the practice will interface. Patients, physicians, and nonphysician referral sources in the area, hospitals, outpatient clinics, psychologists, optometrists, dentists, chiropractors, public and parochial schools, industrial nurses, extended care facilities, and nonprofit speech and hearing centers represent many of the people and referral sources that will interconnect with the practice by virtue of proximity within the market. The market is also defined by a variety of demographic means including mailing codes or a 20- to 30-minute drive time to each office. Specific demographic information is readily available from a variety of sources. The US Census Bureau has extensive information about population characteristics, age, income, and a variety of other information that might be of importance in better characterizing the market for your practice (http://www.census.gov). Local newspapers and to a lesser degree telephone books as well as media outlets have specific demographic information about their readers, viewers, and listeners. The information is often available as a media information kit for potential advertisers. Examining general demographic information is a good first step in obtaining meaningful information to assess and describe a specific market area. General demographics should be periodically re-evaluated over the course of the practice to ensure that the target population remains large enough to continue to sustain the practice and that the type of media is appropriate for the audience. Strong target market definitions are based on observable characteristics, backed by data and research. This section of the business plan should develop a clear picture of your patients and referral sources—who they are, what they need from your practice, where they are located in relation to your practice, how they perceive the value of your services and why they will come to or refer patients to your practice (see Chapters 5 and 6).

St. Clergy (2010) feels that it in a practice tuned for a new generation of computer literate patients it is essential to have a state-of-the-art Web site marketing your practice to those that do not use telephone books and traditional sources anymore. He further suggests that it is important to work your Web site so that it is high on the list of search engines in your area. Web sites and other electronic media solutions have now become an integral component of the marketing mix and are no longer a fringe exercise. As the business plan is developed, consider that there is a whole new generation of patients that will use their computers to find your practice and often decide where to go by the quality and quantity of electronic information available. There are numerous creative marketing services, such as http://www.educatedpatients .com (St. Clergy, 2011) that can be of assistance in business plan preparation, target market identification, search engine positioning, pay per click ads, and innovative other services that place your practice in the Internet/electronic environment.

Business planning without considering internet and electronic marketing is a disservice to your practice and very expected in today's planning process. The use of these innovative marketing schemes will demonstrate to investors and funders that the practice is incorporating the newest available strategies to touch a new generation of computer- and Internet-savvy patients.

Competitive Analysis

Potential investors reading a business plan expect to see a comprehensive assessment of the competition in the defined market area. Wherever there is a market for hearing health care services, there is competition either directly from another audiologist practice providing diagnostic and/or rehabilitative services, an otolaryngology practice, or indirectly from commercial hearing aid dealers selling hearing instruments.

To best typify the competition in the market, specific competitors must be listed with an estimate of their market share and a consideration of their advertising in various media including their Web site. Additionally, the competition should be characterized by their clinical offerings, the qualifications of the care providers in the practice and a candid, unbiased assessment of their strengths and weaknesses. The sources of your information will vary but could include former patients or current vendors who have had interactions with them. Qualifications and other information can be gleaned from licensing boards and other agencies that require licensing or registration information that is readily available to the public.

Understanding the offerings and competencies of direct or indirect competitors will better position a new or existing practice to distinguish itself with identify factors that will insure patients and referral sources choose it by responding to needs that are not being provided by competitors. Additionally, this exercise allows the practitioner to figure out specific competitive issues the new or expanded business must overcome to advance and improve the practice's own market share (Abrams, 2005).

Distinguishing the practice from the crowd of competitors is not merely important; *it is the key to both the short- and long-term success of your practice.* For example, offering an assessment and treatment protocol for tinnitus, central auditory disorders, or dysequalibrium can offer a new or expanded practice an important edge in a market where other providers do not offer the service or fail to advise the health care community about its availability and efficacy. Patients with tinnitus, central auditory, and disequilibrium are vexing problems for primary care practitioners. If they have an audiologist in the community who has made known to them that his or her practice welcomes patients with the complaints of tinnitus or dizziness, the referrals will begin and continue as long as the services and treatment exhaust the patient's need for clinical attention, valid diagnostic and therapeutic intervention, or referral for further treatment. Primary care physicians appreciate the fact that their patients undergo extensive testing, competent counseling, and explanations of their particular difficulty and that their patients have some chance of remediation. Even if the outcome produces only a modicum of resolution, most patients appreciate the improvement and the fact that his or her physician has listened to their complaint and has made the referral to an interested health care practitioner who has been asked to become involved in this particular segment of their care.

Personnel/Human Resources

The personnel and human resources section of the business plan must clarify both administrative and clinical positions in the practice, their respective qualifications, specific duties, and expected contributions to the overall success of the practice. Although job descriptions should not be included in their entirety in this section, they should be used as the basis of the information provided. The reader of this section must understand the need for each position, the qualifications required and the work product expectations of each position. Regardless of the number of positions filled at the outset of the practice, every position filled or anticipated should be described. Metrics should be established in concert with timelines to hire additional personnel. For example, the addition of an audiologist may be considered when specific patient bookings exceed a 2-week waiting list on a consistent basis or when fiscal reserves reach a specified point with monthly or quarterly revenues reaching specific levels. Or it could be as simple as when the workload at the front desk exceeds the limits of the patience of the clerical staff, it is time to add another person to the mix. First and foremost, the perceived need should be weighed against financial facts. Does the practice generate enough opportunity for billable time to support another audiologist? Is there a need to hire another front office position to meet increasing billing and reception loads? Will the addition of another audiologist improve the time a patient can be seen for assessment and follow-up? Will the new audiologist increase the numbers of procedures completed and instruments dispensed? Will the addition of another administrative staff member improve cash flow and billing turnaround time? These questions, if answered in the affirmative, represent positive indicators of growth and financial expansion of the practice.

Operational Plan

This section will be the most difficult to write due to the tendency to want to provide expansive information and support about how the practice will perform in the market, what services it will provide, immediate and long-term equipment needs, whether clinical or office equipment will be leased or purchased, and the office environment in which the specified services and treatment regimen will be issued. Brevity must be the watchword of this section: It must include relevant information about suppliers and vendors with an indication of what performance characteristics the practice will demand from each. For example, each hearing instrument manufacturer will supply instruments under condition that the percentage of repairs by years of use will not exceed a specified amount; repair turnaround time limits should be established as should the incidence of re-repairs (see Chapter 17). The consequences of exceeding established limits should be set forth clearly. Both office and clinical equipment replacement schedules should be set forth in a time line accompanied by projected costs.

A brief description of the diagnostic utility and clinical necessity of each service by CPT code should be included to orient the reader to the breadth and importance of the care to be provided. Special procedures linked to specific equipment should be described relative to anticipated use. Hearing instrument fitting and follow-up care should be explained with projected numbers of instruments to be fit over the course of the first three to five years. If you are beginning the practice with limited services, indicate the services to be added and discuss the timeline and/or a decision metric that will permit service expansion.

Business operations to be considered in this section should include both hardware and software necessary for billing and tracking patient accounts, business equipment necessary to facilitate cash flow and patient satisfaction, as well as office furnishings, patient-comfort, and staff-comfort items. Items necessary for informational security and compliance with HIPAA regulations must be included. The reader of this section should develop a picture of the equipment necessary to provide all clinical services, now and in the future. The reader should understand the business operations from equipment, software, and patient-interface aspects. The office space, furnishings, and business related supplies and services should be clarified in this section—a complete view of what it will take to support the clinical side of the venture by providing state-of-the-art equipment, billing software, and methods of information as well as financial management of the practice. It is best to involve all those involved in the practice, including the practice attorney and accountant, to read and comment on what ultimately defines how the business and clinical sides come together for the patients and referral sources being served in the practice.

Financial Components

This section requires rigorously realistic and objective projections with the inclusion of as much factual information as possible. Do not overstate or inflate revenue projections or numbers of services to be provided nor numbers of instruments to be dispensed. Revenue projections should be based on anticipated referrals and self-referred patients over a specified time. Incremental numbers of patients should be seen as a function of proposed marketing efforts. Break-even points (see Chapter 8) should be defined based on numbers of referrals, procedures completed, and instruments dispensed over a specific timeline. Projected revenues should be tied to the amount to be borrowed or the credit line draw dates to be established. Include realistic estimates of known overhead, expenses, and salary projections to the break-even point—what it will take to fund all operations until the practice is at least paying for itself including all personnel wages. Common sense should prevail: If it is unlikely you will have the referrals to support an auditory evoked potential system in the beginning of your practice, there is no need to allocate funding for its purchase until such time that anticipated referrals can support its use.

Summary

Lenders reviewing the business plan of start-up practices want to be convinced that the proposed venture will reach the financial projections detailed in the plan. In short, they want to be convinced that their participation as a financial partner will result in a successful practice. If the plan is done well, it will provide readers with a measure of confidence and an incentive to lend all monies needed to fund the venture. The document should be straightforward, as short as possible, and offer realistic financial data supported by comprehensive due diligence about the opportunities for success in the market.

As a vital and changing document, the business plan should be revisited periodically and updated accordingly. If the plans for the practice change, the business plan should reflect that change. Consider sending a copy of the revised business plan to your lenders, attorney, and accountant. It keeps them informed and confident that you are managing the business portion of your practice as diligently and with the same level of completeness that you manage your patients.

A checklist for a business plan developed for an audiology practice is offered by Keller (2011) in Sidebar 2–3. It provides an extensive reminder of items of importance to lenders and investors to be applied to your business plan prior to its submission or during the course of your successful practice.

Sidebar 2–3
AUDIOLOGY BUSINESS PLAN CHECKLIST (Keller, 2011)

Executive Summary

- Audiology business plan in brief
  Practice concepts
  Marketing strategy
  Products/ services,
  Business management
  Financing requirements
  Role of investors

Practice Overview

- Historical background
  Founder(s) of the practice
  When founded
  Development of the practice
  Achievements

- Situation today
  Legal structure
  Key financial figures
- Additional background information depending on financing situation
  Financing for start-up
  Financing for expansion
  Financing for acquisitions

Products/Services

- Products/services
  Detailed description of
    products/services
  Benefits for patients
  Patient needs
  Advantages/disadvantages
    compared with competitors
    audiology practices

- Research and development
  - Developments/refinements in the practice
  - Innovations in products and services
- USPs
  - Unique selling points of the practice
  - Competitive advantages

Markets

- Market overview
  - Market analysis
  - Patient analysis
  - Service and product purchase motivation
- Practice market position
  - Market segments addressed
  - Target patient groups
  - Referral channels
- Market assessment/market research
  - Market trends
  - Market entry barriers
  - Estimated patient market growth

Competitors

- Competitor companies
  - Name
  - Location
  - Patient structure
  - Patient Motivation
- Competing products
  - Range of services
  - Products available
  - Differing features of services and products

- Supplementary services/products
- Competitor pricing
  - Price points
  - Price comparison of key products and services

Marketing

- Market segmentation
  - Target markets
  - Target patient groups
- Marketing
  - Product and service sales
  - PR/advertising/promotion
- Packaging of products/services
  - Range of products/services
  - Pricing bundled/unbundled
- Sales targets
  - Budgeted sales volumes for each market segment in the next 5 years
  - Targets for market share in each market segment

Location/Production/Administration

- Location
  - Practice domicile and offices
  - Benefits and limitations of chosen location
- Production
  - Internal and external production
  - Procurement of goods and materials (if products are manufactured in the practice)

- Administration
    - Structure of administration
    - Organization of accounting function
    - Information technology capabilities

Organization/ Management

- Management team
    - Individual members
    - Responsibilities
    - Compensation
    - Special qualifications
- Clinical team
    - Individual members
    - Responsibilities
    - Compensation
    - Special qualifications
- Biography of each member
    - Training and education
    - Professional experience
    - Previous positions

Risk Analysis

- Internal risks
    - Management
    - Responsibilities
    - Compensation
    - Special qualifications
- External risks
    - Economic
    - Environmental
    - Legal
    - Social

SWOT Analysis

- Strengths
    - Strengths of the practice
    - Customer base
    - Skills
    - Location
- Weaknesses
    - Current weaknesses of the practice
    - Capacity
    - Know-how
    - Financial or human resources
    - Succession planning
- Opportunities
    - Sales opportunities
    - New communities
    - New customer segments
    - New products and services
    - Geographic expansion
    - Third-party reimbursement
- Threats
    - Market threats
    - Competitor activity
    - Declining purchasing power
    - Alternative distribution channels

Financial Planning

- Short-term and long-term planning
    - Determining financing requirements based upon forecasts for the balance sheet, profit, and loss (or income) statement and cash flow statement
    - Liquidity plan

Supply contracts
Loan agreements
Leasehold contracts

■ Investment case
   Purpose of financing request
   Investment plan
   Role of investors

Financing

■Financing concept
   Meeting financing require-
      ments through injection of
      new capital

Sidebar 2–4
SAMPLE EXECUTIVE SUMMARY

New Practice

Mission Statement

The mission of Southwest Hearing Care, Inc. is *to always make decisions in favor of the patient or referral source at every opportunity knowing that we cannot be wrong if we are trying to be right by those whom we serve.* Southwest Hearing Care, Inc. is dedicated to working honestly and diligently everyday to exceed the expectations of our patients by providing the highest quality possible hearing and balance care.

Practice Overview

Southwest Hearing Care, Inc. is a private Audiology Practice located in Gulch, Texas that will provide hearing care products and services to the estimated 400,000 individuals in Gulch and the surrounding three county region. The practice will concentrate on providing diagnostic and rehabilitative hearing care to patients of all ages. Patients will be accepted as self-referrals and from primary health care providers as well as nonphysician health care practitioners. Hearing instruments will be dispensed as part of a rehabilitation effort and will include full range digital technologies, assistive listening devices and a full range of support items to maintain the instruments.

Market Assessment

The estimate of patients in need of our clinical and rehabilitative services ranges from 40,000 to 65,000 within the defined demographic area. At this time, those seeking hearing care in this market area travel 75 miles to El Paso for services. That produces a hardship on these patients especially for important follow-up care necessary after a hearing instrument fitting. There are no other professionals offering these services in the area described beyond commercial hearing aid dealers providing occasional visits to patient's residences for hearing aid sales and service. Recent data from the Better Hearing Institute suggest that only about 16% of the hearing impaired that could benefit from amplification devices actually own them, leaving a market of about 84% to be considered eligible for services provided and instruments dispensed in our practice. The funding requested will include marketing to primary care physicians, nonphysician health care providers, and directly to prospective patients.

Competition Analysis

In Gulch and the 3 county areas there are 3 itinerant, commercial hearing aid salesmen selling hearing aids in patient's homes. None have an established office. They do not pose a significant competitive threat. Commercial hearing aid dealers have no formal degree and are licensed to assess hearing solely for the purposes of fitting a hearing aid according to Texas laws governing their practice.

Their focus in the area has been high-pressured hearing aid sales only. They may not engage in diagnostic testing and, therefore, pose no threat to that particular emphasis of the practice.

In contrast Southwest Hearing Care, Inc. will offer full-range diagnostic hearing services and management of nonsurgical hearing impairments for all ages in a rehabilitation-centered program of hearing care. All services will be provided by doctoral level audiologists who are certified by the American Board of Audiology.

Personnel/Human Resources

Southwest Hearing Care, Inc. will begin with a staff of 2 full time administrative employees and Jason Jones, Au.D. Dr. Jones received his Doctor of Audiology Degree from the University of Florida and has worked as a technically competent audiologist for 12 years in various professional capacities. He was most recently employed for the past five years as the Director of Audiology at Adams General Hospital, El Paso, Texas. The proposed staff has worked in the other medical practices and audiology clinics for periods ranging from 4 to 10 years and offer substantial business and patient management experience.

Operational Plan

Immediate objectives for the practice are:

1. To obtain adequate funding for the project including salaries for an 18 month start-up period.
2. To obtain business and clinical equipment for start-up
3. To lease space in a demographically sensitive area of the defined market
4. To decorate the space with appropriate business, clinical and patient-related furnishings
5. To develop a marketing plan including visits to primary care physicians and nonphysician health care providers in the demographic area
6. To establish and fund an appropriate marketing campaign in the local newspapers
7. To secure and/or retain legal counsel to draw appropriate documents for the start-up venture
8. To secure the services of a Certified Public Accountant to establish a chart of accounts for the proposed practice and to establish the accountant's role in the fiscal management of the practice
9. To break even at the 12- to 16-month mark from start-up date with consistent profitability occurring after the 18th month of operation.
10. To secure equipment and instrument vendors with at least a 45 day payment schedule and an understanding that they must stand behind their equipment or instruments and repairs on behalf of the patients to be served in the practice.

Financial Components (Figure 2–2)

Based upon the preliminary referral commitments, anticipated numbers of instruments to be dispensed, numbers of procedures to be completed and billed to third-party payers and business and clinical overhead costs coupled with the analysis of competition within the defined market area, Southwest Hearing Care, Inc. is projected to achieve an annual revenue of in excess of $1 million within 36 months of operation with projected net profit after

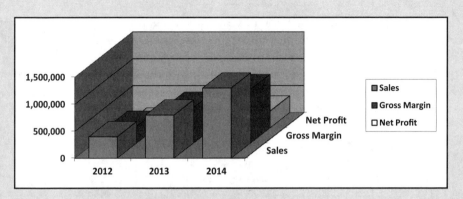

Figure 2–2. Southwest Hearing Health Care, Inc., projected sales, gross margin, and net profit for 2012, 2013, and 2014.

tax of $450,000. The company will turn profitable within the first year with after-tax earnings of $40,000 and $100,000 in year two (2013).

Existing Practice for Expansion

Mission Statement

To demonstrate to the professional community and the communities at large that we are the best source of hearing and balance assessments, hearing instrument fitting and follow-up care, and patient-centric practice operations in the Phillips County area.

Market Assessment

After 30 years of operation, Audiology Associates has stabilized profitability without growth in our current market. This has been due to population and referral sources moving to nearby markets, specifically the Horseshoe and Pinto Platte, Colorado areas. Whereas markets in Horseshoe and Pinto Platte have been steadily increasing by 15 to 25% per year over the last three years, our immediate demographic area has had a 10% decline in the same period.

Competition Analysis

Although there are 3 competitive hearing aid dealers in area, R/R Hearing Aid Center, HearMeNow and Bert's Hearing Barn, these competitors pose little competition in that they focus on high pressure sales rather than professional services, rehabilitation management and follow-up care. The referral sources that have moved into these markets recognize our practice name and understand the need for comprehensive hearing and balance services provided by audiologists in a professional setting. Re-establishing referral relationships will require personal marketing efforts and we have a plan in place and personnel resources to complete that important task. Importantly, several of our former referral sources have agreed to re-establish a referring relationship as soon as we open our office in their area.

Personnel/Human Resources

Audiology Associates has been successful in Horseshoe, Colorado for over 30 years under the direction of John Fedders, PhD. It is the addition of an Audiology colleague that is the key to continued success in the immediate market and in the new market area for the proposed office space. Jenny Keller, AuD, has joined our professional staff and will be managing the proposed new office. She will be merging her practice into ours and will bring approximately 4,000 active patients within a 30-minute drive time to the proposed office in Horseshoe.

Operational Plan

Over the past 12 months Audiology Associates has been in a preliminary planning process to open a new location in the Crossroads Center professional office complex in Horseshoe, just east of Wray, Colorado. This will permit self-referred patients and those referred by practitioners access to comprehensive hearing and balance diagnostic and rehabilitative services in close proximity to the new Scotch Pines Medical Center (SCPMC) in Wray. With the expansion of a 3,000 sq. ft office, now under construction in the McKinley Station area just adjacent to Crossroads Center, Audiology Associates is well positioned for a new opportunity. The presence of our brand of Audiology in this area will be dramatic and profitable by offering state of the art clinical services in hearing and balance diagnostics, high technology hearing instrument fitting and follow up care as well as operative monitoring services at SCPMC.

Financial Component

As requested herein, we are in need of capital infusion funding, in the amount of $100,000, with a return in a renewable 12-month period. Audiology Associates also requests interest-only monthly payments with a balloon payment at the end of this term and an option for a portion of the balance to be renewable for another 12 months. Based upon our market research, our conservative estimate of increased revenues will be an income ratio increase to 80%. The funding requested will enable Audiology Associates to establish a professional presence and thereby capture significant market share in areas populated with affluent people who are more likely to spend money on health-related matters affecting the quality of their lives.

The note will be secured and personally guaranteed by Dr. Fedders.

Sidebar 2–5
COMPUTER-GENERATED BUSINESS PLANS

Business Plan Computer Programs

In this new century there is a computer program for virtually everything. Business planning is no exception and, as a first step, practitioners should consider the use of a software program, such as Business Plan Pro (www .paloalto.com) or any one of a number other programs. There are many of these programs available and most can be downloaded from the Internet for an investment of $80 to $200 or so. There are also some very good Web sites that work to develop business plans, such as www.liveplan.com where the site fee is reasonable and the writer of the business plan may go in and out of the site as necessary to work on the plan. The site offers instruction in the development of plan as the plan progresses from one section to another. While the differences in costs among various programs and Web sites are for extra features and more detailed assistance in planning, they all make the final business plan solid, accurate, and meaningful by presenting realistic milestones for assessment that are expected by lenders and other stakeholders. A good business planning computer program should be easy to learn and expedite the business planning process. If the learning curve is too time consuming, the software can simply add to the frustration of creating the business plan, so choose the program wisely. If possible, software for business planning should integrate with the accounting software and provide templates for charts and graphs that can be customized for the presentation of the financial specifics of the practice. These programs can organize the whole planning process from start to finish, turning the business plan of straw into one of bricks in a relatively short time. In 2012, there are web sites where clinicians can subscribe such as www.liveplan. com. These sites allow the audiologist to subscribe and then use their skills in the development of their business plan. These sites are an alternative to the purchase of a computer program and are extremely beneficial to developing a complete and appropriate plan.

References

Abrams, R. (2005) *Business plan in a day.* San Diego, CA: The Planning Shop.

Berry, T. (2004). *Hurdle: The book on business planning.* Eugene, OR: Palo Alto Software.

Berry, T. (2006). 15 reasons you need a business plan. Entrepeneur.com. Retrieved February 15, 2007, from http://entrepreneur.com/startingabusiness/businessplans/businessplancoachtimberry/article83818.html

Berry, T. (2011). Bplans: Your business plan starts here. Bplans.com. Retrieved July 9, 2011, from http://articles.bplans.com/financing-a-business

Brassil, M. (2007). Six important functions of a business plan. Website Marketing Plan.com. Retrieved February 16, 2007, from http://www.websitemarketingplan.com/bplan/functions.htm

Cohen, W. (2010). *Drucker on leadership.* San Francisco, CA: Jossey-Bass.

Hamilton, D. (2011). Top ten company mission statements. Dr. Diane Hamilton.com. Retrieved May 5, 2012, from http://drdianehamilton.wordpress.com/2011/01/13/top-10-company-mission-statements-in-2011/

Harrison, J., & St. John, C. (2004). *Foundations in strategic management* (3rd ed.). Mason, OH: Thomson Southwestern.

Keller, B. (2007, 2011). Business plan checklist. Presentation to the International Distributor Forum, March 20, 2007, Bernafon A/G sponsor, Lucerne, Switzerland. Updated, September, 2011.

Small Business Administration (SBA), (2011). Essential elements of a good business plan. Retrieved June 20, 2011, from http://www.sba.gov/category/navigation-structure/starting-managing-business/starting-business/writing-business-plan/essential-elements-good-busines

St. Clergy, K. (2010). Phonak practice development seminar. Phonak, Naperville, IL.

St. Clergy, K. (2011). What can Educatedpatients.com do for your practice. Retrieved August 9, 2011, from http://www.educatedpatients.com/services.php

Tracy, J. (2005). *Accounting for dummies.* Hoboken, NJ: John Wiley.

Traynor, R. (2008). Strategic business planning. In R. Glaser & R. Traynor (Eds.), *Strategic practice management.* San Diego, CA: Plural.

Ward, S, (2012). Writing the executive summary of a business plan. About.com. Retrieved May 5, 2010, from http://sbinfocanada.about.com/od/businessplans/a/execsummary.htm

3

Legal Considerations in Practice Management

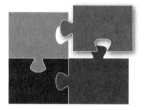

GLENN L. BOWER, JD AND MICHAEL G. LEESMAN, JD

Usual Caveat

The statements and suggestions in this chapter should not be construed as legal advice or opinions. Readers should not act upon information contained in this chapter without professional guidance based on specific facts and circumstances and then-current applicable law.

Securing Professional Advisors

Establishing an audiology practice involves an array of business considerations that can be addressed by any entrepreneur aware of them. However, not all such issues are intuitive. Therefore, it is helpful to engage legal counsel and other appropriate professional advisors early in the process to identify issues, to provide alternatives to address specific or unique concerns, and to recommend preferred solutions.

Attorneys

When selecting legal counsel, the easiest path is usually to retain someone known personally, or at least known to friends or family. This approach may yield a qualified attorney, but a more systematic search, casting a wider net, enhances the probability of finding the most appropriate attorney. Currently practicing audiologists may have suggestions, and the local chapter of the Medical Group Management Association—American College of Medical Practice Executives may also have recommendations. The State of Florida currently certifies health care lawyers as specialists; other states may also add that area of practice as a certified specialty, which could help narrow a focused search. Referral services offered by local bar associations, and other professionals such as accountants, bankers and insurance agents are also good resources for identifying qualified candidates to be considered as legal counsel for a new audiologist.

Desired qualities for legal counsel, as with any professional advisors, include chemistry and value. The "chemistry" element of the relationship can be very important and requires affirmative answers to these critically important questions:

■ Does the attorney understand my legal, business and professional requirements?
■ Does the attorney understand my approach to problem-solving and my preferences regarding how to address relevant issues that have been identified?
■ Does the attorney relate to me well enough to anticipate questions I have not asked, and to provide access and advice if needed outside of normal business hours?

The "value" component consists of quality and cost. Quality legal services derive from several pertinent attributes:

■ Relevant experience;
■ Industry insight;

■ Analytical ability; and
■ Diligence in providing timely advice and appropriate work product.

Significant years of practice dealing with health care professionals and associated business issues would constitute relevant experience. A meaningful degree of interaction with other health care providers, would serve as a basis for industry insight. This can include interaction with other practitioners and institutions, and involvement in relevant professional organizations, such as the American Health Lawyers Association, and health care law committees of local and state bar associations as well as the American Bar Association. Analytical ability and diligence are not characteristics easily ascertained during an introductory meeting or even necessarily by looking at biographical information on an attorney's website. Such characteristics are best determined by speaking with clients the attorney has worked with, so references are quite helpful in this regard.

The cost of legal services can be very significant. Attorneys usually charge fees based upon hourly rates, with expenses passed through to varying degrees. Research and other significant and identifiable out of pocket costs are often added to invoices for legal services, but less significant costs (document delivery, phone, etc.) are more frequently absorbed into the hourly rates these days. Attorneys are generally more willing recently to negotiate fixed prices for specific tasks, so it is worth discussing an alternative fee arrangement to make budgeting easier. Fees are often a function of geographic area, normally mirroring to some degree the regional cost of living, as well as size of the law firm. On the coasts or in major cities fees are usually greater than in the

Midwest, smaller towns and rural areas. Although large firms normally have higher fees than smaller firms, they are also more likely to have attorneys with greater expertise and experience in more focused specialties and greater technical resources within the firm. Reasonable value in legal services, considering the referenced aspects of quality and cost, can be found in any size firm, from solo attorneys to multioffice mega-firms, and should not be presumed according to the size of the firm.

Accountants, Bankers, and Other Advisors

Certain other professional advisors can be very useful in establishing and maintaining an audiology practice. Selection of an accountant, a banker, and an insurance representative should follow a systematic search process similar to securing legal counsel. An accountant normally helps with cash flow projections and budgeting, as well as with tax and other financial planning, and payroll. A banker can establish a line of credit to fund initial operations, as well as set up checking and other relevant accounts. A meaningful line of credit or other type of loan will normally require a carefully prepared business plan and some type of collateral. If the tangible assets to be owned by the practice do not suffice, a personal guaranty and/or home mortgage may be necessary. Insurance agents make recommendations regarding professional malpractice insurance; liability, property and casualty insurance for the business; and health and life insurance for the owner and any employees. As the practice becomes more profitable, an investment advisor may be helpful to deal with personal investments of the audiologist, as well as investments associated with pension and profit sharing plans for the owner(s) and other employees.

Employee, Independent Contractor, or Business Owner?

Now that you have found the critical advisors with whom you intend to consult, it is necessary to determine your place in the scheme of business operations. There are three basic options, with some overlap, that you can choose from and each one has advantages and disadvantages. The three options are employee, independent contractor, and/or business owner.

Life as an Employee

The freedom to control your business, and in many cases your schedule, is not typically one of the advantages of being employed by someone else. Rather, an employee is the person who does the necessary work, collects a paycheck, enjoys their fringe benefits, and calls it a day. This category of people is just as willing to work, but the last thing they want is to run a business, take risk, and deal with payroll. For an employee, the key benefits that professional advisors can help with are employment contracts (attorney) and personal financial planning (accountant/financial planner).

The Independent Contractor

If you want to take some of your entrepreneurial spirit and put it to work, but you do not want to deal with every aspect of owning your own business, the role of an independent contractor might be right for you. The upside here is the freedom you have to make your own schedule, pick and choose from potential work options, and handle your practice like a personal minibusiness. The downside is that you have to individually generate your own fee business and if you do not keep busy, then no money is coming in the door. Typically, independent contractors have to find their own insurance (health, professional liability, etc.) and they need to be comfortable dealing with some basic business and tax issues. As an independent contractor you will rely much more heavily on your attorney and accountant to make sure you are complying with the law and protected.

So, You Want Your Own Business?

The focus of a decent amount of this chapter deals with issues mostly pertinent to independent contractors and business owners. For the purposes of this analysis, these two categories are distinguished by the fact that an independent contractor is in business by him or herself and a business owner, while perhaps the sole owner, has employees of the business. Once that first employee comes on board, the dynamic and complexity of the business operation changes dramatically. As a business owner, you have the most flexibility of any of the options disclosed in this chapter. This is mostly because you now have other people to rely on for work and therefore you can leverage your time and effort to focus on other aspects of the business. The downside is that the "buck"

and the risk of investment stop with you and similar to the independent contractor, you will rely heavily on your attorney and accountant to deal with all sorts of issues that your audiology training did not teach you.

Operation of an Audiology Practice

In the event that an audiologist decides not to become an employee of an established practice, but intends to establish a new practice or practice group, the formal organization of the practice must be determined after alternatives are considered. Whether the practice will be owned by one or multiple audiologists, the following basic issues must be evaluated:

- How to provide compensation and benefits to professionals and other employees;
- How to deal with anticipated contractual issues; and
- How to comply with laws and regulations applicable to the practice of audiology.

Choice of Legal Entity

Forming a legal entity in which to operate the practice can insulate the personal assets of the owner-audiologists from at least the nonprofessional liabilities associated with the practice. Examples of nonprofessional liabilities that would not put personal assets of the owners at risk, if the practice were properly conducted within an entity with limited liability, include real estate and equipment leases, bank loans, and other contractual obligations not otherwise personally guaranteed by the audiologist owner. Nevertheless, landlords, lenders, hearing instrument and equipment suppliers, and others often require a personal guaranty that the owner of a start-up practice will maintain responsibility for all debts incurred until such time that firm credit is established, thereby minimizing the benefit of forming the legal entity. Over time, such third parties may feel more secure and release such personal guaranties (at least upon request), enhancing the benefit of such formal organization of the practice.

"Tort" claims resulting from business operations, such as someone slipping and falling at the office, would also be a type of liability from which owners of a corporation or limited liability company (LLC) would be protected personally. Claims relating to professional services would normally be pursued against the individual audiologist, as well as against the practice, so a limited liability form of entity will likely not provide a barrier for such claims putting personal assets at risk. Note that merely organizing an entity with limited liability to own a practice does not per se insulate owners from personal liability. This protection is a presumption, which can be overcome by a showing that the business was really being operated as an alter ego of the owner(s), without its separate existence being respected by the owner(s). This "piercing the veil" concept of holding the owner(s) liable for liabilities of a corporation or LLC most frequently arises when money received or paid by the practice is not properly tracked, documented or properly accounted for, or when contracts are signed in the name of the owner(s) rather than in the business name.

Failure to formally establish an entity to own a practice would result in a sole proprietorship (if a single owner) or a general partnership (if more than one owner). In either such case, all assets of the owner(s) are available to creditors of the practice, subject to applicable bankruptcy laws that vary from state to state but may permit certain categories or amounts of assets to be protected from bankruptcy creditors.

Corporations and LLCs are currently the preferred forms of entity to accomplish insulation of personal assets from creditors of the practice. General partnerships do not as a rule achieve such limited liability, although states now provide for a form of general partnership commonly referred to as a limited liability partnership (LLP) that limits personal liability, at least to some degree that may vary depending upon statutory law in the state of organization. Limited partnerships provide such limited liability to limited partners, but not to general partners or to those limited partners participating in the management of the business.

Accountants and tax attorneys often have preferences regarding the selection of the form of an entity, a threshold question being whether a "flow-through" of tax attributes is desired. "Flow-through" entities include LLCs (unless they elect otherwise), as well as any corporation electing to file with the Internal Revenue Service as an "S Corporation." The flow through entity is not separately taxed for federal income tax purposes and all revenues and expenses of the entity are attributed to the owners in proportion to their respective ownership interests (or as they may otherwise agree in certain circumstances). Accountants for the entity will prepare a Schedule K-1 annually for each owner, which provides the information needed for such owner's personal income tax return. Conversely, a corporation not properly electing "S Corporation" status (known for these purposes as a "C Corporation") would be separately taxed for federal income tax purposes. Income of a C Corporation is not attributed to owners unless they actually receive funds as compensation (which would be deductible to the entity but only to the extent the amounts are "reasonable") or dividends (which would not be deductible to the entity), and expenses would not "flow-through" to the owners and be deductible on their personal federal income tax returns.

Other factors considered in determining the appropriate form of entity for an audiology practice include projected earnings, specifically in the context of applicable federal, state, and local income tax rates and brackets; employment taxes; other state taxes; and the comfort, experience and familiarity of the professional advisors with the various specific forms of entity.

The corporate form is historically more conventional, but LLCs have been around for many years, and provide more flexibility in structure than S Corporations. An LLC operating agreement may provide that allocations and distributions are to be made other than pro rata with equity/capital ownership. Additionally, there is no limit on the number of or nature of owners in an LLC, whereas an S Corporation may be owned by no more than 100 owners including individuals or qualified trusts. Table 3–1 summarizes certain identifying characteristics of various forms of entity. Please note this chart is not an exhaustive list of entity types,

Table 3–1. Identifying Forms of Corporate and Business Entities

	Limited Liability of Owners	Tax Pass-Through	Federal or State Filing(s) Required to Organize
C Corporation	Yes	No	State
S Corporation	Yes	Yes	Federal and State
LLC	Yes	Yes, unless otherwise requested	State
General Partnership	No	Yes	No (but state may require fictitious name filing)
PLL	Yes, to some degree as defined by state law	Yes	No (but state may require fictitious name filing)
Limited Partnership	Yes, except for general partner	Yes	State
Sole Proprietorship	No	Yes	No

and that other potential but lesser used forms of entities, such as unincorporated associations, may exist from state to state.

The state of organization for the legal entity is usually, but not necessarily, the state in which the practice is located. Certain states, such as Delaware, have historically catered to companies relying on the public equities markets by business-friendly laws regarding organization, flexibility in operations and standards of care for directors and officers of corporations. Delaware in particular has significantly more developed, and therefore more established, judicial case law relating to business issues than other states. Since so many major companies have organized there, many cases with claims associated with business operations and activities have been tried there. Many companies view the increased certainty associated with such established case law as beneficial. However, many other states have in recent years developed a more business-friendly legal environment. Closely held professional business entities do not necessarily have the same degree of concern about scrutiny of directors' actions by public shareholders. Thus, Delaware is really not the preferred state of organization for most closely held businesses such as audiology practices that do not commonly rely upon investors to raise capital.

State taxes on business net income or revenues vary from state to state, but generally apply to operations within the state and cannot be avoided by organizing the practice in another state. In view of the foregoing, and the fact that the state in which the practice is located will also be the state with which retained legal counsel will be most familiar, normally that same state will be the logical state of organization. If for any reason

an audiology practice maintains an office or sees patients in a state other than the state of organization, registration in that other state as a foreign entity will likely be required.

Establishing a solo practice clearly avoids a number of issues associated with having one or more "partners," but there is also a perception of safety in numbers for the viability of a practice. Selection of an incompatible professional partner can adversely impact retention of other personnel, profitability and value of the practice, as well as create substantial stress on all owners. But additional owners are often sought to increase capital and enhance the financial foundation of the business or to bring greater talent to the professional or management mix of the practice.

If co-owners are needed, it is very important to establish relative expectations and ground rules for operations and decision making as early as possible. Issues such as respective ownership percentages, associated amounts and form of capital contributions, and allocation of authority for making prospective decisions of varying degrees of materiality should be clearly identified in the organizational documents (bylaws or shareholder or "close corporation" agreements for corporations; operating agreements for LLCs). If one party is not obviously contributing more than another party, in terms of initial capital, inherited practice (from a retiring parent or other acquaintance) or portable practice (bringing an existing practice from a pre-existing solo or group situation), equal rights among the owners would seem to be appropriate. In the event this produces an even number of equal owners, the organizational documents should also provide for a "deadlock" mechanism to establish procedures in the event that the parties cannot agree on how to deal with one or more material issues.

In a multiple owner situation, it may be appropriate to establish one of the owners or a subset of the owners as the LLC's manager or management committee, or as the corporation's chief executive officer or board of directors. Whether management is so centralized or not, there may be certain identified issues that the owners agree are so important that they should only occur upon agreement of some defined supermajority vote of owners, such as 66⅔%, 75%, 80%, or unanimous. Such supermajority issues could include amending the organizational documents, modifying compensation of owners, incurring bank debt, bringing in new owners, terminating an owner, combining with another entity, or selling the business. A supermajority vote by design makes it more difficult to obtain the required authorization than a simple majority vote. An occasionally overlooked corollary is that minority owners have greater power (that being the potential veto power) in such circumstances. In fact, if there is an out-of-step owner, a supermajority voting requirement facilitates potential "tyranny of the minority," and may require the majority owners to make certain related or unrelated concessions to a minority owner in order to proceed with the matter that required the supermajority vote. Supermajority voting requirements can provide certain comfort to minority owners, but may also ultimately be an unhealthy impediment to appropriate actions and organizational evolution.

Compensation and Benefits

Since each owner in a multiple owner scenario is usually concerned about the productivity of the other owners, compensation structures often involve a base salary or draw, with a supplemental compensation formula to reflect the relative productivity of each owner. Occasionally a health care practice will simply allocate compensation on a pro rata basis each year; this works only when each owner takes his or her responsibilities to the others seriously and peer pressure keeps the owners at comparable and positive rates of productivity. However, unless the chemistry among owners makes such an approach possible, agreeing to some productivity and quantifiable measurement standards will be needed to serve as the basis to make at least annual compensation adjustments.

There are a variety of employee benefit plans, many using pretax dollars, which can enhance the compensation arrangements and financial security for owners as well as nonowner employees. Defined contribution retirement plans, such as 401(k) and profit sharing plans, are common for employers of all sizes while Simplified Employee Pension Plans (or "SEPs") and SIMPLE IRA plans may be particularly attractive to employers with few employees. SIMPLE IRAs and 401(k) plans permit employees to contribute up to a certain amount of pretax dollars to their account in the plan. Subject to legal restrictions, these plans as well as profit-sharing plans and SEPs permit employers to match or otherwise contribute to their employees' retirement accounts. Noncontributory defined benefit plans are less common for closely held companies than defined contribution plans, but that is a potential benefit plan as well. Although substantial health care reform changes are scheduled to begin in 2014, health insurance is currently a typical benefit, with some portion contributory by all employees — the magnitude of employer subsidy to be determined by the owner(s).

Flexible benefit plans (sometimes known as "cafeteria" or "Section 125" plans) permit pretax contributions by employees to pay group insurance premiums and otherwise noncovered health costs, including deductibles and co-pays, and child-care expenses. Other employee benefits to be considered include dental insurance, disability insurance, and life insurance. Benefit plans must be carefully designed in order to avoid violating government-imposed nondiscrimination tests that are intended to protect lower paid employees.

Whether subsidized by the employer as an employee benefit or not, estate planning is important for all the usual reasons of making sure desired allocations are provided for and taxes are minimized. It is important to periodically revisit the estate planning process as financial resources, survivor needs and intended beneficiaries evolve. A qualified estate planning attorney (optimally affiliated with the attorney retained for organizational purposes so planning for business succession can be coordinated with estate planning) can make sure wills and associated documents meet desired goals in consideration of applicable federal and state estate taxes, trusts for life insurance, dependents or others, and living will and other health care planning documents, which are generally governed by state law.

Relationships with Patients

The patient relationship is a professional one, as well as contractual. All audiologists should understand the boundaries set out for them by their state's Board of Audiology regarding the applicable Code of Ethics or other similar rules governing the patient relationship. In the State of Ohio, the Board supervising audiologists is the Ohio Board of Speech-Language Pathology and Audiology (http://slpaud .ohio.gov). On the website for your state's applicable board, you should be able to find volumes of materials related to the standard of practice expected in your state. For example, on the Ohio Board of Speech-Language Pathology and Audiology Web site there is a link to the specific rules and regulations that govern audiologists in Ohio. One of those rules provides the applicable Code of Ethics for audiologists. It is these types of rules that audiologists must be very familiar so as not to overstep or violate a rule that could put their license to practice at risk.

Providing new patients with contractual terms upon initia of the relationship, usually as part of the application/ information forms, is important. This is particularly true in the context of establishing primary payment responsibility. Applicability of insurance coverage is often not clearly discernable until after services are provided and claims are submitted, because of employment status and satisfaction of premium payment obligations. Within certain parameters, insurance companies may deny coverage to patients when employment of the primary covered person with the subscribing employer has terminated, or when that employer has failed to pay premiums. At the time of service the audiologist may not know these facts which can substantially impact payment for services rendered or instruments dispensed.

Other Contractual Relationships

Insurers/Payors

An important aspect of any health care practice these days is relationships with insurance companies and other payors. The major national health insurance companies will provide their standard provider agreements. The goal of reviewing such agreements is usually not negotiation since respective bargaining power of the parties is customarily quite disparate. The review is to simply understand the agreement to determine if a specific relationship with a particular provider is desirable and beneficial to the practice. Many states have specific laws and regulations regarding these types of contracts. Resources are available to you on your applicable state's department of insurance website.

ENTs

As an independent contractor or business owner, you need to actively manage your contractual relationships with the ENTs for whom you provide services. Although your attorney will assist you in preparing or reviewing a contract that adequately protects your business, you need to promote your business to make sure the relationships with the ENTs you serve remains strong. To do this, make sure you maintain consistent and open communication with the ENTs with whom you work. Both parties to the relationship will benefit.

Expert Testimony

The role of any professional in a court of law is to provide information to the court for its review and analysis of the matter under review. As an audiologist retained by a party in a lawsuit, you would be asked to review information and/or evaluate a person and provide your professional opinion regarding the issue being discussed. For the purposes of this activity, you will want to keep a few things in mind. First, your work with the person in question, assuming you are not just evaluating written reports or some other documentation, is still a patient relationship and therefore should be treated as such. Second, while you are being paid by the attorney that engaged your services, you are not being paid to say what they tell you to say. Rather, you should approach the engagement as a request for your professional opinion, which must be based on a nonbiased review of the facts. Third, you should always remain committed to your profession and detached from the emotion of the legal proceedings. Remember, you are a professional resource for an educated opinion, not an advocate for a particular result in the legal proceeding.

Facilities

For a start-up practice, the location of the office for the practice will be high on the list of things to do. While purchasing an existing building or constructing a facility on purchased property are alternatives, a conventional start-up practice will simply lease space. Legal counsel with real estate experience will be useful for identifying usual terms and conditions for the lease within the specific geographic area. Material terms to be considered include rent (and provisions for, and any limitations on, increases and expense pass-throughs); respective maintenance obligations of the landlord and tenant, including exterior and common areas; rights of each party to terminate or modify the lease; any limitations on subleasing or assigning the lease; any limitations on use of the facility (even if the practice is permitted, currently inapplicable prohibitions may be a problem for potential future assignees or subtenants); and allocation of risk associated with the facility, as may be reflected by indemnification and/or insurance provisions. It is important for you to inform your legal counsel if your landlord is also a referral source; this information will help your attorney properly identify all relevant regulatory issues.

Events such as a fire, a major water leak or flood, or a power outage or surge can interfere with a tenant's ability to use the leased space and operate the facility. Leases characterized by a landlord as "standard form" often give only the landlord: (i) a right to terminate a lease in the event of a casualty, (ii) a period of time to decide whether or not to restore damaged premises, and (iii) a further period of time to effect the restoration (six to nine months is common). In addition, the landlord's lender, usually the payee of landlord's insurance proceeds in the event of a casualty, may decline to make such proceeds available for restoration. A tenant with some degree of bargaining power may be able to procure a commitment from the landlord's lender, by means of subordination, nondisturbance, and attornment agreement described below, that insurance proceeds will be made available for restoration if certain conditions confirming the lender's security are met. In any event, a tenant should consider what (if any) portions of the leased space are essential to operation of the practice, and options for alternative temporary space if the need arises.

The subordination, nondisturbance, and attornment agreement mentioned above provides that even if the landlord defaults on its financing arrangements with the lender, including a mortgage on the leased premises, the tenant may continue to occupy the premises as long as the tenant continues to comply with its obligations, including payment of rent, under the lease. Without such an agreement, such a lender may evict a tenant of a defaulting landlord in certain circumstances. Most tenants do not ask for such an agreement, but in cases where substantial improvements are being made to the premises, or other suitable space is difficult to find, it is worth requesting.

If a need for additional space is reasonably anticipated in the foreseeable future to accommodate expected growth in the practice, it is not unusual to ask for an option or at least a right of first refusal in the lease, on identified space adjacent to the currently leased space. Additionally, the lease can be written to include the right of first refusal regarding the sale of the building.

If improvements to the leased space are required before occupancy, the landlord and tenant must agree upon what improvements will be made, who will secure the contractors to make the improvements, and who will finance the improvements. The landlord may agree to give the tenant an allowance or to finance the cost over the lease term with the tenant making periodic payments to the landlord. If the tenant is responsible for construction of the improvements, the tenant will need to obtain all necessary governmental approvals (e.g., building permit), and confirm that the improvements will comply with applicable legal requirements (e.g., zoning, Americans with Disabilities Act). These issues can be dealt with in the lease itself, or in an incorporated and mutually signed side letter.

Depending upon the local real estate market, there may be opportunities to successfully negotiate more favorable terms and conditions to some degree. At least with input from an experienced real estate attorney there will be a baseline for validating that requested revisions to the landlord's proposed terms and conditions are reasonable. If this process is not satisfactory and there are otherwise desirable alternative locations available, more favorable terms might be negotiated with a more reasonable, or at least more flexible, landlord, with either a more even-handed standard form, or a willingness to negotiate more bilateral terms and conditions. Note that even if a lease does not contain obviously problematic restrictions on use of the premises, local zoning laws may have such restrictions, so a look at the local zoning map and related definitions and regulations may be prudent but usually reserved to cases where the property is being purchased.

Risk Management and Dispute Resolution

Risk management for an audiology practice, like most businesses, is addressed primarily by complying with applicable professional standards of care, and by procuring appropriate insurance. Malpractice is an obvious risk, but insurance to cover nonprofessional liabilities of the practice, as well as property or casualty losses, life, health and disability of owners and/or employees must also be considered. The most important action you can take is to implement a process and procedure for reviewing treatment and outcomes and modifying your practice accordingly.

Sometimes, events lead to disputes with third parties that cannot be resolved informally by an insurer or otherwise, in which case selection of the method of, and venue for, dispute resolution can be very important. Contractual arrangements described above can be structured to require mediation and/or arbitration as alternatives to litigation in a judicial setting. Even in situations where the dispute is not governed by mandatory alternative dispute resolution, the parties can agree at the time of the dispute to utilize such alternative methods.

Mediation is nonbinding, but mediators are quite often former judges who can help the parties see the weaknesses of their respective arguments, as well as likely results of a prolonged and costly formal litigation process. This in turn often yields a compromise that is mutually advantageous (compared to proceeding with litigation) and mutually acceptable.

Arbitration can be binding, with the decisions enforceable in court. Although arbitration has historically been promoted as less expensive than formal litigation, that is often not the case, since their standards for conducting arbitration, the rules of evidence, discovery and other matters (that are well defined in the judicial process) can take significant time and energy to negotiate during the arbitration process. Arbitration does have the benefit of being a confidential process, which is usually desired by health care professionals. Lawsuits are generally available for public access and publicity in the media if deemed newsworthy by media outlets.

The location or venue for any dispute to be heard, whether judicial, arbitration or mediation, can be preagreed if the parties to the dispute have an underlying written contractual arrangement. This may be of limited relevance to audiology practices because patients customarily reside in the same jurisdiction as their audiologist and insurance payers usually are unwilling to negotiate to modify their standard contractual terms which include having the venue and area of judicial proceedings in the location of their principal office.

Regulatory Compliance

The practice of audiology is subject to state licensure or registration. Since criteria vary from state to state, it is very important to become familiar with the requirements of the state(s) in which a license is likely to be desired, to ensure that such requirements are met before application for a license is made. A careful review of the state law and administrative rules should provide the information needed; all such information should be available on the applicable state board website. If not, contact the executive director at the licensing board for specific clarifications.

In addition to state licensure, the practice of audiology is subject to a various federal, state, and local laws and associated rules, some unique to the health care industry, and some applicable to businesses generally.

Federal laws that specifically apply to the practice of health care, and therefore impact the practice of audiology directly or indirectly include, without limitation:

- The Health Insurance Portability and Accountability Act (known to its friends and others as "HIPAA"), as further amended by the Health Information Technology for Economic and Clinical Health Act ("HITECH"), sets certain standards relating to confidentiality and protection of patient health information;
- The federal Anti-Kickback Statute ("AKS"), which prohibits and makes criminal any offer, payment, solicitation or receipt of value for influencing referrals to health care providers for services or items covered by Medicare or Medicaid;
- The Stark laws, which prohibit referrals by physicians in which the referring physician has a direct or indirect financial interest, for certain "designated health services" covered by Medicare or Medicaid; and
- The False Claims Act, which dates back to the Civil War and creates a private right of action—any citizen can bring a claim—for fraudulent billing of the federal government.

The various states have laws that contain a variety of similar and parallel restrictions.

HIPAA and HITECH

In 1996 HIPAA was promulgated by Congress to "improve portability and continuity of health care when there was a change of jobs, to combat waste, fraud and abuse in health insurance and health care delivery . . . to simplify the administration of health insurance, and for other purposes" (American Academy of Audiology, 2006). There were several titles that comprised the Act that are pertinent to audiologists: Transaction and Code Sets, Privacy, and Security. More recently, the stimulus package that was signed by President Obama on February 17, 2009 created many new and significant HIPAA privacy and security requirements on covered entities, business associates, and other entities. These changes all fall under HITECH.

Privacy Rules and Business Associates

A key portion of HIPAA, the Standards for Privacy of Individually Identifiable Health Information of HIPAA, sets forth the standards for the protection of certain health information. This portion of HIPAA addresses the use and disclosure of individuals' health information ("protected health information" or "PHI") by organizations subject to the HIPAA, which are known as "covered entities." If a covered entity uses the services of another entity to, for example, perform a function or activity involving the use or disclosure of PHI, the other entity will be considered a "business associate" under HIPAA. Originally, under the HIPAA regulations, a business associate was not directly regulated by HIPAA or subject to HIPAA's civil and criminal penalties (but, the business associate could have been contractually liable via a business associate agreement). Under HITECH, the HIPAA requirements apply directly to business associates in the same way that they currently apply to covered entities. In other words, a business associate of a covered entity would be subject to the same penalties as a covered entity, even though it is not a health plan, health care provider, or health care clearinghouse.

Disclosure Exceptions for Treatment, Payment, and Healthcare Operations

The primary exception to the HIPAA privacy rules relates to routine disclosures of a patients PHI for the purposes

of treatment, payment, or health care operations (often referred to as "TPO"). The general rule covering these disclosures is that a covered entity must issue a general privacy notice explaining what types of disclosures they make for routine purposes. An example of an application that pertains to audiology would be a clinical audiologist and an educational audiologist exchanging information on a mutual patient. For all other disclosures of a patient's PHI, a specific exception must apply or an authorization must be signed by the patient. In order to be a valid authorization, it must, amongst other things, specify the patient's name, address, date of birth, the name of the requesting facility, what information/test results are requested, the expiration date of the authorization request, and the name/address of the recipient. The patient's right to revoke the authorization as well as notification if the PHI may be redisclosed by the recipient need to be addressed in the authorization as well.

Permission to Evaluate and Treat

You will inevitably encounter the patient who does not seek audiologic treatment under their own volition, but by that of a well-meaning relative or friend. The patient has the ultimate right of determining treatment. When that patient is incapacitated and unable to make his or her own decisions, you may rely upon a person who has been designated as the patient's attorney-in-fact under a power of attorney (POA) to make decisions on behalf of the patient. It is suggested you include a place for the patient or attorney-in-fact signature on your practice registration form, indicating the patient or attorney-in-fact is granting you permission to provide the necessary audiologic diagnosis and treatment options. For those 18 years or younger, a note granting permission to evaluate and treat is required from the parent or guardian to provide audiologic services in that parent or guardian's absence.

Privacy Officer

Every office providing health care in compliance with HIPAA has specified on their Notice of Privacy Practices (NPP) the name of their privacy officer. The privacy officer is to be used if a patient has a complaint that can then be addressed in-house. Should a patient wish to exercise their right to review their chart and request a change or otherwise amend their records, they will do so in accord with the designated privacy officer. The change or amendment to the record will be accepted or rejected by the privacy officer who will document the full transaction in the record. The patient may file a complaint if they disagree with the ruling of the privacy officer.

Disclosure Exception for Reporting Abuse

In daily clinical operations, audiologists will see evidence of child abuse or neglect and domestic violence. These situations require careful consideration and appropriate action. Referral to appropriate authorities in cases where abuse, neglect, or domestic violence is seen or suspected may be mandated by state licensing laws governing the practice of audiology or in other sections of laws pertaining to health care practitioners. Privacy concerns are not completely suspended in these cases, but HIPAA allows the covered entity to disclose the minimum amount necessary to protect

the individual. Therefore, these patients may be reported to the appropriate authorities, including law enforcement, children's services and/or domestic violence shelters. This should be addressed in your NPP.

Enforcement and Penalties

Both civil and criminal penalties are possible for violations of HIPAA. Specifically, the Secretary of Health and Human Services may impose civil fines up to a maximum of $25,000 per calendar year and the Department of Justice has the ability to assert criminal penalties ranging from a $50,000 fine and one (1) year in prison to a $250,000 fine and ten (10) years in prison. Notwithstanding those potential penalties, HIPAA does currently provide exceptions for lack of knowledge or where the violation was cured within thirty (30) days.

Under HITECH, the Secretary of Health and Human Services is required to audit covered entities and to investigate any covered entities if a complaint has been submitted. In certain circumstances, when a covered entity did not know of a violation (and by exercising due diligence would not have known), the Secretary of Health and Human Services may allow voluntary corrective action. Furthermore, the civil penalty amounts are distinguished by the type of violation. For example, when a covered entity is not aware of a violation (and would not have been aware exercising due diligence), the minimum penalty is $100 per violation, with a cap of $25,000 for violations of an identical requirement during a calendar year. The maximum penalty is $50,000 per violation, with a cap of $1.5 million for violations of an identical requirement during a calendar year. Notably, HITECH provides that penalties may not apply if the violation is corrected within thirty (30) days of the date the covered entity became aware of (or by exercising due diligence should have been aware of) the violation.

In addition to the federal agencies that may bring actions, HITECH gives authority to state attorneys general to bring civil actions against covered entities for violations of HIPAA and to obtain damages on behalf of the residents of their state. Notwithstanding, if the secretary of Health and Human Services has instituted an action against a person with respect to specific violations of HIPAA, no state attorney general may bring an action. Damages for an attorney general action can amount to $100 per violation, with a maximum of $25,000 for violations of an identical requirement during a calendar year, and include attorney's fees for the state.

The Anti-Kickback Statute (AKS)

The federal Anti-Kickback Statute (42 U.S.C. §1320a-7b) was enacted to prohibit transactions that are intentionally designed to exploit federal health care programs. The AKS is an intent based law that makes it a criminal offense to knowingly and willfully offer, pay, solicit, or receive any remuneration to induce or reward referrals of items or services reimbursable by a federal health care program. Where remuneration is paid purposefully to induce or reward referrals of items or services payable by a federal health care program, the AKS, and likely the applicable state law equivalent, is violated. Notably, for the purposes of the AKS, "remuneration" includes the transfer of anything of value, directly or indirectly, overtly or covertly, in cash or in kind.

The Department of Health and Human Services has promulgated safe harbor regulations that define practices that are not subject to the AKS because such practices would be unlikely to result in fraud or abuse. The safe harbors set forth specific conditions that, when met, assure entities involved of not being prosecuted or sanctioned for the arrangement qualifying for the safe harbor. However, safe harbor protection is afforded only to those arrangements that precisely meet all of the conditions set forth in the safe harbor. If all conditions of a safe harbor are not met, the activity or arrangement is not automatically illegal. Rather, the particular safe harbor does not apply and the intent of the parties may be examined to determine applicability of the statute.

Stringency of compliance will vary from audiology practice to practice. Many hospitals and otolaryngology offices have adopted policies of no gifts, including pens, note pads, or anything of substantive value as it may be considered as remuneration as well as being construed as buying loyalty. The Ethical Practice Committee of the American Academy of Audiology has advised that "[a]cceptance of gifts of any value from any company that manufactures or supplies products that he or she professionally uses or recommends . . . should be avoided" (American Academy of Audiology, 2011).

The Ethical Practice Guidelines on Financial Incentives for Hearing Instruments position statement adopted by the American Academy of Audiology (http://www.audiology.org) and the Academy of Dispensing Audiologists (http://www.audiologist.org) in 2003 defines, for the members of these organizations, the ethics and legality of the acceptance of trips, cash, and other gifts in exchange for recommending items that may be paid for by a federal health care program. Abiding by these guidelines protects the audiologist from inadvertent violations of the AKS. It is recommended that all audiologists read these guidelines as well as adopt them in their clinical practices.

The Stark Law

Section 1877 of the Social Security Act, also known as the Physician Self-Referral law or "Stark": (1) prohibits a physician from making referrals for certain "designated health services" (DHS) payable by Medicare to an entity with which he or she (or an immediate family member) has a financial relationship (ownership or compensation), unless an exception applies; and (2) prohibits a physician from filing claims with Medicare (or billing another individual, entity, or third-party payer) for those referred services. Since the inception of Stark, the Department has provided rules and guidance applicable to Stark. To date, there have been three phases, each of which provide some level of guidance as to how Stark applies to particular situations. Within these phases there are a number of specific exceptions to Stark, but in order for an exception to apply all the applicable elements must be met.

Since referrals and a financial relationship are the triggers for a violation of Stark, the definitions of these terms are integral to this analysis. Section 1877(h)(5)(c) defines "referral" as a request by a physician for an item or service for which payment may be made under Medicare Part B, including a request for a consultation and any DHS ordered or performed by the consulting physicians or under the supervision of the consulting physician, and the request or establishment of a plan of care by a physician that includes the furnishing of DHS. Section 1877(h)(1)(A) defines "Compensation Arrangement" generally as any arrangement involving any remuneration between a physician (or an immediate family member of such physician) and an entity. Section 1877(h)(1)(B) states that "Remuneration" includes any remuneration, directly or indirectly, overtly or covertly, in cash or in kind.

Stark is a civil, not a criminal, law. Violations may result in denial of reimbursement, mandatory refunds of federal payments, civil money penalties, and/or exclusion from federal and state health care programs. To violate Stark, there must be a referral by a physician (or his or her immediate family member) to an entity in which the physician (or his or her immediate family member) has a financial interest for the furnishing of DHS. In this context, audiologists are not considered "physicians," so Stark generally does not apply to referrals by audiologists to other providers. The only audiology services that fall within the definition of DHS are audiology services furnished as hospital inpatient or outpatient services. However, as the entity furnishing DHS is the entity that receives payment from the Center for Medicaid and Medicare Services or CMS), and as CMS reimburses the hospital for inpatient and outpatient services, it is the hospital (not the audiologist) that must comply with Stark.

The False Claims Act

Under the False Claims Act (18 U.S.C. §287) it is a criminal offense to submit false claims to the federal government. A separate law (31 U.S.C. §3729 *et seq.*), also known as the False Claims Act, provides a civil cause of action against anyone making a false claim to the federal government. Violations include the following types of actions:

Submitting claims for services that were not rendered;

Submitting claims for services not medically necessary;

Not billing with the appropriate provider number;

Billing for services known to be noncovered;

Falsifying a patient's diagnosis;

"Upcoding" or billing for a service at a higher rate; and

"Unbundling" bundled codes.

In addition to criminal and civil penalties, violations may result in the revocation of privileges to provide services to a private insurer, and revocation of state license(s). The key point to take away from this section is to accurately bill for only services that are necessary in the quest to determine the diagnosis. The Office of the Inspector General, in its pursuit of fraud and abuse, is on the lookout for false claims, especially claims submitted for services not rendered.

State Regulations Licensure

Audiologists are regulated by state licensure or registration in all 50 states. These laws and administrative rules set forth minimum qualifications, competencies, and continuing education requirements to practice audiology. It is incumbent on every licensed or registered health care practitioner to understand their respec-

tive laws and rules, which can be found on the website for your applicable state board.

If you are registered or licensed as a health care practitioner, you are burdened with the implied acceptance that you have read and understand all tenets of the laws and rules governing your professional involvement with patients under your care. Should a licensee or registrant violate the laws or rules, the consequences may include restriction or loss of the license to practice. This also applies to those who come under your direct supervision in the practice. Licenses and registration certificates carry the weight of law: billing for services performed without a license is fraud and subject to criminal penalties.

Certification

There is a significant difference between obtaining and maintaining a license to practice and being a participant in a program of certification. State laws require health care practitioners to be licensed to practice their specialty within the broad range of opportunities that comprise the delivery of health care in their respective states. Certification is voluntary. By submitting to a process of certification, usually offered in accord with a professional organization, the applicant indicates their specific credentials and preparation to meet the requirements for the certificate. Certification is an affirmation awarded to an individual by a body of his or her peers. It recognizes specific accomplishments and may define an area of specialty preparation or advanced study. The American Academy of Audiology endorses and supports board certification and specialty certification through the American Board of Audiology (ABA). The ABA has a managing director and an elected board of directors that manages the certification process from application to granting of general board certification and recently developed opportunities for specialty certification.

Employment Law Concerns

Relationships with employees constitute another significant category of legal issues, governed by federal, state, and local laws, as well as contractual arrangements. An employee handbook is always a good idea, even if there are few employees, to establish a basis for many otherwise unstated, ambiguous and/or misunderstood aspects of the employment relationship. When permitted by state law, confirmation on the employment application or in an employee handbook that an employee is an "at will" employee can be key to the right of the employer to terminate employment for any or no reason (unless termination is for an illegal reason such as age, race or sex) and without prior notice. Such language can be invaluable if an employee alleges that an otherwise verbal employment arrangement was for an initial term of one year, and one-year increments thereafter, where the employer during the hiring process referred to salary in an annual amount. Furthermore, an arrangement not reflected by an employee manual or other written document permits an employee to assert that the parties understood there would be no termination by the employer without "cause." Obviously, such default or alleged parameters of an employment relationship may be inconvenient and costly to an employer that may have to spend time and energy to

prove a valid "for cause" reason for termination, rather than simply using the "at will" concept to rid the practice of an otherwise incompatible or unproductive employee. Although formal employment agreements for key employees may be an unnecessary cost, an operational practice with more than one professional may be well served by written agreements with the professionals and perhaps other key employees to specifically cover duties, base salary, bonuses, benefits and termination transition issues, among other things.

Other topics covered by employer-employee documentation normally include confirmation and acknowledgement of the ownership of patient records, as well as financial, personnel, and other proprietary business information of the employer. The terms usually confirm the employee's agreement that such information is confidential and proprietary and not to be used other than in the normal course of the employer's business, and is not to be removed from the employer's premises. Required compliance by the employee with identified standards of care is often set forth in such documentation as well.

Retirement, Sale of Business, and Other Exit Strategies

Audiologists, like attorneys, physicians, and other professionals, often retire only with reluctance. It is perhaps the love of the practice and/or perhaps the lack of desirable alternative activities. Nevertheless, planning for retirement may be most effectively accomplished years in advance by anticipating postretirement financial needs in the context of investments (personal and deferred plans) and liquidity of ownership interest in the audiology practice. The liquidity of the ownership interest in the practice is also relevant if practicing with the practice group turns out to be unsatisfactory and a change in practice environment is desirable.

In circumstances where a practice has co-owners, it is logical and usual to have a buy-sell arrangement in a shareholder or operating agreement that contemplates triggers for retirement or other exit strategies from the practice, as well as an agreed valuation method and payment terms for the price. In a solo practice without a co-owner, similar transition upon retirement arrangements can be made with a nonowner employee audiologist, or the owners of another practice. In a sale to an unrelated party, be prepared for a due diligence process during which the prospective buyer thoroughly reviews and assesses the legal and business records of the practice; if they are in order, the process will cause significantly less angst.

To cover situations where the goal is not retirement, but rather voluntary or involuntary withdrawal from an incongruous practice group, the same sort of buy-sell arrangement, or an employment agreement if one exists, can be used to address comparable issues associated with the departure. Customarily, this mechanism involves a sale of the equity interest directly or indirectly to the remaining owners (often via redemption by the practice entity) on a valuation basis that takes into account three major areas of interest:

■ Existing cash and cash equivalents of the practice;

■ Receivables associated with the departing professional; and
■ Existing debt of the practice incurred to facilitate generation of such receivables.

If the departing audiologist is a recent graduate leaving a group practice after a relatively brief period of time, the event can be more simply structured as a "walk away" with no payment for the proportion of receivables, and no offset for existing pro rata debt.

In any retirement transition, issues to be considered include accounts receivable attributable to the efforts of the retiring owner. Patient transition is a major issue since consideration needs to be given for the continuity of the patient's care, how best to retain the patient in the practice and how the patients will be advised of the transition.

Liabilities of the practice are also of significant concern. If the transition involves a sale of assets, a buyer might assume known liabilities, but usually will not assume unknown liabilities. Liabilities not assumed by a buyer of assets will remain with the seller. If the practice is conducted within an entity with limited liability, the entity generally may be dissolved and remaining assets distributed to the owner(s), as long as sufficient assets are retained by the entity to cover all known liabilities.

Tax effects of any such transition must also be considered. General rules include that sale of a capital asset, such as shares of corporation or interest in an LLC, yields capital gains, while the sale of an entity's assets yields tax consequences based upon the nature of the assets sold. Note that assets sold by a C Corporation will be taxed at the corporate level and that any subsequent distribution to shareholders may be nondeductible to the corporation and taxable as ordinary income to the shareholders. Finally, payments to former owners may not be deductible to the entity, depending upon the structure and terms of the buyout. This can leave the continuing owners with the burden of funding the buyout with after tax dollars.

The term "tail" malpractice insurance covers claims made after expiration of "claims made" insurance coverage, but which relate to events occurring during the coverage period. Alternatively, "occurrence" coverage by definition covers events occurring during the coverage period, regardless of when the resulting claims are ultimately made. Since most currently sold malpractice policies are "claims made" rather than "occurrence" based, tail insurance is usually an important (albeit potential costly) safeguard and should be considered whether simply leaving an existing practice or retiring from practice. It is important to make sure your insurance agent explains to you the alternatives and implications of tail coverage as you purchase or modify insurance coverage prospectively.

Record retention is another retirement consideration. This is less of a concern if the practice and associated obligations are assumed by co-owners or by a buyer of the practice. However, if practice-related obligations are not assumed by others at the time of retirement, and patients are simply referred to alternative providers, existing records should be retained as may then be required by previous contracts with payors, applicable law and relevant professional standards.

One hopes that, by the time retirement ultimately arrives, the audiologist will have achieved most of the professional and personal goals established over the years, will have anticipated legal issues to minimize adverse consequences to the practice, and will have found the practice to be the gratifying, rewarding and professionally satisfying experience that caused selection of this career path in the first place.

Suggested Reading

For further information on the foregoing topics, we recommend the following online resources:

Ohio Board of Speech-Language Pathology and Audiology (http://slpand.ohio.gov)

American Academy of Audiology (http://www.audilogy.org)

Academy of Dispensing Audiologists (http://www.audiologist.org)

Medicare Fraud and Abuse (http://www.madicare.gov/frauda-buse/overview.asp)

CMS Fraud and Abuse (http://www.cms.gov/MLNProducts/downloads/Fraud_and_Abuse.pdf)

HHS Information Privacy (http://www.hhs.gov/ocr/privacy/)

HIPAA (http://www.hipaa.com)

Bureau of Labor Statistics—Audiologists (http://www.bls.gov/oco/ocos085.htm)

References

American Academy of Audiology. (2011). *Ethical practice guideline for relationships with industry for audiologists providing clinical care*. Retrieved on January 14, 2012, from http://www.audiology.org/about/volunteer/committees/Pages/ethicalpractices.aspx

American Academy of Audiology's Coding and Practice Management Committee. (2006). *Capturing reimbursement: A guide for audiologists* (pp.1.4–2.4, 3.1–8.6). Reston, VA: Author.

4

Ethical Considerations in Private Practice

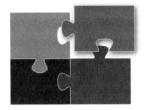

JANE M. KUKULA, AuD

"All that a man does outwardly is but the expression and completion of his inward thought. To work effectively, he must think clearly; to act nobly, he must think nobly."

William Ellery Channing

Introduction

Daily the need for autonomy is present to the private practice audiologist. Over the past 15 years, the profession of audiology has worked diligently to establish itself as an autonomous profession. Self-regulation and adherence to a Code of Ethics (COE) are among the characteristics of a self regulated, autonomous profession (Loh, 2000). Since a unified code of behavior is a key to achieving self-regulation, part of the journey involves a close examination of the ethical behavior of the profession of audiology. The American Academy of Audiology (AAA) has taken a leading role in this self-examination process by establishing ethical standards that are reflective of current public perception and in the education of audiologists.

While most entering the healing professions are good, caring individuals seeking to be of service to others, practicing according to one's personal moral code is not always professionally appropriate. A professional COE guides the moral behavior of a profession. Freeman (2006) describes audiologists as "a mix of practitioners with diverse personality characteristics." It is easy to view audiologists as group of individuals with various personal characteristics being more successful at meeting the needs of a diverse patient population, would also hold diverse ethical opinions. Although diversity in clinical practice is good and necessary, diversity in ethical behavior among a group of professionals is not appropriate. There are good people who line up on both sides of issues creating controversy surrounding the many issues facing our society. Consider how good people are on both sides of issues such as abortion, death sentence, physician assisted suicide, and other controversial concerns. Just as a people live by personal moral codes, so must professionals. When one enters a profession and assumes the skills, knowledge and clinical behaviors of the profession, they also assume the profession's "moral" behavior. Consider the ethical behavior expected of an attorney versus a butcher or a pharmacist versus a hairstylist. Each occupation involves an expected skill set and behavior. As hearing and balance professionals we are expected to assume the entire persona of the profession, not just the clinical skill set required to perform assessment and treatment.

Following is a discussion of business ethical practices in audiology, relevant legislation, professional COE, and ethical guidelines. Good business practices include seeking legal opinions on many issues with an attorney familiar with business, medical law, medical codes, and consumer protection laws. The intent of this chapter is to raise issues, stimulate thought regarding business ethics and to look at the role of legislative requirements and our professional COE.

Professional Behavior

Walden (2009) reported that professional ethics was fundamentally about building a trusting relationship. Consumer trust is built by always placing the patients' interests ahead of those providing the treatment. The trust relationship is based in the consumers' need for services in an area of expertise they know little about. As professionals, audiologists have a specialized body of knowledge and skills needed by the consumer (Loh, 2000). As professionals generating personal income from services provided and products dispensed, it is important to constitute unclouded decisions and recommendations that avoid even the appearance of placing personal and/or financial interests ahead of the patients'. Audiologists cannot afford to be seen through the lens of "consumer beware." As Walden (2009) states, "[U]nethical practice negatively impacts our patients and negatively impacts our profession."

Standards of Professional Behavior

The standards for professional behavior are based on consumer interest, federal and state regulation, and ultimately the best interest of the profession. Licensed professionals are first bound to uphold the standards of professional behavior set forth in state licensure statutes, since the state COE is usually tied to state law. Adherence to the state COE is not optional as an ethical violation can result in revocation of a license putting a rapid end to an audiology career. As members of a professional organization, such as the American Academy of Audiology, audiologists agree to adhere to the organization's COE. An extreme violation of the organization's COE could result in expulsion from the organization, but not necessarily revocation of a professional license. Professional organizations' COE, that speak for the profession can have impact beyond that of the organization by influencing a state licensure board's COE. Furthermore, when evaluating a potential violation of the state COE, a licensure Board may consider how professional organizations view the behavior.

Professional behavior is derived from three general sources; legislation, both state and federal, professional organizations, and employers. Law makers are concerned about public health and containing costs of health related services, while members of ethical practices boards care for the interests of consumers and the profession. When establishing standards, both law makers and ethical practice boards, look to the interests of consumers and empirical evidence. It is important to recognize that although practicing within state and federal statutes is ethical, ethical practice encompasses more than just legal practice.

Employers and business owners are also stake holders in enforcing ethical behavior. Their interest rises from the need to ensure quality care within the facility and to protect the business from malpractice allegations, substantial fines related to violation of statutes, and bad publicity. Unethical and/or illegal practice of an employee can have serious impact on the owner of the business. For example, if an employee bills Medicare for services not rendered, the owner could be required to repay not only the amount incorrectly billed, but may be required to repay the total amount Medicare paid to the practice for the past year or even more. Many facilities have corporate policies that set a standards of professional behavior within the facility. Often, employers require employees to sign contracts attesting to an understanding of and an adherence to the organizational ethical policies. It is recommended that the private practice audiologists employing professionals establish clinical corporate policies regarding a COE for their professional behavior, educating employees regarding these policies, and requiring employees to attest to the adherence of established policies as a means to protect their practice.

State Licensure

The first step to ethical practice is abiding by the requirements of the state license. The main mission of licensure is that of consumer protection as it defines the profession and provides protection for the general public, licensees and the profession. Kukula and Thornton (in press) reported that through state licensure regulation consumers are assured of at least entry level care. State licensees present themselves to the public as the qualified providers of the service, while simultaneously, protecting the profession from those who would provide the services without having met entry level standards for practice. Licensure sets standards in education, clinical training, continued competency, and ethical behavior. The right to practice is tied to all of the state requirements including professional behavior as set forth by the COE incorporated into state law. Although ethical requirements established by states often vary to some degree, all reflect the golden rule of ethical practice, *to do no harm.*

Licensure also supports legal practice by requiring adherence to all pertinent regulations including state and federal health care as well as consumer protection laws. Kukula and Thornton (in press) reported on how state licensure, at times, supports other regulations by reiterating them in the state practice statutes; not all the legal requirements regulating health care and consumer protection are specifically stated in state statutes.

Sidebar 4–1
SAMPLE STATE CODE OF ETHICS

Ohio Revised Code Chapter 4753-9 Code of Ethics

4753-9-01 Code of Ethics

(A) Preamble: Licensees shall hold tantamount the health and welfare of person(s) served.

(1) Licensees shall respect and protect the inherent worth, integrity, dignity and rights of each person served including his/her right of self-determination.

(2) The relationship between the professional and the person(s) served or supervised makes it imperative that the professional is aware of the vulnerability of the person(s) served or supervised, licensees shall not:

(a) Discriminate in his/her relationships with person(s) served or supervised, colleagues, students, and members of the allied professions on the basis of race, ethnicity, gender, age, religion, national origin, sexual orientation, or disability.

(b) Engage in sexual or intimate relations the person(s) served or supervised.

(c) Harass or abuse person(s) served or supervised.

(d) Engage in the evaluation or remediation of speech, language, or hearing disorders except in a professional relationship.

(e) Participate in activities that constitute a conflict of interest.

(3) Licensees shall use reasonable precautions to protect the health and welfare of person(s) served in the delivery of professional services and in research.

(4) Licensees shall be proficient in areas of treatment, objective in the application of skills, and maintain concern for the best interests of person(s) served or supervised, colleagues, and society as a whole.

(5) Licensees shall practice within the established standards of practice and training recognized by the American Speech-Language-Hearing Association or the American Academy of Audiology.

(6) To protect the public confidence, public behavior shall reflect a high level of moral and ethical behaviors.

(7) When making public statements, licensees shall:

(a) Provide information about professional services and products that do not contain misrepresentations or claims that are false, deceptive, or misleading.

(b) Provide accurate information about the nature and management of communicative disorders, the professions, and services rendered to persons served or supervised professionally.

(c) Announce services in a manner consonant with the highest professional standards in the community.

(8) Licensees shall not mislead or limit services with person(s) served or supervised based on professional or commercial affiliations.

(9) Licensees shall subscribe to these principles and the code of ethics adopted by the board and agree to abide by the rules of the board and Chapter 4753 of the Revised Code.

(10) Licensees shall report to the board any violation of the board rules or any breach of the code of ethics that he/she is aware of.

(B) Fundamental rules considered essential. Violation of the code of ethics shall be considered unprofessional conduct.

(1) Licensees shall maintain professional behavior.

(a) Licensees shall not engage in dishonesty, fraud, deceit, misrepresentation, or illegal conduct that adversely reflects on the profession or the individual.

(b) Licensees shall not practice under the influence of illegal substances, alcohol, or other chemicals that may impair decision making or quality of care.

(c) Licensees shall maintain a professional relationship with the board.

(i) Licensees shall conduct their practice according to Chapter 4753. of the Revised Code and agency-level 4753 of the Administrative Code.

(ii) Licensees shall cooperate with all lawful requests of the board within thirty calendar days.

(iii) The denial or revocation of licensure in another state, or from another board in this state, may result in denial or revocation of licensure by the board.

(d) When patients from a primary employment setting are seen in another setting, the person(s) served professionally shall be fully informed of services available from the licensee's primary employment setting as well as those from the private practice and given freedom to choose whether and from whom they will obtain professional services.

(i) The costs associated with obtaining services from the licensee's primary employment setting versus those associated with the private practice shall be made clear.

(ii) Practitioners accepting cases in a private setting from their primary place of employment shall inform the administrator at their primary employment setting of the intent.

(2) Licensees shall maintain records and keep confidentiality of person(s) served, including:

(a) Maintaining adequate records of professional services rendered.

(b) Providing appropriate access to records of person(s) served professionally.

(c) Not disclosing to unauthorized persons any confidential information obtained from any person(s) served or supervised professionally without the written consent of person(s) served or his/her legal guardian unless required by law.

(d) Being compliant with all state and federal laws and regulations relating to records keeping, records access and patient confidentiality.

(3) Licensees shall exhibit professional behavior in the delivery of services by:

(a) Accurately represent his/her training, credentials and competence.

(b) Provide only services for which he/she is properly trained.

(c) Continue their professional development throughout their careers.

(d) Accept for treatment, persons:

(i) Who can reasonably be expected to benefit from services and continue with treatment when there is reasonable expectation of further benefit.

(ii) Following the exercise of independent professional judgment, regardless of referral source or prescription.

(e) Fully inform person(s) served of the nature and possible effects of service

(f) Secure all reasonable precautions to avoid injury to persons in the delivery of professional services including but not limited to the following:

(i) Established guidelines for infection control.

(ii) Established procedural techniques.

(iii) Safety guidelines for equipment.

(g) Provide only services and products that are in the best interest of person(s) served.

(h) Evaluate services rendered and products dispensed to determine effectiveness.

(i) Ensure that all equipment used in the provision of services is in proper working order and is properly calibrated.

(j) Not guarantee the results of any speech or hearing consultative or therapeutic procedure.

(i) A guarantee of any sort, express or implied, oral or written, is contrary to professional ethics.

(ii) A reasonable statement of prognosis is appropriate, but factors, hence, any warranty for services and outcomes is deceptive and unethical.

(k) Use every resource available, including referrals to other specialists as needed, to effect maximum improvement in person(s) served. Licensees shall:

(i) Identify competent, dependable referral sources for person(s) served professionally.

(ii) Include referrals to other audiologists and speech-language pathologists when the scope and nature of the indicated evaluation and/or treatment is beyond the training of the licensee.

(iii) Not order excessive tests, treatment or use of treatment facilities when not warranted by the condition of the person(s) served.

(l) Licensees shall be compliant with all state and federal laws and regulations governing the practice of speech-language pathology and audiology and the dispensing and selling of products.

(m) Licensees shall not disparage the goods, services or business of another by false representation of fact.

(4) Licensees supervising conditional licensees, aides, and students: shall prohibit anyone under their supervision from engaging in any practice that violates Chapter 4753 of the Revised Code or agency-level 4753 of the Administrative Code including the code of ethics.

(a) Supervisors of clinical practice shall:

(i) Provide direct and indirect clinical supervision.

(ii) Maintain adequate records of direct and indirect supervision rendered.

(iii) Not supervise the clinical practice of a student or aide, while completing the supervised professional experience required for licensure under section 4753.06 of the Revised Code.

(b) Supervisors of supervised professional experience shall:

(i) Not delegate any service requiring the professional competence of a licensed clinician to anyone unqualified.

(ii) Limit conditional licensees to providing services pursuant only to a specific plan approved by the board.

(c) Aide supervisors shall:

(i) Ensure aides provide services pursuant only to a specific plan approved by the board.

(ii) Assume full responsibility of services provided by the aide.

(iii) Not offer clinical services by aides for whom they do not provide appropriate supervision.

(iv) Ensure aides do not represent himself/herself to the public as a speech-language pathologist or audiologist.

(v) Ensure aides abide by Chapter 4753 of the Revised Code and agency-level 4753 of the Administrative Code.

(5) Licensees performing research shall:

(a) Ensure persons selected for research be informed of their free choice to participate and guarantee their right to privacy.

(b) Inform person(s) served and research subjects about the nature and effects of research activities.

(c) Use established methods and techniques in research.

(d) Exercise all reasonable precautions to protect the health and welfare of person(s) and their rights.

(e) Assign credit to those who have contributed to a publication and development of materials in proportion to their contribution.

(f) Credit reference sources.

(g) Honestly and accurately report findings in a non-misleading manner.

(h) Enter into agreements with those funding research that allow the researcher to honestly and accurately report findings even when results of research do not positively reflect on the funding source and/or the funding source's services or products.

(i) Disclose funding sources of research resulting in publications, presentations, products, and/or clinical procedures, and/or cited in presentations.

(6) Business practices shall be compliant with regional, state and federal laws.

(a) Licensees shall:

(i) Charge fees commensurate with services rendered.

(ii) Not charge for services not rendered.

(iii) Abide by federal, state, and regional laws regarding billing for services and products rendered.

(iv) Not enter into relationships, which pose or appear to pose a conflict of interest.

(a) Licensees shall not accept compensation from a manufacturer, dealer, distributor, or sales person of prosthetics or other devices for recommending a particular product or service, including but not limited to, monetary, gift or travel incentives.

(b) Licensees who are faculty at meetings and/or consultants who provide instruction may receive reasonable honoraria and reimbursement of travel, lodging and meal expenses from manufacturers, dealers distributors and sales persons of prosthetics or other devices or services.

(c) Licensees who are faculty at meetings and/or consultants who provide instruction shall disclose to participants potential conflicts of interest.

(d) Kickbacks in violation of federal and state statutes shall not be accepted.

(e) Licensees owning stock or having financial interests in a company whose products he/she sells, dispenses or recommends shall disclose to person(s) served the relationship and financial or consultative interest.

(v) Not engage in commercial activities that conflict with the responsibilities to person(s) served or supervised by him/her professionally or to professional colleagues.

(b) Licensees shall be compliant with state and federal laws and regulations regarding business practices, sales practices, including safe harbor and antitrust laws.

(7) Licensees may practice via telecommunications within the state where not prohibited by law.

(a) Support personnel in off-site locations assisting in clinical care, shall be licensed aides under Chapter 4753 of the Revised Code.

(b) Evaluation and/or treatment shall not be solely by correspondence.

Professional Organizations

Professional behavior is further defined by professional organizations. For example, the mission of the American Academy of Audiology (AAA) is to advance the profession of audiology through leadership, advocacy, education, public awareness, and support of research (AAA, 2012). Among the many committees, the primary role of the AAA, Ethical Practices Committee (EPC) is to educate and increase member awareness of the Academy's COE as well as the practical application of the code, rules, and advisory opinions (AAA, 2012). The EPC, with input from the Academy Board of Directors and the membership, periodically reviews and updates the COE. Knowing that behavior accepted by each clinician is the first step in adopting the behavior of the profession, the COE established by an organization, such as AAA, may or may not be as strict as a COE within particular state statutes.

Areas of Business Ethics

The various COE applicable to audiologists addresses all areas of ethics including clinical, educational, research and business practices. Business practices to be addressed include: billing/coding, relationship with industry, marketing, documentation/record keeping, and employee compensation.

Billing and Coding

Billing for services not rendered is unethical and illegal. Government regulations, including the False Claims Act, Medicare and Medicaid, and AAA COE Rule 4b prohibits charging for services not rendered. This pertains to everything, such as "padding a statement" by billing for extras not provided or services of another provided using your provider identification number.

Coding and reimbursement must be conducted according to ethics, government regulations, and appropriate medical definition. Regulations that govern coding methods and reimbursement values include federal and state prohibitions of false claims and false statements to United States government agencies, such as Medicare and Medicaid and the False Claims Act (Hahn, Abel, & Kukula, 2005). The False Claims Act makes false claims and fraudulent billing illegal with language that specifically prohibits claims for uncovered services, services and/or products in excess of what was necessary or less than needed (Liang, 1999). The statute makes it illegal to submit a claim for a service that was not performed or for an item not dispensed. For example, the Ohio Medicaid program reimburses a monaural analog hearing aid for an adult. Based upon the statute, an audiologist is in violation of the law if they provide a digital instrument even if it is difficult to obtain analog instruments or that they are providing a better product.

Government agencies also define who can submit claims for specific services. For example, under Medicare, audiologists are not recognized providers for cerumen removal and, therefore, cannot submit reimbursement claims to Medicare reimbursement for cerumen removal. Under certain circumstances, an audiologist may even need to submit a modified claim to inform Medicare that the procedure was performed. Medicare, Medicaid, and other third-party providers will, however, cover certain services when billed with specific diagnosis codes but it is illegal and unethical to bill a service with an inappropriate diagnosis code. For example, caloric irrigation with a diagnosis of vertigo, when using water to flush a cerumen impaction causing dizziness cannot be legally or ethically billed. Government regulations can be tedious and difficult to read and understand and may require legal counsel and/or seeking information from the Practice Compliance Committee of the American Academy of Audiology. For more detailed information on coding and reimbursement, see Chapter 9.

Conflicts of Interest

Although professionals are in agreement that conflicts of interest (COI) are unethical and often illegal, what constitutes COI in audiology has come under great discussion. Merriam-Webster (1981) defined COI as a conflict between the private interests and of the official responsibilities of a person in a position of trust. A COI is comprised of all endeavors related to the practice of audiology in which professional advice, actions, or judgments may be compromised *or appear* to be compromised by financial or other professional factors (Liang 1999). Kukula (2006) related COI exists when the personal interests and the professional duties of a person are at odds; when the potential for personal gain is in conflict with professional decision making. Put simply, a COI is present when the financial interest of the audiologist is or appears to be at odds with the best interest of the patient. The dispensing audiologist faces this dilemma every day as personal income is generated from revenue created by the provision of services and the

fitting and dispensing of hearing instruments. Although consumers recognize that professionals generate income from the services and products provided, they expect audiologists to recommend the best instruments for them not the best instruments for the financial health of the practice.

As practitioners, the question then becomes how is this conflict best managed?

- Is financial stability of the practice paramount to the best interests of the patient?
- Are untended financial necessities resulting in practices closing in the best interest of the patient?

The answer to both of these questions is no. Whereas one negotiates best pricing to secure the bottom line, the freedom to choose instruments in the best interest of patients must be reserved.

Relationships with Manufacturers

The audiologists' relationship with industry is one of the most discussed and heated ethical issues in audiology. Since audiologists partner with manufacturing to provide quality hearing care, these relationships can be quite complex. Audiologists depend on manufacturers for quality equipment and products, manufacturers look to audiologists to purchase their equipment and products. On the surface a rather simple relationship becomes complex over the manner in which audiologists choose one product over another.

Typically, manufacturers offer financial incentives or gifts to encourage the purchase of their products over others. These financial incentives to purchase more products may be offered as a reward program, business support program, perks such as free product, extra warranties, or other incentives that would otherwise cost extra. Reward programs may offer a free hearing aid after specific number of instruments are purchased or a dollar amount contributed to a business support program that can be used for marketing, new equipment, continuing education and other incentives. Perks may include extra product or benefits for your patients, but they have also included personal gifts such as TVs, DVD players, iPods, gift cards, pens, pads of paper, mugs, and food. Gifts are often freely given by a manufacturer, for example when the representative stops in the office bringing lunch, or the audiologist visits a booth at a trade show receiving a gift. Although these financial incentives and gifts create good will between an audiologist and a manufacturer, ultimately, on the part of the manufacturer, they are offered to encourage the purchase of more products. Financial incentives and gifts create COI, they benefit the audiologist personally or professionally, while clouding clinical judgment or at least appearing to cloud clinical judgment as to if the product offered to the patient is the best for them (Margolis, 2012).

The private practice audiologist needs to be ever vigil of cost effective financial incentives for the management of their practice as they can assist in offsetting costs of products and other incentives that can be beneficial to their patients and the practice, while mindful of COI or the appearance of a COI that can occur in accepting these favors. For example, at the end of the month an audiologist realizes he or she needs to dispense two more premium products from manufacturer X, to achieve the next level of discount for the month. COI arises from a number of fronts when this dilemma is presented.

Is a premium product the best for this particular patient? What if the patient does not have any difficult listening situations? They may be elderly, under hospice care, living at home, where premium instruments may not be necessary. If a premium product is appropriate for this particular patient the question becomes, is manufacturer X's premium product the best for the patient? If manufacturer X's premium products are the best for the patient, would the patient feel confident in the recommendation if he/she knew the audiologist was gaining free hearing aids or some other perk from their purchase? The best way to avoid these dilemmas is to not enter into a restrictive financial agreement with manufacturers.

Some audiologists feel participating in buying groups removes the COI by becoming part of a larger network where they receive better pricing, access to several manufacturers' products while simultaneously receiving other incentives for purchase, such as marketing, management assistance, or other benefits. A COI still exists if the buying group has the same type of incentives, that is, dispense two more premium products to receive a greater discount or free hearing aids at the end of the month.

Bribes are defined as anything bestowed, with a view to influence judgment and conduct. Although gifts may be presented "without strings directly attached," it is the implied expectations received with the gift that create the COI. Studies have shown that gifts, large or small, influence the receiver's behavior in favor of the presenter (Katz & Caplan 2003; Margolis 2007, 2012; Reist & VandeCreek, 2004; Wanaza, 2000; Zipkin & Steinman 2005). Furthermore, they found that when gifts are accepted, the receiver has a strong need to reciprocate the favor. Katz et al. (2003) found that even gifts of little value such as note pads, pens, and sticky notes can and do influence the behavior of the receiver. Wazana (2000) conducted a systematic review of medical literature and discovered that accepting gifts had a negative impact on patient care. Loewenstein (2003) indicates that those receiving gifts are often unable to remain objective, reweighing the relationship in light of the gift. Brennan et al. (2006) found the rate at which a physician write prescriptions for a particular drug is increased following a visit with a sales representative.

The disclosure of manufacturer relationships with manufactures is not sufficient to resolve the COI (Brennan et al. 2006). Concerns with the physicians in their study included:

- Physicians in their study did not agree on what constituted a COI resulting in incomplete disclosures.
- Patients are not experts in the field and are not able to see the bias.
- Physicians felt that disclosure could be used to "sanitize" a COI, leading them to believe there is no problem once disclosed.

Brennan et al. (2006) called for zero dollar limit on gifts including education, training and associated meals.

An area of continuing concern regarding COI has been that of obtaining loans from manufacturers. At this writing, bank loans for any purpose are difficult to obtain as recent government regulations for banks have drastically changed how these institutions do business. Many banks are currently required to use more of their own capital assets to make loans than prior to the past recession. In fact, bankers can actually have a better return on their investment with less risk by *not* loaning money to small businesses such as audiology practices.

Bankers often want to grant a loan but these new banking regulations make it extremely difficult to for practitioners to even qualify for the loan, whereas a loan from a manufacturer is readily available at a favorable interest rate and often closed in a very short time. For these and other reasons a loan from a manufacturer is extremely tempting to practitioners securing funds to begin or expand their practice and/or to obtain working capital to keep the clinic going. As a practitioner, these frustrations and the financial pressure to find funds for the clinic can make a good excuse to consider manufacturers as a source of funding.

Ethically, it is about more than the terms of the loan, that is, the agreement to purchase a particular number of hearing aids per month as part or all of the payment. Not only are there problems with a commitment to purchase hearing aids as part or all of payment, but the favor or the "gift" of a loan when others would not grant one may create a COI. Audiologists should convey to lenders in a well prepared business plan the wisdom of investing in a practice that predominantly caters to seniors. There are private investors, state and local programs offering support to begin a small business. Some cities even offer low interest loans to local businesses or offer small business grants for marketing. In these tough times funds can be difficult to find, but by being creative, there may be some other unusual sources that offer audiologists some choices other than manufacturers.

Professional Organizations and COI

Scrutiny of health care providers' relationships with industry has increased awareness of the dangers of COI (AAA

EPB 2004a, 2004b, 2005a, 2005b, 2005c; Abel et al., 2005; Hahn et al., 2005; Larkin et al., 2005; Ray, 2006). Decker (1999) recommended the AAA establish a task force to look at the relationship between audiologists and manufacturers. The result of this task force investigation has led to much scrutiny of the financial relationships between audiologists and manufacturers. In 2003, the AAA and the Academy of Dispensing Audiologists (ADA) published *Ethical Practice Guidelines on Financial Incentives from Hearing Instrument Manufacturers* to assist audiologists in understanding how to conduct appropriate relationships with manufacturers. Following publication of the guidelines, the AAA EPB issued several Advisory Opinions on COI (AAA EPB, 2004a, 2004b, 2004c, 2004d, 2005a, 2005b, 2005c) to aid audiologists in understanding these conflicts. The AAA updated their guidelines in 2011 issuing *Ethical Practice Guideline for Relationships with Industry for Audiologists Providing Clinical Care*, further outlining their rationale restricting the receipt of gift and other perks. These guidelines were based upon available scientific evidence, best practice, and/or expert opinion (AAA EPC, 2011).

Over the past few years many audiologists have suggested that the guidelines are too restrictive and impractical. Some practitioners felt that EPC was meddling in the business of their practice and unnecessarily limiting their profitability. The practitioner's position was that loans, gifts, trips, and other incentives do not influence their decisions as to product choices for their patients. While audiologists may feel that they are not influenced by these incentives, evidence does not support that opinion as it's really not about the audiologist's perception of being influenced, it is about consumer and governmental perception. The AAA recommendations provide clear instructions as to the preferred methods for interaction with manufacturers and do not put specific limits on the profitability of a practice. Adherence to these AAA guidelines can assist audiologists in circumventing issues with COI in their relationships with manufacturers.

Scrutiny of healthcare providers' relationships with industry goes beyond audiology involving anyone that recommends, prescribes or otherwise offers products to patients. Stanford, Yale, UCLA, and Boston University have all implemented no gift policies due to evidence of negative influence (Margolis, 2011). Veterans' Administration and military audiologists have long been prohibited from accepting any gifts since all of their patients are involved with federal programs. Implementing a no gift policy may be the easiest way to stay and maintain a legal and ethical practice.

At the time of this writing a copy of Ethical Practice Guidelines on Financial Incentives from Hearing Instrument could be obtained at: http://www.audiology.org/about/membership/ethics/Documents/ea2004_financialincentives.pdf and a copy of the Ethical Practice Guidelines for Relationship with Industry for Audiologist at: http://www.audiology.org/resources/documentlibrary/Documents/201107_Relationships_Industry_Guideline.pdf, and a copy or the AAA Code of Ethics at: http://www.audiology.org/resources/documentlibrary/Pages/codeofethics.aspx

Anti-Kickback Statute

The federal Anti-Kickback Statute (AKS) was enacted to limit fraud and abuse in healthcare. Passage of the AKS makes gift giving and receiving illegal under certain conditions. Although AKS primarily focuses on payment for referrals, it has significant implications for audiologists (Liang, 1999; Ray 2006). Under the AKS, it is a felony for any person to knowingly and willingly solicit or receive any remuneration, directly or indirectly, overtly or covertly, in cash or in kind, in return for purchasing, leasing, or ordering (or recommending the purchase, lease, or ordering) of any item or service reimbursable in whole or in part under a federal health care program (Abel & Hahn, 2005). The AKS prohibits kickbacks in the forms of incentives and/or perks so as to reduce the over utilization reimbursable services, the distortion of medical decision-making, and unfair competition by freezing out qualified providers who are unwilling to pay kickbacks (Abel et al., 2005). Liang (1999, 2006) reported that some of these financial arrangements between audiologists and industry that may be unethical and illegal under the AKS. The AKS includes safe harbors; specific relationships that have been predetermined to not violate AKS. Hahn et al. (2005) reported that it was doubtful that the typical hearing aid manufacturer incentive plan would fit into any of these safe harbors.

Worth special mention in the AKS is the *quid pro quo r*elationship. The quid pro quo is a relationship where businesses receive or accept rewards in exchange for purchases. The actual meaning of quid pro quo translates to *what for what* in Latin and has evolved in English to a meaning more like *you scratch my back, and I'll scratch yours*. The quid pro quo concept has serious unethical and possibly illegal implications particularly for reward programs that result in money or gifts earned based upon the number of instruments purchased. Some audiologists have argued that these programs assist in reducing business expenses and, in turn, the cost of hearing instruments down for consumers. Although this is a reasonable rationale for use of these funds, it does not change the quid pro quo relationship which has serious COI implications.

When considering these issues Liang (1999) offered the following as a guide in determining COI, ask yourself:

- Would accepting the benefit compromise, or be regarded by others as likely to compromise, the independent exercise of professional judgment?
- Would the provider be willing to have these benefit arrangements generally known by patients and the public?

If the answer to either of these questions is a "yes," the clinician, Liang (1999, 2003), and Metz (2007) feels that the behavior likely results in a COI.

Penalties for violations of the AKS are severe and include; exclusion forever from participation in Medicare, Medicaid, and other federal programs as well as, heavy fines up to $100,000 per violation and imprisonment. The AKS statute has numerous implications for audiologists and their relationships with manufactures. Reward programs, accepting gifts, or other perks from manufacturers may be in violation of the AKS and legal counsel probably warranted for those who enter into these programs. Specific issues that cause COI for audiologists include meeting a specific sales quota to obtain any of the following:

- Free instruments
- Gifts
- Cash
- Trips

- Continuing education
- Backend discounts
- Business development programs
- Reward banks
- Free instruments
- Loans
- Marketing programs.

Even if legal opinion indicates that the practice falls into a safe harbor or other legal exemption applies, legality does not mean there is not a COI. Professional ethical standards usually go beyond that which is legal as it deals with what is in the best interest of the patient. Hahn and Grimes (2006) state that audiologists are guided and governed by two sets of principles: legal and ethical. The mark of a professional is that practice is guided not only by the law, but also by a code of ethics.

Marketing

There are ethical and legal standards for audiologists to consider when marketing and advertising. The Code of Ethics of the AAA, many state licensure statutes and other professional organization dictate professional behavior standards for honesty and clarity in advertising. The goal of marketing is to bring new patients into the practice and a potential source of new practice referrals are local physicians. The AKS regulates the manner in which an audiologist or any healthcare provider interacts with physicians by restricting the use of gifts, cash, or other incentives to entice referrals or for recommending a service reimbursable in whole or in part under most federal health care programs. This AKS rule has ramifications for audiologists that provide services or products covered by Medicare and Medicaid.

Hahn et al. (2005) noted that one reason for this restriction is to level the playing field for those who do not enter into gift giving as a means of seeking referrals.

The Stark laws have implications when seeking referrals from physicians. The statute prohibits physicians and immediate family members from referring patients for designated health services (DHS) to an entity in which the physician or an immediate family member has a financial interest. It also makes it illegal for the entity to bill for services or products provided to the referred patient. DHS impacted by the Stark law statute include:

- Clinical lab services
- Physical therapy, occupational therapy and speech-language pathology services
- Radiology and certain other imaging services
- Radiation therapy services and supplies
- Durable medical equipment and supplies
- Parenteral and enteral nutrients, equipment, and supplies
- Home health services
- Outpatient prescriptions drugs
- Inpatient and outpatient hospital services.

Although audiology is not listed here, audiologists are impacted since hearing aids are defined as durable medical equipment. Additionally, some audiologists offer home visits to their patients and the inclusion for home health services could apply to audiology. Violate of the Stark law involves a physician or immediate family member referring to an immediate family member or an entity in which the physician or immediate family member has a financial interest. A referral is a request, a written order, certification or recertification of the need for DHS (Hahn et al., 2006).

Some audiologists feel that the Stark laws also apply to the relationship physicians use to exploit audiologists when they are employed to dispense hearing instruments as part of an ear, nose, throat, or otology practice. On one side of this argument it appears that an otolaryngologist referring to his audiologist for durable medical goods such as hearing aids is referring to their own entity that they own significant financial interest. Although this appears to be suspect, the physician is legally recommending and providing a medical device for their patient. As for their audiologist that is dispensing the products for physicians they are covered by the Safe Harbors within the AKS legislation. Hahn and Grimes (2006) state that the safe harbor protects any amount paid by an employer to an employee for employment in the furnishing of items and services reimbursable under a federal health care program, provided a bona fide employment relationship exists between the parties. Thus, commissions or bonuses paid by an ENT to an audiologist employee for the prescribing of hearing aids do not violate the AKS, even if the payments are based on the volume or value of hearing aids sold by the employee.

Federal and state consumer protection laws, licensure, and professional organizations' COE require advertisements to be truthful and not misleading. Statements regarding product features and benefits, as well as how audiologists represent themselves must be truthful and not misleading. AAA EPB (2004c) prohibits advertising to exploit consumers by providing inaccurate information about the performance of devices, providing results that cannot be substantiated, are dishonest or illegal, and/or misrepresent credentials.

Gonzenbach (2007) reported that an audiologist's credentials are an important factor to consumers and stated that paramount in presenting one's credentials is the responsibility to assure that there is never an implication of meaning or value that does not exist. Rule 6a of the AAA COE supports this statement and indicates that clarity when presenting titles and credentials to the public is essential (AAA EPC, 2004c). In this spirit honesty and transparency, the advisory also promoted the use of clarity when representing the title of *doctor* to patients. The following were offered as recommendations for the use of titles in printed media including business cards, signs, letterhead, and other communications:

Jane Doe, AuD, Doctor of Audiology

or Jane Doe, AuD

or Jane Doe, PhD, Audiologist

or Jane Doe, PhD.

Documentation and Record Keeping

Documentation and record keeping is another area where ethical and legal requirements overlap. Ethically, we are required to document our services and to maintain those records. Federal and state governments also require health care providers, including audiologists, to document services, maintain and secure records, and keep records confidential. The federal Health Insurance and Portability Accountability Act (HIPAA) 1996, is far reaching and impacts every step of record keeping in healthcare. HIPAA requires adoption of national standards for electronic health care transactions and code sets, unique health identifiers, security, and adoption of federal privacy protections for individually identifiable health information. Violations of the HIPPA are also a violation of the COE and can result in devastating fines. Audiologists are required to adhere to HIPPA regulations and special training on these regulations and implementation can be very helpful. Participation in a seminar Practice Compliance Committee by the American Academy of Audiology on HIPPA requirements can provide updates on the statute and current guidelines for interpreting the law and applying it in one's practice.

A discussion of record keeping would not be complete without at least a mention of the importance of records in a case of malpractice. Keeping accurate and complete records of services, test results and procedures is imperative. Simply put, if a service or result is not recorded, then for all practical purposes, a court would treat it as if it did not occur. For example, a patient complains that a dome came off a hearing aid and is still in the canal. Otoscopy is performed and the canal is clear, the tympanic membrane is visible and the landmarks are noted but this exam is not documented in the patient's record. Later, the patient develops an ear infection and believes it was related to the dome coming off and takes legal action against the audiologist. The audiologist would have a much stronger defense if the evaluation and results had been recorded. Then, accurate and complete records are also necessary to support that a service or procedure was performed or a product was dispensed if

audited by Medicare, Medicaid, or other third-party payers.

Employee Compensation

There are no specific statements in law or codes restricting compensation of audiologists, but compensating or incentivizing audiologists solely on the number of hearing instruments dispensed is a COI. Furthermore, compensation based on simply the number of hearing aids dispensed may be a violation of the AKS, if dealing with a federal or state reimbursement program. This does not mean incentives cannot be used with employees. Liang (2006) discussed incentive systems that reward all forms of productivity equally were ethical. In 2007 the AAA EPC published *Advisory Opinion: Hearing Aid Commissions*. This document further emphasized the need to not incentivize audiologists based solely on the number of hearing aids dispensed. The *Advisory Opinion* recommended more complex incentive systems that use other and or several benchmarks such as number of patients served, patient satisfaction surveys, number of returns and patient outcomes.

Ethical Dilemma Solving

Fleisher (2006) reported that most of the time we know what is morally right and that true ethical dilemmas are rare. Finding oneself deciding between equally weighted moral issues is uncommon, that is, a physician may need to decide between saving the life of an unborn child or that of the mother. When presented with a true moral dilemma, one of the obligations will not be met. To resolve a true moral dilemma, Fleisher recommended the following process:

1. Identify the dilemma
2. Collect and analyze relevant information
3. Frame the issues
4. Deliberate on the issue and information
5. Evaluate and reflect.

With a true ethical dilemma there may be no one correct answer. As a professional you are not alone in ethical decision making. Information gathering and deliberation does not have to be unilateral. Consult with a colleague, ask for an opinion from the licensure board, and or seek input from the AAA EPC.

Summary

Ethical behavior is determined by legislation, the profession and employers and is a requirement of all professionals. It is the hallmark of professionalism and becomes the duty of each and every practicing professional. There are many reasons for professionals to adopt the Code of Conduct for a profession: some are lofty or esoteric, and others are practical. COE informs professionals, consumers and others of the conduct of the profession and announces to the public what type of behavior to expect from those that practice the profession. Self-regulation of professional behavior is a step toward achieving autonomy and reduces the likelihood that other professions or the government will regulate

There are many statutes, both state and federal, impacting audiology and the

behavior of audiologists. The legal penalties can be great and can result the end of a well-earned career as an audiologist or healthcare provider as well as substantial fines. Unethical practice can have a negative impact on the profession as a whole damaging the bond of trust between healthcare providers and the public that can harm all those practicing audiology. Ethical practice and familiarization with the Professions Code of Ethics is the responsibility of each member of the profession.

References

104th Congress. 1996. Health Insurance Portability and Accountability Act of 1996 (HIPAA), Public Law 104-191.

AAA. (2012). Mission. Retrieved December 12, 2011, from http://www.audiology.org/about/information/Pages/default.aspx

AAA EPB. (2003). Ethical practice guidelines on financial incentives from hearing instrument manufacturers. *Audiology Today*, *15*(3), 19–21.

AAA EPB. (2004a). Advisory: To party or not to party? That is the question. *Audiology Today*, *16*(2), 43.

AAA EPB. (2004b). Advisory: Buying groups, rewards and conflicts of interest. *Audiology Today*, *16*(3), 49–50.

AAA EPB. (2004c). Advisory: Misrepresentation of qualifications. *Audiology Today*, *16*(5), 3.

AAA EPB. (2004d). Clarification of EPB buying group advisory. *Audiology Today*, *16*(5), 38.

AAA EPB. (2005a). Marketing support and cost of instrument guidelines. *Audiology Today*, *17*(1), 46.

AAA EPB. (2005b). Advisory opinion: Audiologists beware! . . . and be aware of conflicts of interest. *Audiology Today*, *17*(4), 34.

AAA EPB. (2005c). Ethics or professionalism. *Audiology Today, 17*(2), 44.

AAA EPB. (2005d). Statement on use of the term "Doctor" in advertising. Retrieved January 4, 2012, from http://www.audiology.org/about/membership/ethics/Pates/ea2005c.aspx

AAA EPC. (2007). Advisory: Hearing aid commissions. Retrieved February 12, 2012, from http://www.audiology.org/about/menbershop/ethics/Pages/ea2007a.aspx&PF=1

AAA EPC. (2011). Code of ethics. Retrieved February 12, 2012, from http://www.audiology.org/resources/documentlibrary/Pages/codeofethics.aspx

AAA EPC. (2011). Ethical practice guidelines for relationships with industry for audiologists providing clinical care. Retrieved February 12, 2012, from http://www.audiology.org/resources/documentlibrary/Documents/201107_Relationships_Industry_Guideline.pdf

AAA EPC. (2012). Purpose of the EPC. Retrieved February 12, 2012, from http://www.audiology.org/about/volunteer/committees/Pages/ethicalpractices.aspx

Abel, D., & Hahn R. (2005). Practice management and ethical issues. Ethics in audiology. *Audiology Today.*

American Speech-Language-Hearing Association. (2011). Conflicts of interest. Retrieved December 14, 2011, from http://www.asha.org/docs/html/ET2011-00320.html

Brennan, T. A., Rothman, D. J., Blank, L., Blumenthal, D., Chimonas, S. C., Cohen, J. J., . . . Smelser, N. (2006). Health industry practices that create conflicts of interest. *Journal of the American Medical Association, 295*(4), 429–433.

Decker, T. N. 1999. Conflict of interest in professional practice. *Audiology Today, 11*(4), 28–29.

Freeman, B. A. (2006). Ethics and professionalism. In *Ethics in audiology guidelines for ethical conduct in clinical, educational, and research settings* (pp. 7–9). Reston, VA: AAA.

Fleisher, C. 2006. Approaches to analyzing ethical dilemmas. In *Ethics in audiology guidelines for ethical conduct in clinical, educational, and research settings* (pp. 11–23). Reston, VA: AAA.

Gonzenbach, S. (2007). Audiologists, credentials and consumers. *Audiology Today, 19*(3), 43.

Hahn, R., Abel, D., & Kukula, J. 2005. Audiologists beware! . . . and be aware of conflicts of interest. *Audiology Today, 17*(4), 34–35.

Hahn, R., & Grimes, A. (2006). Risky business: What you need to know. *Audiology Today, 18*(5), 16–19.

Katz, D., Caplan, A. L., & Merz, J. F. (2003). All gifts large and small: Toward an understanding of the ethics of pharmaceutical industry gift-giving. *American Journal of Bioethics, 3*(3), 39–46.

Kukula, J. M. (2006). Ethics 101. In *Ethics in audiology guidelines for ethical conduct in clinical, educational, and research settings* (pp. 133–135). Reston, VA: AAA.

Kukula, J. M., & Thornton, G. (in press). Leadership in regulatory matters: The professional's role on the Ohio Board of Speech Language Pathology and Audiology. *Seminars in Hearing.*

Larkin, M., Walden, T., Hahn, R., & Members of the EPB. (2005). A question of ethics. *Audiology Today, 17*(5), 35.

Liang, B. (1999). In trouble with the law and the profession: Fraud, abuse and professional ethics in a world of provider distrust. *Audiology Today, 11*(4), 25–27.

Liang, B. (2003). *In trouble with the law and the profession: Fraud, abuse, and professional ethics in a world of provider trust: An update.* University of Florida Doctor of Audiology Program, Gainesville, FL.

Liang, B. (2006). *Ethical issues facing audiology: Law and professionalism.* American Academy of Audiology Annual Convention, Minneapolis, MN.

Loh, K. (2000). Professionalism, where are you? *Ear Nose and Throat Journal, 79*(4), 242–246.

Loewenstein, D. A. (2003). Social science perspective on gifts to physicians from industry. *JAMA, 290*(2), 252–255.

Margolis, R. H. (2007). Conflicts of interest in audiology. *Audiology Today, 19*(4), 32–34.

Margolis, R. H. (2012). Influence of gifts in healthcare. Retrieved January 8, 2012, from http://audiologyincorporated.com/articles/influence-of-gifts-in-healthcare

Ohio Board of Speech Language Pathology and Audiology. (2012). Ohio Revised Code Chapter 4753-9-01. Retrieved March 19, 2012, from http://codes.ohio.gov/oac/4753-9

Ray, G. (2006). Ethics at AudiologyNOW!, 2006. *Audiology Today, 18*(3), 54–56.

Reist, D., & Vande Creek, L. (2004). The pharmaceutical industry's use of gifts and educational events to influence prescription practices: Ethical dilemmas and implications for psychologists. *Professional Psychology: Research and Practice, 35,* 329–335.

Walden, B. 2009. Professional ethics: Back to basics. *Audiology Today, 21*(3), 56–60.

Wazana, A. (2000). Physicians and the pharmaceutical industry: Is a gift ever just a gift? *Journal of the American Medical Association, 283,* 272–280.

Webster's New Collegiate Dictionary. (1981). Springfield, MA: G. and C. Merriam.

Zipkin, D. A., & Steinman, M. A. (2005). Interactions between pharmaceutical representatives and doctors in training, a thematic review. *Journal of General Internal Medicine, 20,* 777–786.

5

Fundamentals of Marketing the Audiology Practice

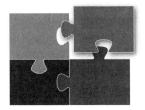

ROBERT M. TRAYNOR, EdD, MBA

Why Market?

Students of audiology are now educated on the AuD model ensuring that new clinicians are ready to practice their profession immediately upon graduation. Audiology has now evolved into a fully accepted professional discipline joining colleagues in optometry, dentistry, chiropractic, and other professions as independent practicing professionals. Along with this professional commitment comes the intense competition among competent colleagues seen in these other professional venues. On the cusp of direct access, audiology now stands as a viable profession with many well-qualified professionals competing in a single market.

The days of complacency in presenting the clinic to the market are gone forever. In the past, audiologists could simply establish a few referral sources and make a rather good living by offering good reports and customer service to their patients. Now that intense competition exists among highly qualified colleagues marketing an audiology practice is absolutely essential to business success. Competition from audiology

119

colleagues presents a significant challenge for all practices as they must find a method to ensure that their clinic stands out from the crowd. It is necessary to establish how this practice is different from the audiologist "up the street" or "on the other side of town." This does not mean that patient care is compromised or that audiologists need to become high pressure salespeople; it does mean that without proper marketing the patients will go to the another doctor of audiology in town and not *you*. The challenge is to differentiate your brand of audiology all the other brands of audiology in the market place. *Practitioners should keep in mind that in order for them to offer the best possible hearing care, the patients must first be attracted to the practice by an organized marketing program.*

Marketing is conducted to increase traffic and subsequently increase the units of service provided and numbers of hearing instruments dispensed. Marketing is not simply ads in the paper, a senior guide, or other local publications. It is more than an isolated presentation at the Rotary Club or a marketing trip to physician's office, it involves an organized, targeted effort to present the practice brand to the marketplace. As indicated above the challenge of marketing a practice is to differentiate the practice's brand of audiology from all the other clinics in the marketplace. In a classic differentiation discussion, Levitt (1980) felt that the way a company [or practice] manages its marketing and the methods used against competition within the same industry can be a major form of differentiation.

Commonly, marketing in many audiology practices peaks when office traffic slows down and is frequently a disjointed process incorporating little evidence-based information on what works best

within the specified geographic and demographic area of the practice. When practitioners respond to a lull of activity in their practice by pulling together a *marketing-after-fact plan*, they will find their reflexive marketing response to be inefficient and costly relative to the meager outcome of their actions.

To properly brand a practice in a community it is necessary to conduct market research and link information about the market to a simple or comprehensive marketing plan. The purpose of this chapter is to not only present basic traditional marketing principles but to also discuss the critical elements of market research that are essential to a marketing plan that will brand the practice in the marketplace. Although advanced, progressive marketing principles and Internet marketing concepts are specifically presented by St. Clergy in Chapter 6, and pricing is specifically discussed in Chapter 7, the intent of this chapter is to present the basic principles of Marketing.

Professional Marketing Defined

Marketing, as defined by the American Marketing Association (2012) is the activity, set of institutions, and processes for creating, communicating, delivering, and exchanging offerings that have value for customers, clients, patients, partners, and society at large. Kotler and Armstrong (2012) have described marketing as a process of identifying and meeting human wants and needs profitably. It is a process by which companies create value for customers, and build strong customer relationships in order to capture value from those customers. Although it may have a social or managerial purpose, marketing is the creation of demand for a particular product or service by establishing public awareness. Oblinger (2012) presents marketing as the process of planning and executing the conception, pricing, promotion, and distribution of ideas, goods, and services to create exchanges that satisfy individual and organizational goals. What do these definitions mean to audiologists? It means that marketing encompasses everything necessary to come up with a needed product or service, making potential patients aware of it, making them want it, and then selling it to them. Put simply, marketing is basic communication between a collection of sellers (such as audiologists) and a collection of buyers of services or products (such as hearing-impaired consumers), presented in Figure 5–1. This collection of sellers offer goods and services to the market consisting of a collection of buyers who pay money for those goods and services. Although this concept is how the system works, in marketing the goal is to get this collection of buyers to choose one seller over another. One of first decisions that must be made in

presenting the practice to this collection of buyers is to *how* it will be branded. Since branding is the key to the image that will be presented to patients, it must be considered as the first component of any marketing exercise.

Branding Your Practice

Hansen (2006) presents that each day brand promises are made to perspective patients and prospects. These promises are made through literature, signage, airwaves, print advertising, and other means of communication. While promises are certainly easy to make, the key to winning new patients and keeping existing clientele loyal to the practice is delivery on those promises. Delivery is exhibited through the practice, in the attitude of the team as well as the products offered and services that accompany them. This connection between promises and their delivery is what leads the consumer to choose a particular practice from the crowd.

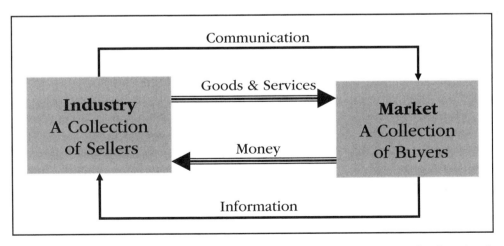

Figure 5–1. Marketing is basic communication between a collection of sellers (such as audiologists) and a collection of buyers of services or products (such as hearing-impaired consumers).

A marketing program distinguishes a particular audiology practice (a brand) from the other practices (other brands) that appear similar to patients in the market place. The goal should be to present a particular practice or "brand of audiology" so that it stands out from all other possible options that could meet the patient's wants and needs for hearing care. This involves "branding the practice" with a marketing campaign that establishes in the consumer's minds that this particular practice is *the* place for them to receive hearing care above all the other possible options or brands.

Branding, according to D'Alessandro (2001), is an old business practice that can be described as whatever the consumer thinks of when they see or hear a company's name. For example, what comes to mind when thinking of BMW, Apple, or Harley-Davidson? Some of the best products worldwide have built strong brands so that in consumer's minds, the thought is of quality, image, reliability, and customer service. Audiology practitioners build their brand every time they see a patient, report back to a physician, present a market offering, participate in a public relations activity, or simply interact with the community. Hansen (2006) further indicates that it is not just what is done with the patients that build a brand; it is the office environment, location, and atmosphere. Marsh (2012) states that in today's audiology clinic even the smell of the office can be part of the clinic's brand. Since purchase rates and satisfaction ratings are connected, negative in office experiences can lead to a loss of 10 to 30% of a clinic's business and create negative branding in the community. If, for example, Audiology Associates is to be branded successfully as *the place* for hearing care; market offerings to the community must be ethically directed toward generating in the minds of perspective patients and others, that the Audiology Associates's "brand of audiology" makes it the *best place* in the market area to receive hearing care. From the first phone call to the greeting upon arrival through the completion of the hearing care experience, the clinic must deliver on the promise presented their marketing communications.

Prior to the age of digital hearing aids, most of the amplification products were essentially the same and the real difference among them was simply the *place* they were obtained and/or the hearing aid *brand name*. In today's high technology world, there are substantial differences among products and consumers are bombarded constantly with market offerings via print media, radio, direct mail, television, and even via the Internet. This constant interaction of the market presenting their brand to consumers makes it even more difficult to brand a particular practice as the special place to receive hearing care.

As indicated earlier, the doctor of audiology (AuD) degree has forever changed the landscape of audiology private practice. Similar to the medical doctor (MD), doctor of dental surgery (DDS), doctor of psychology (PsyD), the doctor of chiropractic (DC), and other professional degrees, the AuD as a universal brand for audiology generates images of high-quality hearing care in the minds of consumers. Consumers can generally feel more comfortable in the knowledge that a professional branded with the AuD is an audiologist educated to certain standards and offers the typical skills that are commensurate with a doctoral level profession. Although the AuD has branded the audiology profession to consumers, the unique designator for audiologists makes it increasingly more difficult to distinguish one audiologist's practice from another. When all AuD professionals are branded the same, how does one practice stand out among the others? Consider that audiologists generally conduct similar diagnostic evaluations and sell (more or less) the similar products from a closed set of manufacturers as well as offer similar aural rehabilitative services to the public at large. Thus, in a world where all practitioners have the same credential, the AuD, how are these professionals and their practices different? Under conditions where all clinicians look the same, it may be the personality of the practitioner, the convenience or physical environment of the practice, and/or the atmosphere created by the staff that can make the difference. In a world of intense competition among audiologists and other hearing healthcare providers, there are a number of competitors simultaneously attempting to brand themselves through market offerings to the same population. All of these competitors may be formidable and it is essential that a specific practice present the difference between their "brand of audiology" and other "brands of audiology" or hearing care offered elsewhere. To better understand the nature of competitive branding, four distinct categories of branding competition have been offered by D'Alessandro (2001):

- *Brand Competition.* All competitors that *are like me*. This category represents all AuD audiologists that offer hearing care in the same market area. These competitors look exactly alike to the consumer, as they have the same "brand" for their credentials. In the consumer's mind,

without proper market offerings differentiating the clinic from other clinics in the area, patients would presume that products and services could be obtained from *any* AuD branded professional. Thus, it is not enough to brand the credential; branding of the particular clinic and the individual audiologist is necessary to insure success.

- *Industry Competition.* All competitors that *look like me* offering hearing care. Pertaining to the field of audiology, this would include doctoral level audiologists (PhD, EdD, ScD) other than the AuD or otolaryngologists. Similar to "brand competition," many professionals and "doctors" appear to be the same in their capability to provide products and services to the hearing impaired. Since often these professionals have established a relationship with their patients providing professional hearing care, it is essential that the new clinician market to obtain their share of the patients seeking services or products. Again, it is the intensity and the direction of the market offerings that ensures the branding of the practice and causes a particular clinic to stand out as the facility or audiology professional of choice.

- *Form Competition.* All those *in the same business*. This category would include audiologists of all brands, master's degree audiologists, hearing aid dealers, drug stores, wholesale warehouse corporations (Walmart, Costco, Sam's Club), Internet offerings, insurance company offerings, or other establishments that offer hearing care or sell similar products. Form competitors are those where considerable diversity may exist in the capability to serve consumers. Branding a practice by a tasteful and ethical market offering that presents the type of hearing care offered, can often provide the differentiation of hearing care providers desperately needed by consumers. Indeed, it may also be an ethical responsibility to present market offerings that direct consumers to the most qualified professional.

■ *Generic Competition. All products that cost the same as hearing care.* In this instance, patients weigh the costs of hearing care against other (possibly more desirable) recreational activities, required services or products; such as, cars, foreign vacations, cruises, appliances, or, on the service side, office visits, physical therapy, eye exams, dental reconstruction, and so forth. This is simply an application of the basic economic principle of "opportunity cost." This principle suggests that there is only a finite amount of funds and if the funds are utilized to purchase an item, then those funds are not available to use for another purpose. It is a simple fact that the products sold in audiology practices, especially hearing instruments, are expensive for most consumers, and compete for attention with other products of similar value. Furthermore, it is also well known that consumers want these other competitive products or services more than those offered in audiology clinics. As it is more fun and, sometimes of more mental health benefit, to take a cruise, a foreign vacation, or purchase a car rather than obtain amplification. Thus, there are many products in competition for the same funds, It

is often the marketing campaign or a specific market offering, that may convince the patient to make the more prudent decision.

While marketing is what builds a particular brand of audiology in the consumer's minds, D'Alessandro (2001) indicates that it is not easy to build a great brand. He states that it takes an artistic sense of proportion and timing as well as a ruthless willingness to distinguish yourself from competing brands (others that are "like you" or "look like you" to the consumer) and, one hopes bury them in the process.

Branding a new practice poses challenging decisions for the practitioner. Kotler and Armstrong (2012) indicate some major decisions necessary to develop a brand that is to be presented to the market.

■ *Brand Positioning.* At this level the product (the practice) is presented with its attributes, such as the benefits of an AuD versus other credentials, a particular insurance affiliation, or a particular brand of hearing instruments offered by the clinic. Generally, patients are not interested in the specifics of the attribute (features of the practice) but more interested in what the attribute will do for them (the benefit to them). These attributes can be many things from a "younger" clinician (attribute) that has the most recent information (benefit), to the reliable clinician (attribute) that has a long and trusted relationship with the marketplace (benefit). Patients relate to brands by "what will this brand insures in terms of benefit for me"; perceived benefit by perspective patients is what will determine the brand's value relative to other brands in the market. When a perspective patient considers a particular clinic's brand, it should suggest that there are certain benefits that stand out relative to the other brands in the market.

■ *Brand Name Selection.* While a difficult task, choosing a good name for the practice can greatly add to the success of the clinic. Ultimately the chosen name will become the brand name for type of audiology offered. Choosing a name involves careful introspection into the type of clinic that is being considered (see Chapter 2). Careful review of the product that will be offered, its benefits to patients and referral sources, the target market, and marketing opportunities available, should be seriously considered as the name is chosen. After these issues are considered, Kotler and Armstrong (2012) suggest that naming your brand of audiology becomes part science, part art, and a measure of instinct. They present that desirable qualities for a brand name include: (1) a suggestion of something about the product's benefits and qualities, such as audiology or hearing; (2) be easy to pronounce, recognize, and most of all remember, such as Audiology Associates or Hearing Solutions; (3) the name should be distinctive, different from other brands within the marketplace; and (4) the name should be legal and protected against infringement by others in the market.

Although essential to success, branding a practice is hard work but when conducted properly promises great benefit.

Marketing Research

Marketing research is conducted for many purposes. It can be used for planning, problem solving, pricing, or control purposes to provide insight and serve as the basis for a simple or comprehensive marketing plan. Kotler and Armstrong (2012) define market research as the systematic design, collection, analysis, and reporting of data relevant to a specific marketing situation facing an organization. Clinics use marketing research in a variety of situations. For example, marketing research offers insights into patient motivations, purchasing behavior, and satisfaction. It can assist in the assessment of market potential, market share, measure the effectiveness of pricing (see Chapter 7) or product, distribution, and promotional activities. Market research is typically used for planning and deals largely with determining which market opportunities are viable for the practice. When a viable opportunity is uncovered, marketing research can provide an estimate of the size and scope of the opportunity so it can be better managed. The use of market research for problem solving focuses on making short- and long-term decisions relative to the mixture of market communications to be used in presenting and branding the practice to the community. For example, one of the major problems of audiology practice can be the rise and fall of demand for products and services. The example presented in Figure 5–2 summarizes the problem that a practice may have with the seasonal demands for products and services. Although the demand for hearing aids and other audiologic services varies by the where they are offered, Figure 5–2 indicates that demand is less early in the year with

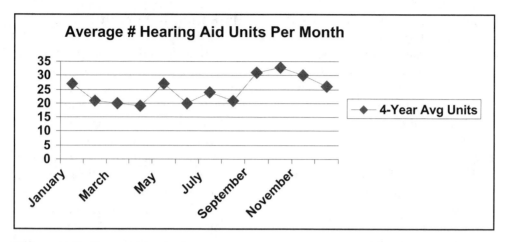

Figure 5–2. Demand analysis.

a demand spike in May followed by a downturn in the summer. It also presents that the greatest demand for hearing aids is in last part of the year. Since the product demand changes throughout the year, it must be stimulated at certain times of the year by an organized marketing plan that is based upon sound market research. This pattern of demand or, *demand analysis*, would suggest that the marketing plan would require more funds when the demand was low (early in the year and summer) and a bit less funding when demand was high (September–December). A demand analysis can be conducted for all products and services offered in the clinic, including hearing aids, routine audiometric evaluations, OAEs, ABRs, VNGs, operative monitoring, and ALDs as well as small accessories. Additionally, these product and service analyses can be as detailed and many even describe patient demand for the specific brands of products or components of audiometric evaluations. Since marketing is an expensive process, successful practices spend their valuable funds presenting their brand of audiology to the community based upon their demand predictions and market research.

Marketing Plans

A good marketer will communicate their brand to the market and receive feedback that can be used to stimulate demand for products and services. Planning a successful marketing program involves conducting marketing research to know how, when, and where to wisely expend that hard earned marketing budget.

Berry and Wilson (2001) offer that marketing should be a set of planned activities designed to positively influence the perceptions and purchase choices of individuals and organizations. Know This. com (2006) states that a marketing plan is a highly detailed, heavily researched, and well written so that many inside and some outside the organization will be able to understand it. Although there is no one format for the marketing plan, it is an exercise that essentially forces the practitioner to look internally into the practice. This is done to fully understand the results of past marketing decisions, the market in which the practice operates, as well as a direction for future. As with business plans (Chapter 2), marketing plans can be a key component in

Sidebar 5–1
OUTLINE OF MARKETING RESEARCH (Churchill & Brown, 2004)

I. Planning

A. What kinds of people buy our products? Where do they live? How much do they earn? How many of them are there?
B. Are the markets for our products increasing or decreasing? Are there promising markets that we have not reached yet?
C. Are channels of distribution for our products changing? Are new types of marketing institutions likely to evolve?

II. Problem Solving

A. Product
   1. Which of various product designs is likely to be the most successful?
   2. What kinds of packaging should we use?
B. Price
   1. What price should we charge for our products?
   2. As production costs decline, should we lower process or try to develop higher quality products?
C. Place
   1. Where, and by whom, should or products be sold?
   2. What kinds of incentives should we offer to push our products?
D. Promotion
   1. How much should we spend on promotion? How should it be allocated and to geographic areas?
   2. What combination of media, radio, television magazines, and the Internet should we use?

III. Control

A. What is our market share overall? In each geographic area? By each customer type?
B. Are customers satisfied with our products? How is our record for service? Are there many returns?
C. How does the public perceive our company? What is our reputation with the trade?

obtaining funds to pursue expansions, equipment, or other operational modifications but is, generally, pursued for any of the following reasons:

■ The plan is required as part of the yearly budget planning process.
■ The plan is required for a specialized strategy to introduce new products, enter new markets, generate a new strategy to fix an existing problem, and other issues.
■ The plan is a component within an overall business plan, such as a new business proposal to the financial community (see Chapter 2).

Marketing research is usually conducted for three distinct purposes, planning, problem solving and control. Planning is the key to successful marketing programs and marketing research must be conducted to know how to wisely direct marketing funds. Market research is also used for problem solving when reviewing issues of product, price, place and promotional (McCarthy, 1960). Control-oriented marketing research assists the practice manager in the isolation of trouble spots within the practice and promotes knowledge of how the clinic is performing. In Sidebar 5–1, Churchill and Brown (2004) outline these three general categories of marketing research into questions used in successful businesses. Although some of the questions are more applicable to general business, many of these market research questions can be directly or indirectly applied to an audiology practice. The application of Churchill and Brown's marketing research outline to audiology practice greatly organizes and simplifies the marketing process.

Generating the answers to the questions is a great place to start in the marketing of a practice. In the planning phase, the answers to the questions vary substantially from one service or product to another. For example, the demand may be constant for hearing evaluations, but rise and fall for hearing aids, or vestibular evaluations. There may be one overall marketing plan for the practice, another for specific products, and still another for specific services.

The answers to these planning questions also develop an understanding of the market in which the practice operates. In the business world, the answers to these questions are obtained through the use of a *target market segmentation*. Traynor (2006) describes the target market segmentation as the identification and profiling of consumers into categories or different components of the market. The target market segmentation answers the questions generated by Churchill and Brown's outline, but can be very simple or quite complex. To conduct a target market segmentation, market segments are divided into major areas such as:

■ Geographic
■ Demographic
■ Psychographic
■ Behavioral.

These general categories of the market can then be further delineated to identify a specific population or segment of individuals that are the most likely candidates for the market offering or the product. The geographic category can be reduced from a large area such as a state to a region, a city, a neighborhood, or even segmented for seasonal offerings to offset the rise and fall of product or service demands.

Demographics are a large category often utilized to target the product or service offering into categories of individuals. These categories identify specific groups or segments of the market by age, income, race, family size, occupation, generation, family life cycle, education, nationality religion, gender, social class, and others. For example, the demographic target market for an audiology practice that offers hearing aids is usually individuals above age 55, mid to upper incomes, any race, one or two in the family, retired or employed person, any occupation, without children at home, of any education level, nationality, religion, or gender from any social class.

Psychographic segmentation usually refers to lifestyle or personality. For example, all of those individuals at an assisted living center or that have a particular personal style might be singled out for a specific marketing campaign.

Behaviorally, segments can be made from occasions or events, such as birthdays or anniversaries; from a status, such as warranty expiration; or battery use. One very useful segment in audiology practices can be the readiness stage, such as when the patient reaches a certain hearing loss level that begins to affect their interactions with family members, or when their attitude toward the product changes. Although accessing a consumer in this stage can be difficult, patients that have been seen a year or so before can be targeted for access when they may be more psychologically ready for treatment. It is helpful to have segmentation for those patients that have been "tested not sold."

The real benefit of target marketing is when these general segments are further delineated and utilized together as multiattribute segmentation in the presentation of the marketing material. These multiattribute segmentations create a population composed of individuals that have a need and want for your products or services. Generally, the better the seg-

mentation, the better the response to the market offering. Although it is necessary to find a portion of the segmentation that requires audiology goods and services, a common mistake is to identify too broad of a market. Thus, it is essential to be accurate in your target market segmentation as segmenting too broadly will minimize the efficiency of the marketing program while increasing the costs and too small of a market will reduce the number of individuals presented with the market offering.

The problem-solving portion of the outline in Sidebar 5–1 focuses on the short- and long-term decisions that must be made with respect to the marketing mix. The *marketing mix* is the specific combination of how the basic marketing elements are used to present the practice. Often called the *Four Ps* of marketing (McCarthy, 1960), product, price, place and promotion are put together to make up the overall marketing plan for the practice. The marketing mix concept is presented in Figure 5–3. Since the purpose of marketing is the creation of value for patients where value is the difference between perceptions of the benefits received from the using the products and services, and the costs incurred.

Patients are usually willing and able to make exchanges of value (usually money) when: (1) the benefits of the exchange exceed their perception of the cost and (2) the products and services offer a superior value compared with the alternatives. Kotler and Armstrong (2012) amplify this purpose in a discussion of customer wants, needs and demands. They feel the most basic concept in marketing is that of human needs. Human needs are states of felt depravation. These states include basic physical needs for food, clothing, warmth, safety, and hearing. Most audiologists realize

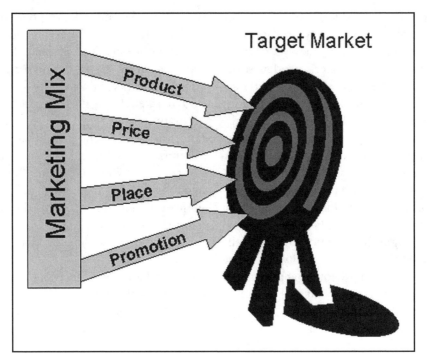

Figure 5–3. Marketing mix.

that good hearing brings social needs for belonging and affection and provides for individual needs such as communication. Wants are the form of human needs that take shape as they are shaped by the culture and individual personality. Patients *need* hearing aids, but *want* to go on a cruise, or to obtain a new car. According to Kotler and Armstrong (2012), wants shaped by one's society and are describes in terms of objects that will satisfy those needs. They feel that when these needs are backed by buying power, *wants* become *demands*. Given their wants and resources, people demand products with benefits that add up to the most value and satisfaction.

Churchill and Brown (2004) indicate that marketing managers, in their attempts to create customer value, generally focus their efforts on the Four Ps, namely the product or service, its price, its placement or channel in which it is distributed, and its promotion. These Four Ps are closely related to the four customer or patient-related variables that Lauterhorn (1990) has called the *Four Cs*. The Four Cs look at the marketing mix from the patient benefit point of view and suggests that products are the *customer solution*, price is the *customer cost*, place or channel is the *customer convenience*, and promotion is the *customer communication*. Thus, the Four Ps should be considered in light of the Four Cs to provide perspective to the marketing process. The questions in the second portion of the Churchill and Brown outline deal with how to market the practice, given the specific mixture of product, price, place, and promotion. A further expansion of the Four Ps of marketing are the Six Ps offered by St. Clergy in Chapter 6.

Product

Product Tangibility

Murphy and Ennis (1986) describe three classic characteristics of products that must be understood for effective marketing. These include durability, tangibility, and consumer use. Durability and tangibility include both nondurable and durable goods.

In an audiology practice, batteries are an example of a nondurable in that they are purchased and used for a period of time when another battery is required to power the hearing aid again. The marketing strategy for nondurable goods is to usually make the item available in many locations and charge only a minimal markup, with some advertising and/or demonstrations to build brand loyalty and preference (see Chapter 7). An example of a durable good is the hearing aid itself since it is, one hopes, used each day for several years. Durable goods are tangible products that require more personal selling and service. Since there is greater involvement in time and attention, durable goods require a higher margin to offset the audiologist's education, research and development, and the necessary warranties. Services, however, are intangible, inseparable, variable, and perishable products and as such require more quality control, supplier credibility, and adaptability. Thus, audiologic services are highly influenced by the provider, their credentials and how well they can adapt to the variables of the evaluation and offer other necessary services.

Product Mix

Most audiology practices sell basically the same mix of products and services. They offer hearing instruments, nondurable goods in support of the hearing instruments, rehabilitative treatment as well as a mix of other services including diagnostic hearing and balance assessment. Some practices offer additional items to the mix such as cerumen management, intraoperative monitoring and various levels of hearing conservation programming. When the patient looks to find a solution to a problem, it is the product mix, both goods and services, tangible and intangible; offered by the practice that meets their want or need.

In a business sense, Berry and Wilson (2001) describe a product offering as something that offers benefits or satisfaction to the target group. Although product mix is part of the practice's image, Kotler (2001) and Kotler and Armstrong (2012) offer that there are specific factors about certain products that cause them to be chosen. The following are some characteristics that can be a part of choosing the products for the product mix:

■ Product variety
■ Quality
■ Design
■ Features
■ Technology
■ Brand name
■ Packaging
■ Sizes
■ Services
■ Warranties
■ Return policy.

A hearing instrument manufacturer must have the correct technology mix in their product line to make them appealing to an audiology practice (see Chapter 17). Certain brand names have a reputation for quality and functionality. Above and beyond a manufacturer's respective technological offerings are peripheral factors such as packaging, utility of the fitting software, warranty, access to inside support personnel, low repair rates, quick repair turnaround time, and well-informed field representatives are a few important components that add to (or detract from) a product's attractiveness to practitioners.

Ethics notwithstanding, product manufacturers, especially hearing instrument companies, are very willing to give audiology practitioners marketing assistance in both advertising and public relations. Many hearing instrument manufacturers offer funds to assist in marketing costs incurred for a campaign that features their products. Although these campaigns are effective and usually available for simply the use of the manufacturer's product during the marketing effort, these product marketing efforts should be accompanied by offers that present the specific practice's brand of audiologic expertise. Many Audiologists use the same brands of hearing instruments so it is best to market your brand of audiology rather than the manufacturer's brand of product that the patient can obtain from many different sources. Of course, these various benefits of loyalty to a manufacturer are subject to the ethical implications (see Chapter 4).

From the patient point of view, the want or need for hearing can be met by the simple acquisition of a hearing instrument but not necessarily from your practice. If they perceive that they do not need the value added by audiology expertise, then they will simply attempt to acquire the hearing instrument at the lowest possible price. Hearing instruments and some related products are in the process of becoming commodity products (see Chapter 1). Commodity products are those products that are perceived as the same by patients no matter where they are purchased. Since they are the same, then consum-

ers tend to purchase them at the lowest available price, no matter the location. Until recently, hearing instruments have only been generally available through audiologists and commercial hearing aid dealers. Many patients, especially those seeking these products for the first time, do not understand the differences among instruments or the services that are required to dispense them properly. This lack of understanding the complexity of hearing instruments, fitting techniques, and rehabilitative intervention, causes consumers consider mail order, the Internet, and discount stores as realistic options (see Chapter 7).

Kochkin (2009) indicated that about 7.4% of hearing instrument sales are completed on the Internet and through discount stores. Although patients consider traditional delivery systems, they seriously consider saving funds by going to the discount store, or an Internet purchase. The products look the same, sound the same, but usually do not have services included with them or the included services are generally inferior to those offered by a private practice audiologist. In markets where discount stores or the Internet are major concerns, market messages should be about audiologic services and follow-up. Patients may not immediately appreciate the value added benefit offered by the audiologist to their use of the device. Practitioners are uniquely qualified by their academic and practical training to provide both the necessary diagnostic studies as well as developing a beneficial rehabilitative treatment plan.

It is the position of the American Academy of Audiology that every person seeking treatment of hearing disorders through the use of amplification devices receive a comprehensive audiological evaluation prior to purchasing a hearing instrument . . . The comprehensive audiological evaluation must be performed by an audiologist who is licensed or registered in the state wherein the evaluation is completed. The diagnostic evaluation is not conducted for the purposes of selecting or fitting a hearing aid, but to rather assess the functional status of the auditory system, and to assure that amplification or other assistive listening devices are an appropriate treatment strategy. (American Academy of Audiology [AAA], 2012)

The focus on a specific product for a marketing campaign is usually not a good idea since patients will review their alternatives to acquire the same product a lower price. It is far better to focus on the branding of the practice so that consumers come to expect a specific brand of hearing care rather than to spend valuable marketing funds branding the manufacturer's product. Since it is the benefits of the product *and* the added value of the audiologist that the patient purchases, the marketing program should focus not only on product features, but also the expertise required to fit and maintain the device to achieve full benefit from these product features.

Price

Nagel, Hogan, and Zale (2011) indicate that setting correct pricing for products and services is a great challenge. It could be that pricing is one of the biggest keys to success as it has such an affect of profit. If the price is high, the number of sales are usually lower but with higher profit, while if the price is low, the number of sales are high with minimal profit. Traynor (2006) presents that from a business standpoint; the goal is to price the product mix where the most products

are sold for the highest price possible without discouraging the consumer as to its cost. Although this seems a simple process, the development of this delicate balance between practice profit and the patient's willingness to pay is difficult affecting profitability of the practice.

Once the product has been chosen then it is simply how much the patient is willing to give up for the product or their willingness to pay. Nagel et al. (2011) suggest that pricing is a game because success depends not only on a practice's own pricing decisions but also on how patients and competition react to them. They further present that pricing decisions should always be made as part of a longer term marketing strategy to generate and capture more profit contribution. Otherwise, it is possible to win many individual battles for market share and still end up losing the war for profitability. For a comprehensive review of pricing fundamentals and procedures as they directly apply to the audiology practice the reader should review Chapter 7.

Once the manager has followed the steps in the calculated the product prices, the components of the "pricing mix" can then be established. These would include:

- List Price—full retail price as determined by a particular method.
- Discounts—a discount from the full retail price.
- Allowances—cash allowances on the trade-in of valuable products.
- Payment Period—period of time allowed for the consumer to pay for the product taking into account the amount put down at the time of order and how much deposit is lost if the product is returned.
- Credit Terms—terms for financing of goods and services by internal and external financing programs.

Place

Place is where the services are offered, the atmosphere, and the image in which the product mix is provided. In any business, a product is anything that can be offered to a market to satisfy a want or a need but the product not only includes the physical goods, but also the services, experiences, events, places, properties, organizations, information, and ideas.

Indeed, part of the product that is presented to the market is the practice's image. From the first phone call until referral or dismissal of the patient the whole experience is part of the product branding of the practice. The more centrally located the clinic is in the community, the easier it is for patients to find and sets up a relaxed situation for them as they arrive. Parking should be easy with a number of handicap spaces provided, as well as wheelchair and walker accessibility, or if possible, even a handicap door allowing easy, convenient accessibility for those with disabilities. Although it is helpful to have a number of convenient locations, the viability of multiple locations must be weighed with the expansion costs incurred from a business standpoint.

The practice should offer a clinical, but not stuffy atmosphere, so as to allow for relaxation and comfort, reinforcing that they have come to the right place for hearing care.

Generally, the clinic should have a neat, uncluttered waiting room with a tasteful décor considering all details, even the smell of the area (Marsh, 2012). The front office staff begins setting the brand image on the phone by their demeanor while scheduling the appointment. Greetings upon arrival must be courteous, interactive, and sympathetic to the patient's hearing impairment. The audiologist should dress to see patients by wearing a clean lab coat that presents a professional image. Simply dressing for image is a good start toward branding the product image that will coexist with the clinicians, personality and the quality of services offered by the practice. In the past, even many doctoral level audiologists did not use lab coats. These were the days before the profession was a doctoral level profession and this attire was considered an unnecessary by some professionals. The profession has totally changed in that more audiologists are in private practice, working for themselves, branding their practice at the doctoral level. Thus, the use of a lab coat promotes the image of a doctor offering services in a professional environment and presents the professional as an individual with credentials to ethically recommend further testing or rehabilitative products that will be of benefit to them.

Image is so important to success in practice that McCall and Dunlop (2004) suggest that it is a good idea to check the brand that is being presented to the community. Clinicians need to check their brand by calling the office using the main number and try to make an appointment, checking on the elements of the experience:

- How were they greeted?
- Was it easy to make an appointment?
- How long did they have to wait for an appointment?
- Were they put on hold?
- Were they advised of what to bring for the first appointment?
- Were they made to feel important?

They also suggest that every so often the professional should park where the patients park.

- Is the signage easy to read?
- Is the entrance to the practice clearly designated?
- Is the parking lot clean?

Professionals should also walk into the practice through the front door and see the practice's first impression from the patient's eyes.

- Is the entrance easily marked?
- Is the entrance inviting?
- Is the waiting room pleasant and comfortable?

McCall and Dunlop also suggest that it is a good idea to check the brand presented to consumers by asking the patients a few good questions. First, they will appreciate being asked and it will convey to them that these details are of concern and that their satisfaction is important.

- How were they treated when they called in for an appointment?
- Did they visit the clinic Web site or the Facebook page? Was it helpful? If not what can be done to make it better?

Product brands are built by "doing the homework" necessary to make a particular brand of audiology or stand out from the other brands already offered in the community. Once your brand is known as the most competent, professional, relaxed and convenient clinic most of the marketing is already done and the goods and services almost sell themselves.

Promotion

Audiologists must communicate with the market to take advantage of the ever-changing market conditions that may be beneficial to the presentation of products or services. There are three specific types of consumers that require promotional intervention:

- Referrals from medical colleagues
- Existing patients in database
- Patients recruited from the general public.

The first consumers that need attention are those that are referred by medical colleagues. The best source of patient referral for general diagnostic and rehabilitative audiology services is from family practice, internal medicine, and occupational medicine. While general surgeons are a good source of referral for operative monitoring, otolaryngologists usually have their own service providers and often dispense hearing instruments. Kochkin (2004) states that the greatest influence on a patient is their family physician and, if hearing instruments are recommended, patients, are *five times* more likely to purchase amplification than if directed to the clinic by someone else. Since marketing to referral sources requires these medical colleagues to entrust *their* patients to you, this is a special relationship requiring a different interactive marketing approach, presented in detail in Chapter 13. Once the referral is made it is responsibility of the audiology clinic to support the referral source and deliver the expected brand of audiology services or products presented to them. Second, are existing patients included in the clinic database. An established practice will benefit from the consumers knowledge of their brand of audiology and often minimal marketing to existing patients nets a rather large return. This is done by generating special promotions through a newsletter, Web site or other communication. In established practices, ensuring the existing database is satisfied is extremely important as 60% or more of new hearing instrument sales are to the existing database.

The third and most expensive source of patients is from the general public. St. Clergy (2012) estimates that it costs $250 to $300 to bring a new patient into the practice using market communications and it costs about $50 to keep a good patient in the clinic. Since the lifetime value of each patient is about $30,000 it makes some sense consider some of these expensive marketing options but smart clinicians use experience, market knowledge and restraint to control costs. Market communications to patients are called a *market offering* which can be in the form of advertising in newspapers, radio, television, direct mail ads, newsletters, on line ads, Facebook, pay per click or other communication media (see Chapter 6). Since these media require the purchase of space, time and other expensive commodities market offerings to the general public can use large amounts of marketing funds. Any of these specific advertising mediums may be used in isolation, but the best result is usually achieved by an organized marketing effort that incorporates a number of these modalities simultaneously. Coordinated market offerings allow multiple exposures that gain maximum interaction with the audience by stimulating a number of senses. In addition to advertising to the general population, a marketing program should also include a coordinated public relations or awareness campaign, conducting presentations to service groups as well as interaction with physician's offices. The demonstration of products, services, and profes-

sional expertise to these groups can be a great (and inexpensive) source of new patients either from the audiences themselves or their family and friends.

General Considerations in Promotional Activities

Promotions can be easily over or under used in marketing the practice. A practice with no promotions will have a difficult time competitive markets. No matter what specific promotional method is incorporated it is better to begin the discussion with some evidence based themes woven into promotions that ensure success. Staab (1992) offers some classic tips that ensure success with promotional programs:

- Try to add value, rather than discounting products
- Put the practice's imprint on promotions; to make them exclusive and identifiable to the specific office.
- Focus on the future; look for repeat business, not just new business.
- Give promotions a theme to help reinforce other promotional efforts.
- Target promotions as specifically as possible to obtain measureable results.
- Attempt to find methods to reward the best patients as they are life blood of your business.
- If the promotion does well, look for cross-promotional opportunities.
- Find ways to make the patient feel good about choosing this particular clinic.
- Promotions should be presented in a quality manner within an affordability range.
- If you have sales staff involved, the promotion should be exciting and

rewarding for them to participate, or it will not perform as well.

- Make promotions fun and easy to execute.
- Keep testing different promotions, even if specific promotions are working well.
- Design the promotion asking the question, "What do hearing impaired patients want us to do for them" or rephrased, the patient should be able to ask, "What's in it for me?"

Many general areas can be included in direct marketing efforts differentiate the practice. These marketing efforts can achieve results by diversifying the message or offering into a number of specific areas such as goods, services, experiences, events, persons, places, organizations, information, ideas, or technology. Kotler and Armstrong (2012) leads practitioners to believe that all of these areas can be considered and varied in their marketing programs:

- *Marketing Through the Goods.* These are products such as hearing aids, batteries, accessories and other physical products for sale in the clinic. The selling of goods can use manufacturer produced or practice generated ads and discuss technology, product changes, and/or product features but should emphasize their benefits to the patient.
- *Marketing Through the Services.* Depending on the audience for the marketing campaign, evaluations and other services offered in the clinic can be presented as an alternative to the traditional testing services. Highlighting other services besides audiometric evaluations such as ABRs, OAEs, balance testing,

programming of hearing aids, aural rehabilitation classes, and cerumen removal, presents the practice as a facility that can help the whole patient. Consumers often view the offering of these other services as an indication of a "patient-oriented" facility and may not only seek services at this clinic, but may also be inclined to refer others.

- *Marketing Through the Experiences.* Although audiologists are aware of how new products can change the quality of life for the hearing impaired individual, the patient is most likely unaware of the broad range of benefits that they will receive from items such as, new technology amplification, a special telephone, or from just reprogramming their current hearing aids. Offering services "beyond the basics" in the form of focus groups and aural rehabilitation classes can also set a practice apart from the competition. These unique offerings are, in fact, a form of informal marketing as it encourages the sharing of experiences among patients with similar problems. Good first-hand experiences are probably the best form of advertising and testimonials are a good inexpensive source of advertising not only for new hearing aid fittings, but also for refits, reprogramming, and audiologic services.
- *Marketing Through Events.* Sponsoring or offering screening services at special events, such as health fairs, will foster awareness of hearing loss and treatment and thus draw people into the practice. Additionally, offering community lectures on hearing impairment to service groups, such as the Lions

Club, Rotary, or Sertoma, is a good marketing tool for visibility. Other events, such as "open houses" must be conducted at strategic times and coordinated with multimodality advertising to insure success.

- *Marketing Through People.* This can be the marketing of a special individual, the practice owner/ audiologist, or other expert, such as a manufacturer's representative as a spokesperson for the practice. Events that market a specific individual are usually more successful when combined with a special market offering with a timed response.
- *Marketing the Place of Service.* The promotion of a specific location, such as rural, conveniently located, accessible by public transportation, plenty of available parking, or other relevant aspects pertaining to the locale of the practice can be a special marketing edge.
- *Marketing Through Organizations.* It is possible to gain recognition by building a strong, favorable image relative to organizations such as senior centers, church groups, or other local groups for the elderly, or hearing impaired.
- *Marketing with Information.* Information, such as explanations about hearing loss, hearing instruments, assistive devices, middle ear disease, and so forth, can be disseminated in brochures made available in displays in the office or through direct mailings.
- *Marketing the Benefits.* Patients really do not care much about the features of a product; they are interested in the benefits that the features create for them. Benefits that are often utilized liberally relative to hearing aids are that they help with

speech understanding, reduction of background noise, elimination of feedback, and comfort among others. Although these "catch phrases" are substantially overused, it is necessary to present the same ads as the competition occasionally so that the practice is seen as offering the same benefits as others are in the surrounding area.

There are many marketing firms that advertise in professional journals to develop specialized mailing lists for practices. Often, these marketers are very knowledgeable but just as often they may know less about the appropriate market segment than the practitioner. Many Internet sites offer assistance in designing multiattribute market segmentations allowing the practitioner to design a direct mail list targeted for their specific market at about one-third the cost of a list generated by professional marketing services.

McCall and Dunlop (2004) present a 1-year marketing map in Sidebar 5–2 that can be used for a small practice in conjunction with the Churchill and Brown (2004) outline. These are simply suggestions and may vary from one practice and community to another.

Detailed Marketing Research and Marketing Plans

Berry and Wilson (2001) present information about the development of detailed marketing plans. They indicate that a marketing plan must fit a need and a particular situation, yet recognize there are common elements to most marketing situations. While the rudimentary

---

Sidebar 5–2
1-YEAR MARKETING MAP

Month 1. Develop a two-page marketing to-do list for the year.

Month 2. Improve practice signage (inside and out).

Month 3. Enhance the Web site; add patient education links and directions to the practice.

Month 4. Hold customer service training for staff on how to be a brand ambassador.

Month 5. Hold a patient education event.

Month 6. Contact local reporters; offer the audiologist as a source for hearing health care stories.

Month 7. Send out direct mail piece to potential patients in market area.

Month 8. Improve waiting room décor, install a computer for patient use.

Month 9. Participate in local health fair or other "show."

Month 10. Contact local civic organizations or speaking opportunities.

Month 11. Sponsor a community event, preferably health-related event.

Month 12. Place an ad in a newcomer publication.

---

marketing plan offered by Churchill and Brown (2004), presented in Sidebar 5–1, may likely suffice in the first early years of practice, a more detailed marketing plan will be necessary as the practice grows or if the practice is expanded. The plan will be required to supplement the business plan when seeking loan funding from your banking partner for that new office, new equipment. or the hiring of that new employee.

Detailed marketing plans are often a component of a good business plan and sometimes stand alone in established practices. These plans are best conducted with either a market planning Web site, such as Live Plan (2012) at http://www.liveplan com, which does both business planning and market planning computer software, or Sales and Marketing Pro offered by Palo Alto Software (2012). Among others on the Internet, another site that offers a free online six-part marketing plan instruction using video tutorials is http://www.knowthis.com/marketplan ning (Know This, 2012). Since these programs and Web sites are readily available and relatively inexpensive, usually about $100, they are an inexpensive method of organizing and presenting your detailed plans for marketing the practice. These software programs and online sites "walk" the first time marketing planner or the seasoned veteran through the step by step market planning process. Figure 5–4 presents examples of the calculations and figures created by the software in these marketing software packages.

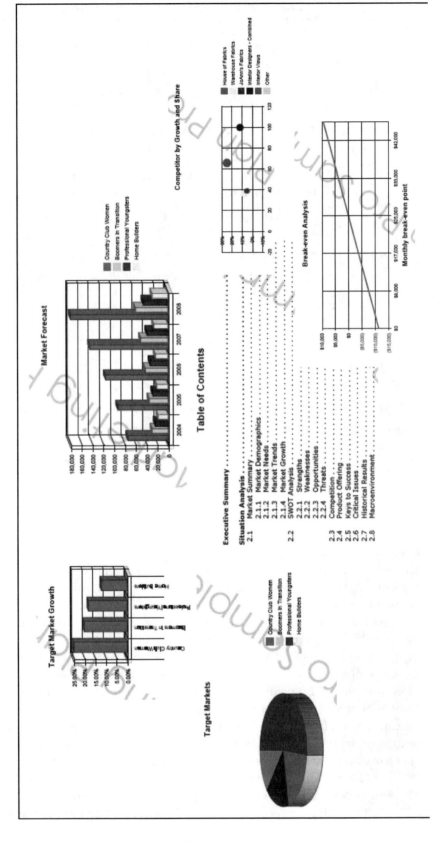

Market Forecast

Country Club Women
Boomers in Transition
Professional Youngsters
Home Builders

Competitor by Growth and Share

House of Fabrics
Warehouse Fabrics
JoAnn's Fabrics
Interior Designers - Combined
Interior Views
Other

Break-even Analysis

Monthly break-even point

Table of Contents

Executive Summary . . . .

Situation Analysis . . . .
2.1   Market Summary . . . .
       2.1.1   Market Demographics . . . .
       2.1.2   Market Needs . . . .
       2.1.3   Market Trends . . . .
       2.1.4   Market Growth . . . .
2.2   SWOT Analysis . . . .
       2.2.1   Strengths . . . .
       2.2.2   Weaknesses . . . .
       2.2.3   Opportunities . . . .
       2.2.4   Threats . . . .
2.3   Competition . . . .
2.4   Product Offering . . . .
2.5   Keys to Success . . . .
2.6   Critical Issues . . . .
2.7   Historical Results . . . .
2.8   Macroenvironment. . . . .

Target Market Growth

Country Club Women
Boomers in Transition
Professional Youngsters
Home Builders

Target Markets

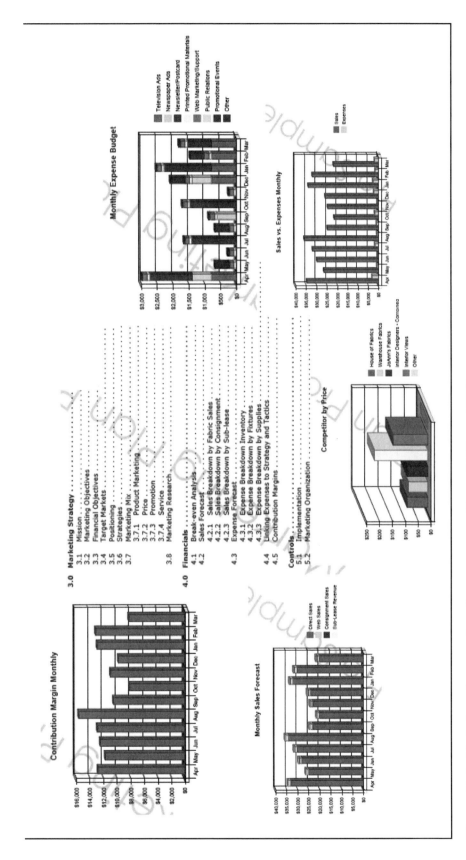

Figure 5–4. Marketing plan sample software program (Berry & Wilson, 2006).

141

These programs can greatly assist the practitioner in analysis of the market, developing a marketing strategy, setting the financials and organizing the controls of the marketing program (Palo Alto Software, 2012). For minimal costs the audiology practitioner with virtually no marketing experience can have years of "user-friendly" marketing expertise.

Organization of the Plan

Most marketers agree with Oblinger (2012) that there are four major components to developing a marketing plan:

- Researching and analyzing your business and the market
- Planning and writing the plan
- Implementing the plan
- Evaluating the results.

Research and analysis are critical because they lead you to the identification your product's target audience. Researching and analyzing the market is a detailed analysis of the situation in which the marketing will take place. The situation analysis consists of a market summary or review of demographics, the target market segmentation; and a review of the needs, trends and possible growth of the market for the products and services offered by the practice. Although similar to that presented above in the Churchill and Brown (2004) outline, data for detailed marketing plans are substantially more specific and often reviewed over a 5-year period to understand the historical trends of each analyzed component. Specific charts and graphs should be presented for each of the trends reported within the plan so as to explain and depict the target market segmentation, needs, trends, and market growth.

A review of the market situation is enhanced by a self-analysis. A self-analysis consists of a review of various issues the clinic should consider as the plan. These can be developed by the professional, or obtained on line. Sidebar 5–3 offers a marketing questionnaire prepared by a professional marketing expert in the hearing industry (Marsh, 2012). The use of professional marketing experts familiar with audiology practice can be a good investment in the future of the clinic and spur growth.

SWOT Analysis

A review of the market situation is enhanced by a self-analysis (Oblinger, 2006). In an audiology practice, a serious look at the strengths (S), weaknesses (W), opportunities (O), and threats (T) —SWOT—leads to the identification of the practice's target audience and usually involves both a qualitative and quantitative review. The qualitative component is simply the audiologist's own opinion of the situation, while the quantitative is an actual review of data. A SWOT analysis is a valuable step in the evaluation of the clinic's situation. Assessing a practice's strengths, weaknesses, market opportunities, and threats through a SWOT analysis is a very simple process that can offer powerful insight into the potential and critical issues affecting a venture. The SWOT analysis begins by conducting a general inventory of internal strengths and weaknesses in the practice (Figure 5–5).

Then the external opportunities and threats are considered within the constraints of the overall market environment.

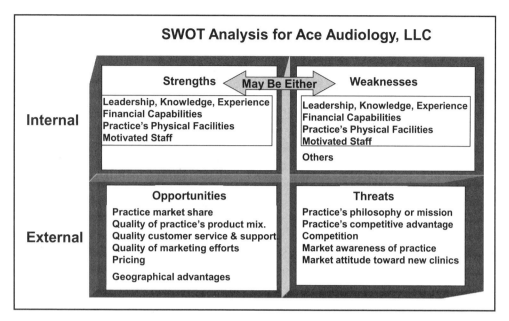

Figure 5–5. SWOT analysis for an audiology practice (adapted from Berry & Wilson, 2001).

Sidebar 5–3
PROFESSIONAL MARKETING ANALYSIS OF THE PRACTICE

These days there are many professional marketers in the hearing industry. Some are affiliated with hearing instrument manufacturers or buying groups, and others offer independent evaluation of practice. These professionals offer great experience and can be of great assistance in facilitating a deep review of the practice's marketing plans and offer suggestions that will insure growth and stability to the clinic. One independent marketer, Marsh (2012), offered the following questionnaire to practice owners so as to obtain an understanding of their operation and insure enough knowledge to present reliable suggestions. The results of these questionnaires are kept confidential by the marketer.

Marketing Questionnaire

1. How many years have you been in business; how many offices and staff do you have?
2. Tell me about the ethnic/economic makeup(s) of your market(s).

3. How are you positioned (i.e., technology, service) in your marketplace?

4. Tell me about your competition; what sets you apart?

5. What is the % mix of high/low end products; 1st time/repeat patients?

6. How large is your active database; how and how often do you communicate with them?

7. What types of marketing (i.e., newspaper, direct mail) have you used?

8. Which have been the most successful, which have been the least successful?

9. Can you provide some of your and your competitors' marketing materials?

10. What is your Web site address; are you also using any social media?

11. What would you want a new marketing program to accomplish?

12. Please provide any other information that also would be helpful to know.

Database Questionnaire

1. Approximately how many names of active patients do you maintain in your database?

2. How many "tested-but-not-solds" or other prospects do you also have?

3. What types of mailings have you conducted to these names; how often?

4. With a "Yes" or "No" answer, can you extract the following information?
   Date of Most Recent Purchase
   Cost of Most Recent Purchase
   All Purchase Histories, including:
   Extended Warranties/
   Batteries/Other After-Market Items
   Median Age of Database Names
   Male/Female Mix of Database Names
   Hearing Loss Profile
   Patient Referral History
      Personal Information:
      Marital/Family Status
      Memberships, Hobbies
      Personal Histories

5. Do you enter Patient Referral history into your database records?

6. Please provide any other information that also would be helpful to know.

As the SWOT analysis begins, it is best to not elaborate on the topics so bullet points are used to capture the major relevant factors in each of the four areas. The primary purpose of the SWOT analysis is to identify and assign each significant factor, positive and negative, to one of the four categories, allowing you to take an objective look at your business. The SWOT analysis will be a useful tool in developing and confirming goals and setting the marketing strategy. Marketers suggest that as the detailed SWOT begins, review the opportunities and threats first, and then move on to the strengths and weaknesses (Berry, 2012).

SWOT: Threat Assessment

While conducting the SWOT analysis, Oblinger (2006) suggests some general areas of investigation that can direct the assessment of threats facing the practice. When reviewing the threats at least the following should be considered:

- Practice's philosophy or mission?
- The practice product (both goods and services) features, benefits or quality?
- The competitive advantage of the practice? (Is there a competitive advantage?)
- How the services are conducted, patient and referral source satisfaction.
- Practice pricing structures? Are the goods and services of this practice priced much higher or lower than the competition?
- Target market's awareness of your practice and its services?
- Target market's attitudes toward audiology, hearing aids, and new referral sources?

- Target market's brand loyalty to your practice?
- Competition's activities? (New product launches, price changes, new companies, etc.)

Reviewing these areas offer the audiology practice manager a good start in the review of the practice, its place in the market, and the possible threats to be encountered.

SWOT: Opportunities Assessment

The analysis of opportunities includes a review of problem solving, product use cycles, creative methods of providing services, or ideal scenarios. Since opportunities are external to the practice analysis. A review of the practice's opportunities should center on market oriented factors such as:

- Practice market share
- Practice's ability to meet the needs and trends of the market.
- Value the practice brings to the target market.
- Quality of the practice's product.
- Quality of the practice's customer service and support.
- Quality/effectiveness of past promotions and other marketing efforts
- Pricing in the practice compared to others for the value obtained.
- The practice's geographic service advantages

Both the threats and opportunities should utilize as much data as possible since they are external factors to the practice. These are concerns that may or may not arise, but they can be a major problem if not considered as part of the analysis.

SWOT: Strengths and Weaknesses Assessment

Strengths and weaknesses are internal factors and important to determine how (or if) the practice can manage the opportunities and threats. Strengths can be anything that will increase market share or financial performance while weaknesses are internal problems that can reduce the market share or the financials. Strengths and weaknesses are more of an internal qualitative analysis, but consist of issues which the practitioner is more familiar. Especially in marketing, closeness to the issues sometimes clouds judgment. Often, the practitioner is too close to the issues and has difficulty seeing some of the marketing issues. Caution must be exercised that this closeness to the issues does impact upon the analysis and presents a clear picture of the strengths and weaknesses. Analysis of these internal factors is essential and should center on:

- The practice's operational leadership, how the practice effectively operates in the community.
- The financial strength of the practice to combat the threats and take advantage of the opportunities observed.
- Practices physical capabilities, large enough facility, equipment, etc.
- Responsiveness of workforce in the practice, enough people, motivated, and so forth.

SWOT planning is conducted to gain knowledge of the competitive environment and to facilitate a plan of attack for going after the competition's business as well as the new business that might go either way. How is the competition different from the practice to be marketed? What is offered by the practice that is not available in the competitive clinic? What does the competition do better or worse than your practice?

The Competitive Analysis

When reviewing the practice and its ability to stand up against the competition, Harrison and St. John (2004) indicate that there are four distinct areas that can lead to competitive advantage (Figure 5–6).

1. *Financial Resources.* This includes areas such as excellent cash flow, a strong balance sheet, and superior past performance.
2. *Physical Resources.* These would include the physical premises of the practice, the atmosphere, location, parking, equipment, and other physical parameters of the practice.
3. *Human Resources.* Human resources include management capability, well-trained and motivated staff, and doctoral-level professionals with certification to ensure the best possible experience for patients.
4. *Organizational Resources.* The organization that has been around for a time will have a reputation or a well known "brand" that has been presented to the community in the past. The clinic might be known for its competence, products, excellent customer service, flexibility, and other specifics of operation that cause them to stand out.

Other components of the situation analysis involve developing some specific keys to success while reviewing critical issues that must be considered, analyzed and surmounted. Additionally, situation

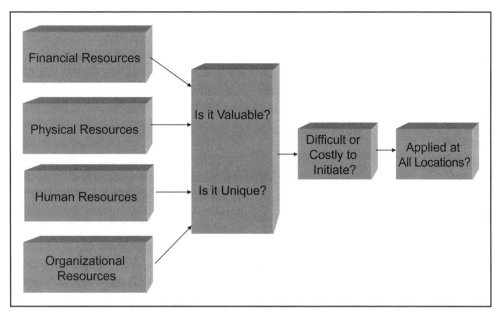

Figure 5–6. Competitive advantage considerations (adapted from Harrison & St. John, 2004).

analysis involves the specific media channels in which these issues will be addressed as well as macro environment or economic conditions of the area in which the practice resides. Foster's Five Forces is another method of assessment of the situation that can be used to assess the competition (see Chapter 1).

Developing a Marketing Strategy

Marketing is most successful when priorities are established and focus is sharpened toward specific targets. If there are too many priorities, the marketing objectives and the branding of the practice will never be accomplished. The limited resources of an audiology practice make it necessary to maximize the profit generated by the marketing effort. An example

of this focus is defining a demographic of interest then identifying a specific audiometric configuration, degree or type of loss for a specific hearing instrument with new technology is focusing the marketing effort for maximum attention. No matter what the media, when a message goes to those that are most ready to hear it, the results are much greater. In the development of a focused marketing strategy, it is essential that audiologists understand the difference between features and benefits. Kotler (2001), Krarup (2001), and virtually every other marketing reference indicate that consumers purchase benefits, not product features. For example, a hearing evaluation is not simply an assessment of hearing; the patient is purchasing information about their hearing difficulties. Patients do not buy the superb signal to noise ratio of directional microphones, they seek the benefit of better hearing capabilities in noisy environments due to the benefits of directional microphones or microphone arrays.

Generally, Oblinger (2006) summarizes the critical components of a marketing plan as:

- Research and analysis are critical because they lead to identifying the target audience, as well as its strengths, weaknesses, threats, and, most importantly, opportunities.
- Knowing the threats and opportunities the practice faces helps to realistically set sales goals and objectives.
- Knowing your opportunities, target audience, and sales goals will present the information required to set marketing goals to take advantage of the opportunities and meet the sales goals.
- Knowing the marketing objectives will net the information necessary to set positioning, pricing, distribution, and other marketing strategies.
- Having marketing strategies set will deliver a road map to set up the tactical elements of your marketing plan, such as advertising, promotions, branding, packaging, and so forth, items that must be tailored to specific markets.
- Once tactical elements are determined, creative elements, budgets, and calendars can be organized.

Probably the most important component of any marketing effort is to track its effectiveness. This is an evidence-based section that requires assessment of the marketing program by defining the important items to be tracked and evaluated. For example, numbers of instruments dispensed in the first 90-day period after implementation of a partic-

ular section of the marketing plan can be tabulated and compared to a similar period prior to instituting the new marketing plan. Another evidence-based example would be to ask each patient at the reception desk if they had heard about the practice before their friend or physician referred them for hearing care. Patients are willing to relate their experiences. If they had read an ad or heard about the practice from another source prior to their referral, they will be forthcoming in their response to your inquiry.

Advertising Options for Audiology Practitioners

Audiologists can choose from a number of methods of advertising that are appropriate to the specific makeup of a particular practice. The following are methods of advertising that have been used in audiology practices.

Advertising Specialty Item

These specialty items are often great awareness reminders for your patients and others. They can be issued after the hearing examination or included in promotional mailings. Specialty items include items such as refrigerator magnets, rolodex cards, coffee cups, and pens or pencils with logos and practice information.

Articles and Columns

Articles in the newspaper and local magazines are important for image, brand awareness of the practice and they provide a forum for your specialized expertise as an audiologist. The practice manager should take every opportunity to place the name of the practice in front of the public at all times. A method of obtaining this type of advertising is to offer routine press releases to the local press or by talking with your newspaper advertising representative and have him or her seek insertion of your article into the main body of the newspaper or in a special advertising section. Audiology practitioners have leverage with the paper if a regular advertiser. Since May is Better Hearing and Speech Month, newspapers are looking for articles about communication disorders and hearing loss in the months of April, May, and June. Other months or weeks are devoted to specific yet related topics. Hearing and cognition are closely intertwined; National Alzheimer's Week would be a good opportunity for an article on the effects of hearing loss in dementia. Christmas time brings noisy toys and an article about noise-induced hearing loss and prevention would be appropriate.

Billboards

Although not for everyone and extremely local, billboards represent an expensive but innovative advertising opportunity for the practice. Billboards are most frequently used in isolation for the awareness of a particular practice. Personalizing the billboard with staff pictured in white coats near equipment will lend to the branding of the practice as a professional and technologically advanced site for hearing and balance care. Strategically placed billboards can be quite expensive but effective when presented

correctly and in addition to other marketing efforts.

Brochures and Circulars

Practice brochures should form the advertising and public relations cornerstone of your practice. Brochures must be well done and printed on high quality, glossy paper. Although these can be done on the practice's computer, professional designers usually maximize the message and imagery to be included in your practice brochure and weave these messages into the marketing mix offered by the practice. Practice brochures should be issued to every new patient coming into your office. They will serve as calling cards and sources of information for potential patients, potential referral sources, and when a reporter calls inquiring about a story. They should be "high end" and displayed in as many referral source offices as possible throughout the practice service area. Many primary care providers will simply hand the brochure to their patients and instruct them to call the office for an appointment. Practice brochures are powerful tools. Health care professionals and other referral sources will judge your practice on what is most immediately available making the practice brochure extremely important to the marketing mix. The practice will be judged as to its quality by the message and images incorporated in in practice brochure.

Web sites

Web sites are an essential component of contemporary audiology practice. As the "baby boomer" generation reaches age 65, visibility on the World Wide Web has become fundamental to success. Although the baby boomers are the new generation of audiology patients, their children Generation X (born 1965 to 1981) and Generation Y sometimes called millennials (born 1982 to 2002) are those that may bring them to the clinic. Reine (2010 compared Internet use among baby boomers to millennials and found that baby boomers use the Internet almost as much as this younger generation. His results showed the following:

- E-mails: Boomers 91% vs. Millennial 94%
- Search Engines: Boomers 88% vs. Millennial 89%
- Health Info: Boomers 78% vs. Millennial 85%
- Get News: Boomers 74% vs. Millennial 83%
- Research Products: Boomers 81% vs. Millennial 83%
- Buy Goods: Boomers 70% vs. Millennial 81%
- Travel Reservations: Boomers 68% vs. Millennial 62%
- Banking: Boomers 55% vs. Millennial 58%
- Auction: Boomers 27% vs. Millennial 26%
- Video Sharing Sites: Boomers 45% vs. Millennial 85%
- Use of Social Network Sites: Boomers 39% vs. Millennial 81%
- Rate Product/Services: Boomers 27% vs. Millennial 38%
- Read Blogs: Boomers 26% vs. Millennial 51%
- Post Comments: Boomers 25% vs. Millennial 33%
- Share Creations: Boomers 23% vs. Millennial 38%
- Have Web sites: Boomers 11% vs. Millennial 18%
- Twitter: Boomers 10% vs. Millennial 29%
- Boomers that write Blogs 8% vs. Millennial 18%.

It is obvious from Reine's research that it is essential to have an online marketing presence if clinics want to attract baby boomers or their children that may bring them to the practice.

Virtual marketing should present an image of the practice, clarify the services and products available, as well as introduce the professional and clerical staff. Professional staff information should include information such as degrees and experience, particular areas of expertise, and items that will "personalize" staff participation in the practice. Clerical staff should also be introduced as they are the first people encountered at the clinic.

The Web site should set forth the menu of clinical services provided, information about hearing instruments, and the hearing aid fitting process from initial hearing examination to instrument fitting, as well as subsequent follow-up visits. Additionally, the messages on the site should be woven into the marketing program with the same messages and visuals that are offered elsewhere, that is, the practice brochure, print media ads, and so forth. The practice Web site should also offer educational information about the ear, hearing loss, its assessment and treatment of balance disorders (if these procedures are part of the practice). Testimonials are also very helpful as they add personal recommendations of the clinic's services and allow the new patient to feel more comfortable as they begin what is hopefully a long and mutually beneficial relationship. If the practice has a referral base from physicians, it might even be beneficial to have a physician page where information of interest to referral sources is relayed efficiently. There is an increasing number of clinic Web sites that offer products on line, such as batteries, RIC tips, and other accessories. These "shopping carts" offer convenience and add to the benefit and utility of the Web site but do add to the cost to set them up.

The Web site also should be easy to remember and provide the viewer with an image of the practice as the site is the practice's distinct location in cyberspace. Since Web site registration has increased at a phenomenal pace, creative Web site addresses using terms "hearing," "care," "aids," "associates," "professional," and the like are less available but new Internet portals are opening with the issuance of newer suffix locations such as ".net" or .biz so may be beneficial to check with various domain providers for an appropriate practice URL.

The site should be custom designed by designers that can capture the "feel" of the practice and make it stand out from the competition. While there are Web site hosting groups, such as Audiology Online, buying groups, and others that provide server hosting and a similar design strategy for everyone and most of these Web sites look very much alike and do not set the practice apart from the competition. Although these sites are less costly and provide an organized place for patients to find audiologists, it is important to stand out in cyberspace and be unique.

Those coming to the Web site address for the first time (unique hits) must be quickly motivated to deepen their search for the information they are seeking or they may be lost forever. Web site designers are experts in arranging the topography of the Web site to maximize unique hits and to keep the patient at the site

long enough to entice with various pages to ultimately schedule an appointment. They will design the site relative to the practice goals and objectives. The site can be informational, educational, or geared to getting new patients in the door for hearing evaluation. The site developers may visit the practice, review practice brochures, and provide recommendations for integration of the messages offered to the market for better use of the eCommerce format. They may even suggest that you put a virtual tour or video on the site to offer some personalization to the experience. They may also suggest that the site offer cleaning tips, counseling, and other procedures in online videos with the practice owner as the star of the show. After a few iterations and modifications, the site will become a space that is unique to your practice.

Until recently Web sites needed to be updated using a computer language called HTML, a special language of the Internet that was difficult to learn and cost extra funds if updates needed to be contracted. Current technology exists for Web sites to be configured in programs such as Wordpress that allow the any authorized person to update the material on the site using a regular word processing format. This keeps the Web site up to date without any extra charges and it can be updated at will as necessary.

Social media is the fastest growing segment of the Internet. Facebook and similar programs are essential to a Web presence and should be included in every practice's marketing program. Although Facebook and other social medial are essential, they are less formal than the practice Web site, a place to demonstrate friendliness, present family, notable developments in the clinic expertise, course attendance by professionals, and other more relaxed interactions with the patients. The clinicians should offer blogging as part of both the Facebook and Web site programs. Offering a weekly blog is a bit like an electronic newsletter, but it also raises the practice level in Google and other browser searches. This allows the practice to come up first or second in a search for "audiology clinics," Greeley, Colorado, or "hearing aids," Dayton, Ohio, and so forth. Twenty years ago, if you were not in the "yellow pages" you were not in business; in 2013, if you are not online, you are not in business. Further discussion of online presence is offered in Chapter 6.

Classified Advertising

Although classified advertising sections are not usually the place that consumers go for audiologic services. They can be used for retrieving a few hearing-impaired consumers for the trial of a specific product, or if the clinic is conducting a true research project. Classifieds may offer an inexpensive option, but is not generally a successful placement of marketing materials to obtain new patients to the practice.

Coupons

Clinics need to be careful when using coupons to reduce the price of hearing instruments or services. Patients may suspect that the original price was set too high so that the promotional coupons could be used, but the prudent use of coupons can be effective. For example, if a goal is to have members of the practice's existing hearing instrument patient

database return for a visit, coupons offering a pack of batteries, hearing instrument cleaning and hearing screening (to assess changes in sensitivity that might need re-evaluation) for a nominal fee will likely produce surprising numbers of returnees. To be optimally effective, coupons should be tied to a reasonable marketing goal and have an expiration date. Possible outcomes from coupon-based promotions presented to the existing database could be increased sales of hearing examinations, hearing instrument repairs, or offer the opportunity to present the need to consider new hearing instruments.

Product Demonstrations

Demonstrations generally work best in a place where prospective patients are already gathered such as trade shows or health fairs. This offers a chance for the patient to see what the device can do for them in a relaxed, social environment. Demonstrations within the practice, as in a trial period of amplification use for a specified time period, are not uncommon and enable the patient and those around him to evaluate the efficacy and communication improvements to be expected with advanced hearing instrument technology. As we see more baby boomers in the clinic these demonstrations are often essential to the sale of hearing devices and they tend to build trust with this generation of patients.

Direct Mail

Direct mail marketing generally has a response rate of 0.5 to 1% of the number mailed directly to a specifically tailored list of segmented recipients. The key to direct mail solicitation is in defining the demographic of the intended group (market segmentation) and the offer that is presented in the piece sent to the list. Although direct mail has worked relatively well with the previous generation of patients, these tactics do not work very well with the baby boomer population as they tend to be skeptical of these mailers offering some "deal" for the day or week. They have seen these before and generally look to these mailings as a "sales operation," interested more in selling product than providing aural rehabilitative treatment.

Internet and Direct Mail Hearing Aid Sales

With the rise of the Internet, direct mail sales of over-the-counter hearing instruments have significantly increased. It is more common today than in any other period in audiologic history to have a patient schedule an appointment for an earmold impression to be sent with their check to a mail order house. While direct mail or Internet sales are highly restricted, illegal in some states, and a topic of some controversy among audiologists; Web sites such as http://www.HearingPlanet.com (now owned by Sonova) and others offer hearing instruments at serious discounts are very much competitors to private practice clinics. Although many of them would like audiologists to become part of their network for the fitting and follow up of products sold to patients, it is up to the audiologist to decide if they choose to accept the minimal reimbursement offered by these

sites. On these mail order sites the wrong product is often obtained for a particular hearing impairment or the lifestyle of the patient and it is difficult to obtain a refund or an upgrade to a higher level product.

Another controversial Internet/direct mail enterprise is now offered by United Health Care (UHC). This semiethical scheme offers patients hearing instruments by mail as a benefit of their insurance program for a nominal cost. Patients send in their audiogram to UHC. UHC then sends the patient a programmed hearing instrument with written instructions on how to use the device(s), not exactly aural rehabilitation. UHC has also established a separate company, Hearing Innovators (HI), to handle these fittings, but offer only nominal reimbursement to audiologists to support these patients. Although it is up to the audiologist and their office manager to decide if they will offer support to these frustrating new models of practice; many clinics have opted to not support this practice. In a private practice clinical situation, working with too many of these high maintenance patients takes time away from full-fee patients that contribute significantly to the cash flow of the practice.

Direct-Response Radio and Television

Unless the audiologist is an invited guest, sponsorship of these shows are effective but very expensive for the usual results. Sponsorship of a Saturday morning hearing health care talk show every other week for five to six months can cost upward of $20,000.00, depending on the broadcast market. If television is the medium, costs are much higher than radio. In many markets, however, talk show hosts are often looking for a professional they can invite to generate interest in their show. These invitations are almost always free and well worth the time, generating good questions from the listeners and great exposure for the clinician and the practice.

Exhibits and Fairs

Exhibitions and fairs are a good source of prospective patients but the selection of the correct, beneficial exhibition or health fair is critical and involves a review of the demographics of the attendees. These fairs are an opportunity to present the professionals and the practice to the public face-to-face and eye-to-eye. Be prepared to offer some sort of demonstration, presentation or give-away to get attention and draw participants to the booth space.

Magazine Advertisements

Local magazines are a good place to present a high end message. It is a good idea to try to get an article in the magazine and place the ad in close proximity to the article. This reinforces the fact that you wrote the article and refers to your brand of audiology to the consumers.

Newsletters

Newsletters are effective tools to communicate with your patients and prospective patients and referral sources. They should contain updates on hearing instrument technology, highlight important regulatory issues, changes in insur-

ance coverage, and provide information about the front office and professional staff. In audiology practice, marketing to existing patients is major source of revenue and the newsletter is one of the most efficient methods of communication. It not only breeds good communication but also substantial word of mouth advertising. Some clinics offer a newsletter occasionally, others monthly, but quarterly newsletters tend to maximize the benefit for the costs involved.

Newspaper Advertisements

Long a staple in practice advertising, the focus of the newspaper ad has centered around two distinct topics; price and time-sensitive deadlines for "call to action," but not all newspaper ads have those goals. Getting the practice branded in the community as a center of excellence, a location where professional services prevail and primary care providers send their patients will also have an impact on newspaper readers. Of course, price shoppers will respond to "special pricing offers" and if those are patients you would like to drive to your particular practice then newspaper ads pushing price is the way to go. If, however, you would like to have patients coming to your office to participate in a continuum of professional, rehabilitative care, your advertising presence in the newspaper will look vastly different than price-based ads. At least initially, it is good to have a marketing consultant assist in the generation of a few good ads that can be placed strategically, no matter your marketing strategy. Marketing consultants vary in their expertise in marketing hearing instruments and to older patients, so choose them carefully. These consultants can be very expensive and sometimes offer little expertise above what is known by the practice owner, the office manager, and the professionals within the clinic.

Personal Letters

Personal letters are appropriate to referral sources, prospective patients and those previously evaluated but who have decided not to act on your recommendations to consider the use of amplification (the so called "tested not sold"). The initial mailing should be accompanied by your practice brochure or specific brochure about hearing instruments or hearing rehabilitation. The letters must be brief, no longer than three short paragraphs. Topics could include, but are not limited to, new products, routine letters for a new evaluation, special offers, moving of the practice, and other timely and appropriate issues.

Radio Advertisements

Radio is an expensive, yet strong medium that can brand your practice in a very short time. It is best used for a short time, usually two weeks to 30 days for a short time. Patients get tired of our ads rather easily and the effectiveness of this expensive medium is short lived. Using clever, humorous, and testimonial spots, the listener can develop an image of your practice and what to expect from a visit. Since consumers spend a lot of time in their cars and offices, the expense is sometimes worth the exposure. In radio, the station will usually assist the clinic orga-

nize a radio marketing program, preparing spots and suggesting communication formats that have worked in the past for other businesses. Testimonials work particularly well in radio advertising where a locally prominent person discusses their experiences in the practice. These testimonials further brand the practice as the place to go for hearing care.

Educational Seminars

No obligation seminars are another form of advertising that can be used effectively. The concern with this type of advertising is that it must be conducted in an environment conducive to presenting the material in a non-obligatory way in a classroom-style arena. These can be organized seminars that are advertised to the public or to a segmented patient base audience, but should be in an upscale venue, a hospital, or other environment that offers an atmosphere of professionalism.

Signage

Sounds simple, but signs are a true form of advertising. Each time the consumer passes the practice, or looks for the practice good signage is necessary. The sign outside the practice is basic communication with a wide expanse of potential consumers. It presents what is practiced at that location and should be professional in the truest sense of the word to reinforce the professional "brand" of service delivery available at that particular location. Signs should be chosen carefully as they are the best example of a "sunk cost" (see Chapter 8).

Telemarketing

Although used in the hearing industry, it is typically incorporated in high pressure sales operations. Telemarketing is the offering of information by paid individuals using a script about products or services via the telephone to special targeted lists of consumers. Berry and Wilson (2001) indicate that more and more people view this as an invasion of their privacy. With increasing public resistance and the advent of "no-call" lists, telemarketing is not a technique that should be considered as a viable marketing alternative.

Television

Much less expensive than in the immediate past, television, especially local cable channels, offer an opportunity to visually engage potential patients. Local channels have become rather affordable in past few years and the station and their producers can assist greatly in the production of the advertising. These programs tend to work best when they are incorporated with other media, such as direct mail and print media as well.

Internet Advertising

Although coming up first in a Google search for hearing care services may not seem important to your practice in your local market, you must recognize that those in your local area seek out information pathways via Google and other search engines in greater numbers that those reading papers, listening to the radio or watching television. Mothers interested in having their child's hear-

ing evaluated or seniors wondering what is available for the communication difficulties they are experiencing will be pleased to see your practice come up on their Google search. See Chapter 6 for more detailed information on Internet and social media advertising.

Yellow Pages

In the past, yellow pages were the primary advertising location for hearing care. If you were not listed, patients would not know that you existed. Although not nearly as necessary as in the past, smaller less display advertising is now the trend as less people consult the yellow pages with the advent of cell phone, and Internet access. One trend that helps the yellow pages ads is the tying of the yellow pages to the Internet with Web pages, phone numbers and other specifics only offered by the various phone companies to keep their Yellow Page customers. In 2012, however, the use of the "phone book" by baby boomers to look for a practice is minimal opting for a Google search to find their providers for many disciplines, including audiology.

Experiential Marketing

This is a new marketing concept that allows the consumer to experience the product before they take it home. For example, in the audiology practice, this would include a room that has a capability to project large images of manufacturer's audio/video presentations that attempt to have the patient involved in the listening experience. These programs are readily available and can be utilized in conjunction with the mounted speakers and amplifiers to create a place where the patient can see if they can hear well, before the ever leave the practice.

Kotler's 4 Steps of Promotional Mix That Communicate Patient Value

Advances in communication technology are causing remarkable changes in the ways that practices and patients communicate. The digital age has spawned a myriad of new information and communication tools, from smart phones and iPods to satellite and cable television systems as well as the Internet, e-mail, social networks, blogs, brand Web sites, and others. Kotler and Armstrong (2012) feel that just as mass marketing once gave rise to a new generation of mass-media communications, the new digital media has given birth to a new marketing communications model, called the "marketing communications mix." The marketing communications mix is a blend of advertising, public relations, personal selling, sales promotion, and direct marketing tools that the practice uses to persuasively communicate patient value and build relationships. Their 4 major promotional tools that should be coordinated and used together are defined as follows:

- *Advertising.* Any paid form of non-personal presentation and promotion of ideas, goods, or services by the practice. Advertising includes broadcast, print, Internet, outdoor, and other forms.
- *Sales Promotion.* Short-term incentives encourage the purchase or sale of products or services offered in the practice. This area includes discounts, coupons, and incentive programs.
- *Personal Selling.* Personal presentation by practitioners for the purpose of making sales and building patient or referral source relationships. Personal selling includes sales presentations, shows, and incentive programs.
- *Public Relations.* Direct connections with carefully targeted individual patients to obtain immediate response and cultivate lasting customer relationships. Public relations involve press releases, sponsorships, noncommercial special events at the clinic, and Web and social media pages.

In summary, Kyle (2006) reminds practitioners that a marketing plan is more than something you "have to do" each year. It is the framework upon which the company's marketing success depends and a guide to follow until it is time to re-plan. As the planning process begins, it is necessary to keep the following elements in mind:

- *Be strategic.* There are many good marketing programs that will be offered to the practice. The job of the practice manager is, through a planning process through to determine which of those marketing programs make tactical and/or strategic sense. The marketing plan can assist the practitioner in staying focused throughout the year resulting in achievement of the business's goals. It is a good idea to start with the big picture objectives then define general strategies and tactics that support those goals. The correct actions and programs for a particular clinic can vary dramatically, depending on the goals and strategies. Consequently, strong strategic analysis behind your marketing plan can make a dramatic difference in the success of your marketing efforts.

■ *Understand that feeling uncertain is normal.* Feeling overwhelmed or incredibly confused at the beginning of the planning process is expected. The purpose of planning is to find the way to the best actions for the business. As the clinic progresses toward completion of the analysis, the best programs to include in the marketing plan to grow a particular business will become obvious. Consider seeking the advice of a practice management specialist or marketing consultant who can assist in focusing your efforts relative to the goals you have established for your practice.

■ *Be realistic.* Optimism is a plus in marketing the practice but understand the clinic's physical and financial limitations. A small or one-person practice can implement only a fraction of the marketing programs of larger operations. So, choose programs carefully and concentrate on seeing them through as the year progresses.

■ *Stay focused.* The marketing plan is only as good as its implementation. Keeping an "eye on the ball" rather than spreading too thin and implementing the plan poorly can make the difference between profit and loss.

■ *Watch the budgets.* For each marketing program included in your plan, spend some extra time collecting real-world costs to use in the budget. At implementation, stick to the budget and the marketing plan to avoid the temptation of throwing more money into the mix, should a lull in traffic occur in the middle of the plan schedule.

■ *Put measurements in place.* Evidence-based practice management requires that assessment dictates the direction of many clinical and business actions in a practice. Certainly, evaluating marketing programs is a prime example of evidence-based management. If your plan is not performing well based on your measurements, the plan should be recalled, reconsidered, and re-appropriated.

■ *Don't forget all four of marketing's Ps.* Promotion gets a lot of attention but pricing, place, and product are equally important to the bottom line. Consider adding new or improved products/services to the mix, evaluating pricing strategies, and improving distribution, along with advertising and promotional campaigns.

References

American Academy of Audiology. (2012). Internet hearing evaluations for the purposes of fitting and dispensing hearing aids. Resolution 2012:16. Retrieved October 29, 2012, from http://www.audiology.org/advocacy/publicpolicyresolutions/Documents/InternetHearingEvaluations_Fitting_DispensingHA.pdf

American Marketing Association. (2012). Definition of marketing. Marketing Power.com. Retrieved October 14, 2012, from http://

www.marketingpower.com/AboutAMA/Pages/DefinitionofMarketing.aspx

Berry, T., & Wilson, D. (2001). *On target: The book on marketing plans*. Eugene, OR: Palo Alto Software.

Berry, T., & Wilson, P. (2006). Market Pro Plus (6.0). Palo Alto, CA: Palo Alto Software. http://www.biz.plan.com

Berry, T. (2012). How to perform a SWOT analysis. Palo Alto Software. Retrieved October 25, 2012, from http://articles.mplans.com/how-to-perform-a-swot-analysis/

Churchill, G., & Brown, T. (2004). *Basic marketing research*. Mason, OH: South-Western.

Churchill, G., & Peter, J. (2002). *Marketing: Creating value for customers* (2nd ed.). Burr Ridge, IL: Irwin/McGraw-Hill.

D'Alessandro, D. (2001). *Brand warfare: 10 rules for building the killer brand*. New York, NY: McGraw-Hill.

Hansen, K. (2006). Successful practice branding. *Advance for Audiologists, 8*(1), 53–54.

Harrison, J., & St. John, C. (2004). *Foundations in strategic management*. Dayton, OH: Thomson Learning.

Knowthis.com. (2006). How to write marketing plans. *Know This, LLC*. Retrieved April 30, 2006, from http://www.knowthis.com/tutorials/marketing/marketingplan1/0.htm

Knowthis.com. (2012). Website for instruction in market planning. Retrieved October 25, 2012, from http://www.knowthis.com/principles-of-marketing-tutorials/how-to-write-a-marketing-plan/

Kotchkin, S. (2004). BHI physician program found to increase use of hearing healthcare. *Hearing Journal, 57*.

Kotchkin, S. (2009). MarketTrak VIII: 25-year trends in the hearing healthcare market. *Hearing Review, 16*(10).

Kotler, P. (2001). *Marketing management*. Upper Saddle River, NJ: Prentice-Hall.

Kotler, P., & Armstrong, G. (2012). *Principles of marketing* (14th ed.). Boston, MA: Pearson Prentice-Hall.

Krarup, N. (2001). Personal communication. September 11, Bern, Switzerland.

Kyle, B. (2006). Tips to calm marketing panic. *Websitemarketingplan.com*. Retrieved May 7, 2006, from http://www.websitemarketingplan.com

Lauterhorn, R. (1990). Marketing litany: 4Ps passé; C-words take over. *Advertising Age*, p. 26.

Levitt, T. (1980). Marketing success through differentiation. *Harvard Business Review*, Jan–Feb.

Live Plan. (2012). Web site for business and market planning. Retrieved October 25, 2012, from http://www.liveplan.com/

Marsh, D. (2012). *Marketing to the mature marketplace*. Presentation to the Annual Convention of the Colorado Academy of Audiology, Vail, CO.

McCall, K., & Dunlop, D. (2004). Marketing a practice. In B. Kaegy & M. Thomas (Eds.), *Essentials of physician practice management* (pp. 394–409). San Francisco, CA: John Wiley & Sons.

McCarthy, J. (1960). *Basic marketing: A managerial approach*. Homwood, IL: R. D. Irwin.

Murphy, P., & Ennis, B. (1986). Classifying products strategically. *Journal of Marketing, 7*, 24–42.

Nagel, T., Hogen, J., & Zale, J. (2011). *The strategy and tactics of pricing: A guide to growing more profitably* (5th ed.). Upper Saddle River, NJ: Prentice-Hall.

Oblinger, L. (2006). What is marketing. *How Stuff Works*. Retrieved May 1, 2006, from http://money.howstuffworks.com/marketing-plan1.htm

Oblinger, L. (2012). What is marketing. *How Stuff Works*. Retrieved October 14, 2012, from http://money.howstuffworks.com/marketing-plan.htm

Palo Alto Software. (2012). Sales and marketing pro. Palo Alto, California. Retrieved October 25, 2012, from http://www.mplans.com/sales_marketing_software/

Reine, L. (2010). Pew Internet and American life project. Pew Research Center. Retrieved October 29, 2012, from http://pewinternet.org/experts/Lee-Rainie.aspx?typeFilter=0

Staab, W. (1992). Sales promotion for office traffic control. In W. Staab (Ed.), *Applied hearing instrument marketing* (pp. 201–254). Livonia, MA: National Institute for Hearing Instrument Studies.

St. Clergy, K. (2012). Effective marketing: Developing and growing the practice. In R. Glaser & R. Traynor (Eds.), *Strategic practice management* (2nd ed.). San Diego, CA: Plural.

Traynor, R. (2006). The basics of marketing for audiologists. *Seminars in Hearing, 27*(1), 38–47.

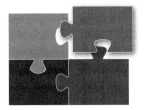

Effective Marketing: Developing and Growing the Practice

KEVIN D. ST. CLERGY, MS

Introduction

To achieve success in today's challenging business world, you must be adept at playing two very different roles. As a skilled, well educated hearing professional, you must follow best practice protocols for counseling and recommending the appropriate treatment to your patients. As a business owner or manager, you must effectively apply the principals of advertising, marketing, and sales so your practice will thrive and grow.

Often misunderstood, the terms "advertising, marketing and sales" are sometimes viewed negatively by those who enter the hearing profession with the oversimplified mission of "helping those who can't hear." It's as if "selling" as a means to that end is distasteful. *The truth is the patients you care so very much about will be best served only if you can sell enough products and services to stay in business.* For if you are "out of business," to whom will your patients turn for help?

Therefore, your ability to implement a results-driven marketing strategy and adhere to a patient-focused selling protocol, in combination with the skills you have as a professional Audiologist, will result in not only your business success, but a long-term relationship with those patients who depend upon your expertise.

This chapter is not intended to make you a marketing expert. Instead, it outlines proven action plans that incorporate traditional and Internet-based marketing methods that, when executed properly, will grow your practice by bringing more people through your doors, helping you convert them to happy, loyal patients, increasing your revenue stream and building your customer and referral bases.

By incorporating these recommendations into your knowledge and attitude about business, you will increase the likelihood that you will be sought out to fill a position in an existing practice or capably develop a plan for success in your private practice venture. In the pages that follow you will learn how to:

■ Prepare yourself and your organization for marketing *before* it begins;
■ Create and implement a simple marketing plan and budget;
■ Attract the right patients to your practice;
■ Measure the success of your overall marketing to ensure success over time.

But first, let's begin with some definitions.

Advertising Versus Marketing Versus Sales

According to Webster's dictionary, *advertising* is the "action of calling attention to one's products or services through paid announcements." The end result of successful advertising is grabbing the attention of the customer.

Marketing is the total of all activities involved in the transfer of goods from the producer or seller to the buyer, including advertising, shipping, storing and selling. The end result of successful marketing is the *sale*. The perfect sale results in the short and long-term revenue that comes from happy and loyal patients who are willing to refer family and friends.

Today's Marketing Must Include an Online Presence

What a difference five years can make. In 2007, a typical marketing plan for an Audiology practice allocated most funds for direct mail, newspaper ads, and Web site development, with a heavy emphasis on word-of-mouth marketing. Today, professional online marketing has replaced traditional word-of-mouth efforts and is vital to your business success.

Statistics show that the majority of your customers (and their decision-making children) are online. McGee (2010) reported that a recent Kelsey Group study discovered that 97% of all consumers currently use the Internet to conduct local searches for businesses in their area. Ninety percent use search engines, 48% use Internet Yellow Pages, 42% use comparison shopping sites, and 24% use vertical sites. Additionally, statistics from the NM Incite (2011) Nielson State of the Media: Social Media Report Q3, 2011 show that:

■ Nearly 4 in 5 active Internet users visit social networks and blogs.
■ There are currently 126 million blogs on the Internet. (Did you know that companies that blog produce twice as many leads as those who do not?)
■ YouTube is the second largest search engine in the world. (That means if you don't post informational videos

about your business and testimonials from your patients on YouTube, you are about to be left in the dust.)

- Ten billion Tweets have been sent on Twitter since 2006.
- Americans spend more time on Facebook than they do on any other U.S. Web site . . . and there are more than 500 million of them!
- Internet users over the age 55 are driving the growth of social networking through the mobile Internet.
- Sixty percent of consumers researching products online learned about a specific brand or retailer through social networking sites.

This means you must use a multi-pronged approach to your marketing strategy by combining the best of traditional methods with social media marketing (Facebook and Twitter), interactive Web sites, online videos (YouTube), blogging, writing articles and press releases, podcasting and social bookmarking to create a strong online presence.

You and your staff must learn to implement all the components of a strategic marketing plan based upon the principles outlined in the next few pages. If, after reading this chapter, you come to the conclusion that you do not have time to execute such a comprehensive marketing plan yourself, you have two choices. You must delegate the job to someone else on your staff or hire someone to do it for you. It is as simple as that.

The 3 E's of Marketing: Educate, Execute, Evaluate

Research by EducatedPatients.com (St. Clergy, 2010a,b) shows that most suc-

cessful marketers adhere to a proven three-step process designed to ensure their marketing efforts and monetary investments reap desired results. The process can be summarized with these three words: *educate, execute, and evaluate.* The material set forth in this chapter is presented with this process in mind.

Educate

"Learning is not a product of schooling, but the lifelong attempt to acquire it."

Albert Einstein

Educate Yourself

Your professional success begins with a lifetime commitment to continuing education. This personal pledge will help you avoid the common pitfalls (ineffective marketing, underestimating the competition, poor execution, failing to change with the times), cited by Dun and Bradstreet (2012) as some of the common reasons most businesses fail. Don't let the lack of business knowledge and skills become your nemesis. Set educational goals for yourself. Read two to three business related books per quarter. Develop relationships with experts in marketing. Keep up with the times. Watch what your competitors are doing. Before you know it you will be an expert yourself.

Educate Your Staff

Did you know that traditional marketing efforts (newspaper, direct mail etc.) of the average audiology practice cost anywhere from $250 to $1000 per call? That's why it is so important your staff is well trained and prepared to respond professionally to every call received. Your front desk manager must be able to consistently convert calls into appointments. You and/or your providers must be able to convert those appointments into sales and you, as an owner or manager, must convert those sales into lifetime raving fans who will tell everyone they know how great you are. Invest in training programs that meet these needs and that can deliver measurable results.

Educate Your Patients

Ensuring that your patients have the information they need to make a good buying decision will go a long way to establishing yourself as the expert in your local community. And there are so many ways to do this. Inform your patients through online blogging and by creating videos featured on your Web site, on YouTube or Facebook. Write articles and press releases. Don't forget the more traditional methods either. Your office brochure and patient newsletter are also tools you can use to ensure your patients know how to shop for hearing aids, are aware of the types of professionals they should seek and are aware of all the latest news and information about your staff.

Let's begin your personal education now with an overview of marketing and how to develop a comprehensive marketing plan for your practice.

Laying the Groundwork for an Effective Marketing Plan

Benjamin Franklin once said, "Failing to plan is planning to fail." That's very good advice when it comes to marketing. A good marketing plan begins by laying some groundwork. Before you decide to commit any of your hard-earned dollars to promoting your practice, you must first identify who you are as a company; do some market, demographic and psychographic research; and complete a business climate and competitive analysis. Only then will you be ready to put together a marketing strategy and action plan.

Unique Selling Proposition (USP)

One of the most important components in any successful business and/or marketing plan is your *unique selling proposition (USP)*. Without a USP, your practice will struggle to compete and will fail to leave a lasting, positive impression in the minds of your patient base.

Defined by Murray (2012), USP is a term that designates the primary focus of a business. The USP of a business is what makes it unique and different from all other businesses. A USP for an hearing healthcare practice, for example, is what makes this particular practice different from all other hearing health care practices. The USP can underscore product benefits, unique services, customers served or other unique aspects of the business. It should describe the greatest and most exclusive benefit your products and services have to offer. It is at the very center of why someone should choose you over a competitor. Your USP can make or break your business. Make it a memorable one.

Once you identify your USP, use it in every marketing campaign so it becomes linked with your overall brand.

To begin your search for your USP, start by asking yourself:

- How can my business improve someone's life?
- How can my business help my future and current patients?

■ What does my business offer that other services and products fail to provide?

As you go through the process of discovering your USP, be sure to consider all of the benefits you may provide to your customers, such as:

■ Enhanced Training Tools
■ Additional Support Options
■ Guarantee and Warrantees
■ Price Discounts (Be careful. See section entitled *The Dangers of Not Having a USP*)
■ Special Offers
■ Auxiliary Components
■ Exclusive Features and Options
■ Valuable Bonuses
■ Faster Delivery
■ Patient Access
■ Better Overall Service
■ Better Education.

To create your USP, you must thoroughly understand your potential patients. What do they want? What services do they value? Try thinking from your customer's perspective to discover what will motivate them to come to you. Master marketing guru Dan Kennedy (2009) recommends you do this by asking as a customer, "Why should I choose to do business with you versus your competitor?" Once you know the answers to these questions, you will know what your patients are passionate about and what will make them decide to choose you.

A well-known example of an effective USP is one that has been used by Wal-Mart. "Always Low Prices. Always." set Wal-Mart apart from others and was so effective it was also used as Wal-Mart's slogan. Their new USP is equally powerful. "Save money. Live better." is featured on their Web site.

Such successes can be accomplished at the local level as well. Just make sure your USP is sincere and is believable. A couple of sentences will do and if you succeed, your USP will be permanently associated with your brand. Two examples of USPs that have been successfully used in Audiology practices are:

Sample USP #1

Finally—A Simple, Professional Delivery Model For Hearing Aids That Does Not Involve Getting Ripped Off Or Dealing With Any Sales Pressure . . . Guaranteed. 100% of our patients thank us for our professional service. 100% of our patients are also guaranteed results or their money back (Hearing and Dizziness Wellness Center, Clermont, FL).

Sample USP #2

Education + Knowledge + Service = 100% patient satisfaction . . . guaranteed (Audiology and Hearing Aid Center, Scottsdale, AZ).

When you have decided on a USP for your business, incorporate it into your marketing message. Include it on your business cards, practice brochures, your Web site, educational tools, print and direct mail advertising, and social media advertising.

Integrating Your USP into Your Practice

Once you have determined what your USP will be, you and your staff will need to live up to what you have stated, even if that means you have to change the way you do things. For example, if your USP says your customers are always satisfied and your return rate shows something else is true, how can you honestly promote your business around the USP you have chosen? You must deliver what you have promised.

The Danger of Not Having a USP

If you choose not to develop a USP for your business, your potential patients will have no choice but to compare your practice to your competitors based on price and price alone. This is not something you want to happen.

Think about it. If you were shopping for a new cell phone, knew nothing about the product, and the sales person told you the two phones you were looking at were similar, how would you determine which one to buy? You might choose the most expensive one or you may choose the least expensive one, but the result would be you made your decision based solely on price. You should never compete on price alone, because you lose what little control you have over your competitor. There is absolutely no benefit or long-term growth associated with practices who compete on price in a local market.

USP Flexibility

Keep in mind; you always have the option to change your USP to meet the changes in the marketplace. Sometimes your competitors try to emulate your success and will copy the services and benefits you provide that make you unique, causing your original USP to be less effective. Never become so complacent about your business that you don't ever see the need for changes.

Market Research

An effective marketing plan requires you to thoroughly analyze your market to determine information about prospective patients, business competitors and market trends. Do not make the mistake some Audiology business owners have done and simply flip open the Yellow Pages and say, "WOW, there is nobody else in this market. I should open a practice here." Perhaps there is a reason for the absence.

Market research is also necessary to launch new products and services, reposition existing products and services or to expand the reach of your business. After an analysis of the targeted market, in which age, gender, location, and income level are reviewed, you can determine who will most likely purchase your product.

Other factors to consider in your market research, in addition to the demographics mentioned above, are psychographics, business climate, competitive analysis, and SWOT analysis in which the strengths, weaknesses, opportunities and threats are thoroughly analyzed (see Chapter 5).

Using Internet Market Research to Understand Your Target Market

Conducting market research on the Internet is a reasonably-priced way to carry out your market research. Best of all, there are organizations available to do the research for you and access to these groups is often available via manufacturers, buying groups and other Audiology business resources.

Internet market research has become more reliable than ever before due to the sheer volume of growth in the number of Internet surfers (providing a larger sample group) and the technological advances made in the methods used to collect data. The "do-it-yourself" approach can also reap great results if you begin your research with the Census Bureau site and have time to devote to the search engines.

Benefits and Drawbacks of the Internet as a Research Source

The distinctive characteristics of the Internet create benefits and well as drawbacks according to Chander Prabha (2010). Not only is Internet research fast and timely, benefits include new sources and volume of information, views other than those expressed by the mainstream population, unusual or hard-to-find information, government information, searchable databases, and digitized versions of primary sources. Many libraries are making electronic versions of official government documents, treaties, photographs, and some video and audio files available online.

On the other hand, because virtually anyone can publish their thoughts online, information found on the Internet may be incorrect or lack context. Off-limit sites can require passwords or fees. Additionally, search engines have limitations that prevent you from finding all that is available about a topic. Worse yet, Web pages can disappear, a headache for students who need to cite references.

Demographic and Psychographic Research

Understanding your market is a very important aspect of any business and should be the next item on your agenda for developing a marketing plan. Michael Gerber (1995), author of *E-Myth Revisited: Why Most Small Businesses Don't Work and What to Do About It,* refers to demographics and psychographics as the "two essential pillars supporting a successful marketing program."

Demographics is defined as the statistical data of a population based upon selected descriptors such as age, income, education, employment status, and so on for the purpose of the study of consumer behavior, usually to support marketing or opinion research. If the demographics indicate your market is an extremely poor area or there are not many people over the age of 65, then chances are your Audiology and hearing aid business may not be as successful as you desire.

Psychographics, on the other hand, define your market's attitudes, tastes, lifestyles, values, opinions, interests, etc. Harder to determine than demographics, psychographics are considerably more useful when it comes to gaining meaningful insight into your target market. You can learn more about the psychographics of your customers by posing questions to them about their wants and needs, reading their comments on your blogs and forums, listening to what they say about your service and products and by observing other hearing health care practices in your market.

While not as valuable to online businesses who sell products and services on a worldwide scale, demographics are still very important to traditional 'brick and mortar' locations.

Demographic Variables

Marketers often group consumers into segments based on demographic variables such as age, gender, family size, family life cycle, occupation, income, education, sexual orientation, home ownership, socioeconomic status, religion, and nationality.

Demographic Profiles

Demographic profiles are determined when several variables are combined to: (1) identify what subgroups exist in the overall population and (2) create a complete mental picture of a typical member of each subgroup. For example, a marketer may speak of a married male of upper middle income, age 55 to 64.

Demographic Trends

Due to the predictability of many demographic relationships, many demographic trends are easy to determine. If, for example, the unemployment rate steadily increases, we can predict there will eventually be a decrease in the demand for luxury items like jewelry and furs.

If there is an increase in the birth rate, there will be an increased demand for items for infants. As those infants grow up, there will be an increased demand for toys, video games, music CDs, and eventually an increased demand for universities and colleges, cars, houses, insurance, weight-loss centers, hearing aids, assistive living services, and ultimately funeral services.

Demographic trends have been used to give rational for everything, from the popularity of racquetball in the 1970s to stock market and election results. Of course, in reality, nothing is that simple. Yet demographic trends can explain a lot. This is the meaning of professor D. Foot's (1996) often quoted claim that "demographics explains about two-thirds of everything."

Generational Cohorts

A generational cohort is a group of people bound together by the sharing of the experience of common historical events. Understanding these cohorts can have a profound effect on the success of your marketing. Generational cohorts have been identified by various sources in several ways. In an article by Gandolf and Hirsch (2011) the following groupings were identified.

Depression Cohort (born from 1912 to 1921). This generation together experienced the Great Depression, poverty, financial insecurity and high levels of unemployment. Key characteristics of this group include striving for comfort and financial security.

WWII Cohort (born from 1922 to 1927). This group experienced the personal trials of war, women working in factories and a focus on defeating a common enemy. This group is characterized by patriotism, the belief in the nobility of sacrifice for the common good. They are team players.

Postwar Cohort (born from 1928 to 1945). The Cold War, McCarthyism, economic growth, and sustained tranquility are what bring this group together. Key characteristics are conformity, conservatism, and traditional family values.

Baby Boomer Cohort #1 (born from 1946 to 1954). Defined by the assassination of John F. Kennedy, Robert Kennedy, and Martin Luther King Jr., as well as political unrest, the walk on the moon, the Vietnam War, antiwar protests, social experimentation, sexual freedom, drug experimentation, the Civil Rights movement, and the environmental and women's movements, baby boomers are free-spirited. They have the characteristics of being experimental, social cause oriented, and individualistic.

Baby Boomer Cohort #2 (born from 1955 to 1965). This group experienced Watergate, the Nixon resignation, defeat in Vietnam, the oil embargo, raging inflation, and gasoline shortages. They are less optimistic, are cynical and have a distrust of government.

Generation X Cohort (born from 1965 to 1976). Those born during these years witnessed the Challenger explosion, Iran-Contra, Reagonomics, AIDS, safe sex, social malaise, the fall of the Berlin Wall, and single-parent families. They are independent, informal, and search for emotional security.

N Generation Cohort (born from 1977 to date). Joined by the rise of the Internet, the 9/11 terrorist attack, cultural diversity, and two wars in Iraq, members of this generational cohort share an extreme sense of patriotism, a quest for physical security and safety and are willing to accept change.

Business Climate and Competitive Analysis

A business climate analysis examines the economic, social, cultural, political and legal environment of a given market. Again, the local Chamber of Commerce is a good place to start your search for information.

A competitive analysis assesses the strengths and weaknesses of potential and current competitors. This analysis focuses on key competencies and the unique selling propositions of business rivals. Having this knowledge of business opportunities and threats can make a significant contribution to your development of a marketing strategy. The methodology of creating a competitive analysis involves many steps, which are presented below.

Competitor Profiling

Competitor profiling provides an objective analysis of a competitor's projection in the market and separates strong rivals from weak ones. It allows you make lists of what they are doing well and how they position themselves in a given market (see Chapter 1).

Media Scanning

Make it a habit to study your competitor's advertisements on a regular basis. You will gain invaluable knowledge about their marketing strategy. Watch for changes in that strategy and you may be able to gain a business advantage.

New Competitors

When there is unmet demand or high profits, there will be new competitors that enter the market. Monitor them carefully as they could pose a significant threat to you. Customer loyalty will ensure your customers do not "abandon ship."

SWOT Analysis

SWOT is a well-known strategic planning tool credited to Albert Humphrey who led a convention at Stanford University in the 1960s and 1970s. Today SWOT analyses are done by academics and business consultants alike to evaluate the *strengths, weaknesses, opportunities and threats* that may affect projects or business ventures. SWOT analysis can be effective, but only if used properly. Sometimes obvious problems receive attention while others are overlooked (see Chapter 5).

To perform a SWOT analysis, David E. Coffman (2007) recommends using a structured approach:

> Strengths and weaknesses relate to internal factors, while opportunities and threats cover external ones. The internal factors can be divided into five categories: management, workforce, sales and marketing, operations, and financial. The external factors are also divided into five categories: threat of new entrants, bargaining power of suppliers, bargaining power of patients, threat of rivalry from competitors, and threat of substitution.
>
> To approach the analysis in a structured way, prepare a checklist using the categories mentioned above. Identify factors within each category that are important to your practice. Under management for example, a major weakness for virtually every small practice is relying too heavily on the owner. What would happen to the practice if something happened to the owner? In the workforce category a factor could be employee turnover and the availability of new hires. The threat of new entrants might include the possibility of a corporate consolidator opening near your business. The bargaining power of suppliers and customers categories should consider the possibility of losing a major supplier. Come up with several factors for each category to complete the checklist. It is important that you do not try to rate or solve each issue as you identify them. If you do, you will get bogged down on each factor and never complete the analysis.
>
> Once the checklist is complete, you should rate each factor based on its importance to your business. Use an alphabetical scale from A to E, where A = very important, B = important, C = some importance, D = little importance, and E = not important. Next rate each factor based on proficiency (internal) or vulnerability (external). Use a numerical scale from 1 to 5, where 1 = very proficient or not vulnerable, 2 = proficient or little vulnerability, 3 = average proficiency or some vulnerability, 4 = poor proficiency or vulnerable, and 5 = deficient or very vulnerable.
>
> The factors with the lowest letter and highest number (A5) are the biggest weaknesses or threats. The ones with the lowest letter and lowest number (A1) are the biggest strengths or opportunities.

View your results with a critical eye. Fix the worst problems first and take advantage of the best opportunities.

Marketing Strategy, Budget, and Goals

A marketing strategy is a plan that will show how your marketing objectives will be fulfilled. The strategy and action portion of your marketing plan is where you outline specifically what you will do to attract *paying* patients to your practice.

A favorite planning tool that can help give your plan some structure is centered around the P's of Marketing, originally broken down into 4 P's by marketer E. Jerome McCarthy in 1960. Today, the Marketing P's have been adapted and expanded by other marketing experts. This version incorporates 6 P's.

Marketing P #1: Price

If you decide you want to consider price as part of your marketing strategy, you will have to decide whether or not to price your product and services lower or higher than the same products and services your competition provides (see Chapter 5 and 7). The results of your demographic and psychographic analyses will help you to make that decision. Just remember that pricing has a big impact on the long-term sustainability of your practice. In other words, you need to charge enough to be able to turn a profit. If you have multiple locations in multiple markets, decide whether or not your products and services will have the same price in every market.

Effective pricing strategy in an Audiology and hearing aid practice involves service pricing and product pricing. Depending on the model you are creating, service pricing can be obtained with help from your governing organizations or consultants that work for those groups. Products such as hearing aids should be priced by using a cost of goods formula. Good practices price their hearing aids with a 25 to 40% cost of goods (i.e., if a hearing aid costs $500, you sell it for $1800). This should give you the margins you need to sustain your practice.

Payment terms may cause problems down the road unless you work with insurance companies who pay in a timely manner. Hearing aids are usually a cash business and most practices make sure the hearing aid is paid for before being dispensed. This process allows for a good cash flow for the practice.

Financing should be an option in all practices because that is how people like to buy today. You can opt to use an outside agency to finance hearing aids, but do not ever be afraid to offer in-house financing. If you do offer in-house financing, make sure to receive at least one-half of the total owed as a down payment. You can finance the rest over time.

Marketing P #2: Product

A product strategy can help you determine how to introduce new products into the marketplace effectively in order to achieve the highest impact possible. When you launch a new product or service, make sure you brainstorm the features, benefits and end benefits of the product. Develop a plan to communicate those benefits to potential patients and make sure the packaging of the product matches the quality of services you provide.

Such a strategy can also help you determine what to do if you notice your products are not selling as well as they once did. Having a plan to turn public opinion around or finding alternative uses for your product will help you stay on target to reach your revenue goals.

Marketing P #3: Promotion

Promotion refers to traditional and nontraditional advertising. Traditional advertising includes television, radio, billboards, newspaper, direct mail, community networking, and outreach, as well as referral marketing. Nontraditional advertising, sometimes referred to as digital advertising, includes Web sites, search engine marketing (SEO), video marketing, article marketing, mobile marketing, podcasting, and social bookmarking. We discuss advertising in detail later.

Marketing P #4: People

Make sure you invest in good, highly-trained support staff members as well as Audiologists who work in your practice. Without the right people in place, you risk losing sales by *not* converting calls into appointments and appointments into sales and referrals.

Invest in training systems that make sure your people are highly trained. Don't expect a front office assistant to convert calls into appointments after 1 to 2 days of training.

Marketing P #5: Persuade

Once your potential patients notice your advertisement (headline), take the time to read your ad (irresistible offer), decide you're the company to work with (USP), contact you so they don't miss out (sense of urgency and contact information), you must be able to persuade them to take the next step to keep the sales process moving forward. Now is the time to persuade the caller to make an appointment, spend money and refer their family and friends. Unfortunately, most practice owners do not think this way. It is the most important of the "6 Ps" of marketing and also the most ignored in our profession.

Marketing P #6: Place

Your location is also important to your business success. If your business relies on medical referrals, space within a medical complex makes the best sense. If your business is a retail organization focused on selling hearing aids, a medical mall setting is a good option. Additionally, your place of business should be easy to find, have ample parking, and show up on Google Maps and Google Plaxo.

Budget and Measurements of Success

Depending on what stage of business you are in will determine how much you should spend on marketing in your practice. For newer practices, the recommended marketing budget can be as high as 25 to 45% of net revenues to get their name out into the local market. More established practices can get away by budgeting 6 to 15% of net revenues for marketing.

Determine the goals you want to achieve through your marketing efforts. Once you identify the specific amount of sales you want to produce, write it down, in the past tense, as though you have already reached that goal. You can use this goal to help you create your marketing budget. For example, if your goal is $500,000, write:

I produced $500,000 in net revenues by December 31, 2020.

Now we can put together a strategy and action plan as well as a budget based on this goal. Most importantly of all, your marketing plan should be S.M.A.R.T., a mnemonic (Doran 1981) used to set objectives. Each letter stands for a value that should be applied to the goal or plan. In this case, each letter stands for the following.

S-Specific. Identify the specific group the ad or marketing medium is attempting to target.

M-Measurable. This means you must be able to track all calls, appointments, sales etc. to determine whether or not the marketing effort worked. If it did not, do not repeat the ad or event verbatim again.

A-Action-Oriented. Identify everything that must be done and assign a staff member to perform the activity.

R-Relevant. Does the ad or marketing event support the vision of the organization and its team members?

T-Time Bound. Establish deadlines to ensure all tasks will be executed or accomplished.

Execute

> *"Quality is never an accident; it is always the result of high intention, sincere effort, intelligent direction and skillful execution; it represents the wise choice of many alternatives."*
>
> William A. Foster

No matter how well you plan, the results you want lie in your ability to execute those plans. As you put your marketing plan into action, review it often with the awareness that business climates often change, requiring you to respond quickly. Everything you do should be done with the goal of building a presence to establish yourself as an expert and to position your practice as *the* place to go for hearing health care.

Crafting an Effective Message

The message you've chosen to deliver to your target market must be carefully constructed to be effective. There are five critical components that must be included every time you craft your message, no matter what medium you use to deliver it. Make sure your message includes:

Critical Component #1: USP (Unique Selling Proposition)

As stated earlier, your USP is your way of branding your practice as a unique place of business. It is your opportunity to say to your potential patients, "Come to me for your hearing loss treatment and you will receive *this* benefit."

Critical Component #2: An Engaging Headline

Grab the reader's attention with the headline that appears at the top portion of any newspaper article, Web page, or sales letter. It defines the type or nature of the content written below it.

Usually, headlines are written in bold-face type, using a larger sized font as compared to article text or body copy. Headlines appearing on the front page are usually in a different color or in all caps. This helps the visitor become engaged in what you have to say.

Headlines should be written in present tense and should not use "to be" forms of verbs or articles such as "the" and "a." Words used for the headline need to be short, active, place emphasis on the content and grab the reader's attention. Add a curiosity factor to your headline and your reader will want to read more, especially when inserting a numeric value to heighten the impact. Here are some examples:

Headline Example #1: Discover 5 Simple Ways to Overcome Hearing Loss!

Headline Example #2: Avoid a Costly Mistake with Hearing Aids by Following Three Easy Steps!

Headline Example #3: Discover What You Need to Know Before You Even Consider Buying Hearing Aids by Following Three Simple Steps

Critical Component #3: An Irresistible offer

An irresistible offer is a call to action in any advertisement that gets a patient to say, "WOW! I need to respond to this ad to take advantage of it." The offer could be add-on benefits or products, battery offerings, trade-ins, discounts (although not a favorite), or any number of offers that will articulate additional value to your offering.

Critical Component #4: A Sense of Urgency

By including in a deadline in your ad you are letting the reader know that quick action is required or the irresistible offer will be missed. The deadline date needs to be clearly stated more than once.

Critical Component #5: Clear Contact Information or Next Steps

Tell the reader what he must do next. If you want him to call and make an appointment, say so and include a phone number in large, bold type.

Traditional and Nontraditional Media

There are many media you can use to deliver your message to your audience. Some are more suited to your targeted audience than other, but positives and negatives of each advertising channel are reviewed below.

Traditional Media: Not Dead Yet

Television, radio, newspaper, magazines, books and most print publication are considered traditional media. While traditional media aren't as strong as they used to be, they still occupy an important place in your overall marketing plan in which seniors represent a high percentage.

Television

Just 17% of TV ads generate a positive return on investment (Qualman, 2011), even though 97% of homes have a television. Despite the fact that the average use per day is 7+ hours, ads are expensive to produce, receive brief exposure time and have very poor viewer retention rate. Many new TV commercials drive their viewers to a Web site to take action.

Radio

Radio is not the best medium to use if you are trying to attract new patients. A better use may be as a vehicle to brand your practice. As with TV, those who use radio will sometimes drive people to a Web site as a call to action.

Billboards

Billboards can be extremely expensive, especially if you want to change your message frequently. Overall, they are not very effective.

Newspaper

Newspaper advertising has grown more expensive as readership declines. Its benefits include a long life span and multiple readers per household. Running multiple and consistent ads can affect ad prominence and brand recognition but is very expensive to do this. Newspaper advertising works best when used simultaneously with a direct mail piece.

Direct Mail

Direct mail response rates have continued to decline, but this medium is still the most successful secret weapon Audiology and hearing aid practices depend upon. Common direct mail pieces used in the industry are sales letters and patient newsletters. Mailings should be sent consistently to the patient database.

Community Networking

Although difficult to do, it is necessary that you get out of your office on a regular basis to build a network of community members. Join your local Rotary Club or other local groups to build relationships with people.

Community Outreach

Volunteering or sponsoring programs that give back to your community let your potential customers know you care about the neighborhood you share. Further your efforts at community outreach by becoming a member of the local Speaker's Bureau or by presenting public educational seminars.

Referral Marketing

Make it a habit to ask every single patient for a referral. For absolutely no expense and very little effort, you may find that the old adage, "those who ask sometimes get" is true.

Nontraditional Media and Methods: Creating an Online Presence

Web presence is defined on Wikipedia as being "the appearance of a person or organization on the World Wide Web. The amount of Web presence can be measured in the amount of sites an organization or individual has, which can include their own Web site, social network profiles, and their site's search engine ranking, traffic, popularity, and backlinks."

Nontraditional media and methods, when used together, can help increase your Web presence.

Web sites

Your Web site is a window into the soul of your practice and should match the high quality of care you provide. It should be professionally designed, interactive. and evoke a sense of trust. Even if you are a new business, you can have the look and feel of a more established business if your Web site is well done.

Web sites can be relatively inexpensive to build if you use online vendors who can supply you with the basic layout, color scheme and outline for your content, graphics, and images. Your Web site can even be ready to go within one weekend.

If it fits into your budget you can have your Web site custom built to give you a unique presence online, one that is uniquely different from the Web sites of your competitors. You can have a professional Web site developer plan and build a quality Web 2.0 Web site for anywhere from $2,000 to $5,000.

Not sure what Web 2.0 means? According to Wikipedia, Web 2.0 is a buzzword describing changing trends in the use of World Wide Web technology and Web design that aims to enhance creativity, information sharing, and collaboration among users. These concepts have led to the development and evolution of Web-based communities and hosted services, such as social-networking sites, video-sharing sites, wikis, and blogs.

As you begin to develop your Web 2.0 site, it's important to take the time necessary to determine a good domain name. When considering name choices, your focus should be on the products and services you provide, not on your company name. This will ensure visitors will associate the domain name with what you sell and make it much easier for your target audience to find your Web site during engine searches.

The name should not be peculiar, funny, or cute. Rather, it should be short and easy to remember as you will want your customers to readily share it with their friends and family. It is also important to look for ways to incorporate key words (like hear, hearing, or hearing aids) into the domain name, such as http://www.yourtownhears.com or http://www.yourcityhearing.com.

A title tag is the descriptive name of a page that is shown by browsers as the page name in the browser window. Your title tag should *never* look like this:

<TITLE>Welcome to Our Web site</TITLE>

Greeting your visitors is not necessary and the title tag is way too important to waste. Your goal is to quickly grab their attention, within ten seconds or less, and tell them what you have to offer. If you have a great title tag, they may stick around and read a little more. If that happens, you will most likely show up higher on many search engines.

Search Engine Marketing

Although it is always nice when patients come to you, the fact is you will starve if you take the attitude that your wonderful Web site is going to have people lining up to make appointments to buy hearing aids. If the right people don't know your Web site exists, it will take forever for you to build up a steady patient base. You must make it easy for your patients to find you. That's where search engine marketing comes in.

If you have a Web site that doesn't show up on the search engine results pages, it is like having a billboard on a dirt road. Everyone is using Google to find information online. If they don't find you when they search, then you are missing out on leads. To capture the leads you need to survive, you must use local listings, pay-per-click advertising, blogging, and search engine optimization (SEO).

Blogging. At the core of a good Internet presence is your ability to build and consistently maintain a blog (Web log). For whatever reason, consumers don't associate blogs with selling and are much more likely to surf a blog when researching.

A blog can be about any topic. It can be about your audiology and hearing aid practice, your customer service philosophy, industry news and the community service you do. Or it can be about new products where you spotlight their features and benefits. It's totally up to you.

Structuring your blog is also up to you. You can organize it any way you want. Design it as a place to write articles about hearing loss and hearing aids. Along with the main article section, you can create a Question and Answer section that will allow current and potential patients to ask questions or make comments on your articles, your product line, or your services. These types of features can encourage visitors to come back often and regularly, since a Q & A or comments sections usually feature new reading material quite frequently. In fact, you might even receive inspiration for some great new articles from your visitors' comments and questions, making your blog interesting and something that will be bookmarked and read every day.

Of course, you will want to include links to your Web site. Imbed them in your articles or feature them sidebars on your blog's main page. Making sure your readers always have convenient access to your practice Web site may tempt them to click on the link, call to ask for more information or better yet, call to make an appointment for a hearing test.

Make your blog visually appealing with the use of graphics and color. Just don't use too much animation or you may prevent your pages from loading quickly. This would be especially irritating if some of your target audience is still accessing the Internet with dial up connections. Remember, most people will not wait more than 10 seconds for pages to load.

There are many resources online that will help you set up your own blog. Check out Blogger.com or do an online search for "blog setup." There are also many online vendors who will create a customized blog for you.

Do some research by looking at some popular blogs. Ask your friends and family what blogs they like to read so you can review a wide variety of blog sites. Look at the content and how it is arranged. Notice how the pages are laid out, the use of white space, the graphics and pictures, and ad space. This will help you lay out your own blog space and give you a few ideas on hosting ads for other Web sites related to your own should you choose to do so after your blog is up and running.

Pay-Per-Click Advertising (PPC). Available since the late 1990s, pay-per-click advertising is an easy way to drive traffic to your site and has been the online advertising choice for many types of businesses with presence on the Internet.

Its appeal comes from the fact that the owner of the ad only pays for that ad when someone clicks on it and is taken to the linked Web site. Ads are seen on various Web sites that forward the interested party back to the advertiser's Web site. Best of all, the cost per click is low and is based upon the bidding amount the advertiser has finalized. Bid prices can be less than a dollar and can go up from there.

An effective pay-per-click ad will feature key words most likely to take the "clicker" to relevant Web sites. The rationale is that people who visit those sites would most likely be interested in the content of your site as well. Find the right Web sites for your ads and your chances increase for generating clicks to your site.

In addition to generating clicks through key words, you can also create clicks through content pay-per click. As the name says, the main difference is that rather than basing the search on key words, the results are based on the content. For example, as an owner or manager of an Audiology and hearing aid practice, it would be natural for you to want to place ads on local sites dedicated to medicine, health related issues, or hearing loss sites. When used together, key word and content matching create a well-rounded component of your marketing strategy.

The Google AdWords program makes placing pay-per-click ads simple. Start with a list of your top key words to aid you in writing the ad and use online tools to help with the look of your PPC advertisement. There is even a tool available that will keep track of the number of completed hits you receive so you know exactly how much pay-per-click advertising costs each month. Compare these numbers to the leads, appointments and sales that result from these hits each month to see how well the program is working for you.

Pay-per-click is not exclusionary, allowing you to contract with several key word services. It is recommended that you try out several key word services to determine the company that does the best job for you.

If your budget is limited, start with Google, and then add more key word services as you can afford it. Be patient. It may take some time to see positive results, usually about six months to a year to see a significant increase in traffic that can be correlated to a sales increase.

Each time a visitor clicks the ad linked to your Web site, you pay for the click. The cost per click is based on bidding and the amount you pay for each click is determined by the amount of your finalized bid. Bid prices can be less than a dollar and go up from there.

Pay-per-click advertising programs include the very popular search engine program of Google AdWords, Yahoo!, and Bing. Google AdWords is the most popular with a 50% market share in the United States, with Yahoo! coming in second and MSN third.

Local PPC. Local PPC advertising targets potential patients in your specific geographic area, putting you in touch with those who are currently searching for the products and services you have to offer. In other words, local PPC will give you hot leads.

Local PPC helps you specify your advertisement in relation to its geographical reach and key phrase (audiologist or hearing aids or find an audiologist). To maximize results try running a national ad with key words being the name of your city and hearing aids, that is, Houston Hearing Aids or any combination that you can think of with the name of the

area or your city in the phrases you set up. You can run a local campaign at the same time, but don't forget to setup the national campaign as well.

Local PPC ads provide you the chance to fine-tune home pages and landing pages on your Web sites. Landing pages are specifically designed to give a visitor the information they were seeking. It is not your home page. You can also utilize PPC to analyze varied versions of your Web site to know what lures your local potential patients. Benefits of PPC advertising are numerous. It:

- Attracts traffic: PPC advertising has the power to generate traffic instantly. It is also extremely responsive and a fast paced method to create some buzz for your professional Web site.
- Has simple principles: PPC dictates that any company that is ready to place the highest bid for a specific key word will get the highest rank on the page of search results.
- Has great flexibility: You can easily adjust the key words as required and even add or delete key words as per the demands of the current market conditions.
- Is affordable: PPC is very affordable when compared to most of the other traditional advertising.
- Is ideal for short-term campaigns: PPC advertising is tailor made for short-term advertising campaigns. You can change advertisement copy to reflect any changes that have made to the key word.
- Provides instant investment return: PPC advertising provides you with instant investment return if your Web site is designed to encourage

phone calls that can lead to appointments being scheduled or leads generated.

■ Makes budgeting easy: PPC advertising allows you to come up with a daily budget that can be adjusted based on your results.

■ Is targeted: PPC provides you the best of control over your Web site traffic via your personal choice of key words. This is really crucial when it comes to reaching the local audience.

■ Is flexible: A PPC campaign is very easy to measure and adjust. If a key word doesn't work, you can easily revise the content without much difficulty.

■ Allows you to pay only for success: PPC advertising assures that you pay only for those who are genuinely interested enough to click through to your Web site. Each click is a potential sale.

■ Provides for easy analysis: PPC advertising measures and monitors the speed at which traffic visits your site. This is helpful in analyzing the demand for your service or products.

■ Creates brand awareness: PPC advertising helps create brand awareness in addition to a direct response to your ad.

■ Gets results: When a PPC advertising campaign is managed correctly, it produces relevant results in a short period of time . . . sometimes within minutes!

■ Targets your local customers: PPC advertising targets local customers, ensuring you have targeted the right audience.

■ Connects online customers: PPC advertising allows you to connect with your customers who are online and who may be missing your traditional advertising messages.

■ Prequalifies customers: With a PPC campaign you can connect with customers who are genuinely interested in the products and services you offer. They have already visited your Web site and have been "presold" on the value of what you have to offer.

■ Tracks ad success: With PPC advertising, you receive instant feedback on the number of visitors clicking through without manual tracking methods. Monthly metrics allows you see who is clicking on your ad allowing you to alter your strategies if necessary.

Search Engine Optimization (SEO). The quality of your Web content will directly affect how well your pay-per-click program works and this is where search engine optimization (SEO) comes into play. In the book *Search Engine Optimization: An Hour A Day* (Grappone & Couzin, 2008) search engine optimization is described as a "diverse set of activities that you can perform to increase the number of desirable visitors who come to your Web site via search engines. This includes things you do to your site itself, such as making changes to your text and HTML code. It also includes communicating directly with the search engine, or pursuing other sources of traffic by making requests for listings or links."

When people think of search engine optimization, they first think of key words, those all important words related to your business that help those who are interested in what you have to offer find your site. But don't use key words without careful thought. Use them naturally in your content instead of focusing on the volume of usage. Key word density should be kept at 1 to 5%. You may also use bold or italics on certain key words. Just be careful to avoid using bold or italics in a repetitive pattern.

It is important to use as key words the same words your customers use to conduct a search. Many hearing professionals in private practice do not like to use the words "hearing aids." Instead they prefer terms like "hearing instruments" and "hearing devices." Like it or not, people use the search term "hearing aids" when looking for information online, so it is very important that you use those words in your Web site.

Along with the usage of key words in your content, you should register your Web site with each of the various search engines. As part of that registration, you can include all sorts of key words that will add your site to a search command. You can use terms that have a direct relationship to the content and purpose of your site, as well as key words that have some indirect relationship to your content.

It costs nothing to register on all the search engines, but it will take some time. Complete your list of key words and key phrases before you begin each registration process. It is best to have the list in an electronic format, so you can cut and paste it into the registration form. This will reduce data entry time and allow you to more quickly complete each registration.

Begin with well-known search engines like Google, Yahoo, and MSN first. Generally, it takes somewhere between 24 to 48 hours to deploy information about a Web site into the search engine files. By taking care of major search engines first, you will have an Internet presence very quickly. Once these are taken care of, you can move on to some of the smaller search engines.

Don't dismiss the smaller search engines as part of your search engine project. While the major engines will cover just about all the Internet, you never know when one of the minor engines will yield some results. Since it costs nothing to register, one sale would more than a make up for your investment of time. (TIP: Try one or two of the search engines first, just to get a feel for how much time and effort is involved. Then, you will be able to decide if registration is something that you want to do on your own, or farm out to a service.)

There are numerous methods of Web site optimization. However, these depend on the Web site's type, purpose, competition, and content. Let's review a couple of specific techniques.

It is very important to understand the placement of key words in the coding of a Web site. Key words must appear in the TITLE section of the source code in a Web page initially. These key words need to appear in the META (which is the technical word for page description section) as well. The META key words portion can also contain key phrases or key words that describe your content, product, or services.

Other useful tricks for enhancing the effectiveness of SEO include giving names to image files and anchors with key words. Anchors are also known as cross-links. These serve as references to other pages within your Web site.

Backlinks are also very important when it comes to optimizing a Web site for search engines, as they link other Web sites to yours. This can affect how relevant the search engines consider your Web page to certain search terms.

SEO is not a difficult task, just a time consuming one. There are affordable solutions available if you can learn to perform key word searches on your own. If you choose to hire someone else to do it for you, make sure the company you choose is geared for local Audiology and hearing aid practices.

In summary, let's review the benefits of utilizing SEO:

- Patient acquisition made affordable: Unless you pay for someone to set it up, you don't pay anything to the search engine for being indexed. This is especially crucial for phrases that are of high volume and low intent. These phrases can be quite expensive in the paid search process.
- Fixed prices: The cost for using SEO technique is fixed. It does not vary with the volume of click. The cost for each click from SEO usually decreases with time, especially after initial optimization costs are absorbed.
- Brand visibility: SEO optimization helps you to get brand visibility that you want for your Web site to get desired volume of traffic.
- Repeat business: SEO strategy is vital for getting consistent business online. It makes sure that your customers stick to your Web site for a long time or they can find you quickly if they need you again.
- Targeted prospects: With SEO, the search conducted by the users is demand-based. Anyone that hits your Web site via a search engine wants to get a Web page that fulfills his or her demand. If you optimize your Web site for search query, you will get customers who would like to

visit your Web site and interact with you again and again.

- Visitors: Apart from increasing the number of visitors on your Web site, an effective SEO strategy is capable of directing quality and interested visitors to your Web site.
- Savings: When your Web site ranks well in organic search results, it becomes possible for you to save a considerable amount of money.
- Advertising costs: Traditional advertising costs are huge. Web site owners can choose to optimize their Web site for search engines in order to save money on traditional advertising.

E-mail Marketing

Beware of ready-to-use e-mail lists as the e-mail addresses may not have been acquired legally. Too often lists are sold that consist of e-mail addresses "harvested" from the Internet. The use of these unsolicited e-mails is called spam and no responsible marketer would ever use one of these unqualified lists. Why run the risk of ruining your reputation by having irritated consumers who received your unsolicited e-mail turn you in to a spam reporting Web site?

A qualified e-mail list will only include e-mail addresses for those who have chosen, or opted in, to receive communication regarding certain products and services. You can build an e-mail list on your own by offering free information, like reports, guide or white papers on your Web site. Try to use double opt-in methods where a visitor inputs his name *and* e-mail in a form on your Web site. In response, an automatic e-mail is generated asking for a confirmation for the request. That way you are always protected if someone does report you as a spammer. As a courtesy, you should also promise that you will not share or sell the list to a third party. As a result, you will be seen as an honest professional.

Article Marketing

Article marketing generates traffic by improving your search engine position through an increase in backlinks; by Web masters publishing your article with its link on their own Web site; and by people clicking your link when they see your article listed in the article directory.

It works like this. When you write an article, include a resource box at the end of the article that contains a link to your Web site. Web publishers go to these sites searching for articles they can use on their Web sites for free. And when they publish your article, your link goes along for the ride. That's free advertising.

To see how it works, go to this link: http://ezinearticles.com/?Audiology-Marketing---Exclusivity-Sells&id=2254639. Now scroll down to the bottom. The resource box is at the end and, in this case, gives a biography of the author:

> Kevin D. St.Clergy is the author of "The Death of Audiology"—Discover what is killing our industry at http://www. DeathOfAudiology.com.

Here's another example: http://www.hearingreview.com/issues/articles/2009-08_05.asp. This example shows how great the resource box looks with a picture.

Your articles should be well written and should appeal to the reader as well as the search engine. Follow these guidelines when writing articles to make sure they get the results you want.

Do Key word Research. Since people use key words to search for information in the search engines like Google, you'll want to target appropriate key words if you wish to show up at the top of the results pages. The easiest way is to find relevant key words is to use Google's research tool at http://adwords.google.com/select/keywordtoolexternal.

Simply type in a key word for your Web site and Google will give you many key word ideas. Google also gives you the numbers that tell you how often people search for each term. That way you know the key words you're targeting are worth your efforts. Another important piece of the puzzle is figuring out how much competition there is for each key word. If you are targeting words that have too much competition, it's going to be harder for you to reach the top of the search engine results pages. Don't worry about that happening, because it's easy to figure out how much competition there is. Go to Google and type in your key word surrounded by quotation marks. The results that pop up are the other sites that are specifically targeting that term. Now that you have these key words you can use them to give you a basis for your articles. It's easiest to choose one key word per article and focus the topic around that key word. Remember to put the same term in your title as well.

Write Articles for the Reader—and the Search Engines. Provide good content your readers will enjoy and follow the previously suggested guidelines for key word density.

Submit to the Best Article Directories. All article directories are not created equal. The best directories are EzineArticles.

com; GoArticles.com; ArticleDashboard. com; and Buzzle.com. Regular article submission to any of these directories will bring more visitors to your site. Conversion rates should be high as the people coming to your site are looking for what you sell.

Make Your Author's Resource Box Compelling. Your author's resource box should contain a compelling reason for people to continue on to your Web site. For example, if your Web site is offering a solution for hearing loss, let the reader know you have the answer they are looking for if they visit your Web site.

Submit Multiple Articles. How many articles will you need to submit to an article directory to increase the number of visitors who come to your site? One or two is not enough, that's for sure. But you don't have to spend your life writing articles. You just need to submit articles on a regular basis over a long amount of time. One per week would be good. But if you have time constraints, try for two articles per month, every month. The key is consistency.

Repurpose Your Content. Maximize the value of your content by submitting the same article to more than one article directory. Many people report that submitting the same article more than once actually increased their rankings. Others, however, debate this. If you have your own doubts, you can make a few changes in your article before submitting it again. This would still save you some valuable time.

You should also place the article you submitted to article directories and feature it on your own site. Search engines love to see new content and as a result, you might get visited by search engines more frequently. This is called being "spidered."

Don't Give It All Away. The purpose of article writing is to get the person reading it to come to your site. If you give them all the information they need in the article you write, why would they bother to do that?

Instead, give them enough information to peak their interest and let them know you have the information they need. Your article can still be of high quality, especially if you use the AIDA method of writing articles, which can result in a click-through rate of around 40%.

AIDA stands for attention, interest, desire, and action. Capture the reader's *attention* with a compelling headline and a great opening. Then, maintain their *interest* by showing them how important what you're about to say is. Next, increase their *desire* for visiting your Web site by handing out a solution or piece of information, but indicate that you have addressed the rest of the information on your site. Then ask the reader to click on your author's resource box, the *action* you want.

Brand Yourself as an Expert. You will automatically be viewed as an expert if you write a lot of articles. That means you'll get more traffic visiting your site. The more people you impress, the more people who will link you and recommend you as a link to others.

Research the Competition. When you see a competitor's Web site ranking especially high by search engines, wouldn't you like to know why?

You can find out by going to ezineart icles.com and searching for the most viewed articles in your market or in "audiology." Take a look at the key words your competitors use in the titles of their articles. Look at the content and how it is written. Check out their resource box and look at their profile to see how many articles they have submitted. How many Web sites are they linked to?

Pay Attention to Your Profile. Add a picture and information about yourself in your article profile. By doing this you will immediately gain trust in the eyes of the viewer. And the more people trust you, the more they will visit your Web site.

You don't have to write a lengthy biography to make your profile effective. Just provide enough information to prove that you are indeed an expert. Readers who like reading your articles may decide to subscribe, an option that is available at many article directories.

Web 2.0 Web sites

Web 2.0 Web sites are sites that rely on user-generated content to increase the value of the site and enhance readers' experience.

It's only been in the last few years that these types of sites have taken off like wildfire. It's next to impossible to find someone who has not heard of Facebook, Twitter and LinkedIN. But, how can you use them to generate traffic to your site? That's what we're about to cover.

Facebook

Facebook has fundamentally changed the way we communicate. Not only can you find long lost friends and stay connected with family, you can find new friends . . . friends who can become customers.

Use Facebook to make blog entries and describe changes you've made to your Web site. You can join networking groups related to the topic you're focusing on and place a link to your site in your profile.

You can even have a customized business page as well. Be sure to interact with people who visit and "friend" your page in order to get more traffic and make connections. Your Facebook visitors will enjoy seeing what you have to offer.

Facebook also has an array of add-ons available that have been developed by independent programmers. These offer a way to interact with prospective customers and visitors.

Blogger.com

Blogger.com is a free blogging platform owned by Google. When you set up a blog with Blogger, it will be created as a sub domain on the blogspot.com domain (i.e., http://kevinstclergy.blogspot.com/). That means you will get all the "link juice" that comes from an authority site like blogger and that's a good thing. Link juice has the power to increase traffic.

To take advantage of this strategy, you should create a "mini blog" on Blogger that links back to your own site. This is a similar concept to adding articles to an article directory, though you have more control over the blog. The downside is that you don't get the built-in article directory traffic.

The more entries you add, the more likely you are to be found by other Blogger.com users. And you will rank highly in the search engines because your blog is coming from such a respected domain. Since you're linking back to your main Web site you should start to see your traffic and search engine rankings increase over time.

WordPress.com

WordPress.com is another free blogging platform that should not be confused with WordPress.org, which is a self-hosted blogging application. WordPress.com will allow you to set up a blog as a subdomain on their domain. Just like Blogger.com, this is a great way to build links to your own Web site so that your rankings in the search engines increase.

Squidoo.com

Another way to generate traffic to your site is through Squidoo, a community Web site where users can create their own pages called lenses. A lens is not really a blog or a Web site, but rather a hybrid of both. And the great thing is Squidoo offers many different modules that help you add content more quickly and easily than you might think possible.

You can also place your RSS feed from your own blog on your lens, a great, hands-off way to keep your lens updated and fresh with new content. And your blog gets the benefit of a great link.

Squidoo is also very flexible about placing links to your own site, unlike WordPress or HubPages. Google and other search engines also tend to love Squidoo, so you'll find that your lenses will rank highly and send "link love" to your site. You can also join groups within Squidoo in order to get even more targeted people to visit your lens, and eventually your Web site.

HubPages.com

HubPages is a lot like Squidoo in many ways. They have modules that make it easy to add content to create a miniature Web site in a very short amount of time.

The difference between HubPages and Squidoo is that HubPages is a lot pickier about what goes on your hub. You may only have two outgoing links to your site, including any RSS feed links.

Still, HubPages has a very dedicated community behind it that can drive a lot of targeted people to your Web site. They are also very well liked by the search engines so the potential is great. One of the greatest things is that people love to comment on hubs and regularly seek out new ones, so you may get a lot of questions and commentary on your hub. This will help expand your reach as an expert.

Twitter

Twitter is a little bit different from the rest of the Web 2.0 sites we've discussed so far, but that's what makes it so great. It's all about networking with others in what is called a microblogging platform.

When you sign up for Twitter, you'll be given a chance to collect followers and to follow other people. The point here is that you will see the updates of people you follow, and people who follow you will see your updates.

Beware of following people who have tons of followers who in return are only following a few. Realize that they are viewing Twitter as a one-way street, so determine whether that's ok with you or not.

On Twitter, you can talk about the great things you're doing to your site or in your business, as well as the things that are going on in your personal life. You can follow people who are interested in your niche, and they will most likely follow you back. As you update and talk about the helpful content on your Web site, you will begin to receive some very targeted traffic.

Another great thing about Twitter is that your updates, or "tweets," contain links which will show up in the search engines. This gives you a chance to rank for the key words you are tweeting about, as well as adding additional backlinks to your Web site.

Video

Videos are an amazing way to get traffic to your Web site. There are many people who search for videos online to for informational value or simply to entertain themselves. You can take advantage of this by creating your own videos and uploading them to popular video sharing Web sites.

Create a compelling video that captures people's attention, make them interested in what you are talking about, and get more visitors to your Web site. It could be a PowerPoint presentation with recorded audio or a video of yourself or your patients. Check out special software like Camtasia Studio.

YouTube

While there are many video sites out there, the most popular one by far is You-Tube. You can bring traffic to your Web site just by using this one video sharing Web site.

To begin, go to YouTube and make your profile. Don't forget to include a link to your Web site. Just like people who visit article directories are interested in the author, people who visit video sharing Web sites are interested in who made the video. You also get a backlink by including this in your profile.

While you are uploading your video, you'll notice that YouTube allows you to write a description. This is also an excellent spot to insert a link to your Web site.

YouTube will also give you a code so you can place your video on your own Web site. While this won't directly give you more traffic, it will give your site more dynamic content that your visitors will love.

The more videos you have out there, the greater the chance of traffic. You can test and track different methods of video creation to see what visitors respond to the most. You may find that a video you thought would really take off, doesn't, and vice versa.

Press Releases

A press release is a written communication directed at members of the news media for the purpose of announcing something newsworthy. Typically, mailed, e-mailed, or faxed to news agencies to distribute at their discretion, the Internet makes it easier than ever to place your press releases in front of your target market.

The traditional use of a press release is to announce a change, a new company, a new employee, a promotion or a new aspect of your business. The copy is concise, uses key words and employs a journalistic style of writing that describes who is involved, what is happening, when it is happening, where it is happening, and why it is happening. The components of a press release consist of a headline, an introduction, body copy, a call to action, contact information, and a business summary. Templates for writing press releases are available for free online. As always, make use of key words.

Submit your press release to high traffic sites that offer the best benefit. Recommendations include PRWeb, Click-Press.com, PR.com, and PressReleases. com. Additionally, your press release can be picked up by newspapers and other traditional news agencies.

Links

Getting links from other Web sites is one of the oldest search engine optimization strategies in the book. It works because search engines rank you more highly based on the number of links you have. You can increase your ranking by exchanging or buying links from other Web masters.

After your site is up and running, contact Web masters of highly ranked Web sites in your market. Search their site for a links page or area where it is clear that they have sold or exchanged links with other Web masters. Some of them will want to give you a link in exchange for a link on your Web site. Others will just want a straight-up payment to place your link on their site. This latter option is better in the long term because Google often gives more weight to one-way links rather than reciprocal links. Three way links are an option as well, if you have more than one Web site. That way you can add the Web master's link to one of your sites and they can add a link to your other site on their page.

Sometimes people will link to you naturally, if your Web site features some really great content. This is called "link bait" when you write something so amazing or controversial that other people can't help but talk about it. This also works well on blogs.

When you comment on other people's blogs you will often be able to leave a link to your Web site in the comments field. If you are commenting on a highly trafficked blog, visitors will sometimes click through to your Web site right then and there. Regardless of whether or not that happens, a link left in a comments field will be counted by search engines. You can either comment on blogs manually or hire a freelancer to comment with a link for you. Never spam a blog using automated software as Google has ways of figuring this out.

Social Bookmarking

Social bookmarking is an excellent segment of Web 2.0 that you can use to bring more traffic to your Web site and to provide backlinks. These Web sites are basically services that allow users to bookmark their favorite sites all over the Web. You can make use of this by bookmarking your own site along with the sites that you find to be interesting. Digg.com and Del.icio.us are two very popular social bookmarking sites.

Word-of-Mouth Marketing

Word-of-mouth marketing is an excellent way to increase Web site traffic. The idea is to create a campaign that will cause people to pass along your Web site URL, the content you produce and other information, all with a click or an e-mail.

Be prepared to give away something for free or to talk about something controversial to encourage people to pass the word along. You will have to "think outside the box" to get people interested enough to pass the word along, though. This often means giving away things for free or speaking about controversial or important topics.

Blogging to Attract Visitors

Blogging is an excellent way to bring more visitors to your Web site as search engines tend to rank blogs very highly.

To make sure your blog is search engine friendly, add some plug-ins, like All in One SEO, and optimize your content by including a key word(s) in the title, first paragraph, body, and last paragraph. Your content should be relevant to your niche and should link to internal pages in your Web site.

Pinging. Pinging alerts are very important as they tell search engines that you have updated your blog content. WordPress, the most popular blogging platform, automatically pings your blog entries for you if you set it up to do so. Still, it doesn't use every ping site out there by default so you will want to add an optimized ping list to your settings.

Blog Feeds. There are sites dedicated to collecting blog feeds so readers can subscribe to your feed just like they would a newspaper or magazine. They can choose from headlines to get an idea about what they would like to read, then link to the post it describes. These readers syndicate your content by using your RSS feed and they also give you a link back to your blog.

Write Guest Blog Posts. Writing guest blog posts are another great way to bring traffic to your Web site and receive quality links. This is especially true if you're able to post a comment on a blog that is very popular. When your post is published you will get the benefit of their credibility and some of their traffic as well.

Blog Often. The more often you blog, the more often your site will be spidered. This means that new blog posts will be indexed in the search engines quickly and you will begin to become a "favorite." While you won't have to blog every day,

you should post frequently and consistently as both readers and search engines like to see new, updated content.

Evaluate

"One of the great mistakes is to judge policies and programs by their intentions, rather than their results."

Milton Friedman

Evaluating marketing effectiveness doesn't have to be difficult, but it is necessary in today's turbulent economic times. If you are spending money for marketing, you must be able to measure the effectiveness of your efforts. Marketing that produces excellent results should be repeated. If results were poor, do not throw good money after bad and make the same mistake twice.

Traditional Measurements Used to Track Marketing Results

Consistent tracking is necessary to accurately measure marketing results. Use these metrics to look at your overall success for the year, quarter and month. Systems and processes should be in place to ensure every member of your team, including yourself, understands how to track the following:

- Number of Calls Received: The total number of calls you received as a result of a marketing effort.
- Number of Calls Converted into Appointments: The total number of calls resulting from a marketing effort converted into appointments.

- Cost per Call: Marketing cost divided by the number of calls.
- Appointments Generated: The total number of appointments that were kept.
- Cost per Appointment: Marketing cost divided by the number of appointments that were kept.
- Spousal Attendance Rate: The percentage of appointments that had spouses attend an appointment.
- Net Revenue Totals: Total revenue generated minus returns and adjustments.
- Revenue per Call: Net revenue total divided by the number of calls received.
- Revenue per Appointment: Net revenue total divided by the number of appointments generated.
- Return on Investment: Profits divided by investment.

Phone Tracking Systems

You will notice a large percentage of these metrics involve relying on tracking the number of calls you receive. Expecting call tracking measurements to be accurate without also expecting human error is unrealistic. The best way to measure phone calls is to use *special call tracking telephone numbers*. A special phone number is placed in all advertisements, with a different number being assigned to each marketing medium being used. When that particular phone rings it will automatically track how many calls you receive from the marketing medium assigned to that number. Some of the more advanced call tracking systems can also track other valuable information, like point of call origination or the incoming call phone number. You can also use the best of these systems to record calls for quality assurance.

Web Site Analytics

When people visit your Web site they leave a trail letting you know what they are doing, where they are going and where they came from. A computer cookie, small bits of computer code that is automatically downloaded to a visitor's computer when they come to your Web site, allows Web site analytics software to track all sorts of data about your visitor.

At one time this data was only available at great cost and effort, and then Web site owners had to manually make sense of it. Today, Web site analytics programs gather and compile data automatically then convert it to understandable and useful reports you can use to help grow your business.

What Web Site Analytics Can Tell You

Web analytics can help you gain insight into your business that will help you make good marketing decisions. The most critical and actionable data revealed through Web analytics are:

- Key Words: The words and phrases people type into search engines to find your site.
- Search Engines: What search engines were used to find your site?
- Internet Browsers: What internet browser was used to view your site?
- Visitor Count: How many people visit your site per day, week, and year?
- Referring Sites: What other sites sent you traffic.

- Popular Pages: What people were reading on your site and how many visited each page?
- Time on Site: How long people stayed on your Web site.
- Entry Pages: The page on which people entered your site.
- Exit Pages: The page on which people left your site.
- Conversions: The pages that had conversions, which resulted in e-mail sign ups, and so forth.
- Demographics: Countries visitors live in.
- Time: The busiest days and times on your site.

Who Needs Web Site Analytics?

Anyone who is interested in growing their practice, that's who. Whatever you measure tends to improve over time, so measure everything. Web analytics can give you valuable insights into what you need to work on to improve your overall Web presence. It will tell you if you need to change your offer on your home page, if you need better content on your Web site, or if you need to re-design your Web site to get more clicks in the areas that you want people to click.

Failing to use Web site analytics is like opening a brand new practice and never looking at your bills, your profit and loss statements, balance sheets, payroll, sales, returns, exchanges, or even patient satisfaction studies. Without this information, how would you even know if you are making money, have the right people in place, or if your patients are happy? How do you know if your marketing is working or if you even have enough money to pay yourself?

You wouldn't if you didn't measure. Web site analytics allows you to measure your online presence just as you do with your practice.

With an audiology Web site you need to know if the right visitors are coming through your virtual, online practice doors, what they are doing while they stay, what page they leave from, and how long they stayed. There is an enormous of amount of information you can collect online about what your patients like and want, and it's the job of the practice owner or manager to monitor the Web site analytics and see what people are doing. Using the right information can help an owner or manager make the right decision about what comes next.

Web Site Statistic Terms to Learn

Most analytic software uses certain terms to identify traffic and give you the information you need to make informed decisions. Let's go over these terms as you will use them often while analyzing your statistical data.

- Visits: The number of unique visitors to your site or page.
- Pages/Visit: The average number of pages per visit.
- Avgerage Time on Site: The average time a visitor spends on your site.
- Percentage of New Visits: The percentage of visitors who have never visited your site before.
- Bounce Rate: The rate at which people leave your site from the page they landed on, without ever going anywhere else. If you have 100% bounce rate it means that every person who lands on a particular page of your site leaves without clicking through to another page. Obviously, the lower your bounce rate is the better. If sites are sending

you lots of traffic but your bounce rate is very high, that means the traffic is likely untargeted. Consider this rate carefully when looking for more traffic from certain sites.

Referring Sites

Sites that send you traffic are friends indeed. With any business, traffic is life-blood—and the referring sites are your veins. They pump life into your business and allow you to make more money. Don't underestimate the power of your referring sites and the inbound links they use to send traffic your way. As you'll see below, you should adjust regularly to optimize the opportunities already in front of you. Here are some tips about what you can do with your referring site report:

- ■ Visit the Sites: Go visit the site and make sure you are using the traffic and exposure you are currently getting to your maximum advantage. If the site is a blog, comment to further solidify your presence there. If the site published an article of yours, contact the owner to see if you can post more or become a regular contributor. If the site is an article directory, add more articles.
- ■ Look for Patterns: Is there a certain type of site that you get more traffic from? Are you getting a lot of people coming from your social media marketing? Look at what efforts you are currently making to see if they're paying off. For example, if you contribute weekly to a blog in your niche but you're getting little or no traffic, then it may be time to trim nonproductive activities.

- ■ Look for Additional Opportunities: While you're visiting referring sites, take note of any opportunities for additional traffic from related sites. See who else they're linking to and check them out. You never know when you'll find another great source of traffic.
- ■ Contact the Site Owners: If you have not yet been in contact with the owners of the sites that are sending you traffic, establish a business relationship and send them a message to introduce yourself and let them know they are a top referrer for you. Say "thank you" and leave the discussion open. Ask what you can do to help them achieve their site goals.

Key Words Report

The key word report show terms your visitors searched with to find your site. The number of key words listed in your report depends on how much your site is currently loved by the search engines. If you have a new Web site, then you'll most likely have a low number of key word terms to analyze. If you have a very large site that is well established you may have hundreds or even thousands of key word terms in your report.

- ■ Top Key words: Study your top five key words. These are the key words that are giving you the most traffic. Are these the words you want to be known for, or are visitors just randomly finding you through some old page you put up without a second thought?
- ■ Web site Navigation: Is your site navigation in line with the words that people are using to find your Web site? Can you reword some of

your links in order to make them more attractive to the visitors who are finding your site?

■ "Information" Words: There are some key word phrases that clearly indicate someone looking for information, rather than looking to make a purchase. They are not in a buying state of mind while searching, and are clearly telling you so, so there's no sense in trying to sell them something directly. Two examples: "Hearing aid reviews," or "choosing an audiologist." It's not likely you're going to convince either searcher to buy anything from you immediately.

■ "Potential" Words: Some words are "information" words on the surface, but they express an underlying need or potential need to make a purchase. An example might be "What kind of hearing aid is the best?"

■ "Money" Words: Some words on your key word list will be "money" words, meaning that the people searching are looking to make a purchase. Examples might be "Where to buy hearing aids" or "buy hearing aids." These searchers are telling you they're ready to make a buying decision.

■ Potential Articles: Can you use some of the key word phrases as jumping off points for great articles? Do it! Even "information" words can make great blog posts that will help develop a relationship with your target market. High-quality information gives those who read your articles and blog posts a reason to come back again. Perhaps you can even use these key words to create a report, a product, videos, or

other marketing materials that will continue to boost your business.

Over time you'll develop other ideas for what you should do with your key words. In the meantime, keep pulling those reports and looking for patterns. A final tip for you on the key words is to make sure you don't put too much pressure on yourself. Use what you can and leave the rest. You won't be able to implement every idea or suggestion immediately. Start with your top five key words so you can target your efforts where they'll have your biggest payoff.

Content by Title

This part of the report will show you the most popular pages and posts on your Web site listed by title. Use this information to improve your content. Begin with the pages most visited and make them even better. Optimize your content by giving it a purpose. If you've written a page to get people to sign up to your newsletter, invite them to do so. If you've written a page to share your expertise, point them to additional content. If you've written a page to lead a prospect towards a sale, tell them how to get there. If there's a way to make your existing content work better for you— your highest traffic pages are the place to start!

Conclusion

What better way to end this review of modern audiology marketing strategies than to look at a couple of case studies conducted by EducatedPatients.com

(St. Clergy, 2010a,b) to demonstrate how important it is to incorporate the Internet into your marketing calendar along with traditional media?

Practice A is a medium-sized clinic in a small-sized town. From June 1 to December 31, 2010, they decided to scientifically track all their lead sources by using unique tracking numbers on each marketing medium. The results were pretty dramatic. Forty-two percent of the leads they received during that time period came from their Web site and Internet marketing efforts. By comparison, direct mail produced 24.6% of the leads, radio generated 18.6%, and newspaper was responsible for 10.1%.

Using the same tracking techniques over the same time frame, Practice B, a small practice in a fairly large town, generated 79.3% of their leads from the Internet, compared to 11.7% produced by direct mail and the 5.4% as a result of the health fair and home shows staff attended.

Results like these are not accidental. The owners of Practice A and B applied the marketing principles set forth in this chapter.

Will you?

References

Coffman, D. E. (2007). Using SWOT analysis to improve your business. Retrieved March 6, 2012, from Isnare.com, http://www.isnare.com/?aid=15894&ca=Business+Management

Doran, G. T. (1981). There's a S.M.A.R.T. way to write management's goals and objectives. *Management Review, 70*(11), 35–36.

Dun and Bradstreet Credibility Corp. (2012). The top ten reasons why small businesses fail. Retrieved March 4, 2012, from Small Business Dun and Bradstreet, https://smallbusiness.dnb.com/business-planning-structures/business-plans/1440-1.html

Foot, D. K. (1996). *Boom, bust & echo: Profiting from the demographic shift in the 21st century.* Toronto, CA: Macfarlane Walter & Ross.

Gandolf, S., & Hirsch, L. (2011). What is a healthcare marketing plan? Retrieved March 6, 2012, from Healthcare Success Strategies, http://www.healthcaresuccess.com/articles/what-is-marketing-plan.html

Gerber, M. (1995). *E-myth revisited: Why most small businesses don't work and what to do about it.* New York, NY: HarperCollins.

Grappone, J., & Couzin, G. (2008). *Search engine optimization: An hour a day.* Hoboken, NJ: Wiley.

Kennedy, D. (2009). Unique selling proposition vs. dumb slogans. Retrieved March 7, 2012, from Glazer-Kennedy Insider's Circle, http://dankennedy.com/blog/small-business-marketing-tips/unique-selling-proposition-vs-dumb-slogans/

McGee, M. (2010). Two more studies confirm: People research online, buy locally. Retrieved February 10, 2012, from Small Business Search Marketing, http://www.smallbusinesssem.com/two-more-studies-confirm-people-research-online-buy-locally/2901/

Murray, J. (2012). Creating a unique selling proposition for your business. Retrieved March 4, 2012, from About.com U.S. Business Law and Taxes, http://biztaxlaw.about.com/od/businessstartupsteps/a/createusp.htm

NM Incite. (2011). State of the media: The social media report Q3, 2011. Retrieved February 10, 2012, from Nielson Wire, http://blog.nielsen.com/nielsenwire/social/

Prabha, C. (2010). Create benefits and drawback of the Internet as a research tool. Retrieved March 5, 2012, from Articlesbase.com, http://www.articlesbase.com/education-articles/create-benefits-draw

backs-of-the-internet-as-a-research-source
-1322461.html

Qualman, E. (2011). Social media revolution 2011. Retrieved March 7, 2012, from http://www.youtube.com/watch?v=3Su
Nx0UrnEo

St. Clergy, K. (2010a). Audiology marketing/ E3 educate. Retrieved March 3, 2012, from EducatedPatients.com, http://www.edu
catedpatients.com/blog/

St. Clergy, K. (2010b). Audiology marketing/ E3 evolve. Retrieved March 6, 2012, from EducatedPatients.com, http://www.edu
catedpatients.com/blog/

7

Optimizing Pricing Strategies for the Practice

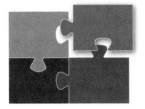

ROBERT M. TRAYNOR, EdD, MBA

Pricing is a component of the marketing mix. Crafted by McCarthy (1960), the classic marketing mix consists of price, product, promotion, and place. Smith and Nagle (1994) and Smith (2012) both refer to pricing as the process of arriving at that delicate balance between the profitability of the clinic and the patient's willingness to pay. While proper pricing is essential to the success of the practice, Smith (2012) feels that it is a combination of educated guessing, reality, and a bit of luck. Even the most successful audiology practice managers struggle to reach the appropriate prices for products and services. On the one hand, they realize that

they must cover their costs, consider the competition, and the patient's willingness to pay; and on the other, the general concepts and specific procedures for setting prices are somewhat of a mystery. Specifically, the pricing process involves an integration of concerns for practitioner costs and overall value offered to and perceived by patients. Pricing experts, such as Kotler and Armstrong (2012), indicate that in the narrowest sense, a price is the amount of money charged for a product or service. In a broader sense, however, price is the sum of all of the values that patients must give up to gain the benefits of obtaining a product or service provided by the clinic. Although patients view the price for products and services as giving up something of value, generally money; practice managers must view the price charged as essential revenue generation (Know This, 2012). Historically, price has been the deciding factor in patient choices for clinics and/or products, but recently nonprice factors such as service, quality, credentials, experience, relationships, clinical environment, personality, and other issues have gained increasing importance. In audiology clinics where most competitors offer similar (or the same) products and services to the market place, these non-price factors are especially important. The increased competition by competent audiology colleagues, makes mastering these non-price factors as important to success as arrival at the correct price. Although the other components of the marketing mix are specifically discussed in Chapters 5 and 6, proper pricing is so essential to success it deserves a separate discussion to present fundamental concepts and practical guidelines for developing a pricing strategy. Although there are evaluative services and accessories, such as batteries, ear care products, telephones, and other items in the clinic that must be priced, hearing instruments present the most complex pricing decision that can drive the practice either positively or negatively. Thus, most of our discussion involves the pricing of hearing instruments.

Factors That Influence Price

Staab (2000) presented the factors that influence prices. These factors not only influence prices for audiology clinics but for most other products. His concept of these factors is presented in Figure 7–1. Although portions of this chapter discuss most of these issues in detail, each of these factors is important to success and influence the price of everything we purchase.

Our Customers Are Patients

As we move through our discussion of the pricing process customers are referred to as patients. By definition one who seeks treatment and advice is a patient, while one who simply seeks advice is a client, and those who purchase from a business are customers.

Most experienced audiologists realize that audiology patients are mostly older individuals. The purchasing habits of older people are deeply affected their life experiences and the current generation of patients, baby boomers, is quite different from that of the previous generation. Previous generations of older patients were significantly affected by the Depression, World War II, and other life experiences which caused them to "get by" when presented with health issues. Baby boomers, however, have quite different purchase behaviors and an attitude toward health issues and products that keep them active and participating in life. Thornhill and Martin (2007) indicate that this attitude was created by the affluence of the 1950s and 1960s and that the world has revolved around this generation all of their lives. Shopping malls were created to accommodate this generation, schools were built for them, the Mustang among other products were targeted to meet the wants and needs of baby boomers. Although some baby boomers are frivolous and

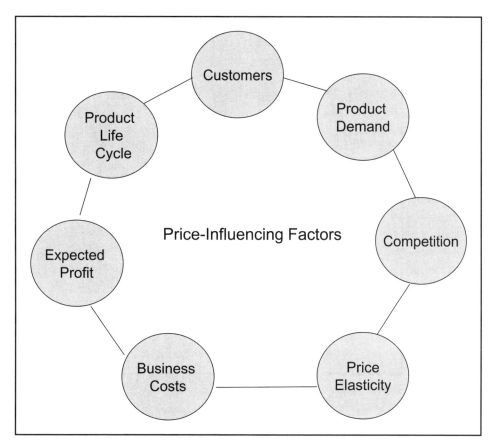

Figure 7–1. Price-influencing factors (adapted from Staab, 2000).

others are cautious with their finances, their tendency is to meet their needs immediately. As a group, they may not wait the typical 5 to 7 years after they know there is a hearing problem before seek audiological services and products.

Pricing and Demand for Products/Services

Pricing is a major factor in the demand for the product and services. If products are priced too high, demand will be low but margins are high reducing the necessity for volume. When pricing low, the clinic typically sells a higher volume of product. Figure 7–2 visually presents the concept of demand according to price, the higher the price the less volume, whereas the lower the price nets a higher volume. It follows that pricing also reflects the actual value added to the products by the audiologist and the clinic that provides the support. Higher volume clinics where prices are low generally do not have the capability to offer high service and follow up to their patients as there are many demands for their time thus, less added value to patients. Low volume clinics have the time to offer special follow up and other services as there is less demand for their time, thus more added value to the patients.

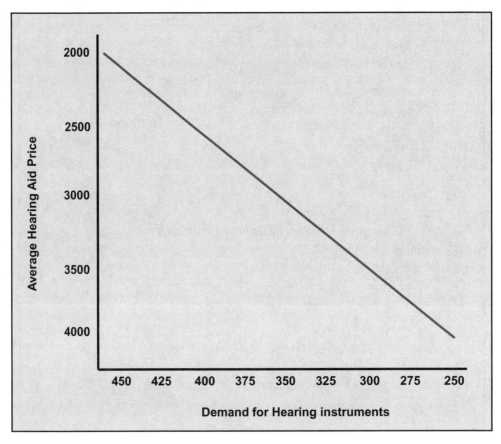

Figure 7–2. Demand for hearing instruments by price.

Cost-Plus and Competition Pricing Philosophies

Although some pricing strategies, such as cost-plus (see Sidebar 7–3) or competition pricing (Table 7–1) are logical and used quite often, the literature does not support their use and they do not create the best pricing options for the patients or the clinic. An old discussion is that businesses either pay too much attention to the competition or not enough. A common pricing strategy is called competition pricing, and is sometimes referred to as the "tail wagging the dog" or "follow the leader" pricing (Hosford-Dunn, Dunn, &

Harford, 1995). Competition pricing is when practitioners lower their prices to gain market share with the idea that the increased volume in sales will offset the lowered prices (see Table 7–1). Nagle and Dolan (2004) hold that prices should be lowered only when they are no longer justified by the value offered in comparison to the value offered by the competition. Although price cutting is probably the quickest, most effective method to achieve a sales objective, it is usually a poor financial decision. Since a price cut can be so easily matched by the competition; it offers only a short-term competitive advantage at the expense of perma-

Table 7–1. Competition Cost Example

Normal Situation		Meeting the Discount Competition	
Current Retail Price	$3,950.00	New Retail Price	$2,850.00
Invoice Cost per fitting (2 yr warranty)	−$1,400.00	Invoice Cost per fitting (3 yr warranty)	−$1,550.00
Fixed Costs per fitting	−$500.00	Fixed Costs per fitting	−$500.00
Incremental Costs	−$300.00	Incremental Costs	−$300.00
Gross Profit/Loss	**$1,750.00**	Gross Profit/loss	**$650.00**
		Extra Warranty Service Cost	−$150.00
		Battery Cost	−$30.00
		Gross Profit/loss	**$320.00**

nently lower margins. Although product differentiation, advertising, and improved distribution do not increase sales as quickly as price cuts, their benefit is more sustainable and therefore usually more cost effective. Hosford-Dunn et al. (1995) indicate that looking to the competition is a dangerous method to select pricing since the competition may have unrealistic prices for their products relative to their business costs which may be drastically different than costs associated with your practice. As the value added pricing strategy is employed it is necessary to be aware of competitive prices within the immediate demographic area of the practice but using prices set by your competitors is not sound business strategy.

Price Elasticity

Price *elasticity* is a basic concept of pricing that refers to the amount patient demand for a product or service fluctuates according to rises or reductions in price. Amlani (2007) summarized price

elasticity as the sensitivity of the consumer to the price of a product. Prices that are *inelastic* are not sensitive to price modifications while products that are sensitive to price changes are considered to be *elastic*. Figure 7–3 demonstrates consumer price sensitivity in that sales volume or consumer demand (D) is reduced as the price of the product is increased. For example, if the price of a hearing instrument is raised, how much will the sales volume go down or with price reductions how much will sales increase. Riley (2006) demonstrates this in Figure 7–4. In the graph on the left of Figure 7–4, price at P1 yields patient sales (demand) at Q1. As prices go up at P2 or down at P3, sales or patient (demand) is at Q2 and Q3, respectively, demonstrating that patient sales (demand) for the product does not change much with modifications in the price. This is an example of a product that has an *inelastic* price elasticity of demand as might be found in hearing instrument sales which tend to be relatively inelastic or not very sensitive to changes in price.

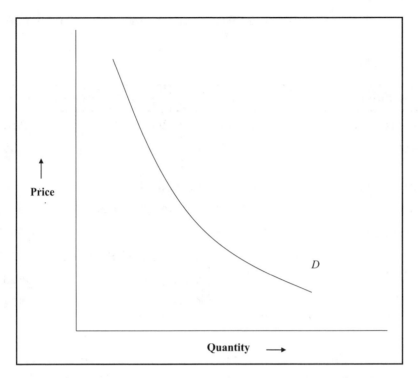

Figure 7–3. The relationship between price and quantity for a hypothetical demand function (*D*).

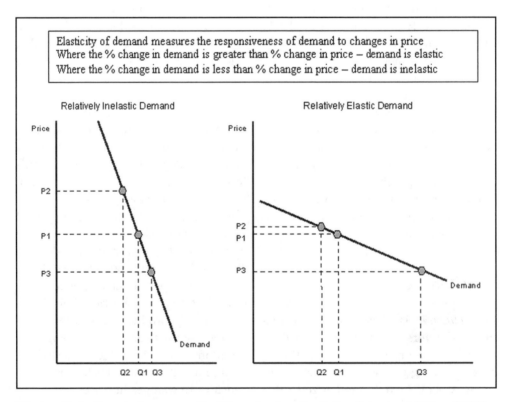

Figure 7–4. Demand curves with different price elasticity of demand (Riley, 2006).

The graph on the right of Figure 7–4 presents price at P1 that yields patient sales (demand) for product at Q1. As prices go up to P2 and down at P3, patient sales (demand) for product is at Q2 and Q3 respectively. This is an example of a product that is *elastic* as might be found for hearing aid batteries which tend to be relatively elastic or sensitive to changes in price.

Price elasticity (E), according to Kotler and Armstrong (2012), is figured as a ratio of the percentage change in demand or sales volume (SV) to the percentage change in price (P) as expressed in the formula below:

$$\text{Price Elasticity of Demand (E)} = \frac{\%\ \text{Change SV}}{\%\ \text{Change P}}$$

Nagle, Hogan, and Zale (2011) indicate that price elasticity (E) is usually a negative number, since positive changes in price (price increases) produce sales (demand) declines and negative changes in price (price cuts) generally produce sales (demand) increases. Thus, the greater the absolute value of E (usually >1), the greater the elasticity or change in the sales volume (demand), whereas the smaller the value of E (usually <1), the more inelastic or the less fluctuation of sales volume (demand). The slope of the sales volume (demand) curves in Figure 7–4 are directly related to the elasticity of a product. Practitioners should realize that their product sales are subject to some fluctuation relative to price elasticity. If the price elasticity is known for a specific type of product, the practitioner can make an intelligent decision as how to price these products, which ones to be discounted, and those that should be discontinued. Since price elasticity can assist

in predicting how many sales will reasonably occur if prices are modified by 10, 20, or 30%. The prediction of demand for stock items such as assistive listening devices (ALD), open fit and receiver in the canal hearing instruments, and other popular items can reduce over or understock situations.

Demand can be estimated by three general methods. First, if the practice has been in place for a substantial period of time, demand can be reviewed historically. A historical demand analysis reviews the number of specific products, evaluations often by CPT code, and other specific procedures that were completed over a specified period, usually 1 year. The historical review is a reliable method of evaluating demand throughout the year unless there are substantial changes in market or economic conditions. Second, demand can also be estimated by direct experimentation, purposely increasing the price and reducing the price to determine the price elasticity. For example, raising and lowering the price of hearing instrument batteries and carefully observing the percentage that sales goes down with the price increase and the percentage that sales go up with price reduction. Once the elasticity is known prices may be modified according to knowledge of demand that is generated by the experimentation. Direct experimentation is, however, a dangerous method as it compromises profit to obtain information. A third method of predicting demand is that of asking the patients what they would pay for a specific service or product. Although this is a well-known method of predicting demand for products and services, Nagle et al. (2011) cautions its use since buyers often underestimate what services or products they will purchase at higher price.

Sidebar 7–1
PRODUCT PRICE ELASTICITY IN THE AUDIOLOGY PRACTICE

According to Kotler and Armstrong (2012) as prices are adjusted up and down there is less change in product or service demand (price inelasticity) when:

- The cost of a product is low relative to income.
- The product is unique.
- High quality.
- High prestige.
- Exclusive.
- Substitutes are difficult to find.
- When it is difficult to compare the quality or performance of the various competitors or substitutes.
- When the costs are shared by another party.

Using hearing instruments as an example, today's technology make these devices unique to most patients and they are amazed by their size, performance, and flexibility compared to older products that were used by other family members. Although hearing instruments are not a product coveted by most individuals, the instruments themselves are considered by most to be of very high quality. Depending on the market focus, the clinic or the particular doctor where the devices were obtained may be considered exclusive in a particular city as well as carry some prestige. Often, the capability to afford the costs of amplification, well known to be expensive, may also offer some form of prestige and exclusiveness. The comparison of various products by consumers is difficult as these comparisons require multiple visits to various audiologists in numerous clinics so the review of products, hence, performance assessment of many brands and models is not readily available. Although not funded by Medicare, in today's market many supplemental third-party payers are available to share or totally pay the costs of hearing instrumentation offering consumers assistance in the purchase of these devices. These factors contribute to minimal price elasticity in amplification products so small to moderate changes in product prices, at least currently; have minimal effect on product demand (price inelasticity). As the number of private practices, manufacturers outlets, and other dispensing operations expand via Internet, television, and patient mailboxes, there is a threat that price elasticity could become greater over time for these products.

On the other hand, Kotler and Armstrong (2012) also present that price elasticity is high when the product can be readily available at a number of price points from many different sellers. Consider hearing aid batteries at

Costco or Walmart, where, for example, batteries are sometimes featured for $0.30 each, whereas in typical clinical audiology practice batteries are about $1.00 each. Although there may be some slight differences in brand and performance, patients perceive these products as commodities, suggesting that all batteries are essentially the same, thus, it makes no difference as to the brand of batteries used or where they are purchased. Since there is no perceived uniqueness by consumers, all brands are perceived as high quality that will power their hearing instruments equally. Since there are many different price points and places to purchase; there is no reason not to accept the lowest price obtainable. For products such as batteries and some other readily available hearing aid accessories, the price is very sensitive to small changes (elastic), unless it can be demonstrated to the patient that there is a higher quality battery available only through an audiology practice.

Business Costs

No matter what philosophy is used for pricing, an essential component of most pricing structures is business costs (see Chapter 8). Audiology practices incur numerous costs associated with doing business and understanding these costs is a challenging component of pricing. Once these costs are appreciated it is easy to comprehend why the price for a product or service, at a minimum, must cover **all** relevant operational costs. Costs that must be covered when considering the price to charge for a product or service include:

- Opportunity costs
- Fixed costs
- Incremental or variable costs
- Avoidable costs
- Sunk costs.

Opportunity Costs

Hall and Lieberman (2013) discuss the fundamental economics of opportunity costs as that which is given up when the choice is made to offer a service or product in the practice. Since there is a limited amount of assets in the practice there are a finite number of procedures and activities that can be accomplished profitably. Decisions to offer a particular procedure in the practice can sometimes generate a tradeoff involving financial resources, personnel, or other assets within the practice. The efficient use of these assets to generate income becomes the question. What profitability will not be realized if the opportunity is not seized and the procedure(s) is/are not offered? Consider the decision to offer a new procedure in the practice, such as videonystagmography (VNG)(see Sidebar 7–2). There are overhead costs if the procedure is offered in the practice and opportunity cost that is part of the conscious decision not to offer VNG examinations in the practice. If the choice is **not** to offer VNG in the clinic, there will be income lost (opportunity cost), but also the overhead of the equipment purchase, personnel to conduct the examinations, and space allocations will not be necessary. As presented later in Table 7–3, the decision is not how much it costs to offer or not to offer VNGs, but if the finite assets of the practice could be utilized the more efficiently to make higher profit for the practice by using them elsewhere.

Fixed Costs

Fixed costs, sometimes known as overhead, are those incurred each month. Examples of fixed costs include bank loans, rent, telephone, utilities, salaries, payroll taxes, and other expenses that

---

Sidebar 7–2
THE OPPORTUNITY COST OF VESTIBULAR ASSESSMENT

A good example of opportunity cost is in the offering of vestibular assessment in the practice (Traynor, 2006). When considering instituting vestibular services in the practice it is important to estimate the number of procedures that will be conducted per month to arrive at the appropriate decision regarding the use of practice assets to conduct the procedure. Basically, the concern is if the same assets can produce a larger profit by conducting another procedure or if offering the procedure costs more than the opportunity for profit. For example, if the practice will conduct 7 VNGs per month at $300 each, the practice would forfeit $2100 (7 × 300) per month or $25, 200 per year in income. If the practice chooses *not* to pursue the VNG opportunity, the expense of $23,000 for equipment and payment of the audiologist (someone else or the practitioner) to provide the service would not be necessary. If the personnel costs per month would be $850 and the equipment costs were $500 per month the total costs of doing VNG business (the cost of the opportunity in overhead) would be $1,350 per month. When the income of $2,100 per month is considered against the expenses of $1,350 each month; then the opportunity cost of *not* offering VNGs would be $750 ($2100 to $1,350) or $9,000 year. Although there is an attractive opportunity to add an extra $25,200 to the practice income per year, the question of if the opportunity is worth the assets required to acquire the additional income remains. It is possible that a more profitable service that can be added to the practice which will generate more profit with the same asset investment.

On the other hand, if the VNG procedure is offered and there were 14 referrals per month with an income of $4,200 per month or $50,400 annually there could be substantial income opportunity lost. Even with the doubled personnel time of $1,900 and the $500 equipment payments there would be a substantial gross profit each month $4,200 to $2,400 or $2,550 per month or $30,600 each year. If the practice can make more than $9,000 per year by using the funds for another procedure, then this opportunity cost is offset by the profit on the other procedure.

must be paid even if there is no business conducted. These expenses are a "hurdle" that must be cleared each month before any profit is created. In the breakeven analysis presented in Figure 7–5, the practice must dispense 13 hearing instruments to cover fixed expenses each month, before reaching profitability. High fixed expenses commonly generate cash flow issues that can, if left unchecked, become a primary cause of financial collapse resulting in failure of the practice.

Incremental or Variable Costs

Variable costs are those that are incremental to the amount of business conducted. The greater amount of business

transacted, the higher the incremental/variable costs. Incremental/variable costs include the costs of hearing instruments, commissions to employees, warranty support, materials costs (electrodes, probe tips, earmold impression material), and other items that will vary relative to the number of services provided or hearing instruments dispensed: The more business conducted, the higher the incremental/variable costs.

Some examples of methods to control incremental/variable costs include: observing and taking advantage of supplier discounts, modification of supplier arrangements, offering less warranty for hearing instruments with less profit margin, modification of employee relationships,

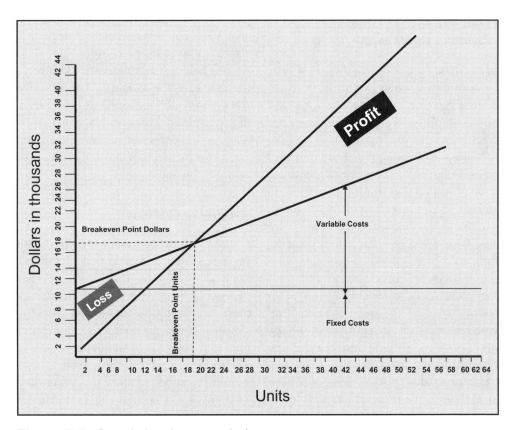

Figure 7–5. Sample breakeven analysis.

credit card merchant fees, and insurance discounts. If a supplier offers a discount of 12% for 2 hearing aids per month, but offers 25% if 4 are ordered each month, it might make sense to consider ordering at least four instruments each month as this reduces the variable costs for the next sale and adds to the profit. Another example of a variable cost is when credit is necessary to dispense instruments and a 12-month "same as cash" financing is utilized. To obtain the 12-month financing program the cost to the merchant (the practice) may be 8.8% of the sales price, but costs for a 6-month program might only 4.9%. It may make sense to use the 6 month program and not use the 12-month program unless absolutely necessary.

Fixed and Incremental (Variable) Costs and Pricing

Accountants argue that **all** costs should be considered when establishing realistic pricing structures. Nagle et al. (2011), however, presents that not all costs are relevant to the pricing decision and the first step is to identify those relevant costs. Dolan and Simon (1996), however, have indicated that the primary concern should focus on **relevant** incremental/variable costs. Relevant incremental/variable costs are those that actually impact the profit of the practice and vary with the services and products offered, pricing philosophy, competition and other factors specific to each location. Previous models for pricing in audiology practices have recommended averaging relevant incremental/variable costs as a basis for product pricing (Hosford-Dunn et al., 1995). The use of average incremental costs to determine pricing often masks the real price point and leads to over or underpricing services and prod-

ucts offered by the practice (Nagle et al., 2011). In principle, the identification of costs relevant to pricing is straightforward but in everyday practice it is often difficult to identify all relevant costs. Smith and Nagle (1994) describe incremental costs that are associated with changes in pricing and sales volume. The distinction between incremental costs and nonincremental costs parallels closely, but not exactly. Sometimes this incremental/nonincremental cost differentiation is a bit confusing in the business literature. A distinction more familiar to clinical practitioners is the difference between *variable* and *fixed* costs commonly involved in the operation of any business. Variable costs, of course, are those that vary with sales volume, such as product acquisition, direct labor, telephone, power, supplies, commissions, warranty exposure, and so forth. Since pricing decisions affect the amount of business that will be conducted, variable costs are always incremental for pricing. Additionally, *fixed costs* such as marketing, advertising, leasehold costs, taxes, and insurance, represent static operational costs are those incurred in the normal course of doing business.

Avoidable Costs

Avoidable costs are those that have not yet been incurred or can be reversed. Avoidable costs are true business costs that could be avoided. In all businesses there are methods to reduce costs by simply incurring less expense. For example, sometimes it is better to have the employees clean the office than to hire a janitorial service, to use less expensive equipment that allows the same procedures to be completed as the expensive brands, employees paying a significant percentage of their insurance costs, not upgrading the mobile phones, and/or by carefully observing the opportunity costs involved in offering new procedures and products. Although these are only a few examples of how to cut costs, more inventive methods may be practical for a variety of practice venues. Nagle et al. (2011) state that many of the costs of selling a product or offering a service to a patient, replacing sold items, or consumables are avoidable. Avoidable costs can be reduced or eliminated with the exclusion of a service, or modification of the products or consumables used in the process of clinical treatment but, in their opinion, it is easy to overestimate the amounts that can be saved through attempts to reduce avoidable costs. For example, it may be possible to reduce the professional employee compensation, but malpractice insurance, continuing education, and benefits do not change that much unless the position is completely eliminated. Another example is to obtain product from another supplier, request a better discount, and procure consumables (insert tips, electrodes, etc.) from another supplier at a lower cost. The funds that are not expended due to the better discounts are costs that are avoided.

Sunk Costs

According to Nagle et al. (2011) sunk costs, are basically the opposite of avoidable costs in that they are expenses to which the practice is irreversibly committed and, once incurred, they will not be recovered. In audiology practices these are costs for equipment, such as the ABR/OAE unit, VNG unit, computers, and peripheral systems. Although it can be argued that when systems such as an audiometer, ABR units, or computer systems are incorporated into the practice for a significant period past their expected life, that some recovery of their sunk cost can be obtained, but the equipment is still substantially reduced in value to other practitioners that might be interested in their purchase. In an audiology practice, a classic example of a sunk cost is a new neon sign for the office that marks and brands the practice. It is a good sign and can be used for years and certainly worth its cost but it is not likely that another audiology practice will want to purchase the sign that has been custom designed to brand the clinic. Similar to some other business expenses, once the sign is obtained, it is a sunk cost that will never be recovered. Chapter 8 offers a detailed discussion of costs and how they affect the practice.

Cost-Plus Pricing

Cost-plus or markup pricing is the most common method for products since it offers an aura of financial prudence to practitioners. Financial prudence, according to the cost-plus theory, is achieved by pricing every product or service to yield a fair return to the practitioner relative to the overall fixed and incremental costs that are fully and fairly covered by the markup of the product. Kotler (2001) feels that this is a popular method of pricing in business because it is easier for practitioners to determine their costs than the patient's capability and willingness to pay a particular price. Since the actual determination of the patient's willingness and their price ceiling involves expensive sophisticated market research that is often beyond the reach of most private practice audiology clinics and this is considered to be a method of pricing that is fair to both the practice and the patients. Cost-plus pricing typically works best when all the practices in the area use this system as it tends to minimize price competition and essentially allows practitioners to simplify the pricing task (Dolan & Simon, 1996) while concentrating on other differences among the practices, such as location, service, and so forth. Even though cost-plus or markup pricing is the most popular method of pricing for products and services Staab (2000) considers cost-plus pricing strategies in Audiology practices the least rewarding. Pricing professionals, such as Nagle and Dolan (2004) even state that cost-plus or markup pricing is a blueprint for mediocre financial performance.

Sidebar 7–3
FIGURING COST-PLUS OR MARKUP PRICES

Five Times Cost Rule of Thumb Pricing Scheme

In the old days of hearing aid sales, the commercial hearing aid dealers would mark up a hearing instrument five times the unit cost from the manufacturer. Although the simplest form of cost-plus or markup pricing, this tended to insure cost coverage and profitability with a simple calculation, presented below:

$$Cost \times 5 = Retail\ Price$$

In the days of analog conventional instruments when costs for these products were $79, retail prices were $395. These were high for the times, considering the value of money, but still affordable and practitioner could be assured that they were compensated very well for warranty service and follow-up for this simple markup. If this simple rule was applied to current digital products it becomes useless as the cost of the products become prohibitive when the 5 times cost rule is considered. For example, if the cost of an entry level hearing instrument is $595.00, then the retail price is $2,975 each or $5,950 for the binaural set, hardly entry level. Similarly, if the cost of a high end hearing instrument is $3,125, then the retail price would be $15,625 each or $31,250 for the binaural set, totally outrageous in most markets. While these are ridiculous prices, versions of the scheme such as 2.5, 3, 3.5, 4 times cost can be used to simply calculate retail prices.

Percentage of Profit Over Cost Scheme

Percentage markup strategies are also utilized to provide a more accurate calculation of real cost coverage and a margin that will bring profitability with an eye toward competitive retail pricing. The use of percentage markup requires that the practitioner establish a percentage markup for the products that will ensure cost coverage and profit on everything sold. In the percentage scheme, the practitioner should have knowledge of about how many products will be sold each month. To cover fixed costs, the number of expected instruments to be sold each month is divided into the monthly fixed expenses to arrive at the per unit fixed expense costs. These fixed costs are added to the purchase price of each unit as part of the purchase price when it is sold. Additionally, the known incremental costs are also added into the retail price to offset the known costs that vary by the number of units sold each month. Once the costs are added into the price, then the profitability is added in to arrive at the final retail price of the device. For example, consider the situation presented in Table 7–2, where the practitioner's goal is to make a 150% profit over the fixed and incremental costs. In this example, the cost of the instrument is $1000 including shipping and handling, the incremental or variable costs are $500 per unit and the fixed costs are $500 per unit. At this point, there are $2,000 in costs that must be made up before the 150% profit is added into the equation. Marking up the costs of $2000 by 150% gives us a retail price of $3000 which will be charged to the patient for the instrument.

Target-Return Pricing Scheme

Target pricing involves obtaining a price for products that will yield a certain return on investment (ROI). This method is often used by large corporations that manufacture automobiles and toasters that look for a return on their investment of 15 to 20%. Although this is often good enough if the corporation sells 50,000 units of a product, it is not very applicable to the audiology practice unless the percentage of return is greater. An ROI of 120% is more

Table 7–2. Cost-Plus Pricing Example

Cost-Plus Markup Pricing Example—150% Over Cost	
Cost of Instrument . . . . Including Shipping/Handling	$1,000
Cost of Dispensing Instrument . . . . Time, Variable Costs, Warranty Costs	$500
Fixed Costs	$500
Desired Profit (150% over costs)	$1,000
Total Retail Sales	$3,000

reasonable for the audiology practice since the number procedures of products is usually extremely low in comparison to looking at the return on investment for a manufacturing process and provides a target pricing scheme that will in give the practitioner reasonable profit for the investment that has been made in the practice. To utilize the target return method for pricing the formula is:

$$TRP = \text{Unit Cost} + \frac{DR \times IC}{\text{Unit Sales}}$$

Where the target return price (TRP) is equal to the total unit cost (including acquisition, incremental and fixed costs) plus the profit which consists of the desired return (DR) times the invested capital (IC) divided by the unit sales. If the target return pricing concept is considered for pricing a videonystagmography (VNG) procedure the estimated cost to provide each procedure must first be calculated and then that sum must be added to the desired profit.

When using the target return method of pricing all costs must be figured per unit. For pricing purposes, all costs are added together including, acquisition, fixed, and incremental/variable and figured as a factor of each unit produced. Although conducting a VNG does not necessarily incur real acquisition costs, there are fixed and incremental costs that must be considered. The real costs of conducting the VNG procedure include an employee cost to cover time conduct and reporting the examination of $6,000 per year ($500 per month), lease payments on the equipment of $6000 per year ($500 per month), material costs of $300 per year (paper, etc.), and allocated space costs of $1200 per year. Other costs that must be included in the initial cost calculation are $2000 for marketing, $1000 for continuing education, and $5000 for insurance discounts. As presented in Table 7–3, the total estimated unit cost, if 180 procedures are conducted per year is $21,500 and when calculated per procedure (180 procedures per year) there are $119.44 of the total retail price simply to cover costs.

$$\text{Total Unit Cost} = \frac{\Sigma \text{ Costs}}{N \text{ Procedures per year}}$$

$$\$119.44 = \frac{21,500}{180 \text{ Procedures per year}}$$

To arrive at the total retail price of the VNG procedure the practitioner's goals for profit must be considered since $119.44 simply covers the: cost of performing the evaluation. Although this covers the costs, the profit component must be added in to allow the return on investment (ROI) necessary to meet the practitioner's goals. In this example, the practitioner's goal is to achieve a 125% ROI of $25,000 that it took to implement the

Table 7–3. Costs Per Year to Conduct VNG

$6,000	Employee time to conduct the procedure
$6,000	Payments of the equipment
$300	Materials
$1,200	Space Costs
$2,000	Marketing Costs
$1,000	Continuing education
$5,000	Insurance discount
$21,500	Costs to conduct VNG for 1 Year

procedure into the clinic. The formula for obtaining the total retail price (TRP) is presented below:

$$ROI = \frac{DR \times IC}{Unit\ (Procedure)\ Sales}$$

Where, the ROI is equal to the desired return (DR) times the invested capital (IC) divided by the unit or procedure sales per year. In this case, the practitioner's desired return on the capital investment of $25,000 is 125%, or $31,250 and will require obtaining $31,250 per year in profit. Using the formula above, the calculation of the total retail price of the VNG becomes simple arithmetic:

$$ROI = 173.61 = \frac{31,250 \times 25,000}{180}$$

The ROI component of the price for each of the 180 VNG procedures per year is $31,250/180 or $173.61 per procedure. By rounding the costs per procedure to $120 and the ROI per procedure to $174 per, these two figures are added together to obtain the total retail price of the VNG procedure at $294, covering both the costs necessary to conduct the procedure and the desired return on investment necessary to meet the practitioner's goals.

If the practice sells 180 VNG procedures per year, then the return on the investment, or profit would be 1.25% at the end of the year. If, however, there were not 180 VNG procedures conducted, it might be beneficial to use a breakeven analysis to determine how many procedures it would take, given the practitioner's costs, to not make a profit, but simply recover costs. It is possible to determine these figures from a breakeven analysis which reveals how many units it takes to break even, and thus, at what number of procedures profit begins.

A review of the problems with cost-plus pricing begins with an assessment of costs. Generally, in cost-plus pricing there is a problem in finding a product's real unit cost before determining its price. That is, product costs usually change relative to the number of units sold. For example, if you order one or two hearing instruments per month there is a minimal discount, but if 20 or 30 per month are ordered a much larger discount is realized. If a true cost-plus or markup pricing system is instituted, there is one price for products that have a marginal discount and another price for those that have a major discount based upon volume sales. If patient demand goes down, then the price goes up, if patient demand goes up the price goes down. Thus, true cost plus pricing is difficult to achieve and leads to overpricing in weak markets and underpricing in strong markets. Audiology practices can use buying groups and other methods to reduce this patient demand/price difficulty but problems still arise in keeping up with actual costs. Costs for products, not only rise and fall across manufacturers, but some clinicians take more time, and some points of product and service delivery (locations) are higher cost than others. Thus, the literature suggests that if cost-plus pricing is used at all, it should only be used as the minimum price to charge (Dolan & Simon, 1996; Nagle & Dolan, 2004; Staab, 2000).

Although cost-plus or markup pricing is not a recommended process as the procedure ignores such issues as current demand, perceived value, and competition components of the pricing equation; it remains the most used pricing system among audiology practitioners (see Table 7–2). As discussed earlier, the procedure is to mark up products and services by some magical percentage or formula to ensure a fair price to the consumer, but also cover business operating costs and to make a profit. In times before programmable and digital hearing instruments, the old time commercial hearing aid dealers had a "rule of thumb" where the retail price of a hearing instrument was 5 times its cost (see Sidebar 7–3). Although the 5 times cost rule does not work these days as costs have substantially increased, many audiologists use some version of this simple system, such as 2, 3, or 4 times cost to price their products. Although this is the most popular method of incorporating of cost-plus or markup pricing strategy, percentage markups are often used as well to allow for cost coverage and profitability. Percentage methods are essentially the same but add a percentage markup to the cost of an item rather than a set amount. A percentage markup may be computed by taking the cost of the instrument, ALD, or other product and adding a percentage to the cost, such as 150%. If the cost is $100 then the retail price in the practice would be $250.

Other than the straight markup procedures there are some other philosophies that can be utilized. First, the practitioner can obtain a price for products that insure a certain "return on investment" (ROI) often referred to in the pricing literature as a Target-Return philosophy. Most businesses price products to insure an expected return about 15 to 25% which provides a target pricing scheme that allows the practitioner a profit for the investment that has been made in the practice.

Another method of pricing according the cost-plus or markup strategy uses the breakeven analysis. The breakeven analysis considers the fixed, variable, and total operational costs and determines the number of units or amount of revenue necessary for the practice to reach a breakeven point—where the practice costs equals total revenue (Parkin, 2005) (see Figure 7–5). Staab (2000) indicates that once this point is exceeded, profits increase in direct proportion to the level of sales achieved beyond this point. The breakeven analysis for the practice can be put into spreadsheet form and various "what if" scenarios can be exercised to determine the necessary prices to cover expenses and to achieve profit goals.

Expected Profit

The expected profit is the amount that the clinic expects to make from the sale of products and services. This is based upon the margin minus any negotiated price discounts or inclusions that were required to make the sale. Margin is based on the value added and the ultimate price for the product and the number of units of product sold.

Product Life Cycle

Generally, the price of any product is based upon its utility, longevity, and the maintenance required throughout its lifetime. In audiology, product utility, longevity, and maintenance requirements change with technologic improvements and, accordingly, the appropriate product or service price must be continually evaluated and adjusted for these updates. Since the advent of digital hearing instruments in the mid-1990s, the product life cycle has been expanded greatly. Manufacturers realized this years ago when they began charging more (double or more) for repairs for hearing instruments

that are 5 years old or more. Digital processing allowed for more modification of a fitting over a longer period of time and accommodation of hearing loss as it progresses. Thus, there may be costs for services incurred by the patient, but they may be able to use the same devices for quite a while. The average life of a hearing instrument varies as there are those that find themselves in bad environments, such as moisture, dirt, and so forth, while other instruments live in a pristine environment. Experience suggests that the average life of a BTE device in a pristine environment may be 8 years or more and an ITE is about 4 to 5 years. Of course, experienced audiologists have seen beneficial instruments that are much older and devices that have run their useful cycle with a much shorter lifespan. Patients have different perspectives on the useful life of hearing instruments, some will use them as long as possible, while others are interested in staying on the edge of technology. Nevertheless, there is a product cycle that puts some years at higher sales than other years. For example if the practice has been in business for 5 or 6 years, then it not only has those patients that would normally be seen for new instruments during the year, but also those patients that need to replace their devices, increasing income to the practice. The key is that pricing for returning should still be reasonable as patients go through the repurchase process.

Fundamental Concepts in Pricing

Pricing decisions have great impact on the profitability of the practice, patient demand for products and services, and the latitude of the practice to adjust its competitive position (Marn and Rosiello, 1992). Price can be the centerpiece of strained relations with long time patients and are often the weapon competitors use to steal market share. Pricing audiologic services and hearing instruments is typically a balance between the patient's desire for a good value and the practice's need to cover costs and earn a profit. Profit, according to Dolan and Simon (1996), is generated by the number of units of service and products (volume) sold times the assigned price for which each unit sells minus relevant costs incurred to secure the sale. A look at hearing instrument dispensing would suggest that profit is dependent on the number of instruments dispensed times the price of the instruments to the patient minus the fixed and relevant incremental/variable costs.

$$Profit = Sales\ Volume \times Price - Costs$$

Though a simplistic concept, pricing is far more involved than arbitrarily assigning how much revenue the practice owner chooses to make, what the competition charges, or the suggested retail price offered by the instrument manufacturer. In addition to understanding the costs in the practice, accurate and effective pricing requires a full perspective of how the patient views the value of the services provided and products dispensed and a reasonable understanding of what price points the targeted market segment will withstand.

Correct pricing is essential to survival as it impacts the profitability of the practice. When products and services are priced too high, many patients will refuse to purchase them. Prices that are too high will cause the practice to relinquish market share to its competitors as perspective patients will move to more reasonably priced alternative clinics within the market place. Unless the environment is ripe for presenting the clinic as the high priced place to go for treatment, the practice will eventually need to lower its prices in an effort to regain attention, hoping that it is not too late to recapture patients due to negative consumer sentiment. Pricing too low also causes difficulty for the clinic as there is a missed opportunity to earn the correct profit proportional to the value offered to patients. Sometimes prices are strategically set low to gain volume or market share (Costco, Walmart, and Sam's Club) but this can backfire in setting incorrect price expectations among patients. Often audiology practices attempt to compete with these low priced operations. While it can be challenging to compete without meeting their prices, it is the wise clinician that realizes it is usually business suicide to compete with these large discount operations on price alone. These operations have totally different cost structures than a traditional audiology clinic and offer competitive challenges to the private practitioner competing with a low price philosophy. Attempts to compete on price will usually result in returning to a more reasonable retail prices or a business closure. Smith (2012) indicates that practices recovering from pricing too low will generally face a headwind of patient expectations for products and services to be priced too low.

Over the years, one of the cardinal rules of pricing has been to cover *ALL costs* but covering costs is only a portion of the pricing equation. Of course covering costs is essential, but it is not the only consideration when pricing products. Nagle et al. (2011) presents that a good pricing strategy not only considers costs but also involves five distinct but very different sets of choices of that build upon one another. To illustrate this concept they offer a strategic pricing pyramid, presented in Figure 7–6. Lower levels of the pyramid are supportive concepts that provide a foundation for each following level until the peak, where the prices are actually set. These considerations are:

- Value Creation—Economic value, offering design, and segmentation
- Price Structure—Metrics and fences
- Price and Value Communication—Communication and value selling
- Pricing Policy—Negotiation tactics and criteria for discounting
- Price level—Actual price setting.

Value Creation

The cash cow of any audiology practice is hearing devices. These instruments are obtained for invoice cost that is assigned by the manufacturer according to the features and benefits of a particular instrument. This is the *wholesale* price representing the product only and no services. The *retail* price is not simply the hearing instruments but the audiology expertise required to evaluate the patient's hearing loss and situation, selection of the appropriate device, programming and fitting, and the follow-up support offered by the physical presence of the audiologist and the clinic. Without the value added by the audiological expertise and the clinical support to

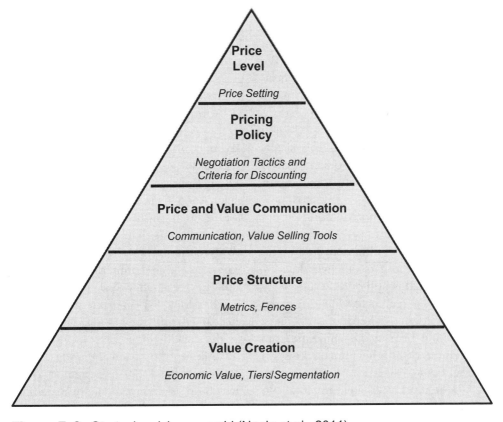

Figure 7–6. Strategic pricing pyramid (Nagle et al., 2011).

the devices, patients would have to figure out what devices to obtain, how to program them, how to use them, send them somewhere when they break, etc. Since the value added to the bare product is created by the audiologist and the clinic, the question remaining is how this added value is perceived by the patient and what is this expertise worth to them?

Nagle et al. (2011) state that most people are unwilling to pay for things that are new to them or for products they do not understand. Hearing instruments are generally new and unfamiliar to most purchasers as most patients do not take the time, energy and effort to become familiar with various devices, unless they are experienced users. Even educated, savvy new purchasers of hearing instruments are often confused by the myriad of styles, brands, methods of purchase, and differences in education standards for those that fit them as well as other variables that must be considered in the acquisition of amplification. Complicating the process is that hearing instruments are usually differentiated by technology where a high technology (higher cost) hearing instrument looks physically identical to entry level products (lower cost), contributing to confusion and purchase reluctance. Additionally, most new patients have heard horror stories about the high cost of these products and that many people have obtained little or no benefit from these expensive devices. Internet searches add additional confusion in that a search for "hearing aids" are likely to net a herd of Web sites, most selling hearing instruments from one vendor or another, but lacking an independent discussion features and their benefits. These sites are likely to offer hearing devices at much lower cost than professional audiology clinics and

patients unfamiliar with amplification and the value added by audiologists are tempted to simply purchase the lowest priced product. The patient's unfamiliarity with these devices and their use makes them even more reluctant to purchase an unwanted product. Thus, the *value* that *clinicians and their physical clinics* add to a hearing instrument is a significant portion of the purchase price.

Economic and Differentiation Value

The term *value* commonly refers to the overall satisfaction that a patient receives from using a product or service offering. Nagle et al. (2011) indicate that economists call this *use value* or the utility gained from the product. They further present that there is significant value in the convenient placement of products. To illustrate this concept they use the example of a hot day on a beach where the *use value* of a cold drink is quite high for most people; perhaps as high as $10 for a cold soda or a favorite brand of beer. Since few people would actually pay that price, knowing the use value is of little assistance to beach vendors selling their wares. The people on the beach know from experience that except in rare situations they would not have to pay a seller all that a product is really worth to them. They also know from past experience that competing sellers will usually offer a better deal at prices closer to what they expect from past experience, maybe $2 for a soda. The people on the beach might also know that a half-mile up the beach the soda can be purchased for $1.50 and a short drive away there is a convenience store selling whole 6-packs for $3.99. Consequently, the thirsty sun worshipers would probably reject a very high price ($10) even when the product was worth that much to them. Thus, the value of pricing strategy is *not use value*, but is what economists call *exchange value* or *economic value*. Using the example of Nagle et al. (2011), not many of the beach people walk up the beach and pay $1.50 and almost none will take the short drive to the convenience store to take the deal at $3.99. They will rather take the soda for $2 delivered to their beach blanket. The vendor adds value to the soda by having it available easily and conveniently, this concept is called a *differentiated product offering*. Differentiated product offerings are the reason that a $5.00 umbrella in a rainstorm it costs $20, a hot dog that costs $1 at the local convenience store is $7.00 at the ball game, and why $3,100 in high technology hearing instruments on the Internet will cost $6,995 at the audiology clinic. *Differentiation value* suggests that there is some sort of differentiation to most products sold that adds value to them. This concept could be selling soda at the beach, hot dogs at the ball park, or the value that an audiologist adds to amplification products and/or the convenience of offering evaluations, amplification, assistive listening devices, batteries, and other ear care products altogether in one place.

Differentiation value has two components, *monetary value* and *psychological value*. Both of these components maybe instrumental in a consumer's choice but there are very different approaches to them. *Monetary value* represents the total cost savings or income enhancements that a patient accrues as a result of the purchase of a particular product. In audiology clinics, this could be funds saved by the use of an entry level device versus the premium product or a device that uses less batteries, such as a rechargeable instrument. Well-fit hearing instruments have a great *psychological value* to our patients. The communication enhancement the patient receives may allow them to keep their job, obtain a better one, save their marriage, allow appropriate social interactions, or other benefits. Sometimes psychological satisfaction is created for patients by the prestige of seeing a particular audiologist, or going to a specific clinic and other times it is being the first with a new type of instrument, such as Lyric or the new IICs. These are differentiations that may or may not be worth a higher price, depending on the competitive environment.

Value-Based Price Segmentation

Each industry has its own quarks relative to pricing. In the airline industry scheduling your flight in advance will net a lower price than finding a flight on a day's notice. Hotels offer discounts on certain nights that they often do not fill, just to get you to stay with them on those empty nights. In the 1980s hearing instruments were usually priced by their size where a BTE cost less than a CIC. Since the1990s, hearing instrument manufacturers have modified their pricing such that devices with the most technology are the highest cost, no matter what the style (ITE, BTE ITC CIC, IIC, etc.). It is well known to audiologists that exactly the same device styles are differentiated by de-featuring (thus, theoretically de-benefiting) the instruments to offer a middle and, further de-featured, entry level technology at lower prices. Manufacturers even offer previous generation technologies for the most price sensitive patients. To accommodate various types of patients, most audiology clinics structure their pricing in tiers according to the technology involved.

To pricing experts, tiers are considered as a *value-based price segmentation*. This concept insures that pricing is commensurate with the actual value perceived and delivered to patients. The goal of a value-based market segmentation is to divide the market into subgroups, often called tiers by audiologists, whose product members have a common criteria to differentiate buying behaviors. The segments or tiers are necessary as some patients are older and sedentary and others are active; some have complex variables in their hearing impairment and others do not while still others are simply cost conscious. The various technology levels which are designated as tiers/segments enable a practice pricing structure that offers a "something-available-for-everyone" strategy. Audiologic variables such as the severity of the patient's loss, speech recognition capabilities and loudness tolerance issues, lifestyle, and other issues become important in the process of selecting a particular tier/segment of instruments best suited for the patient's

particular needs. By discussing the benefits of each instrument group or tier/segment, the patient's clinical status, lifestyle, and financial capability will, by necessity, become the focus discussion. Tiered/segmented pricing structures enable a patient to incorporate both benefit and value in their decision making. If the instruments within each tier/segment are appropriately priced, adequate margins can be expected to be fair and reasonable pricing for both the clinic and the patient. Tiered/segmented pricing reinforces the practitioner-patient partnership where both parties are working together to generate an optimal outcome at the best price possible.

From a business standpoint, a practice will lose patients without a tiered/segmented pricing system. Dolan and Simon (1996) state that heterogeneous customers warrant the cost of administrating multiple classes (or tiers/segments) and differing price relationships. In business it is always better to sell something at a profit, than to sell nothing as demonstrated in Figure 7–7. These figures, adapted from Dolan and Simon (1996),

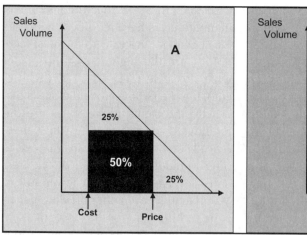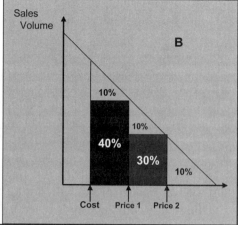

Figure 7–7. Pricing tiers/segments.

present the fact that with a single price for products, such as hearing instruments, sales are limited to about 50% of the patients presenting themselves for treatment as many may have difficulty affording the services or products (Figure 7–7A). Figure 7–7B considers a two tiered/segment system and demonstrates that if there are two pricing structures more patients will opt to purchase since they are more able to afford the instruments required to treat their hearing loss. Although some of the sales from higher priced tier are compromised, the overall profit to the practice will be greater since more of the patient population presenting can afford the hearing instruments. If the tiers/segments are increased to three and four the same benefits to the bottom

line will occur, although the percentage of increased sales for each added tier/segment becomes smaller. Clinics should consider 4 levels of pricing presented in the pricing pyramid in Figure 7–8. First, the *Budget Level* is for those patients that have significantly reduced needs or are extremely resource limited. Virtually all manufacturers offer products from a previous generation of devices, usually priced very favorable in all styles. Second level or *Entry Level* instruments are those products that are the current generation but significantly de-featured. For example, often if the highest level technology has 20 channels, the entry level may have 6 or 8 channels and may have 2 programs that change automatically rather than 4. Still extremely good technology, but not

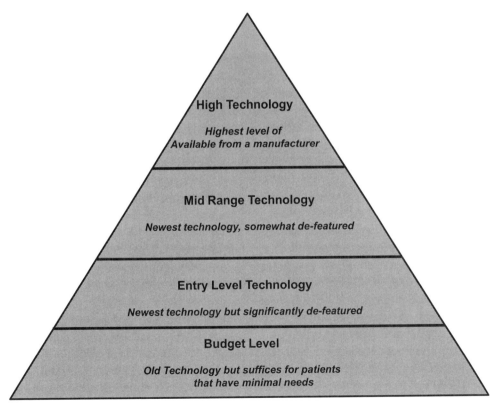

Figure 7–8. Pricing tiers/segments for hearing instruments.

the highest level that the chip may have the capability to offer. The *Mid-Range* technology is de-featured somewhat, but not to the degree of the entry level. For example, these devices may have 16 channels, 3 automatic programs, and other features that differentiate it from both the entry level and high technology instruments. The *High Level* technology is the state of the art chip with all features, such as 20 channels, 4 automatic programs, and many other features accessible to facilitate the best possible, state of the art option for the patient's hearing impairment and lifestyle.

The development of a value price segmentation or tiers, according to Nagle et al. (2011), involves 6 steps:

1. *Determine Basic [Tier] Segmentation Drivers.* The market must be divided into tiers that have common criteria allowing for the differentiation of one patient from another. In audiology this is rather simple as there are patients that require the most technology available, such as physicians, lawyers, high pressure business people, and others. The lowest technology level might include those patients that are financially limited and/or are sedentary. Most clinics now offer 3 to 4 tiers or price segments to facilitate the variable needs of their patients at all cost levels.

2. *Identify the Discriminating Value Drivers or Purchase Motivators.* For each of the tiers/segments, the audiologist needs to obtain information as to the situations that are the most important to the patient. This allows the clinician to offer suggestions and make recommendations as to the appropriate tier/segment of product necessary to meet the rehabilitative goals for each individual patient.

3. *Review Operational Constraints and Advantages.* In this step the practice manager reviews those value drivers that can be delivered more efficiently and at a lower cost than the competition. This could be that a clinic has greater clinical expertise than others, more knowledge of the product benefits and limitations within the various segments, more programming capability than the competition or other competitive operational issues.

4. *Create Primary and Secondary [Tiers] Segments.* This component is already known to audiologists as part of their training and experience, Different types of patients require various levels of product. The application of the auditory, personal style, lifestyle, and communication needs variables can be used to set up the tiers/segments, where the price of specific product tiers/segments are according to the benefits offered. Within some tiers there may be one group or brand of products that will be of more benefit than others for specific types of patients.

5. *Create Detailed [Tier] Segment Descriptions.* Clinicians need to have some idea of which types of patients benefit from each of the tiers/segments, experienced audiologists realize that the tiers/segments adjustment from time to time according to changes in technology and their interaction

with patient auditory variables, communication needs, and lifestyle. Margins, the value added to the bare product should remain the same for all tier/segments as the value added is the same no matter which tier/segment is chosen.

6. *Develop Tier Segment Metrics and Fences.* The metric or actual monetary value is the basis for tracking what patients receive and how they pay for it. It is important for audiologists to recognize that tiering/segmentating is not very useful until you develop the metrics for the value offered by each and devise fences that encourage patients to accept price policies for their specific tier/segment.

Mironov (2003) cautions that the presentation of the various pricing tiers/segments should be simple as most buyers can't handle pricing complexity. Presenting today's amplification products, the various benefits and limitations to a particular patient can be very confusing. If patients are given too many choices, they may panic and, while some will suffer through the sales process, others vanish into a cloud forever. Audiologists have varying levels of sales or rehabilitative skills. Practice managers must decide which clinicians can sell, providing essential rehabilitative treatment and those professionals whose time is best spent conducting diagnostic evaluations. Most patients are very clever when presented with many pricing plans (segments or tiers), they usually figure out which tier will save them the most, so it is essential to carefully develop the pricing tiers/segments.

Price Structure

Pricing structure is the development of a method that reflects the differences in the potential contribution to the practice income of particular tiers/segments. Capturing the best possible price from each tier/segment is essential to maximizing income from sales within each tier/segment. Although audiologists and practice managers understand the differences among patients and the need for various pricing levels, they also must appreciate that to keep the practice profitable in times when low cost products make up most of the sales; margins for these lower cost products tiers/segments must allow profitability.

Fencing

Key to structuring prices is the concept of *fencing*. Fencing is pricing terminology for how the differences between the tiers/segments are presented to the patient. Basically, what are the differences among the various tiers/segments? What do I get with the high end device? What don't I get with the low end device? The fence is the possible benefits that the patient must give up in order to compromise to the next lower priced tier or segment (see Figures 7–7 and 7–8). As discussed by Nagle et al. (2011), fencing is fundamentally the identification and classification of various levels of buyers and is known in pricing circles as the buyer identification fence. Hearing impaired patients have obvious characteristics that allow audiologists to identify who belongs to which tier/segment and what "fences" they need to climb to qualify for the next higher or lower tier. Presenting the differences among the various tier/

segments and the functional application of each product within the tiers, at least in audiology, clearly relies upon the aural rehabilitative treatment skills of the clinician in sorting patients by their rehabilitative requirements. Thus, proper price fencing is really effective aural rehabilitative treatment. A tiered/segmented offering scheme presents the patient with the best options for them, while the simple selling of one high priced product to all patients requires little skill, is probably unethical, and is simple product sales, not aural rehabilitative treatment.

Pricing Metrics

A price metric defines the units to which a price is applied. They define the terms of exchange or, in other words, what exactly does the patient receive in exchange for the price paid? There may be differences in product performance, warranty, and various other inclusions or a special market offering for a limited time only. Pricing literature offers 5 components of a good price metric:

1. A good price metric should have the same value same across the tiers/segments. Since the value added by the audiologist to each tier/segment is essentially the same this component of the metric may possibly remain the same across the various tiers/segments, There may, however, be differences in the features and benefits as well as other inclusions (warranty, batteries, accessories) that facilitate price also facilitate these price reductions.
2. Effective price metrics track the differences in the costs, particularly variable or incremental costs associated with serving patients choosing the various tiers/segments. Basically, the margin or value added should stay the same reflecting a difference in price across the tiers but with an appropriate amount of value added. Patients that are lured by price alone will naturally be served by the discount houses, such as Walmart, Costco, and the Internet. Those that value the extra benefit provided offered by the expertise of the audiologist and the support from the clinic will usually consider the price reasonable. Basically, this second component tracks the differences in the costs to serve the various patients that make up each tier/segment and adjusts prices accordingly.
3. Price metrics should be easy to understand and to implement with no ambiguity as to how much the patient has to incur in expense to obtain the products and services necessary within a particular tier/segment. Both audiologists and their patients should be able to figure out the metric easily.
4. Price metrics should attempt to place the clinic's offer more favorably than competitive offers. Practice managers should consider the price metric in terms of how it positions the practice relative to competitive clinics in the market place. As price metrics are considered clinicians should also respect the impact of patient perceptions of the clinic that will affect the attractiveness of the clinic to specific patients.
5. The price metric should align with the audiologist's experience

of patients using the product or service. The better the alignment, that is, how the metric fits the timing and magnitude of the patients expenditure, the more attractive the offer.

These fundamental components pricing metrics should be considered as the various tiers/segmentations are created.

Bundling/Unbundling

Smith (2012) states that price bundling is a concept that benefits from heterogeneity of demand. Specifically this suggests that when there is demand for two separate products it makes sense to consider putting them together into one product. Thus, by combining a product, such as hearing instruments, with another product, the audiologic services required to add value and benefit to the devices, we have *a bundled* product: Hearing instruments and audiologic services. If the clinic choses to separate those charges with specific prices for each service and product offered the pricing scheme would be considered *unbundled*. Bundled fees often even include batteries, extra warranty, accessories, and other products as part of the bundle. When fees are itemized or unbundled, the price of the hearing aid(s) as well as the fees to deliver the hearing aid(s) are billed and itemized separately. Abel (2011) presents that one of the hottest topics in the current coding and reimbursement arena is whether to bundle or unbundle hearing aid and/or assistive listening device services. Abel indicates that when a hearing aid claim is filed to a third-party payer, reimbursement is more likely to be captured when services are itemized (unbundled); however, many practitio-

ners feel itemized services may result in patients not returning to their office for the necessary follow-up care as it costs them extra for more follow-up visits.

Historically, the distaste by audiologists for unbundling began as part of the process by which the American Speech Language Hearing Association (ASHA) mandated that hearing instruments be dispensed back in the early days of hearing instrument dispensing. In the early 1970s, the sale of hearing instruments by audiologists was prohibited by the ASHA code of Ethics (Staab, 2012). When compared to traditional hearing aid dispensers of the time, it was obvious that audiologist's had the academic background to facilitate increased benefit from hearing devices. This actually showed how little audiologists at that time knew about business. Due to ASHA certification regulations of the time, audiologists would lose their ASHA Certificate of Clinical Competence in Audiology (and many did) if they did not adhere to the strict ASHA regulations in the dispensation of hearing instruments. Thus, most clinicians simply complied with the ASHA mandated regulations or did not sell products. A prevailing view of among audiology professors and influential individuals in ASHA at the time was articulated by McConnell et al (1973) that stated, "It was OK for audiologists to dispense as long as they did not make a profit." As Staab (2012) reviews, as early as the 1971 ASHA convention in Chicago, discussion had already taken place about a plan for hospital clinics to sell hearing aids on a non-profit basis. Proponents of this plan contended that the ASHA plan would reduce the cost of hearing instruments by 300% or more while assuring patients of professional care and fitting. In Staab's opinion, this actually showed how little audiologists

Sidebar 7–4
BUNDLING AND UNBUNDLING OF PRICES

There is much discussion in the literature and at conferences about another method of reducing prices for products. Since there is more to hearing instrument use than the product itself, most hearing instruments are sold with many services bundled into the costs. Ross (2005) indicates that the selection and fitting process takes time and audiologists may spend four contact hours or more with each new hearing aid user. Of course, audiologists still need to interview the person, conduct appropriate audiometric and other tests, take ear impressions, select and fit the aids, reprogramming when necessary, schedule several follow-up appointments, provide all necessary information, and deal with drop-ins when problems occur. Ross views these kinds of services as intrinsic to the hearing aid selection process. Without these services, patients could easily purchase hearing aids through mail order catalogues.

In this concept of unbundling hearing instrument delivery the device is sold as a distinct product and that every evaluation, clinical activity, and follow-up visit are charged separately. The proponents of unbundling point out that some patients take an inordinate amount of the audiologists time, returning often for troubleshooting visits, while others take relatively little time, but that both pay the same price for the hearing aid. Thus, some patients can be said to be subsidizing the visits of other patients. The unbundling approach makes each patient pay only for the services that they receive whereas the opponents of unbundling are convinced that many people would not return for necessary follow-up services, and/ or would not contact the audiologist when problems occur. Often patients require extra assistance with amplification products that repeated visits can give them, but unless these services are part of the original deal they are unable or unwilling to pay for them, or simply unaware of the frequent necessity for follow-up visits. Bundled pricing means that the patient not only purchases the hearing instrument, but they also receive services on the instrument for a period of time, often for the warranty period, sometimes for life.

Harrington-Gans (2006) feels that patients actually respond positively to the unbundling of fees and services from the product costs and when payment was requested for services required, they did not question the charges. The unbundling or separation of product price from the fees and follow up services can also be a strategy for competition in price sensitive markets. This strategy can allow the practitioner to reduce their price for products while maintaining their services separate keeping the cost of the products competitive. Although this appears to be a price cut, it is actually diverting the higher costs to those that use the extra services.

at that time knew about business since these figures totally ignored operating costs, insurance, overhead, equipment purchases, bad debt, and benefits such as medical plans, retirement, and taxes. Although 40 years later this seems like a ridiculous concept to anyone that understands business, it was the reality of the time. To circumvent this frustration, many audiologists found other means to practice their profession, integrating amplification into the aural rehabilitation process. Rather than sell products and lose their ASHA certification, clinicians would have their patients order hearing instruments from a mail order hearing aid sales company. When the instrument arrived at the patient's home, they would then bring the device to the audiologist and charges would be incurred for the fitting and aural rehabilitation services. This would allow audiologists to manage their patient's rehabilitative needs without violation of the ASHA code of ethics. Audiology businesses thrived on this mail order model in the early to late 1970s and it served a real purpose in the need to circumvent the ASHA dispensing regulations, hearing aid licensing, and other issues. After a major anti-trust suit in 1978, ASHA changed the rules and allowed audiologists to dispense hearing instruments fostering the beginnings of the private practice community. Thus, unbundling of product costs, fees has been in the vocabulary of audiologists for quite some time, but has not taken off as a universal model due to a historical distaste for the process and concern about patient benefit. Realistically, as conceived by ASHA, it was a ridiculous model designed and perpetuated by audiology university professors that had never sold products as part of business model and felt that audiologists were scientists not salespeople. Of course these "leaders" of the profes-

sion forgot that attorneys sell their services, surgeons sell surgeries, and engineers sell design and products, why not audiologists selling hearing instruments and offering professional services as part of their practice. Today, even clinicians that advocate an unbundled pricing system for their practice offer quite a different system than that old ASHA model.

Harrington-Gans (2006) studied and used an unbundled pricing system in her practice for a number of years. In her opinion, this model was a solution to the problem that some patients require a substantial amount of time whereas fittings for others are simple and unbundling spreads the costs to those that really need the assistance. Patients that do not need as much rehabilitative treatment save money on their hearing rehabilitation, whereas those that need those extra rehabilitative visits for programming or counseling pay for the extra time required to provide the in depth services. Harrington-Gans (2006) indicates that her program suggested that unbundled pricing has the capability to:

- Differentiate a "doctors" practice from that of commercial hearing aid dealers.
- Reduce price shopping by patients.
- Limit or eliminate the non-income-producing follow-up visits after the sale.
- Increase repeat patients and shortens the time between new hearing instrument purchases.
- Produce strong word of mouth referrals without advertising.
- Control high payables due to vendors as the clinic pays for the instruments immediately.

One side of the bundling-unbundling argument is why should a patient pay for services included that they will never use? Often, there are many things included with a hearing aid purchase, such as unlimited follow-up visits, batteries, or longer warranties all included as part of the price segment (tier). The other side of that argument is that patients really want these things and they are used to purchasing products that have items bundled into them. For example, patients do not simply purchase a basic car, but it usually has power steering, power brakes, automatic transmission, and often has service features bundled into the price of the vehicle. McDonald's meals are a bundle of their products most often ordered with a basic hamburger, for a better price. When a new computer is purchased there is usually software and accessories that come with the purchase.

On the purist's side, it is probably ethical and reasonable to itemize each and every product, the services attached, evaluations, programming, and 1 to 2 follow-up visits. Inevitably, patients will want the product without these itemized services as they do not understand the value added by them. Whereas, if the bundled approach is taken, they will more readily accept the value added to the product and appreciate that there are some services and other products that come with the instruments to facilitate their use. Whatever the clinical decision is about bundling or unbundling it is necessary to incorporate the concept into the overall pricing strategy.

Price and Value Communication

At the next level of the pyramid in Figure 7–6 is price and value communication. At this level, the clinician develops a "willingness-to-pay" within the patient for the products and services offered through communication and sales tools. Pricing literature indicates that development of a patient's "willingness-to-pay" is among the most difficult of all tasks. The clinician's ability to develop this "willingness-to-pay" or value in the patient's mind begins with a thorough understanding of the value drivers for particular patient populations. It is no accident that many of the ads to the hearing impaired feature issues such as communication with the family or "hearing is not understanding" or "invisible hearing aids" as these are all value drivers that grab the patient's attention. Knowledge of these value drivers are based partially on the clinician's education, partially on experience, and to some degree on their personality and the rehabilitative treatment ability. As part of a Doctor of Audiology education, audiologists learn the variables of hearing loss that that drive the value of hearing rehabilitative treatment. For example, a patient that lives alone and does not go out very often has less need (less "willingness-to-pay") for the products and services of audiologists, while those with a moderate loss in a profession that involves communication have more of a handicap (more of a "willingness-to-pay"). For these patients, products and services offered by audiologists are perceived at a higher value. When the needs are significant as in severe to profound losses the value of the restorative products is even higher as these patients cannot interact at all without some rehabilitative intervention.

Nagle et al. (2011) state that the best method of communicating value is when the product can be shown to offer benefits that are not otherwise obvious to potential buyers. Furthermore, they indicate that the less experience a patient has in the market or the more innovative the product's the benefits, it is more likely the patient will not recognize or fully appreciate the value of the product or service. For that reason, automobiles are test driven before purchase, clothes are "tried on" before purchase, and ice cream is sampled before making a full cone purchase. Since most amplification patients have virtually no idea of what they are purchasing, one method of communicating value is through demonstrations or product trials. Working through a demonstration of hearing instruments, like the test drive of the automobile, presents an opportunity to show unknown and unexpected benefits to patients, building value for the products and associated audiologic services. Experienced clinicians usually find that just being able to hear better communicates the value of the product and begins the dialog that develops a "willingness-to-pay."

As clinicians are developing the "willingness-to-pay," patients are attempting to sort this audiologist's offering from the other market offerings that they may be considering. This concept is referred to by pricing professionals as the "*relative cost of search*." The "relative cost of search" refers to the patient's financial and nonfinancial expenditure that must incurred to evaluate the features and benefits of the products under consideration to complete an intelligent purchase. A few patients or their relatives will bring their Internet search and ask questions, whereas others will not have a clue as to one hearing device from another. Most patients will not even know what their amplification needs as often there is even difficulty understanding that they have a hearing difficulty. Thus, it is generally up to the audiologist to differentiate their product offering as part of their rehabilitative treatment program from the other

offerings presented to the patient by the market place.

There are two general components in the communication of price and value, *monetary* and *psychological*. Measureable monetary benefit would include increased productivity or keeping ones job as a result of the use of amplification, while psychological benefit would include comfort, appearance, pleasure of use, status of going to a particular clinic, or other issues. For some patients, a monetary discussion may be how they can obtain the most for the least cost. These monetary discussions should revolve around the features and benefits for a particular amount of cost. Why is this a good deal? What features do you get for the price? While most patients will be interested in the overall costs, when the discussion is primarily psychological the value is usually subjective and will vary from one patient to another. Psychological discussions focus the discussion on the benefits that the patient may not have expected from the device. How will those product's features be translated into actual benefits in conversation and other situations and, what is that worth? Further discussion would carefully raise the patient expectations of the product's performance benefits that are not easily judged until after the purchase. Of course, the clinician does not want to raise expectations so high that the device does not perform, but many patients do not have very high expectations of amplification and this can add psychological benefit. High cost searches are the issue with amplification. As discussed earlier, where will a patient find out information about amplification? The Internet is confusing and often inaccurate and it is a huge inconvenience to go to the audiology clinic and begin the search. Without experience how does the patient know that the information they are given is actually correct? As with most high cost items, Nagel et al. (2011) indicate that patients purchasing amplification will go through a four step purchasing process and the challenge is to adapt the rehabilitative message to each step (Figure 7–9). It is essential to recognize these various stages as patients are in varying stages of purchase and require specific types of information at various stages of purchase. A push for a sale at the wrong time can lead to a returned or unused products. The following stages of purchase for hearing-impaired patients are adapted from Nagle et al. (2011) (see Figure 7–9).

■ *Step 1: Origination.* At this stage the patient becomes aware that there is a need for the amplification products. From experience and the literature it is well known that most patients wait 5 to 7 years from the time that they recognize they need hearing instruments, until they actually purchase. Often the time between awareness and action can be reduced by a physician's examination or an audiological evaluation and/or rehabilitative discussions. As patients get closer to the purchase, they begin to search for a suitable offer in the market to fulfill their need.

■ *Step 2: Information Gathering.* Methods of search for a solution to the problem could involve the Internet, word-of-mouth recommendations, response to advertised offers, or simply a referral from their physician. At this stage the patient is simply obtaining information.

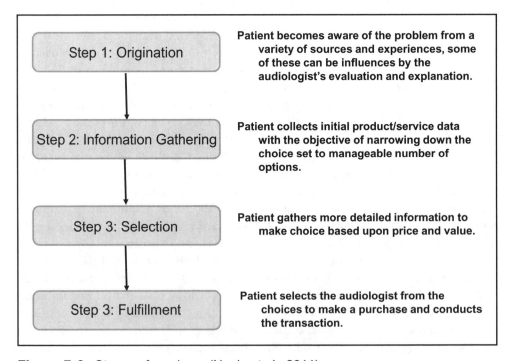

Figure 7–9. Stages of purchase (Nagle et al., 2011).

that will assist them in narrowing down the offers in the market for the device that they need. They may even evaluate one brand relative to another and various styles of amplification products, such as BTE, RIC, ITE, ITC, CIC, IIC, extended wear, and so forth. Patients will imagine what it is like to use these products each day and seek information that facilitates their decision. At this stage, clinicians should not push patients into purchase as they usually do not have enough information to make an informed decision. As in other areas of the purchase process, pushing patients to purchase while they are still gathering information will often lead to returns or unused amplification devices.

- *Step 3: Selection.* After much deliberation, the patient is finally ready to make a decision as to the particular clinic, audiologist, style of product and they sometimes even know the brand of instrument they would like to purchase. At this point, they are involved in the purchasing process and audiologists should present their recommendations for one tier/ segment over another. Clinicians should be aware that the combination of the product, their clinic, and their services are the brand that the patient purchases, not merely the hearing instrument.
- *Step 4: Fulfillment.* Nagle et al. (2011) describe this final stage of the buying process as the selection of a place to purchase and making the actual purchase of the instrumentation. They suggest that the value communication goal in step 4 is to justify price using value to create a favorable framing for the price,

benchmarking the prices against other offerings in the market. The clinician should also provide good fencing for the various tiers (value segmentations) offered by explaining the advantages and limitations of products each of the segments as part of their value communication. The patient is now ready to purchase and listening carefully to the various costs and options presented in the value communication.

It is rare for audiologists simply work with the patient when presenting their value communication. The buying process often involves the family, a spouse, or a friend and these individuals are also in some stage of recommending the purchase to the patient. In amplification purchases, the family, spouse, or other influential individuals often progress through the purchase process faster than that patient. Even though there may be substantial influence from others, it is essential that the patient be ready for the purchase. If the rehabilitative process has patients pushed too fast, by either the audiologist or others the patient will often return their instruments and/or not be successful in their use.

Methods of Price Communication

Pricing literature suggests that patients do not evaluate prices logically. This is especially true for products that have a high psychological value, such as hearing instruments. Patients will often perceive the same price paid in return for the same value differently depending upon how well the value is communicated to them. As in many fields where there is no exact answer to a question there are many suggestions as to how to present prices to purchasers. Pricing literature suggests that there are four components of price perception that are important to the communication of value and essential to the audiologist's knowledge of pricing. These four components are *proportional price evaluations, reference prices, perceived fairness,* and *gain-loss framing.*

1. *Proportional Price Evaluations.* Studies suggest that patients will evaluate prices proportionally rather than on simple amount differences. For example, if a 16 pack of batteries costs $16.00 at the clinic and a patient could purchase exactly the same product at Walmart or Costco for $10.00, there is roughly a 68% chance that they will purchase their batteries at the discount store to save the 40% or so on their batteries. The larger the purchase, however, the less a few dollars difference makes to them. An example of hearing instruments that cost $5,000 in one clinic and are offered for $4,795.00 at another. This would not be enough to make the patient go elsewhere as it is only a 4% difference and it is a larger frustration to go elsewhere than to pay the extra funds for the products and services. The key to the proportional evaluation is to determine what percentage of difference will send the patient elsewhere to shop for products.

2. *Reference Prices.* Recall from earlier discussions that the reference price is what the patient feels is a reasonable and fair price for the product and services. Patients may have a distorted idea of what is reasonable and fair and it is often necessary to communicate the value to them through the rehabilitative discussion. Marketers found long ago that buyers tend to give greater weight to the prices they see first suggesting that it is best to present prices in descending order from the highest to the lowest. Thus, audiologists will want to build value in their communication with patients presenting the prices for the highest tier/segment and, if necessary, work their way down to the lower cost tier/segment. This method in some circles is known as "top down selling," and works to effectively communicate the value of products and services even if the patient eventually chooses a lower cost tier/segment (Rajendran and Tellis, 1994).

3. *Perceived Fairness.* The process of arriving at a "just price" is of considerable mystery to virtually all that price products. When practitioners are making pricing decisions is necessary to simultaneously make some ethical decisions (Martins and Monroe, 1994). Figure 7–10 presents a number of pricing philosophies that can be incorporated into the pricing decision, including the path chosen by most practitioners where high quality is high priced, medium quality is medium priced, and low quality is low priced. Departures from this model may cause either ethical concerns or profitability problems.

The challenge to ethics is when the practitioner chooses the high price for medium or low quality products. Figure 7–10 presents that a possibility is to charge a high price (such as that normally charge for a high end digital

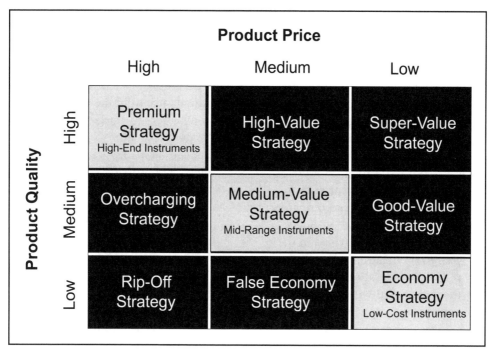

Figure 7–10. Pricing strategies (adapted from Kotler, 2001).

instrument) for a medium quality or low quality product. Charging the high price for a medium quality is simply considered as an overcharging strategy, while Kotler (2001) considered a high price for low quality to be a rip-off strategy. Although this may be part of the overall practice positioning, there are some ethical questions that arise with either of these strategies. The question that with either the overcharging or rip off strategies, the patient could acquire the exact same technology to provide the assistance necessary for much less cost and it is the audiologists responsibility to provide this technology for a *reasonable* cost. To the ethics purest, this "smells" of taking advantage of patients who do not understand the products

they are purchasing while maximizing the profit on each product.

On the other side of Figure 7–10 there is the opposite situation. In this situation, high quality products are presented to the public at a very low price for marking what Kotler (2001) presents as the super value or good value strategies. This strategy compromises profitability to provide the best possible products for a minimal amount of cost. Although this appears to be highly altruistic and a good deal for the patient, it can drastically compromise the profitability of the practice. Ethically, this can also be a problem in that the compromise of profitability may be the reason that that the practitioner will not survive in the marketplace and leave the patient to look for another practitioner before the warranty and other provider responsibilities have been conducted fully.

Patients seem to consider the "just price" by comparing what they think is the audiologist's likely margin. Although patients may not know the actual margin, they compare similar product margins to cost structures that are known to them or compare other medical/dental products they may have purchased in the past to the hearing related product under consideration. Although those that deal with amplification have not necessarily had a pristine reputation over the years, Campbell (1999) indicates that the audiologist's perceived motives can greatly affect patient perceptions of price fairness. Hence, visible clinics or specific audiologists with a high reputation can offer products and services at a higher price and still be considered "fair" by the patients they serve. The perception of a "just price" is further supported by keeping prices high enough that they can be discounted for slow times or to offer special incentives, rather than raising prices when business is slow to compensate for less business. Most patients understand that the clinic is in business to make a profit and that if there is no profit or incentive to the audiologist, then they lose significant value to the product and/or service they are purchasing.

4. *Gain or Loss Framing.* It is well documented (Kahneman & Tversky, 1984; Tversky & Kahneman, 1992); that most patients expect a certain price for an item and tend to judge "fairness" of a price based upon how much higher or lower the clinic's price point is relative to their expectation. While the methods patients use to frame those judgments affect the attractiveness of the purchase, there are methods that can be incorporated to insure the palatability of a particular price for a product or service. One method is to have a high list price and offer discounts. While this can be dangerous in that no one will ever want to pay the list price, the clinic's objective is for patients not to pay the list price, simply the discounted price allowing price adjustments according to various economic or clinical situations. A second method involves the use of adding services (warranty follow ups) or products (batteries, accessories) to the mix of product to frame the fairness of the price to the expectations of the patient (Staab, 2000).

Pricing Policy

If all patients paid the asked price for products and services, pricing policy would be simply that everyone pays the same, no matter what their needs or desires. Of course, there are rich patients, poor patients, those with less needs, those with more needs and those that just plain want a "good deal." If there is no firm pricing policy that determines how negotiations and discounts are offered, the patients will dictate their terms and ultimately they will set the prices for your clinic. The pricing policy (see Figure 7–6) is primarily how departures from the usual and customary price are conducted when there is patient opposition to the price for products and services. It provides direction for the employee or audiologist as to what can be negotiated or discounted and how these departures from the usual and customary price are applied. Nagle et al. (2011) state that pricing policy refers to the rules or habits, either explicit or cultural that determine how a clinic varies its prices when faced with factors other than value and costs to serve patients that threaten its ability to achieve its objectives.

Of course, drafting any policy for a practice is more than merely a task of writing it down and telling employees the rules of the game. It is necessary to insure the pricing policy is value related, suits the chosen business model, and is compatible with the goals and objectives all of the practice stakeholders. Successful pricing policies involve the evaluation, contemplation, and adjustment of a number of variables. Although some of these issues have been discussed under other levels within the pricing pyramid (see Figure 7–6), Cohen (2004) offers seven fundamental factors to consider as a pricing policy is developed:

1. *Determination of market segments.* Consideration of the product tiers/segments that are to be offered to patients. This assists the practice manager in the assessment of the value that the clinical and follow up services add to the bare product. Market tiers/segments are important for positioning and insuring sales will be maximized according to the needs and financial capability each patient. Here is where the practice manager and the clinical staff decide how many tiers/segments to offer (usually 3 to 4), and develop the appropriate academic, practical, and financial differentiations among them.

2. *Assessing the product's availability and near substitutes.* As discussed earlier, underpricing hurts the product offering (the audiologist, the clinic and the instrumentation) as much as overpricing. If the price is too low, potential patients will think that the audiologist, the clinic and the products offered are not really of high quality. Cohen (2004) feels this is particularly true for high-end, prestige brands, such as clinics with a high reputation or amplification products that are known brands to patients. Assessing availability also involve a general assessment of the competition, their credentials and clinical atmosphere to allow for differentiation of the clinic from the competitors. How easily can patients substitute another clinic (product) for the one offered by this clinic and how similar is that to the competition?

3. *Survey the market for competitive and similar products.* Consider whether new clinics, modifications of existing clinics, or new technologies offered in the market place compete with or, worse, leapfrog your offering. Examine all possible methods for patients to work with the clinic, such as referrals, word of mouth, media ads, and other methods. It may be necessary to become creative in your policy to explore the use and modification of all possible situations. If competitors attempt to mandate certain prices, it is possible to develop a

policy where products and services are priced higher as long as patient perceptions is that the brand combining the audiology services and products are significantly better (Erickson & Johansson, 1985).

4. *Examine market pricing and economics.* A good pricing policy is well thought out in terms of the products used to augment the hearing impairment, the value added by clinical and office personnel, and the advantages of a brick and mortar clinic that offers support. Questions that should be considered here include: Is this clinic capable of becoming the high cost facility for patients demanding high end services or should this market have a low cost clinic to meet the needs of the community? Should the clinic attempt to offer all prices to all patients? Should there be prices for adults in all market segments, at all price ranges? Should the clinic offer bundled and unbundled fees? Should the clinic serve pediatric patients and, if so, should the prices be structured the same as for adults? Are there price adjustments necessary due to economic conditions? If these adjustments are necessary, how are they conducted?

5. *Calculate the internal cost structure and understand how pricing interacts with the offering.* Although discussed separately (see Chapter 8), costs must be considered as part of the pricing policy. These would include fixed, avoidable, and sunk costs, but particularly important are the variable or incremental costs since they vary according to product and the services offered. For example,

the more ITE and ITC instruments that are sold, the more impression material is necessary or the more ABRs and routine evaluations conducted, the more tips are necessary for insert headphones. The longer the warranty, the more services that are provided at no charge, adding to the incremental costs. It is difficult to stay in business if the products and services sold are priced under what it costs to sell them and pay necessary overhead. Therefore, the pricing policy should carefully consider the margin in the context of maximizing profit for each tier/segment while considering the incremental and other costs involved in the delivery of products and services.

6. *Test different price points if possible.* Since markets vary in competition, patient income, economic situations, insurance offerings and many other variables, it may be necessary to present some price points to the market in an effort to determine the offering's value to patients. Although current markets change and require updates, test pricing is especially important if entering into a new, possibly untapped market or the offering of a new product or service as it allows the assessment of a many price points to determine their feasibility. Test pricing can be risky as it may be set too low, where patients feel that anything higher is too high or if set too high no product is sold.

7. *Monitor the market and your competition continually to reassess pricing.* Market dynamics and new products can influence and change consumer wants and needs. It is

essential to monitor prices and the market for changes in technology, procedural modifications, patient attitudes and needs as well as the clinic expenses for necessary changes in the pricing policy.

Patient Purchasing Behaviors

A buyer's decision to purchase differs greatly from items such as toothpaste, razor blades, mobile phones to vehicles houses and, of course hearing instruments. In a description of buyer types, Assael (1987) presents that there are four classic types of buyers in the market (Figure 7–11). Assael bases his types of buyers in Figure 7–11 on the degree of the buyer involvement in the purchase and the differences among brands. In audiology, the brands that are in discussion are the various competitive clinics that offering rehabilitative services and products.

■ *Complex Buying Behavior.* Patients will assume this type of behavior when they are highly involved in

a purchase process and perceive significant differences among brands. Kotler and Armstrong (2012) indicate that this behavior tends to be active when the purchase is expensive, risky, purchased infrequently, and highly self- expressive. Consumers often do not know the differences among products. In the general marketplace this behavior may be active for purchase of a computer processor where the computer has 2.68 GHz AMD and 8 GB dual core, 64 bit or, in an audiologic purchase, a Phonak Audeo hearing instrument with as 20 channels, bandwidth from 250 Hz to 9.2 KHz and 4 programs that automatically change according to the environment. This type of a buyer will work through a learning process where they develop product beliefs about the product, then attitudes, and finally, make an intelligent choice. This will be conducted first in the choice of the clinic that is chosen and within the clinical

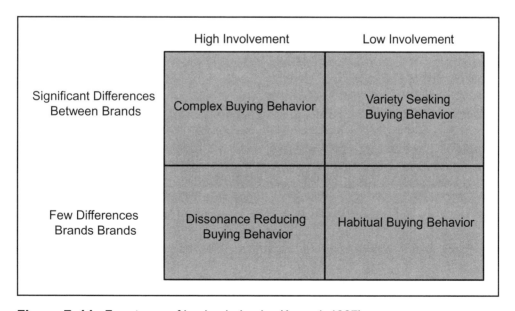

Figure 7–11. Four types of buying behavior (Assael, 1987).

situation another complex buying behavior will ensue regarding the specific brand of product. As audiologists it is the clinical skill, often called aural rehabilitation that is used to assist patients as they learn the various product tiers/segments and the features and benefits of each level. These patients respond well to literature, white papers, and other material as they are in a learning mode, discovering all possible information about the instruments they are considering. Clinicians must understand that, for some patients this is normal component of their buying process, especially when the product is expensive.

■ *Dissonance Reducing Buying Behavior.* Dissonance is a condition of mental conflict. Dissonance occurs in patients that are highly involved in an expensive, infrequent, or risky purchase and where they often see minimal difference among brands, such as in the purchase of hearing instruments. On the one hand the patient really needs the device, but on the other are the costs and the overall benefit. Did they purchase the correct level of product? What if they did not get the correct device? Most experienced audiologists have seen post purchase dissonance behavior. A good example of this is when the patient returns to the clinic with the hearing instruments in a plastic bag along with all the supplemental materials. Often, the dissonance is the result of a bad experience or a friend or relative that had the same brand of instruments and received little or no benefit. Dissonant patients are common in audiology clinics and if this is not handled correctly, the instruments will be returned and/or the patient will move to another clinic for purchase/services. To counteract the dissonance, Kotler and Armstrong (2012) suggest that after-sale communications should provide evidence and support to assist patients in feeling good about their choices. In audiology this is often done by follow calls, and visits designed to facilitate modifications in benefit and support the use of the devices.

■ *Habitual Buying Behavior.* A habitual buying behavior is usually demonstrated for products of low-patient participation and where minimal brand difference is obvious. Although this is not prevalent for hearing instruments it might be obvious for battery purchases. Since patients are often not loyal to brands, they simply go to the store and reach for the product, they may simply look for the right size and the best price. The purchase is inconsequential and, thus, does not justify the time, energy, and effort that it takes to research the best brand of batteries for their device.

■ *Variety Buying Behavior.* Patients will use a varietal behavior when they have a low involvement in the purchase but have a perception of significant brand differences. Often, patients will perceive that there are great differences among hearing instruments and they have used a particular brand for quite some time and are now ready to switch another brand simply because they are bored with the same brand or just to try something different. Usually, a market leader will work to obtain habitual business by dominating the outlets and frequently running advertisements that remind patients of the reasons to purchase their brand. Challenger products or second brand manufacturers will encourage variety and offer lower prices, special deals, coupons, marketing assistance or some other perk that puts their brand ahead of the market leader offering more "value for money."

Negotiation and Discounting

In the world of medical devices such as hearing instruments there are lots of opinions on discounting and negotiation. Staab (2000) indicates that price should never be negotiated, but other inclusions can be negotiated such as warranty, follow-up visits, fitting dates, financing, batteries, and accessory items. Although price negotiation and discounting seems reasonable, it is a two-edged sword. One side of the argument is that price negotiation and/or discounting is part of the buying process for many patients facilitating closure for certain types of buyers. The other side of the question is that if the price is negotiated all the time then the practice compromises their margin and depending upon magnitude of the compromise, can lead to practice financial issues. Additionally, negotiating the price routinely causes patients to feel that the clinic never charges the retail price and makes it difficult to ever obtain full price. If inclusive items are negotiated the question becomes when to negotiate, always, sometimes, or never. When the clinic always negotiates, more sales will probably be made, but at what cost? The cost will be that patients will realize that that the clinic will always give various items for free or at significant discount, which creates an unrealistic value for these items and may place

the clinic itself in a lower esteem. If the clinic never negotiates the margin it is never compromised and a high value is retained for the otherwise included items, but there is usually less sales and often patients will move on to other clinics in the market. Sometimes negotiating seems to be the middle ground in this process as the perception of the clinic is still high, margins are only minimally compromised and their perception of the clinic is still quite high. Additionally, the clinic will have higher sales due to the flexibility. Alexander (2009) lists *five major mistakes* that negotiators make when adjusting prices and/or items that are included with the sale.

- *Not Building Value.* Clinicians must fully understand the value that they bring to the product and their recommendations as a solution to the hearing difficulty. If not well understood the patient then has all of the negotiation power

- *Starting Negotiations with an Already Discounted Price.* Patients cannot come in with an ad from the paper offering a 10% discount and expect to receive more than that off on their purchase. Never offer more than one discount per purchase. The rationale is why give up something when you don't have to? If you have correctly ascertained the value of hearing solution for the patient you never have to begin with a discounted price. Always start at full price, then if necessary negotiate or discount to the lower price or add the inclusions.

- *Negotiating More Than One Price Drop.* A common mistake is to negotiate a discount or inclusion in conjunction with another offer. A firm component of any negotiation or discount situation is to only allow one discount or inclusion at a time.

■ *Not Having A "Drop Dead" Date to Agree to a Price Adjustment.* Price negotiations can carry on forever if you don't provide a date in which your offer is no longer valid. This assists the clinic in delivering on a sale that is seen by the patient as one that only has a limited time offer and prevents the patients from requesting the same negotiated discount for a later transaction at a later date.

■ *Not Having a "Walk-Away" Price Point.* As has been indicated previously, clinicians should never agree to a price that represents a financial loss for the practice. If the clinic chooses to negotiate, know the negotiation procedure and the maximum amount of price or inclusions that can be available to provide the product at a profit.

Once a pricing policy is in place and rules for departure from the routine pricing are established, they should be adhered to by all personnel. Sound procedures for negotiating and discounting that respond to patient demand without much modification in the audiologist or employee's behavior. Poor policies are those that allow price changes in ways that cause patients to have less demand for products and services in the future.

Price Level

Price level in the pyramid in Figure 7–6 refers to the process of actually setting the price. In theory prices should be set at a level within each tier/segment that reflect value differences and maximize

profitability. The process involves three basic steps, establishment of a pricing window, the setting of the initial price, and, finally, communication of the prices to the market.

The definition of a pricing window is the setting of the initial price range based upon the differential value of the product and the relevant costs, discussed earlier. The questions that the practice manager must consider in the establishment of a pricing window for each tier/segment are as follows:

■ What is the appropriate ceiling for this product?
■ How can reference prices be incorporated into this pricing window?
■ What is the role of costs in the setting of the initial price range?

Nagle et al. (2011) indicate that the price window is set for each tier/segment and is defined by a ceiling or the highest allowable price point. It is also defined by a floor or the lowest allowable price point. Once the window is established, then it is necessary to establish where, within the window, the initial price should be set. The ceiling is the economic value of the product for each tier/segment. Recall that economic value is not what the product is worth the patient, but what it costs to obtain the product elsewhere.

As the practice manager sets the initial price window they must consider:

■ Is the price point consistent with the clinic's overall business strategy?
■ What are the nonvalue determinates of price sensitivity?
■ What are the price-volume trade-offs and what is their impact on profitability?

Practice managers operate with various business strategies. While a new clinic may need to undercut prices to establish their market share, an established operation may simply set prices within the tiers/segments according to their operating costs, the volume goals, Prices are not set by altruism, but more on the business needs of the practice and the market in which it operates. Ultimately, the price will affect the volume of the product sold. As the prices are established it is necessary to determine the necessary volume and set prices so that the appropriate amount of product is sold to establish and maintain the business.

Once established, process must be communicated to the market by a plan that ensures the established prices are fair. Questions asked by the practice manager at this stage include:

- What is the best approach to communicate prices to patients?
- What are the implications of implementing significantly higher prices?

Pricing Objectives

Price levels must be set consistent with the goals of the practice. Pricing objectives must be set so that they yield long term, sustainable profitability. As suggested earlier, low price will allow patients to migrate to a particular product or service quickly while foregoing margin but it may be difficult or impossible to raise prices late. There are three philosophies that are useful to the practice manager when setting prices:

1. *Market Skimming.* Market skimming is designed to capture high margins and low sales volume. Skimming is the process of convincing patients to pay more

than most others will pay for the products and services. This strategy optimizes immediate profitability only when the profit from selling to relatively price insensitive patients exceeds that from selling to a larger number of patients at a lower price. While paying for a higher level of product and service, a clinic that uses the market skimming philosophy must be prepared to offer more than impeccable service and support to justify the excessive costs to the patient. The competitive environment must be appropriate and a clinic should have some type of competitive edge to keep competitors from offering the same products and services at a lower price. These differences can be location, product, reputation, education, patient service, equipment, or many other considerations that would warrant a higher price.

2. *Market Penetration.* Penetration pricing involves setting the prices for products and services low enough to attract and hold a large number of patients. This method of pricing is not designed to present the product as cheap, but prices are low enough to attract price sensitive patients. The key to setting of prices for market penetration is pricing so that the patient perceives the price to be at the lower end of the patient's perceived value (Kortge & Okonkwo, 1993). Penetration pricing works if clinic has a significant cost or resource advantage so that competitors could not compete at the same low prices. Penetration pricing is also successful if

the clinic is in a facility that offers numerous complementary products, such as Costco, Walmart, and so forth. Additionally, this strategy can be successful if the clinic is small enough with minimal fixed and incremental costs and does not interfere with competitive sales so as to prompt a retaliatory response.

3. *Neutral Pricing.* Neutral pricing involves a conscious effort not to use pricing as a strategy to gain market share. By its nature it minimizes the role of pricing as a marketing tool in favor of other tactics that may be more powerful and/or cost effective. Often, the neutral strategy is chosen by default as there is not an opportunity to use either a market skimming or penetration. Nagle et al. (2011) indicate that neutral pricing is less proactive that either skimming or penetration pricing, but its proper execution is no less difficult or important to profitability.

Seven Principles of Pricing

1. All relevant costs must be covered
2. The market dictates the changes in prices.
3. Charge the maximum price the patient will pay.
4. Check the price continuously and adjust accordingly.
5. Prices must be established that will ensure sales.
6. If the public perceives a product has significant value they will pay more.
7. Patients purchase products based on benefits, not features.

Summary

The price we charge for our products and services are the financial remuneration for our hard work in school and a reward for putting off of the earning an income while learning our profession as well as for the risks taken in private practice. Often, there is no discussion of pricing and where these values come from in audiology clinics and training programs. Most audiologists forget that the price we charge for a product or service in the practice is simply the economic sacrifice that the patient makes to acquire the product and have us apply our hard learned expertise to their hearing problem. In essence, a patient purchases a product or service only if that product or service's perceived value, in terms of money, is greater than the price. This chapter provides a foundation for practitioners to develop the skills to present that delicate perceived value, fairly, to their patients and themselves.

References

Abel, D. (2011). To bundle or not to bundle? AU Bankaitis's Blog, Oaktree Products. Retrieved September 3, 2012, from http://aubankaitis.wordpress.com/2011/10/05/to-bundle-or-not-to-bundle-guest-post-by-debbie-abel/

Alexander, G. (2009). 5 most common price negotiation mistakes. San Jose, CA: Goeff Alexander and Company. Retrieved September 26, 2012, from http://www.alextrain.com/inside-sales-telesales-tips-blog/bid/7413/5-Most-Common-Price-Negotiation-Mistakes

Amlani, A. (2007). Impact of elasticity of demand on price in the hearing aid market. *Audiology Online.com*, February.

Assael, H. (1987). *Consumer behavior and marketing action*. Boston, MA: Kent.

Campbell, M. (1999). Perceptions of price unfairness: Antecedents and consequences. *Journal of Marketing, 36*, 187–199.

Cohen, H. (2004). Pricing policy: Seven factors to consider. ClickZ.com. Retrieved September 18, 2012, from http://www.clickz.com/clickz/column/1692278/pricing-policy-seven-factors-consider

Dolan, R., & Simon, H., (1996). *Power pricing*. New York, NY: Free Press.

Erickson, G., & Johansson, J. (1985). The role of multi-attribute product evaluations. *Journal of Consumer Research, 12*(2), 195–199.

Hall, R., & Liberman, M (2013). *Macroeconomics principles and applications* (6th ed.). Independence, KY: Cengage.

Harrington-Gans, P. (2006). *Professional dispensing model: Differentiating goods from services*. Lecture from R. Traynor (Professor) CAS 7308 Business and Professional Issues, University of Florida Working Professional Doctor of Audiology Program, Gainesville, FL.

Hosford-Dunn, H., Dunn, D., & Harford, E. (1995). *Audiology business and practice management*. San Diego, CA: Singular. Retrieved from http://www.knowthis.com/principles-of-marketing-tutorials/pricing-decisions/what-is-price/

Kahneman, D., & Tversky, A. (1984). Choices, values and frames. *American Psychologist, 39*, 341–350.

Know This. (2012). Pricing decisions. Know This.com. Retrieved July 24, 2010, from http://www.knowthis.com/principles-of-marketing-tutorials/pricing-decisions/

Kotler, P. (2001). *Framework for marketing management*. Upper Saddle River, NJ: Pearson.

Kotler, P., & Armstrong, G. (2012). *Principles of marketing* (14th ed.). Upper Saddle River, NJ: Pearson.

Kortge, G. D., & Okonkwo, P. A. (1993). Perceived value approach to pricing. *Industrial Marketing Management, 22*(3), 133–140.

Marn, M., & Rosiello, R. (1992) Managing price, gaining profit. *Harvard Business Review*, September–October, 84–94.

Martins, M., & Monroe, K. (1994). Perceived price fairness: A new look at an old concept. *Advances in Consumer Research, 21*, 75–87.

McCarthy, E. J. (1960). *Basic marketing: A managerial approach*. New York, NY: Richard D. Irwin.

McConnell, F., Lassman, F., Lawrence, C., & Yantis, P. (1973). Task force 11: Methods for developing input into ASHA. Retrieved September 3, 2012, from http://www.audrehab.org/jara/1973-1/McConnell%20Lassman%20Lawrence%20et%20al,%20%20JARA,%20%201973.pdf

Mironov, R. (2003). What's your pricing metric? Product Bytes, Mironov Consulting. Retrieved September 1, 2012, from http://www.mironov.com/pb/PBApr-03.pdf

Nagle, T., & Dolan, R. (2004). *Strategy and tactics of pricing: A guide to profitable decision making* (3rd ed.). Upper Saddle River, NJ: Prentice-Hall.

Nagle, T., Hogan, J., & Zale, J. (2011). *The strategy and tactics of pricing* (5th ed.). Upper Saddle River, NJ: Prentice-Hall.

Parkin, M. (2005). *Microeconomics*. Boston, MA: Addison-Wesley.

Rajendran, K., & Tellis, G. (1994). Contextual and temporal components of reference price. *Journal of Marketing, 58*(1), 22–34.

Riley, G. (2006). Price elasticity of demand. Tutor2U. Retrieved July 26, 2012, from http://tutor2u.net/economics/revision-notes/as-markets-price-elasticity-of-demand.html

Ross, M. (2005). Why do hearing aids cost so much? *Hearing Loss: Self-Help for the Hard of Hearing, 26*(1), 32–33.

Smith, T. (2012). *Pricing strategy*. Mason, OH: South-Western Cengage Learning.

Smith, T., & Nagle, T. (1994). Financial analysis for profit-driven pricing. *Sloan Management Review, 35*(3), 71–84.

Staab, W. (2000). Marketing principles. In H. Hosford-Dunn, R. Roeser, & M. Valente (Eds.), *Audiology practice management*. New York, NY: Thieme.

Staab, W. (2012). Hearing aids for profit — from unethical to ethical overnight. Hearing Health and Technology Matters, LLC. Retrieved September 3, 2012, from http://

hearinghealthmatters.org/waynesworld/
2012/audiologists-in-industry-wayne-
staab-part-7/

Thornhill, M., & Martin, J. (2007). *Boomer consumer: Ten new rules for marketing to america's largest, wealthiest and most influential group.* Great Falls, VA: Linx Corporation.

Traynor, R. (2006). The business of audiology. In N. Decker and S. Ackley (Eds.), *Trends in audiology.* New York, NY: Academic Press.

Tversky, A., & Kahneman, D. (1992). Advances in prospect theory: Cumulative representation of uncertainty. *Journal of Risk and Uncertainty, 5,* 297–323.

Fiscal Monitoring: Cash Flow Analysis

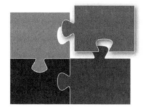

ROBERT M. TRAYNOR, EdD, MBA

Accounting Basics

Audiologists are practitioners, not accountants, but accurate accounting for the revenue and expenditures is essential to the success of the practice and facilitates knowledge of the sources of income and the expenses involved in conducting day to day business transactions. Although it is not essential that practitioners know specific bookkeeping procedures and accounting theory, they should be familiar with the terminology and general procedure allowing for intelligent conversation with the profession-

als that do understand these concepts. Accountants are trained in bookkeeping procedure and in preparation, audit, and analysis of accounts. Practitioners should, however, possess enough knowledge of the vocabulary and language of accounting to effectively communicate with accounting professionals that assist in the management of their practice and in the protection their assets (Tracy, 2008). It may seem to audiologists that dealing with a newborn for a follow-up hearing assessment or the fitting and follow-up of sophisticated hearing instruments constitute challenges in the day-to-day operation of their practice, but the

Sidebar 8–1
AN OVERVIEW OF ECONOMIC EXCHANGES
IN AN AUDIOLOGY PRACTICE

In a perfect world a transaction would simply be between the patient and the audiologist. Tracy (2008) describes six basic types of economic exchanges for which accountants ensure correct business interaction (Figure 8–1). Generally, these economic exchanges involve many others who are part of necessary interactions in daily operations of the practice:

- Patients
- Government
- Equity Sources of Capital
- Debt sources of capital
- Suppliers and vendors
- Employees

These basic exchanges are how the practice interacts with the real world of daily operations. The practice deals with the patients through employees, office and clinical supplies as well as hearing instruments and support items

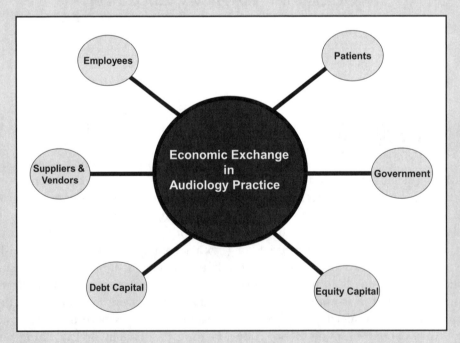

Figure 8–1. Economic exchanges of an audiology practice. (Adapted from Tracy, 2008.)

purchased from suppliers, vendors, hearing instrument manufacturers and repair facilities.

If cash reserves are unavailable to purchase these products or pay the employees and other expenses, the practitioner may have to obtain an interest bearing loan or establish a credit line through their banker. Another option available to the practice owner is to add partners or stockholders who can bring additional financial opportunities in exchange for shares in the practice. These partners or stockholders will own a percentage of the practice and appropriately expect a return on their investment. Additionally, as they are financial stakeholders in the practice; they will likely want a say in the day-to-day operations and management of the business segment of the practice. The attorney for the practice will be involved in document preparation to establish the most appropriate method for adding partner/ stockholders. The accountant for the practice will re-configure the books to include allowances for the partner/stockholders and to make sure the practice meets its financial obligations to them.

real challenge is staying in business over a long period of time. The more a practitioner knows about appropriate accounting methods, the better their capability to understand and execute professional business recommendations for adjustments in procedures and/or policies to ensure profitability.

Accounting in an Audiology Private Practice

Accountants provide the practitioner with internal and external methods for monitoring theft, embezzlement, as well as honest bookkeeping errors by performing internal audits should theft or errors be suspected. Simultaneously, accountants may also offer personal and business financial planning services and business valuations. Accountants not only ensure funds are deposited in the appropriate accounts, they advise the practitioner about the fiscal health of the

practice. They provide information about cash flow and retained earnings relative to the adequacy of funding required to conduct day-to-day business transactions. It is also the responsibility of the accountant (in association with the practice bookkeeper) to insure that expenses are paid on time and that transactions for these payments are recorded properly. In addition, property such as sound rooms; audiometers; VNG, ABR, OAE and other equipment; paper; printers; pens; and all other property are also accounted for so as to control the use of these assets and assess their real value for property tax purposes and in establishing appropriate business expense deductions.

Accountants prepare reports for practitioners to assist in evidence-based decisions about the success or failure of daily operations, a specific procedure, or a new market offering. These reports are fundamental to understanding the reasons for positive or negative changes in the bottom-line performance of the practice.

An accountant's primary responsibilities vary from one practice to another but common areas of responsibility include, but are not limited to:

- Cash into the practice (receivables)
- Cash payments from the practice (payables)
- Inventory and purchases
- Property accounting
- Tax accounting methods: cash or accrual
- Payroll preparation
- Assist in monitoring the bookkeeper/financial manager.

Just as audiologists are licensed to practice in their respective states, accountants are licensed by State Boards of Accountancy. Similar to audiologists that choose to seek certification from the American Board of Audiology (ABA), accountants may seek certification from the American Institute of Certified Public Accountants (2012) (AICPA: http://www.aicpa.org). Their certification title is certified public accountant (CPA). All CPAs are accountants, but all accountants are not CPAs. Just as ABA or ASHA certification is voluntary for audiologists, so too is the certification process for accountants.

Audiologists have specialty certification opportunities through the ABA and ASHA. CPAs have specialty certification available to those seeking advanced credentials as well. For example, the AICPA offers specialty certification for CPAs in the conduction of business valuations. The Accreditation in Business Valuation (ABV) identifies those CPAs with advanced training and certification in assessing and issuing valuations of various businesses including health care practices. The use of an accountant and their services is fundamental to long-term success and

requires a basic business vocabulary that allows for good communication.

Cash and Accrual Methods of Accounting

The core of the cash method of accounting is the flow of cash in and out of the practice. Income is recorded when received and expenses are paid when they occur: Both income and expenses are put on the books and charged to the period in which they are received and taxes are paid based on actual revenue in hand. Historically, accountants have recommended the cash basis for small businesses with minimal inventory, less complex business structure, and only one or two partner/owners involved. From a tax perspective, it is sometimes beneficial for a new business to use the cash basis of accounting so that recording income can be put off until the next tax year, when expenses can be claimed immediately.

The accrual basis of accounting requires that income and expenses are entered into the ledger when a transaction occurs regardless of whether monies have been received for the services or products provided. Expenses are deductible when the practice is billed, not when the expenses are paid. Taxes are paid on the revenue on the ledger with or without the revenue in hand. The obvious downside to this method resides in the fact that the practice might have to pay income taxes on monies that have not been collected in part or in full.

The owner or manager of the practice can minimize the downside of the accrual method by collecting revenue for services and hearing instruments as soon as possible, preferably at the time of service. That may not be such a problem for hearing instruments; however, most patients rely on their insurance carriers to pay their medical bills, including diagnostic studies common to the practice of audiology. Third-party payers who reimburse in a timely fashion (a dwindling lot to be sure) will aid in reducing the tax impact inherent in the accrual method of accounting.

Whether the practice is inclined to go with the cash or the accrual basis, the accountant of record must be involved in the decision process. They can clarify the two accounting methods and recommend the best course of action for your particular practice circumstance and venue.

Generally Accepted Accounting Principles (GAAP)

General knowledge of accounting procedures and good communication skills can ensure an understanding of where and how the revenue is generated and the costs involved in the daily practice operation. Accountant reports and bookkeeping operations are prepared according to internationally accepted accounting rules called the generally accepted accounting principles (GAAP), a universal method of valuing profit and measuring assets and liabilities. Although they vary slightly from one country to another, GAAP rules are used to conduct accounting in all businesses. GAAP describes how transactions for costs, profit, inventory, sales, and other business specifics are recorded and allows a comparison of one practice to another as businesses all use the same procedures for accounting. The Accounting Coach (2012a) describes GAAP as being founded on the following basic accounting principles and guidelines:

- *Economic Entity Assumption.* The accountant keeps all of the business transactions of a sole proprietorship separate from the business owner's personal transactions. For legal purposes, a sole proprietorship and its owner are considered to be one entity, but for accounting purposes they are considered to be separate entities.

- *Monetary Unit Assumption.* Economic activity is measured in US dollars, and only transactions that can be expressed in US dollars are recorded. Since this is a basic accounting principle, it is assumed that the dollar's purchasing power has not changed over time. As a result, accountants ignore the effect of inflation on recorded amounts. For example, dollars from a 2001 transaction are combined (or shown with) dollars from a 2013 transaction.

- *Time Period Assumption.* This accounting principle assumes that it is possible to report the complex and ongoing activities of a business in relatively short, distinct time interval such as the five months ended May 31, 2012, or the 5 weeks ended May 1, 2012. The shorter the time interval, the higher the probability that an accountant needs to estimate amounts relevant to that period. For example, the property tax bill is received on December 15 of each year. On the income statement for the year ended December 31, 2011, the amount is known; but for the income statement for the three months ended March 31, 2012, the amount was not known and an estimate had to be used. According to GAAP, it is imperative that the time interval (or period of time) be shown in the heading of each income statement, statement of stockholders' equity, and statement of cash flows. Labeling one of these financial statements with "December 31" is not good enough: the reader needs to know if the statement covers the one week ended December 31, 2011, the month ended December 31, 2011, the three months ended December 31, 2011, or the year ended December 31, 2011.

- *Cost Principle.* From an accountant's point of view, the term "cost" refers to the amount spent (cash or the cash equivalent) when an item was originally obtained, whether that purchase happened last year or 30 years ago. For this reason, the amounts shown on financial statements are often referred to as historical cost amounts. Due to this accounting principle, asset amounts are not adjusted upward for inflation. In fact, as a general rule, asset amounts are not adjusted to reflect any type of increase in value. Hence, an asset amount does not reflect the amount of money a company would receive if it were to sell the asset at today's market value.

- *Full Disclosure Principle.* If certain information is important to an investor or lender using the financial statements, that information should be disclosed within the statement or in the notes to the statement. It is because of this basic accounting principle that numerous pages of "footnotes" are often attached to financial statements. For example, if a company is named in a lawsuit that demands a significant amount of money. When the financial state-

ments are prepared it is not clear whether the company will be able to defend itself or whether it might lose the lawsuit. As a result of these conditions and because of the full disclosure principle the lawsuit will be described in the notes to the financial statements. A company usually lists its significant accounting policies as the first note to its financial statements.

- *Going Concern Principle.* This principle assumes that a company will continue to exist long enough to carry out its objectives and commitments and will not liquidate in the foreseeable future. If the company's financial situation is such that the accountant believes the company will not be able to continue on, the accountant is required to disclose this assessment. The going concern principle allows the company to defer some of its prepaid expenses until future accounting periods.

- *Matching Principle.* This principle requires companies to use the accrual basis of accounting. The matching principle requires that expenses be matched to revenues. For example, sales commission expense should be reported in the period when the sales were made (and not reported in the period when the commissions were paid). Wages to employees are reported as an expense in the week when the employees worked and not in the week when the employees are paid. If a company agrees to give its employees 1% of its 2012 revenues as a bonus on January 15, 2013, the company should report the bonus as an expense in 2012 and the amount unpaid at December 31, 2012 as a liability. As the future economic benefit of items such as advertise-ments cannot be measured (and thus the ad expense cannot be matched with related future revenues), the accountant charges the ad amount to expense in the period that the ad is run.

■ *Revenue Recognition Principle.* In an accrual based accounting (as opposed to the cash basis of accounting) system, revenues are recognized as soon as a product has been sold or a service has been performed, regardless of when the money is actually received. Under this basic accounting principle, a company could earn and report $20,000 of revenue in its first month of operation but receive $0 in actual cash in that month. For example, if ABC Audiology completes its service at an agreed price of $1,000, ABC should recognize $1,000 of revenue as soon as its work is done; it does not matter whether the patient pays the $1,000 immediately or in 30 days. Do not confuse revenue with a cash receipt.

■ *Materiality.* Due to this basic accounting principle or guideline, an accountant might be allowed to violate another accounting principle if an amount is insignificant. Profes-sional judgment is needed to decide whether an amount is insignificant or immaterial. The principle of mate-riality also suggests that financial statements usually show amounts rounded to the nearest dollar, to the nearest thousand, or to the nearest million dollars depending on the size of the company.

■ *Conservatism.* If a situation arises where there are two acceptable alternatives for reporting an item, conservatism directs the accountant to choose the alternative that will result in less net income and/or less asset amount. Accountants are expected to be unbiased and objec-tive, conservatism assists accountants in "breaking a tie," but does not direct accountants to be conserva-tive. The principle of conservatism leads accountants to anticipate or disclose losses, but it does not allow a similar action for gains. For example, an accountant may write inventory down to an amount that is lower than the original cost, but will not write inventory up to an amount higher than the original cost.

Types of Bookkeeping

Bookkeeping can be either conducted in a single entry or double entry (Quick MBA, 2012). Single entry bookkeep-ing keeps track of revenue against the expenses and offers simplicity, but not enough detail to track the sources and destinations of revenue and expenses. A system that offers detail is the double entry bookkeeping system that is now the standard of accounting (Figure 8–2). Pioneered by medieval Venetians, the double entry system treats a transaction as an exchange between two accounts. The double entry method has two characteristics in that each transaction is recorded in two accounts and each account has two columns. Double entry systems have some distinct advantages over simple single entry systems:

■ Accurate calculation of profits and losses in complex organizations.
■ Inclusion of assets and liabilities in the bookkeeping accounts.
■ Preparation of financial statements directly from the accounts.

Date	Accounts	Debit	Credit
July 8	Cash	300.00	
	Hearing aid Repairs		300.00

Figure 8–2. Double entry bookkeeping.

■ Easier detection of accounting errors, fraud, and embezzlement.

The recording transactions in each account involve two significant items; debits and credits, with debits in the left column and credits in the right column (Lerner & Gokarn, 2007). For each debit there is an equal and opposite credit and the sum of all debits must equal the sum of all credits. The debit/credit principle makes it easier to find errors, fraud, or embezzlement within the double entry bookkeeping system. In the double entry system balanced entries are made that keep the accounting equation in balance so that:

$$Assets = Liabilities + Owners/Stockholders\ Equity$$

Receivables and Payables

The accountant will set up a chart of accounts depicting all transactions necessary to record incoming revenue (e.g., payments from patients or third-party payers) and pay bills necessary to satisfy vendors, landlords, and other providers of services or goods to the practice (e.g., rent, hearing instrument manufacturer). The chart of accounts represents an exhaustive list of important accounts which must be monitored and carefully followed since it is the basis for the general ledger for the practice. The general ledger for the practice is the nuts and bolts of the financial monitoring system. It includes every account on the chart of accounts and contains information about monies received in the practice and money that must be paid to suppliers, vendors, Federal, state, and local taxing agencies.

Inventory Control and Property Tax Accounting

Recording purchases and related acquisition costs of items necessary for daily practice operations is important for a variety of reasons, not the least of which is to establish appropriate tax preparations and deductions. The accountant will establish appropriate guidelines to record all transactions that are important to your practice and works with the office manager/bookkeeper (see Sidebar 8–2) to optimize tax reporting, credits, and deductions. Although accountants can issue quarterly reports, semiannual reporting is less costly. As long as the practitioner is attending to fiscal details, semiannual reporting is usually adequate. A single, end of the year report is not adequate to monitor the overall fiscal health of any health care practice. It is one thing to make up for an error or initiate needed changes in reporting at the mid-year point; it is another to have to retread the path of a full year of business transactions.

Sidebar 8–2
KEY QUALITIES IN A BOOKKEEPER OR FINANCIAL MANAGER

As accounting for the incoming and outgoing funds is essential to a successful practice, special attention must be given to the person that handles the money. The first credential for bookkeepers and/or or financial managers is honesty. Since the practitioner has patient, management, supervisory, marketing, and other responsibilities, there is no time to babysit, second guess, or follow up every transaction of the bookkeeper or financial manager. Practitioners, however, should, be wise to the bookkeeping process as well as accounting methods to recognize when these people are being dishonest. If direct monitoring is not possible, then the practice accountant should monitor these transactions at least monthly to discourage and/or eliminate employee criminal activity. Although this monitoring is costly in accounting fees, embezzlement is substantially higher and can not only affect the office cash flow, but the very existence of the practice and the practitioner's valuable reputation. Believe it or not, bookkeepers and financial managers stealing funds from practitioners is extremely common and, according to law enforcement, becoming routine with all the methods of identity theft available. If the practice does have an issue with embezzlement, it is very difficult to obtain cooperation of the district attorney for prosecution without specific evidence if they will prosecute the case at all. Embezzlement is not only a problem for audiologists, but also physicians, dentists, chiropractors, and other professionals that have significant cash flow in their practice. As the practice manager or chief executive officer (CEO) watch out for changes in the accounting process or procedures, illogical business expenses, spending habits of the person involved, capricious movement, and/or disappearance of funds in bank accounts. *Do not use* a signature stamp for checks as the stamp can easily be used by the unauthorized, duplicated by others, or set as a signature for computerized checks. Additionally, guard the practice debit and credit cards as once someone knows your pin, they can actually pull funds from the practice at the ATM. Daily monitoring of the bank accounts and questions to the bookkeeper/financial manager as to any suspicious expenditure are essential to wise practice management. If possible, have the practice accountant monitor their work and audit the accounts at least semiannually to reduce the possibility of embezzlement.

In addition to being impeccably honest, bookkeepers and financial managers should be knowledgeable of business with a basic understanding of the essential differences among the five basic types of accounts (assets, liabilities, equity, income, and expenses) so that transactions are organized properly. The practice owner or CEO, of course, is ultimately responsible for all that happens with the books, ensuring that expenses, employees, payables and taxes are paid, but a good, honest, bookkeeper or financial manager can make life much easier. Bookkeepers and financial managers should also clearly understand the three basic financial statements including the balance sheet, the income statement (profit/loss statement), and the cash flow statements that are fundamental to tracking the costs by item and procedural detail.

The days of manual bookkeeping systems are gone forever making it essential to find a bookkeeper with a knowledge of the basics of bookkeeping software, Word, Excel, E-mail, and the Internet. They should be committed to enhancing their skills with additional classes or self-study to ensure that they're staying up to date with the accounting skills your business demands. If hiring a part-time bookkeeper, the practitioner should find someone who will make your business a priority, not allowing a part-time bookkeeper to "squeeze" their bookkeeping responsibilities into their personal life as this puts the practice at a low priority.

Newman (2006) suggests an eleven-factor checklist that should to be considered when hiring the bookkeeper, they must possess:

- A basic understanding of bookkeeping/accounting terms
- Be detail oriented
- An understanding of the big picture
- A willingness to follow through on projects
- The capability to have monthly financial statements available by the 10th of the following month
- An understanding of how to do proper job costing
- A basic understanding of your industry
- Good communication skills
- Good computer skills
- An interest in continuing their education
- A willingness to make a strong commitment to your business.

Payroll Preparation

Preparing payroll is extremely important since all employees, including the practice owner or manager, must be paid for their services in a timely fashion. Appropriate Federal, state, and local payroll taxes such as Social Security, Medicare, city taxes, and other deductions from their salary must be accurately calculated, applied and recorded. Although these deductions used to be deposited at the practice's bank each month in a special account reserved for government tax collection, it is now necessary to deposit these funds at a special Web site reserved for this purpose by the Internal Revenue Service (IRS) and other collection agencies. Failure to deduct and deposit these taxes has severe penalties for the practice owner and possible liabilities for the individual within the practice designated responsible for developing the payroll and depositing the taxes. It is the practice owner, however, who bears the ultimate responsibility of insuring all taxes are deducted and that these deducted funds have been directed to the appropriate depository. Even if the practice is a corporation the a tax liability can still be assessed against the owner or anyone individually if that had control over dispersing funds for the practice.

It is cost prohibitive for most practices to have the accountant of record complete the payroll. A reasonable solution is to secure the services of a payroll company. There are a number of companies operating on a national basis specializing in payroll preparation, such as Paycom (http://www.paycomonline.com) or ADP (http://www.adp.com/). Their clients include large and small companies and a variety of health care providers. They follow specific tax guidelines for state (varies from state to state) and federal reporting. Payroll companies will cause deductions to occur as directed, issue payroll documentation, and print payroll checks drawn on the practice bank account. Practitioners should consult with the accountant about payroll services available in the area. They will suggest establishing levels of deductions relative to your specific needs and should review the first two or three sets of payroll checks and documentation to insure appropriate deductions and documentation have been issued and recorded. As presented above there are also many Internet-based payroll systems and software programs that can offer the practice manager and their office personnel some relief from these tasks with increased accuracy.

Financial Statements

There are two primary objectives of every business, including health care practices, are profitability and solvency. Unless a practice can produce satisfactory earnings and pay its debt obligations in a timely manner, all other objectives will never be realized because the practice will not survive. Financial statements are documents typically prepared by the practice accountant that reflect the business' solvency (the balance sheet), its profitability (the income statement), and a view of its financial health (the cash flow statement). Information of solvency, profit, and financial health are essential to practitioners in making informed decisions that reflect the direction of practice operations.

Financial statements are so important that bankers and other lenders depend on them to support their decisions to grant credit opportunities. Additionally, the figures on financial statements are the bases of the calculations for business ratios that offer important, informative metrics and milestones about activity, liquidity, profitability, and debt of the practice.

The Balance Sheet

The balance sheet contains the elemental fiscal components of the practice; information about assets, liabilities, and owner's or stockholder's equity. It presents a snapshot of the financial condition of the practice at a specific moment in time, usually at the close of an accounting period such as the end of the month, quarter, or year (Brealey et al., 2010). Accounting Coach (2012b) indicates that its purpose is to quickly view the financial strength and capabilities of the business as well as answer important questions such as:

■ Is the business in a position to expand?
■ Can the business easily withstand the normal financial ebbs and flows of revenues and expenses?
■ Or should the business take immediate steps to strengthen cash reserves?
■ Do the numbers make sense?

The balance sheet gets its name from the fact that the two sides of the statement must numerically balance. Assets are recorded on the left side of the balance sheet and liabilities and owner's (or stockholder's) equity are recorded on the right side of the balance sheet, as pre-

sented in Table 8–1. Total assets are set to equal 100%, with all other assets listed as a percentage of the total assets. On the right side of the balance sheet, total liabilities and equity is also set equal to 100%. Entries of all liabilities and owner's equity accounts are also represented as the appropriate percent of the total liabilities and equity. The balance sheet must contain all of the practice's financial accounts and should be generated at least once a month. Monthly review of the balance sheet provides a comprehensive overview of the practice's overall financial position at that specific point in time.

Assets

Assets listed on the balance sheet are items of value and represent the financial resources of the practice. Accounts

Table 8–1. Balance Sheet

Audiology Associates, INC. Balance Sheet December 31, 2012	
Assets	**Liabilities & Owners' Equity**
Current Assets:	Current Liabilities:
Cash . . . . 34,000.	Short-Term Debt . . . . 20,000.
Accounts Receivable. . . . . . 80,000.	Accounts Payable . . . . 35,000.
Merchandise Inventory . . . . 170,000.	Other Accrued Liabilities. . . 12,000.
Total Current Assets . . . . 284,000.	Total Current Liabilities . . 67,000.
Property, Plant and Equipment (Fixed Assets):	Long-Term Debt . . . . 50,000.
	Total Liabilities. . . . . 117,000.
Equipment. . . . . 40,000.	
Less Accumulated	Owners' Equity . . . . 203,000.
Depreciation . . . . (4,000.)	
	Total Liabilities and
Total Assets . . . . 320,000.	Owners' Equity . . . . 320,000.

listed on the balance sheet are placed in order of their relative degree of liquidity (ease of convertibility of assets into cash); therefore, cash is always listed first as it does not require an action or an agent to convert cash into cash. Accounts receivable is listed second since it represents cash but must be "converted" into cash by collection. Assets are commonly differentiated into two classes, current assets and fixed or long-term assets; see Table 8–1. Current assets are short lived and expected to be converted into cash or to be used up in the operations of the practice within a short period of time, usually within a fiscal year. Current assets include cash, accounts receivable, hearing instruments, assistive listening devices and accessories in inventory, and prepaid expenses, such as insurance.

Long-term or fixed assets are assets that will not be turned into cash within the practice's fiscal year. Examples of long-term or fixed assets include audiometric and other equipment used in the practice, office equipment and computers, purchased vehicles, purchased buildings, leasehold improvements, telephone systems. These assets are found in the balance sheet (see Table 8–1) listed as "Property, Plant, and Equipment" or as "Fixed Assets." To best conceptualize long-term or fixed assets, consider that most fixed assets are purchased over time and must be in place over a long period of time to foster the day-to-day clinical and business operations of the practice. As equipment ages, it is said to depreciate. This depreciation of the equipment is an expense and can be claimed as a tax deduction. The accountant for the practice will evaluate the appropriate method for calculation and the extent of deductions available for every fixed asset listed on the balance sheet.

Liabilities

Liabilities include all obligations the practice has acquired through daily operations. Liabilities include accounts payable (e.g., hearing instrument acquisition costs), accrued business expenses, interest owed on loans, and other obligations incurred in the daily operations of the practice. Owner's or stockholder's holder's equity includes financial investment by the owner or shareholders and the earned profits that are retained in the business. Presented on the right side of the balance sheet (see Table 8–1), current liabilities are listed as amounts owed to lenders and suppliers and are usually separated by those that are due in the short term and long term. As with the asset categories, current liabilities are delineated into subcategories such as short-term debt, accounts payable, and accrued liabilities. These are referred to as current liabilities since they are due to be paid within a short period of time, usually within the fiscal year. A separate category is for long-term debt, such as bank or other loans payable over a much longer period, usually longer than the fiscal year. All current and long-term liability amounts are then totaled collectively to reflect the total liability of the practice (see Table 8–1). Owner/stockholder equity is also listed on the right side of the balance sheet. This represents funds that were initially invested by the owners/stockholders as well as the profit that was earned and retained in the practice.

The Income Statement

Income statements, sometimes called profit and loss statements or "P and L" statements, depict the status of your overall profits. McNamara (2007) indicates that income statements simply include how much money has been earned (revenue) and subtracts how much has been spent (expenses), resulting in how much has been made (profits) or how much has been lost (deficits). Basically, the statement includes total sales minus total expenses. It presents the nature of the practice's overall profit and loss over a period of time. Therefore, the income statement gives a sense for how well the business is operating (Table 8–2).

In accounting, the practice's profitability is measured by comparing the revenues generated in a given period with the expenses incurred to produce those revenues. The difference between the revenue generated and the expenses created during the generation of the revenue is the profit (or loss) of the practice. In an audiology practice, revenues are defined as the inflow of revenue from providing patient care or the dispensing of products. Expenses can be considered the sacrifices made or the costs incurred to produce these revenues. If revenues exceed expenses, net earnings result whereas if expenses exceed net revenue, a loss is recorded.

As with other financial statements, the income statement, presented in Table 8–2, may be prepared for any financial reporting period and is used to track revenues and expenses for the evaluation of the operating performance of the practice. Accounting Coach (2012c) suggests that managers can use income statements to find areas of the practice that are over budget or under budget and identify those areas that cause unexpected expenditures. Additionally, income statements track increases or decreases in product returns; cost of goods sold as a percentage of sales and offer some indication of the extent of income tax liability. Because it is very important to format an income statement appropriate to the type of business being conducted, the structure of income statements may vary from one

Table 8–2. Income Statement

Audiology Associates, INC. Income Statement Year Ended December 31, 2012	
Net sales	1,200,000.
Costs of goods sold	850,000.
Net profit	350,000.
Selling, general and administrative expenses	311,000.
Income from operations (EBIT)	39,000.
Interest expense	9,000.
Income before taxes (EBT)	30,000.
Income taxes	12,000.
Net Income	**18,000.**

practice to another, depending on the particular mix of business conducted in diagnostics, hearing products, and rehabilitative services.

Net sales on the income statement consist of sales figures representing the actual revenue generated by the business. Marshall, McManus, and Viele (2010) state that the net sales entry on the income statement represents the total amount of all sales, less product returns and sales discounts. Directly below the net sales in Table 8–2, is the cost of goods sold (COGS). COGS are costs directly associated with making and/or acquiring the products. These costs include the acquisition of products, such as hearing aids or assistive devices provided by outside suppliers. If hearing instruments are repaired or manufactured by the practice, COGS could also be materials, parts, and internal expenses related to the manufacturing or repair process, such as faceplates, shells, microphones, receivers, and components. Net profit, sometimes called gross profit, is derived by subtracting the cost of goods sold from net sales. Net profit, however, does not include any operating, interest, or income tax expenses. Just below the net profit entry in Table 8–2 is a category for selling and general administrative expenses. This subcategory is described by Tracy (2008) and Marshall et al. (2010) as a broad "catch-all" category for all expenses except those reported elsewhere in the income statement. Examples of selling and general administrative expenses that are recorded here are legal expenses, the owner's salary, advertising, travel and entertainment, and other similar costs. The actual income from operations, sometimes called *earnings before interest and taxes* (EBIT), is the result of deducting the selling and general administra-

tive, expenses from the net profit. The earnings before interest and taxes (EBIT) is the net revenue generated by the practice but there are still interest expenses and taxes that must be recorded. At this point, the interest expense is deducted and then tax amounts are subtracted to arrive at the net income (or loss).

Account Balancing

Account balancing is primarily for the bookkeepers in the practice, but it is beneficial for the practitioner to know how the procedure works. Simple accounting programs specifically designed for small businesses, such as Quick Books, have revolutionized bookkeeping tasks. These relatively inexpensive programs, some of which are now incorporated into office management systems such as Sycle.net, substantially reduce or virtually eliminate many of the common accounting mistakes that have plagued bookkeepers for decades.

One of the common bookkeeping tasks is the trial balance. The trial balance of the books is usually conducted at the end of the month, quarter or year, but could be done at any time. The purpose of the trial balance is to determine if the total debits and the total credits balance for all of the asset and liability accounts. Occasionally, these accounts do not balance and it is necessary to find errors and determine how to reverse them. Although accounting software programs have safeguards and special routines that will assist in finding these errors it may be necessary to check for the following common causes of trial balance errors:

■ Errors in the recording of a transaction

- Posting errors
- Computation of account balances
- Copying balances to the trial balance.

The Statement of Cash Flows

The cash flow statement reflects the cash position of the practice as well as the sources and uses of cash in the practice during a specified business cycle. It presents how cash flows in and out of the practice. Monthly cash flow statements are useful but quarterly statements of cash flow provide look at trends that might be developing in the overall cash-flow picture. Financially successful practices manage both profit and cash flow well.

Profit and cash flow are intimately related. A practice can be highly profitable yet on the verge of bankruptcy if the profits are sequestered in accounts receivables: *high profit, low cash flow*. This situation results in limited cash to pay the practitioner and other employees and to service the accounts payable. Conversely, if there is substantial cash inflow to a practice with excessive overhead costs strangling profitability, financial difficulties will ensue: *low profit, high cash flow*. This is a situation in which the practice owner has overextended available resources with ill-conceived equipment purchases, exceptional leasehold costs, or extraneous staff salaries and other questionable business decisions. To illustrate how cash flows in and out of the practice, Marshall et al. (2010) indicate that the statement of cash flows is used to identify the sources and uses of cash over time and can be compared to the current period for analysis. In Table 8–3, the cash flow statement is divided into three general sections, cash flow from operating activities, cash flow from investment

activities, and cash flow from financing activities. The operating activity section begins with the net income (taken from the income statement, see Table 8–2) and includes all transactions and events that are normally entered to determine the operating income. These entries include cash receipts from selling goods or providing services, as well as income from income earned as interest and dividends, if the practice has investments. Cash flow from operating activities also includes cash payments such as inventory, payroll, taxes, interest, utilities, and rent. The net amount of cash provided (or used) by practice operating activities is the key figure on a statement of cash flows. The operations section is of the most interest as it presents the specific areas of the practice where cash was consumed.

The second section of a statement of cash flows reviews income generated from investing activities. This section includes transactions and events involving the purchase and sale of securities, land, buildings, equipment, and other assets not generally held in the practice for resale. This area of the statement also covers the making and collecting of loans, if the practice internally finances products and services, these loans to consumers internally. Investing activities are not classified as operating activities as they have an indirect relationship to the central, ongoing operation of the practice.

Transactions in the third section record cash flows from financing activities and deal with the flow of cash between the practice, the owners (stockholders), and creditors as well as the cash proceeds from issuing capital stock or bonds. For example, if there was a need to transfer profit from the practice to the owners or from the owners (or creditors) into the practice, it would be reflected in the financing activities section.

Table 8–3. Statement of Cash Flows

Audiology Associates, INC.	
Statement of Cash Flows Year Ended December 31, 2012	
Cash Flows from Operating Activities:	
Net income.	$ 18,000.
Add (deduct) items not affecting cash:	
Depreciation expense.	4,000.
Increase in accounts receivable	(80,000.)
Increase in merchandise inventory.	(170,000.)
Increase in current liabilities.	67,000.
Net cash used by operating activities	$(161,000.)
Cash Flows from Investment Activities:	
Cash paid for equipment	$ (40,000.)
Cash Flows from Financing Activities:	
Cash received from issues of long-term debt . . .	$ 50,000.
Cash received from sale of common stock	190,000.
Net cash provided by financing activities	$240,000.
Net cash increase for the year.	**$ 39,000.**

Careful review of the statement of cash flows can present valuable information to the practitioner as to where the cash generated actually goes and presents an invaluable opportunity to make adjustments in practice operations for management purposes.

Financial Accounting Ratios

Until the financial data is actually used to track information about the practice, the balance sheet, income statement, and the statement of cash flows are just numbers. These numbers, however, are totals of practice performance in various catego-

ries did during a particular period of time and have valuable information for the management of the practice. Financial accounting unlocks the real information in these statements by conducting some simple calculations on the balance sheet and income statement data that presents the practitioner with the capability to track specific information areas for management purposes.

Performance Comparison

These calculations, called financial accounting ratios, are used in business to compare the practice to other practices or to compare the practice to itself at different points in time. Freeman, Barimo, and Fox (2000) describe cross-sectional analysis and time series analysis as two methods for the comparison of practice performance using these financial ratios.

Cross-Sectional Analysis

Cross-sectional analysis involves the calculation of financial ratios and comparing them to an industry standard usually compiled by a trade organization. A cross-sectional analysis offers an industry standard for financial performance that facilitates comparison of a specific practice to the industry standard. These ratios are calculations on the various totals (from the balance sheet, Table 8–1; income statement, Table 8–2; and the statement of cash flows, Table 8–3). Although cross-sectional analysis facilitates a comparison of a small two-person practice with a large corporate conglomerate in many areas, these cross-sectional analyses are not readily available to practices in audiology. Within the field of audiology, these industry standards are not readily available, except possibly to a few practice appraisers and audiology franchises, such as Sonus, or huge buying groups such as Audigy, American Hearing Aid Associates, and others.

Time Series Analysis

As it is difficult to obtain the data to conduct a realistic comparison of practice performance to an industry standard, the time series analysis is usually of the most value to the practitioners. A time series analysis compares the practice's performance to itself over various periods of time, usually month to month, quarter to quarter, or year to year. This type of analysis involves conducting calculations on financial statements to determine finan-cial ratios, which by themselves, simply present how the practice performed at a particular point in time and have minimal significance in isolation. Although the various statement totals and calculated ratios give some indication of how the practice has performed, the real information in financial statements is unlocked by a comparison of the practice to itself across other financial periods. Although only somewhat informative in isolation, comparing the current totals and calculated financial ratios to those conducted at other points in time, such as monthly, quarterly, or yearly intervals, they come alive with informative data that paints a true picture of success or failure. For example, comparing the totals and calculated ratios of the 1st quarter 2011 with the 1st quarter of 2012, or year ending December 31, 2010, totals and calculations with year ending December 31, 2011, or year to date for this year and last year can reveal a wealth of information to the practitioner or other stakeholders. More specifically, Marshall et al. (2010) offer that these ratio calculations can assist in the determination of a practice's financial position as well as the result of overall practice operations in terms of liquidity, activity, debt, and profitability. These relatively simple measures can be calculated and tracked by spreadsheets to be reviewed over time to demonstrate the health of the practice for obtaining loans, supplier credit, reviewing success and failure for management decisions, or simply general information. Ratios calculated on these statements also provide information regarding the practice's capability to meet its obligations regarding supplier expenses, employee salaries, product returns, loans, leases, and a multitude of other miscellaneous expenses that become apparent in the balance sheet calculations.

Monitoring the Practice with Ratio Calculation

Although there are interesting calculations on the other statements, most of the important ratios are performed on the balance sheet.

There are four general types of financial ratios that are used to analyze the balance sheet. These ratios demonstrate the strengths and weaknesses of a practice for:

- Liquidity
- Activity
- Debt or leverage
- Profitability

Although liquidity ratios are used to measure the short-term ability of a practice to generate enough cash to pay currently maturing obligations, activity ratios measure how effectively the organization is using its assets by specifically analyzing how quickly some assets can be turned into cash. Debt or leverage ratios reflect the long term solvency or overall liquidity of the practice and are typically of interest to the investors and/or the bankers that have loaned money to the practice. Profitability ratios are an indication of practice performance and look at the adequacy of the practice's net income, the rate of return, and profit margin as a percentage of sales.

Liquidity Ratios

Current Ratio and Quick Ratios

Accounting for Management (2012) states that a common liquidity ratio is the current ratio (CR), sometimes called a working capital ratio. The CR is a calculation of how many times the practice's current assets cover its current liabilities. Put another way, the current ratio asks the question; can the practice pay its bills? The current ratio is figured as follows:

$$\text{Current Ratio} = \frac{\text{Current Assets}}{\text{Current Liabilities}}$$

If the result of a CR calculation is less than 1, the practice will not be able to meet its current liabilities, whereas if the CR is 2 or more, the practice can pay its bills with money left over. Usually, most bankers and practice managers like to see this ratio at least between 1 and 2. The CR calculation includes prepaid expenses, such as insurance and inventory, and sometimes presents a cloudy, overoptimistic view, of the real capability to meet expenses.

If the inventory and other prepaid expenses are included in the calculation, it increases the CR offering a higher ratio than if these prepaid expenses are not included. Thus, the current ratio can sometimes offer an unrealistic picture of the practices capability to pay its expenses. This may be especially true as audiology practices move from mostly ordering hearing instruments to stocking open fit products. To figure activity without considering the inventory and prepaid expenses calculation of the quick ratio (QR) also known as the acid test ratio (ATR) can be calculated. The QR or ATR evaluates the practice's liquidity without considering the inventory and prepaid expenses and, in doing so, often presents a more accurate indication of the liquidity of an audiology practice. The QR is figured as follows:

$$\text{Quick Ratio} = \frac{\text{Cash} + \text{Marketable Securities} + \text{Accounts Receivable}}{\text{Current Liabilities}}$$

As with the CR, quick ratio values less than 1 demonstrate that the practice has serious difficulty meeting everyday expenses. Creditors and practice managers also prefer to see this ratio between 1 and 2 (see Sidebar 8–3).

Sidebar 8–3
COMPUTATION OF THE CURRENT RATIO AND QUICK RATIO (ACID TEST RATIO)

The current ratio and quick ratios are activity ratios calculated on balance sheet totals useful in the determination if the practice can pay its expenses. The current ratio formula is as follows:

$$\text{Current Ratio} = \frac{\text{Current Assets}}{\text{Current Liabilities}}$$

Referring to Table 8–2, find the total current assets of $284,000 and the current liabilities of $67,000. Once these figures are found then put them into the formula as presented below:

$$\text{Current Ratio} = \frac{\$284,000}{\$67,000} = 4.2$$

In this example, this practice has 4.2 times the amount of funds necessary to pay its expenses. Stocked items, or inventory, included the CR can often present an over estimate of the practices expense paying capability. If the inventory is included in the calculation it increases the CR offering a higher ratio than if the inventory is not included. To correct for this the quick ratio (QR) is used and calculated with following formula:

$$\text{Quick Ratio} = \frac{\text{Cash} + \text{Marketable Securities} + \text{Accounts Receivable}}{\text{Current Liabilities}}$$

To compute the quick ratio (QR) from the balance sheet offered in Table 8–2, add the cash to the accounts receivable to obtain the current assets (there are no marketable securities) to obtain the total current assets of $114,000.

$$\text{Quick Ratio} = \frac{\$114,000}{\$67,000} = 1.7$$

Once obtained, divide $114,000 by the total current liabilities of $67,000 and obtain a quick ratio of 1.7. Since the QR must be over one to pay its bills, this practice has enough funds to pay their current expenses. In this example the QR offers a more realistic picture of the practice's capability to pay expenses.

Defensive Interval Measure

Another useful liquidity calculation is the defensive interval measure (DIM). Answers.com (2012) defines the DIM as a ratio that measures the time for which a practice can operate without any external cash flow or simply, how long the practice can operate if there is no business. The DIM is determined by the amount of cash or assets that can be used to keep an otherwise healthy practice open if there are unforeseen problems, such as hurricanes, major snow storms, or other situations where business ceases or drastically slows down. In accounting, these emergency funds are called defensive assets (DA). By definition, the DA are those assets that can be turned into cash within 3 months or less, such as cash (savings), marketable securities, or accounts receivable. In order to figure the DIM, based on a specific amount of DA, it is first necessary to know the projected daily operating expenses (PDOE) of the practice or how much it costs to keep the practice open each day. To find the PDOE, simply go to the income statement and find the selling and administrative expenses for the year and divide by 365:

$$\text{Projected Daily Operating Expenses} = \frac{\text{Total Yearly Expenses}}{365}$$

Once the daily operating expenses (PDOE) are known, the DIM is found by dividing the DA by the PDOE:

$$\text{Defense Interval Measure} = \frac{\text{Defensive Assets}}{\text{Projected Daily Operating Expenses}}$$

The DIM calculation gives the practice manager the length of time the business could survive if revenue was substantially reduced or absent (see Sidebar 8–4).

Sidebar 8–4
CALCULATION OF THE DEFENSE INTERVAL MEASURE (DIM)

Although natural and other disasters are rare and often do not create difficulties beyond two to three weeks, there are some that can create issues for longer, such as Hurricane Katrina, Hurricane Sandy, wildfires, floods, snow storms, and other disasters. The possibility of issues that can cause no business for a period of time, makes it essential to know how long your business can sustain itself with no income. The defense interval measure (DIM) is a ratio that determines the time for which a practice can operate without any external cash flow or how long the practice can operate if there is no business. The DIM is determined by the amount of cash or assets that can liquidated to keep the practice open if there are problems, such as hurricanes, major snow storms, or other uncontrollable situations where business ceases or drastically slows down. The formula for the DIM is as follows:

$$\text{Defense Interval Measure} = \frac{\text{Defensive Assets}}{\text{Projected Daily Operating Expenses}}$$

To compute the DIM, however, there are some things that must be known. First, the amount of funds that can be used for defense purposes. In accounting these funds are called defensive assets (DA) and can consist of many different types of assets, but they must, by definition, have the capability to be turned into cash within 3 months. The amount of the DA necessary will vary from practice to practice, but it is suggested that somewhere between a 90 and 120 day capability should be available. To calculate the DIM to determine the length of time that the practice can open its doors in an emergency, it is necessary to consider the projected daily operating expenses (PDOE). The PDOE is calculated by the following formula:

$$\text{Projected Daily Operating Expenses} = \frac{\text{Total Yearly Expenses}}{365}$$

To arrive at the PDOE, simply go to the selling, general and administrative expenses located on the income statement in Table 8–2 and find the total yearly expenses of $311,000. Then divide the total yearly expenses of $311,000 by 365 as presented below:

$$\text{Projected Daily Operating Expenses} = \frac{\$311,000}{365} = 852.00$$

In this example, it costs the practitioner $852 per day to stay open each day. This is if the practice is open 365 days per year, most practices are only open Monday through Friday and thus, the divisor should be much less, on the order of (365–104 [days closed]) or 261 and in this case the PDOE would be much higher at about $1,191 per day. If the practitioner has $50,000 available for defensive assets, then the practice's defensive interval measure would be 58.6 days or with the more conservative measure 41.9 days. To meet the recommended DIM of a minimum of 90 days the practitioner in this example would need $76,680 for the first example of $107,190 for the more conservative example.

Activity Ratios

Activity ratios are calculations that allow the manager to review how efficiently the practice uses its assets to generate cash. Although there are a number of activity ratios that can present the efficiency of the practice, the accounts receivable turnover ratio (ART), the inventory turnover ratio (IT), and the total assets turnover ratio (TAT) are quite useful to practice managers (see Sidebar 8–5 for calculation examples).

Accounts Receivable Turnover Ratio (ART)

Ideally, all patients need to pay when services are delivered but reality is that insurance companies pay slowly, sometimes 60 to 120 days after the services are rendered, may often not even pay the first time the claim is submitted. Additionally, some patients need credit to pay for goods and services they require such as hearing aids, batteries, repairs, and other goods or services. Managers need to monitor the accounts receivable to determine how much is due to the practice and how long, on the average, it takes to collect these credit sales. The accounts receivable turnover ratio (ART) reveals how many times the receivable account is turned into cash each year. To obtain the ART ratio it is necessary to first find the average amount that is due the practice from the receivable account or average accounts receivable (AR) balance. This is obtained by adding the accounts receivable balance at the end of last year (or other period) to the balance of the accounts receivable at the end of the current year (or other period) and divide by 2 (see Sidebar 8–4):

$$\text{Average Accounts Receivable} = \frac{\text{AR (Year 1)} + \text{AR (Year 2)}}{2}$$

Once the average AR is computed, the ART ratio, or the time it takes to convert this account into cash, can be obtained by taking the net sales (sales after returns and discounts are subtracted) and dividing that amount by the average accounts receivable balance:

$$\text{Accounts Receivable Turnover Ratio} = \frac{\text{Net Sales}}{\text{Average Accounts Receivable}}$$

Once known, the ART can tell the practice manager how long it takes, on the average, to collect the amounts in the accounts receivable. In this calculation, the higher the ratio the better; for example, if the ART ratio is 5.3, the practice turns over the accounts receivable 5.3 times per year or every 2.26 months which is about average. To obtain more detail, the calculation of the number of days it takes to turn the accounts receivable can be obtained by simply dividing the average accounts receivable into 365, in this case 68.86 days. Sidebar 8–5 offers a calculation example where the accounts receivable is turned 21 times per year, about every 17 days.

In the above example, the accounts receivable turnover time is very short, but it can often take much longer to receive cash those that you have extended credit. If the accounts receivable only turns two or three times per year it may make some sense to consider factoring your accounts receivable. Factoring is a process specially designed to turn over the accounts receivable and is used in many other professions, including medicine, dentistry,

Sidebar 8–5
AVERAGE ACCOUNTS RECEIVABLE (AAR) AND ACCOUNTS RECEIVABLE TURNOVER RATIO (ART)

Managers need to monitor the accounts receivable to determine how much is due to the practice and how long, on the average, it takes to collect these credit sales. The accounts receivable turnover ratio (ART) reveals how many times the receivable account is turned into cash each year. To obtain the ART ratio it is necessary to first find the average amount that is due the practice from the receivable account or average accounts receivable (AAR) balance. This is obtained by adding the accounts receivable balance at the end of last period to the balance of the accounts receivable at the end of the current period and divide by 2. In this example, our interest is in the average accounts receivable balance from past two years. To calculate this AAR use the following formula:

$$\text{Average Accounts Receivable} = \frac{\text{AR (Year 1)} + \text{AR (Year 2)}}{2}$$

The calculation of the AAR balance comes from the balance sheet. Referring to Table 8–1 (balance sheet), find the current AR balance of $80,000 assume that last year's AR balance from last year's balance sheet was $31,000. Using these figures the AAR would calculate as follows:

$$\text{Average Accounts Receivable} = \frac{\$31,000 + \$80,000}{2} = \$55,000$$

Once the AAR is determined then the accounts receivable turnover ratio (ART) can be calculated using the formula presented below:

$$\text{Accounts Receivable Turnover Ratio} = \frac{\text{Net Sales}}{\text{Average Accounts Receivable}}$$

From the income statement (see Table 8–2) the net sales are $1,200,000, which is divided by the $55,000, the average accounts receivable as follows:

$$\text{Accounts Receivable Turnover Ratio} = \frac{\$1,200,00}{\$55,000} = 21$$

The example above demonstrates that the accounts receivable turns over about 21 times per year of about every 17 days.

chiropractic, and optometry. Factoring companies can give the practice quick cash infusion by purchasing the receivables at a discount. Although this process is a way to increase cash flow without increasing debt, it largely depends on the credit worthiness of your patients and the insurance companies with which you interact as well as the amount of your monthly invoices. For example, if the monthly accounts receivable regularly totals at least $8,000 to 10,000 factoring firms will act as a collection agency for your practice. Although some of these companies have some upfront fees, shop around, as many simply take a percentage of the receivables and often immediately advance as much as 80 to 90% or more of the confirmed amount of the receivables. The factoring firm later collects from patients and companies that owed you when the account is due. If your accounts receivable totals $60,000 or more and it runs 90 to 120 days, it may make sense to pay factoring company to collect it. If there is a 10% fee on the $60,000 it would cost $6,000. In this situation, they would pay the practice $54,000 in cash immediately. If the fee is more or less then the costs the benefits of factoring need to be weighed by the practitioner. Certainly, the accounts receivable is often a tremendous source of cash and if handled correctly can keep the practice from actually needing a loan during business downturns.

Inventory Turnover Ratio

The recent advent of receiver-in-the-canal (RIC) hearing instruments notwithstanding, Audiology practices generally do not have much inventory—a few loaners, some demonstration instruments, batteries, accessories, and some assistive devices. When inventory exists in the practice it is important to understand how fast the inventory turns so that plans can be made for restocking. The inventory turnover (IT) ratio is a calculation that measures how fast the inventory is sold. As in the measurement of the ART, before figuring the inventory turnover ratio, it is necessary to obtain the value of the average inventory on hand in the practice. Thus, the average inventory is found by adding the beginning inventory for the year (or period) to the ending inventory previous year (or period) period and dividing by 2 (see Sidebar 8–6).

$$\text{Average Inventory} =$$

$$\frac{\text{Beginning Inventory} + \text{Ending Inventory}}{2}$$

Once the average inventory is known, the IT ratio is computed by dividing the cost of the goods sold by the average inventory. If, for the year, the IT ratio was 5.9, the inventory will turn almost 6 times each year. As with other activity ratios:

$$\text{Inventory Turnover Ratio} =$$

$$\frac{\text{Cost of Goods Sold}}{\text{Average Inventory}}$$

the turning of the inventory can be further delineated to reflect how long it takes the inventory to sell out in days by simply dividing 365 by the IT ratio. In this example, if the inventory turns about 6 times per year, then it takes about 61 days for the inventory to sell out. These data assist the manager in planning product orders efficiently throughout the year insuring that there is always a fresh, sufficient supply as well as taking advantage of a discount; see Sidebar 8–6.

Sidebar 8–6
AVERAGE INVENTORY AND INVENTORY TURNOVER RATIO

The inventory turnover (IT) ratio is a calculation that measures how fast the inventory is sold. As in the measurement of the accounts receivable turnover ratio, before figuring the inventory turnover ratio, it is necessary to obtain the value of the average inventory on hand in the practice. Thus, the average inventory (AI) is found by adding the beginning inventory for the period to the ending inventory previous period, such a year and dividing by 2.

$$\text{Average Inventory} = \frac{\text{Beginning Inventory} + \text{Ending Inventory}}{2}$$

The calculation of the AI balance comes from the balance sheet. Although the practitioner could look at any period, in this case, the is in looking at how many times the inventory will turn each year. Referring to Table 8–1 (balance sheet), find the current merchandise inventory balance of $170,000 and assume that last year's merchandise inventory from last year's balance sheet was $111,000. Using these balance sheet figures the average inventory (AI) would be calculated as follows:

$$\text{Average Inventory} = \frac{\$170,000 + \$111,000}{2} = \$140,000$$

Once the AI is determined the inventory turnover ratio can be calculated to determine how many times the stock will turn during the year. Inventory turnover ratio is calculated as follows:

$$\text{Inventory Turnover Ratio} = \frac{\text{Cost of Goods Sold}}{\text{Average Inventory}}$$

To arrive at the inventory turnover ratio, it is necessary to refer to the income statement, Table 8–2, and find the cost of goods sold, $850,000. This is the total amount of goods that were sold during this 1 year period. The $850,000 cost of goods sold is divided by the average inventory of $140,000 obtained earlier to present a calculated inventory turnover ratio of 6.

$$\text{Inventory Turnover Ratio} = \frac{\$850,000}{\$140,000} = 6$$

An IT of 6 indicates that the inventory in this practice turns over 6 times per year, every two months, or 60 days. This calculation is useful in ordering stock, such as batteries or stock RIC or open fit hearing instruments in that it is necessary to have a 60-day supply of goods on hand to insure that the goods will not sell out before another shipment can be obtained.

Total Assets Turnover Ratio

An activity measure that presents how effectively the practice assets are turned into cash is the total assets turnover (TAT) Ratio. In practice the TAT ratio looks at the use of the assets, such as employees, materials, space, equipment, and other assets calculating how effectively these assets were turned into cash for the practice the practice. The TAT ratio looks at the sales for goods and services and divides by the total assets to arrive at how many times the practice assets turnover per year.

$$\text{Total Asset Turnover Ratio} = \frac{\text{Sales}}{\text{Total Assets}}$$

Of course, the higher the TAT value the better, as this is an indication that the assets of the practice turn over more times during the year and suggests that the assets are used efficiently; see Sidebar 8–7.

Debt or Leverage Ratios

Two ratios that are beneficial to the practitioner in presenting how much debt the practice has relative to its assets are the debt to assets (DA) ratio and the times interest earned (TIE) ratio. These ratios give indications whether the practice has the capability to support more debt for the purpose of loans, adding equipment, opening another location, or other activities.

Sidebar 8–7
TOTAL ASSETS TURNOVER RATIO

An activity measure that presents how effectively the practice assets are turned into cash is the total assets turnover (TAT) ratio. The TAT ratio looks at the sales for goods and services and divides by the total assets to arrive at how many times the practices assets turnover per year.

$$\text{Total Asset Turnover Ratio} = \frac{\text{Net Sales}}{\text{Total Assets}}$$

To calculate the total assets turnover ratio it is necessary to obtain information for both the balance sheet (see Table 8–1) and the income statement (see Table 8–2). From the balance sheet, the total assets are obtained at $320,000, while the net sales of 1,200,000 is obtained from the income statement.

$$\text{Total Asset Turnover Ratio} = \frac{\$1,200,000}{\$320,000} = 3.75$$

The calculation is simply dividing the total assets into the net sales to determine how many times the practice assets are turned into cash each year. A total asset turnover ratio of 3.75 offered in this example suggests that this practice is efficient in that it will turn its assets into cash 3.75 times per year or about every 94 days.

The Debt to Assets Ratio

The debt to assets ratio (DA) is expressed in percent and offers an indication of how much liability the practice has for every dollar of assets. Creditors can review the debt to assets ratio and obtain insight as to the ability of the practice to withstand losses without impairing the interest of the creditors. Although good and bad debt to asset ratios are different for each industry the general goal for most practices should be to keep the percentage as low as possible. A low debt to assets ratio is a goal for the practitioner as the higher the number indicates that the practice is more dependent on borrowed money in order to sustain itself. Similar to the personal debt to asset ratios familiar for personal loans, Edmonds et al. (2006) indicate that business lenders are concerned if the DA is high, as this suggests that small changes in cash flow might cause serious difficulties in the capability to repay debt. The DA computation is simply the total liabilities divided by the total assets (also presented in Sidebar 8–8):

$$\text{Debt to Assets Ratio} = \frac{\text{Total Liabilities}}{\text{Total Assets}}$$

Times Interest Earned Ratio (TIE)

Edmonds et al. (2006) indicate that the times interest earned (TIE) ratio is an indication of how many times the practice would be able to pay its interest using earnings. The TIE provides lenders with more information as to the success of the company and its capability to repay loans for expansion projects, or other activities. The TIE is computed by taking the earnings before interest and taxes (EBIT) and dividing it by the interest charges.

$$\text{Times Interest Earned Ratio} = \frac{\text{Earning Before Interest and Taxes}}{\text{Interest Charges}}$$

Freeman et al. (2000) indicate that in audiology practices the TIE should be somewhere between three and five, indicating that the earnings are at least three to five times greater than the interest payments. A TIE that is less than 1 is evidence that the practice cannot pay its interest commitments; see Sidebar 8–8).

Profitability Ratios

Although most of the routine calculations presented so far are conducted on the balance sheet, sometimes the ratios that may tell the most about a practice are the profitability ratios. These profitability ratios are clues as to how well the practice has performed and look at whether the practice's net income is adequate, the rate of return achieved, and profit margin as a percentage of sales. The ratios routinely considered in this group are the profit margin on sales (PMOS) using information from the income statement and the asset turnover (AT) Ratio that uses information from both the income statement and the balance sheet discussed earlier in this chapter.

Profit Margin on Sales

The profit margin on sales (PMOS) presents the profit margin achieved after all of the expenses are subtracted and calculates how much of every dollar of sales are profit. The PMOS is important as it can give you an indication of how much margin there is on each sale or service provided. This calculation can establish if the margins are adequate from period to another

---

Sidebar 8–8
DEBT TO ASSETS (DA) AND THE TIMES
INTEREST EARNED (TIE) RATIOS

The DA presents how much liability the practice has for every dollar of assets and provides the creditors with information about the ability of the practice to withstand losses. The DA is simply the total liabilities divided by the total assets from the balance sheet. In this example review of the balance sheet:

$$\text{Debt to Assets Ratio} = \frac{\text{Total Liabilities}}{\text{Total Assets}}$$

Table 8–1 will find the total liabilities of $117,000 and total assets of $320,000.

$$\text{Debt to Assets Ratio} = \frac{\$117,000}{\$320,000} = 36.5\%$$

Dividing the total liabilities by the total assets yields 36.5%, suggesting that for every dollar of assets, the practice has 36.5 cents of debt. Although not serious debt, in practice the debt to assets ratio should be as low as possible.

The times interest earned (TIE) ratio is an indication of how many times the practice earns the amount of interest charged on the money that it has borrowed. The TIE is computed by taking the earnings before interest and taxes (EBIT), and dividing it by the interest expense, both values are obtained from the income statement (see Table 8–2).

$$\text{Times Interest Earned Ratio} = \frac{\$39,000}{\$9,000} = 4.3$$

In the example, the EBIT is $39,000, divided by the interest expense of $9,000 for a times interest earned ratio of 4.3 and these ratios should be, according to Freeman (2000), between 3 and 5 and a TIE less that 1 is an indication that the practice cannot pay its bills.

---

so as to sustain the practice. To compute the PMOS, net profit is divided by sales:

$$\text{Profit Margin On Sales} = \frac{\text{Net Profit}}{\text{Sales}}$$

PMOS results are represented in a percentage that reflects the amount of each dollar that is profit. For example, if the calculation yields 20% then $0.20 cents of every dollar collected is profit. These values can be tracked to determine if there are either up or down changes in the ratios that occur during the year (see Sidebar 8–9).

Sidebar 8–9
PROFIT MARGIN ON SALES

The profit margin on sales (PMOS) presents the profit margin achieved after all of the expenses are subtracted and presents how much of every dollar of sales are profit. To compute the profit margin on sales, net profit is divided by the net sales. For example, refer to Table 8–2 and find the net profit of $350,000 and the net sales of $1,200,00.

$$\text{Profit Margin On Sales} = \frac{\$350,000}{\$1,200,000} = .29$$

To arrive at the PMOS simply divide the net sales into the net profit and obtain 0.29. This figure refers to the fact that 29 cents of every dollar is profit from this practice and this figure can be tracked to determine if there are changes that require attention.

Tying It Together

Unless there is so much cash that in the practice that there is never a concern about where it goes, and this is extremely rare, a fundamental monitoring of the health of the practice is essential. The above ratios are certainly not an exhaustive list and the practice accountant may recommend that other ratios be monitored in addition for special purposes. The ratios presented here should be considered fundamental calculations essential to an overview of financial health. The practitioner should know if the practice is capable of paying the bills and if not, why? Knowledge of how fast the accounts receivable turns into cash is important to the cash flow into the practice and fundamental to paying the bills. Why not know when the inventory will need to be reordered so that cash allocations can be made to facilitate payment?

A look at the debt structure, operating costs, and profitability offers a simultaneous sense of reality and security to the practitioner rather than "seat of the pants management."

Just knowledge of these ratios and what they are today, however, does not present the opportunity to make changes in management decisions to modify the health of the practice. Ratios must be tracked and compared to other months, quarters, or years before these calculations unlock the important information essential for management modifications in the practice. Before you can alter an upward or downward trend you need all the information to make the correct managerial adjustments. By simply creating a spreadsheet and entering data each month, ratio data can be analyzed to manage the practice. Tracking or monitoring ratios allows the practitioner to evaluate the liquidity, activity, debt, and profitability over time to investigate the reasons for successes or failures and make appropriate adjustments.

A classic example of how tracking can be of assistance in the explanation of difficulties in the practice is presented in Figure 8–3. Figure 8–4 presents Quick Ratios for Audiology Associates, Inc. for the years 2008 to 2012. A review of the quick ratio histograms for the years 2008, 2009, 2010, 2011, and 2012 demonstrate that the quick ratios are greater than 1 indicating that the practice could pay its bills and even with money left over in 2008, 2009, 2010, 2011, and 2012. In 2010, however, the quick ratio was less than 1 suggesting that there were problems paying business bills. In 2010, the practice was having difficulty meeting expenses and even had to borrow funds to meet expenses that year.

Although this information is of great benefit, it must be remembered that all financial statements and the subsequent ratios generated represent specific informational snapshots in a specified window of time. These data reflect how business has been in the past and, due to competition, market pressures and other significant factors, may or may not be predictors of the health of the business in the future. Ratios can be very helpful in the evaluation of a practice, however, Freeman et al. (2000), Tracy (2008), and Marshall et al. (2010) offer cautions on the use of ratio analyses. They indicate the best information about a company's financial health is determined from comparisons and analyses of a group of ratios, not a single ratio, and that these comparisons need to be made at similar times of the year to arrive at accurate data on the practice's performance. In the example presented in Figure 8–3, simply tracking the quick ratio across

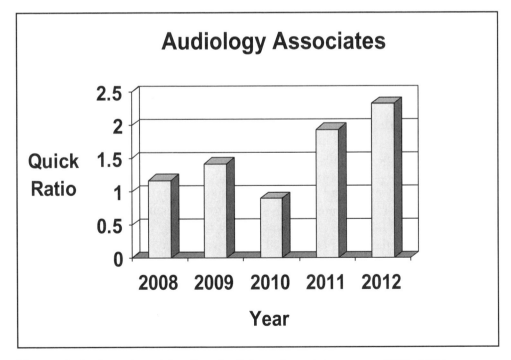

Figure 8–3. Sample quick ratios, Audiology Associates, years 2008–2012.

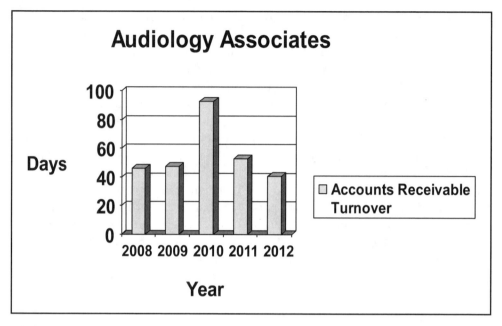

Figure 8–4. Accounts receivable turnover ratio, Audiology Associates, years 2008–2012.

the years provided information as to what the quick ratio was during the good and bad years but it is necessary to review other ratios to explain *why* the quick ratio was less than 1 during 2010. Tracking a number of ratios allows the practitioner to search further for differences between 2010 and the other years to insure that these difficulties are not repeated. By tracking other ratios and comparing them to the quick ratios from 2008 to 2012, the answer to the problem experienced by Audiology Associates, Inc. becomes evident. Figure 8–4 presents the tracking of the accounts receivable turnover ratio (ART) for Audiology Associates, Inc. for the same period 2008 to 2012. Recall that the ART presents how long (in days) it takes for the practice to turn the accounts receivable or credit sales into cash. Figure 8–4 demonstrates that in most years it only takes 40 to 50 days to turn the accounts receivable into

cash. In 2010, however, it took over 90 days to clear the accounts receivable.

By reviewing Figures 8–3 and 8–4 together, the practitioner can see at a glance, one possible reason for the problems in 2010. In 2010, when the quick ratio documented that it was difficult to pay the bills; the accounts receivable turnover ratio indicated that it took over 90 days to turn credit sales in to cash. When compared to the other years, it took almost twice as long to be paid for products and services in 2010 than the other years, offering a possible explanation for the financial difficulties. Obviously, tracking the various ratios and reviewing them over time greatly eases the management burden on practitioners and provides a mirror to reflect the problems in the practice and to fix them before they have had too much impact. These days it is rather easy to obtain software that can easily track ratios in a spread sheet and apprise the manager instantly of the difficulties or successes to make decisions.

The development of an assessment technique most appropriate to the venue and demographics a particular practice should be generated to track various important components of a practice should be developed with the guidance of the practice's accountant. Once established, these calculations and others discussed below can be easily monitored on readily available spreadsheets. Managing your practice with the clarity that data provides represents the highest form of evidence-based practice management.

Finance for Audiologists

Generally defined, finance is a discipline that studies and addresses the ways in which individuals, businesses, and organizations raise, allocate, and use monetary resources over time, taking into account the risks entailed in projects that create wealth. Finance is used by individuals (personal finance), by governments (public finance), by businesses (corporate finance), and so forth, as well as by a wide variety of organizations including schools and nonprofit organizations. The goals of each of the above activities are achieved through the use of appropriate financial instruments, with special consideration to their institutional setting. Finance is one of the most important aspects of practice management for without proper financial planning, a new practice cannot even start, let alone be successful. As cash is the single most powerful liquid asset, managing cash is essential to ensure a secure future, devel-

oping wealth for both for an individual practitioner as well as the practice.

For audiology practice management purposes, the term finance incorporates:

- The management and control of assets.
- Profiling and managing project risks.
- Finding funds for the generation and maintenance of business.

When considering financial operations of the practice a special set of techniques are used to manage financial affairs, particularly the differences between income and expenditure while monitoring the risks of their investments. In a profitable practice where income exceeds expenditure, the practitioner can lend or invest the excess income. Excess profit must be invested to build defensive assets for the practice or for funding expansions, equipment, or other projects that led to more profit. On the other hand, in an unprofitable practice where income is less than expenditure the practitioner may need to raise capital by borrowing, selling shares in the company, decreasing its expenses, or increasing its income.

Investing the Profit

When the practice is profitable, the profit should be invested to provide security for the practice when business is slow. These savings and investments for the practice are, as presented above, called defensive assets to be used when times are difficult to pay employees, accounts payable and other expenses. Typically, a certain portion of these assets will be kept in a place where they can be rather liquid such as a certificate of deposit or a mutual fund that allows for transfers to the business account as necessary. The best method of securing and sustaining the investments to be used as defensive assets, is to consult with the practice's accountant and/or an experienced financial planner.

Borrowing Money for the Practice

All businesses have ups and downs in their lifetime. Although the practitioner would rather not need to borrow money, there is usually a time when this is necessary to pay suppliers, employees and other monthly expenses. Most practitioners know of borrowing from various personal loans, auto loans, or educational loans and other borrowing experiences and loans for the practice work very much the same.

If a financial advisor is used, they should not have access to the practice finances, bank accounts, or books as these individuals can create extreme difficulty for practice managers if they are dishonest. Their credentials should be checked, rechecked, and police records investigated before they have access to any accounts or financial information. In this new century, all a dishonest person needs is the business tax ID number or a social security number along with a birthday and other minimal information to facilitate a major fraud. These frauds can have severe tax implication for the practice, the practice manager, even other employees that may have had control over funds. The fact that the practice is a corporation does not shelter its owners and others against mismanagement of tax filing responsibilities. Advice is to be very careful as to whom has access to financial accounts and sensitive information for the company and the employees.

One of the three most important individuals to the practice is a good banker. Without the financial advice and assistance of an experienced financial advisor the practice will have difficulties. Do not just shop for a bank, shop for the *banker*, an individual that knows you, your practice, and your business plan. The correct banker can help with the investment of profits or supply cash infusions as necessary, but it is the individual relationship that makes the difference. There are always risks involved in borrowing money, so you should carefully analyze your need for it first. Bankrate.com (2012) indicates that the practice's place in the business life cycle will help determine the type of loan you need. There are three basic phases in a company's early years: seed, startup, and growth.

- *Seed money* is used for initial planning. These funds sustain during the time that market research is conducted and is also used to create a business plan. Few small-business owners require a lot of cash for organizing and planning, so this step is typically self-funded.
- *Startup funds* are used to get going in business can vary greatly. This phase may be financed by the owner or a commercial lender. The credibility for the lenders is based on the practitioner's business plan (see Chapter 2). Even though the practitioner is a doctor, banks and commercial finance companies are less likely to lend money to startups unless there is a significant amount of collateral pledged by the owner. If your collateral doesn't meet the standards of a conventional loan offered by a bank, the next consideration should be the Small Business Admin-

istration (http://www.sba.gov). Your bank may even be a preferred lender with the SBA, and can give you a loan under the SBA-guaranteed loan program where the bank's risk is minimized because the government guarantees payment.

■ *Growth financing* is used when the practitioner has a successful practice and wants or needs to expand. This growth point is when practitioners look to banks or large investors for cash to fund new locations, equipment, and other cash need during this growth phase of the practice.

When money is borrowed for a company, the lender (the bank) receives interest and the practice will pay a higher interest rate than the lender (the bank) pays for the money from the Federal Reserve, and pockets the profit (see Chapter 1). The bank charges the interest at a rate that reflects their risk in the transaction. Thus, if a loan is considered for a startup practice with little or no track record, the practitioner will usually pay a higher rate than an established practice that has an established clientele and solid financial history. The purpose of the business plan see Chapter 2) is to convince the lenders that the risk for this specific practice is minimal so that the correct amount of funds can be obtained at a reasonable interest rate.

As borrowing money is expensive, Bankrate.com (2012) suggests some points to consider when deciding whether you really need a loan:

■ Make sure it's capital you lack, not good cash-flow management.
■ Borrow in expectation of needs, not in desperation—or due to the risk,

you may have to accept expensive terms.
■ If your business is in transition to its next life stage, you probably do have a need for cash to foster growth.
■ Have a specific purpose in mind, and be prepared to tell a lender exactly how the money will be used, preferably in a solid business plan.
■ Gauge the health of your industry in your business plan; it will make a difference in how favorably your loan proposal is viewed.
■ Consider establishing a good credit relationship with a banker by opening accounts or taking out small lines of credit, but don't get into debt without a plan for paying it back.

There are two basic kinds of loans available, *short-term* and *long-term*. Short-term loans generally reach maturity in one year or less and can carry you through the doldrum months in a seasonal practice. For example, if your practice is in Arizona and there are no patients in the summer or in northern Minnesota there are no patients in the winter, lines of credit, working capital loans, and accounts-receivable loans that are repaid in a short term can be essential to survival. Long-term loans usually mature in one to seven years, but can be longer for real estate or equipment. These loans are used for major business expenses such as vehicles, purchasing facilities, construction, and furnishings. They also can be used to carry the practice through a depressed business cycle.

Recently graduated doctors of audiology that want to create a start-up practice on their own will have an uphill struggle, despite the accuracy of their well-developed business plan and accurate projections for profitability. Traditional lending institutions will consider the practice, the demographics, and letters of recommendation then, in the end, likely not fund the venture completely. The bank might provide startup funding and create a flexible line of credit at specific times in the practices first three years but even that is a weak assumption. Glaser (2006) refers to the realities of securing conventional financing for new AuD graduates with substantial debt from their education. He states that the note (bank loan) must be secured with assets, not promises of future income, or the note must be co-signed by an individual with the means to repay the note. Especially in a very slow economy and after the recent overhaul of the financial regulations, debt load (the amount of indebtedness) plays heavily in determining loan eligibility.

Couple the above with the fact that bankers, by nature, are conservative and skeptical of practitioners with little or no track record or experience in managing a practice. Bankers are in business to lend money but well aware that often startup businesses, even medically based healthcare practices, are unsuccessful, especially when those requesting these startup funds have little training or experience in business and practice management.

Basic Financial Management

Budgeting

A major error in the financial management of a practice is not planning for the future. One such plan may involve building a budget to use as a guideline for the expenditure of funds. Budgeting is the process of developing and adopting a profit and financial plan with definite goals for the coming period. Budgets are financial plans that include forecasting expenses, revenues, assets, liabilities, and cash flows based upon a plan that is guided by the goals of the practice manager for a particular period, usually a year. Once the budget is determined, the actual performance of the practice can be compared to the budgeted goals to determine progress or the lack of it.

Tracy (2008) indicates that budgeting in business provides some important advantages. First, the budget allows for an understanding of the profit dynamics and financial structure of the practice, and second, it becomes the plan for changes in the coming period. The preparation of a budget forces the practice manager to focus on the factors that must improve in order to increase profit. In most audiology practices, however, it is rare to see a budget planned for more than a year in advance. Although budget preparation can be time consuming and frustrating, it is simply not enough to live day to day in a practice, paying the payables, collecting the receipts and hoping for enough profit to make it next month. In the absence of a budget or a plan for the future it is possible to end up paying higher taxes, overpaying for products, and/or making bad investment choices in equipment and/or in office expansions.

Although budgets for major corporations can be quite complex and take months to complete, for a small audiology practice, the process is relatively simple and can be a painless process if the accounting is conducted accurately. There are many different sources for budgeting software that can be easily obtained online. Before beginning the budget, the practice manager needs to make some assumptions about the industry, the local economy, and other factors such as increased competition that will affect the business (and audiologic) climate as well as the practices' strategy for the particular period in question. These decisions will drive the budget for its optimism or conservatism, depending upon the outlook. Although the budgeting process should be conducted with the assistance of an accountant or other business professional, it may be a complex conservative estimate of expenditure if a new practice in the first year or simply a look at the expenditure from the previous year and allotting an amount for each category based upon your expected increase or decrease in revenue. If it is a new practice, the business plan can be a good source of a budget for the first 1 to 3 years. Whatever the specific procedure, budgeting is well worth the process as it provides a spending plan that is based upon a substantial consideration of the practice and the economic climate.

Lease Versus Purchase

As practitioners are involved in learning how to take care of their patients, the idea that money is worth more today than tomorrow may only be a peripheral concept. Since money *is* worth less tomorrow than today, the practitioner's hope is that by laying out the capital today, there will be business in the future that will more than offset the expenses. In general, the purchase of items that appreciate make sense because as the dollar is worth less each day, the appreciation usually more than makes up for the devaluation that occurs over time. Items that depreciate, however, are usually better paid for with today's dollars and continue to devalue from the date of purchase until the value finally goes to nothing over time. Thus, it may be wise financial management to purchase your office space, as it does not usually depreciate while simply paying to use (rent, lease) equipment and avoid the use of working capital to pay for a

depreciating asset, such as a new VNG, audiometer, or ABR unit.

Leases often have a lower investment at the beginning, as compared to loans that usually require a down payment of 15 to 20%; however, at the end of the lease payment program you will not own the equipment. It must be turned in or you may choose to pay a slightly higher payment and be able to purchase the item at fair market value, sometimes only $1.00, at the end of the lease. For office equipment or audiologic equipment with its constant changes, leasing simply makes good sense but only if your cash flow will accommodate the payment. As the equipment technology is constantly evolving the capability of the instrumentation that was purchased today will change over the next 3 to 4 years, possibly outdating it—why own it? The goal then for rapidly changing equipment is to simply have the right to use it for a specified period of time since it will usually be worthless in 3 or 4 years. On the other hand, if the equipment is a sound room that is less sensitive to technology changes, it makes sense to purchase it and then use the room as long as the practice exists without a monthly expense. Business Spreadsheets (2007) and other companies offer prepared Excel spreadsheets that assist in the calculation of the lease purchase decision. These pre prepared analysis systems can assist practitioners when the decision is not obvious (Table 8–4 and Figures 8–4 and 8–5).

Types of Leases

There are a number of different lease products on the market that apply to various situations and types of equipment. Two types that are often used in audiology practices are the operating lease and the financial lease.

Table 8–4. Equipment Acquisition

Lease	Purchase
Conserves Capital No down payment	**Consumes Capital** Down payment required
Flexibility of Payments Lease payments are fixed and do not change withinterest rate fluctuation	**Specified Payments** According to interest rate, term of loan and may change with interest rate fluctuation
Convenience On the spot financing and immediate delivery	**Inconvenience** Apply for loan, credit application, counts against debt of the practice
Protection Against Obsolescence A lease can be structured to include upgrades and partial or complete equipment swaps either at mid-term or at lease-end.	**Cannot Turn in for Updates** What you bought is what you got . . . forever
Eliminates Risk At the end of the lease it is turned in or bought for $1.00	**More Risk** Must junk it, use it, or sell it at the end of the loan
Off Balance Sheet Financing Can potentially increase borrowing capacity while easing the budgeting process and preserving key financial ratios	**On Balance Sheet Financing** Uses up precious capital and causes debt ratio to be higher
Improved Return on Assets (ROA)	**Less Return on Assets (ROA)**
Paid with BEFORE Tax Dollars	**Paid with AFTER Tax Dollars**

Operating leases, according to Business Victoria (2007), are relatively short-term contracts for the use of an item. As the term of the contract is relatively short is short the payments are lower, the payments made to the leasing company usually are not enough to allow the lessor to fully recover the cost of the asset. As the term of the lease may be less than the economic life of the asset, the remaining value of the item is called a residual value. For example, if you lease a car for two years, the car will have a substantial residual value (or leftover value) at the end of the lease, and the lease payments you make will pay off only a fraction of the original cost of the car. The lessor, in an operating lease, expects the lessee to either lease the car again or purchase it for the residual value, or turn it into the lessor. If turned in the lessor will either lease or sell the car (or equipment) again. Sometimes, in operating leases the lessor is responsible for taxes, insurance, and maintenance of the item, which is usually passed on to the lessee in the form of

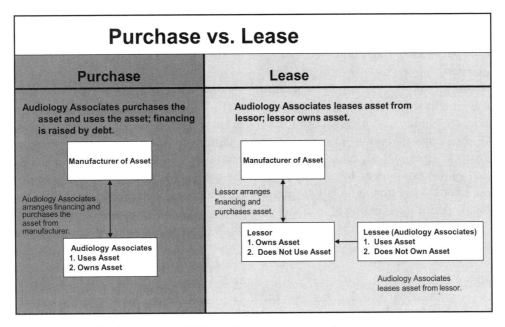

Figure 8–5. Equipment acquisitions, lease versus purchase.

higher payments. Another defining characteristic the operating lease is that the lessee may have the right to cancel the lease with very short notice by turning in the item and ceasing payments, although this option usually requires a higher payment for the cancellation option. Although practices have these operating leases for the automobiles, hearing conservation vans, and other very large items that they will never pay off, there are other types of leases more appropriate to leasing audiometric equipment, computers, and office furniture.

Financial leases are also referred to as capital leases, lease purchase, $1 buyout, or full payout leases and are usually for longer terms involving equipment. Stratus.com (2005) describes a financial lease as being similar to a loan, with the lessee building equity in the equipment as they make each payment. Because of this, the lessee has to account for the asset as a conditional sale and must depreciate the equipment as a capital asset. At lease termination, the lessee may purchase the item at fair market value, fixed price, or for some items, such as equipment or software, a $1 purchase option is usually available for a slightly higher payment. The term for these financial leases must exceed 75% of the estimated economic life of the leased property and the value of all the lease payments must be equal to 90% or more of the cost of the leased property.

Leasing of equipment for an audiology practice can have significant advantages since there are usually major changes in the audiometric equipment over a short time. Audiology is traditionally an "equipment poor" discipline in that our profession is extremely sensitive to changes in technology. For example, it took almost 10 years to replace the 1982 Nicolet CA 1000 ABR unit in our practice. The old beast was a workhorse remembered very fondly as rugged, reliable, and accurate, a device used for years after its lease was fully paid. The Biologics Traveler that replaced it in 1991, however, was replaced in 3 to 4 years due to the changes in software, transducers, and other technological changes that ensued during that time. By the time the lease was fully paid, it was purchased for $1.00 and used occasionally, but it was basically out of date. Obsolescence is part of our profession just as it is part of many other professions that utilize equipment for analysis and rehabilitative treatment of various physiologic difficulties. Leasing of audiometric equipment and computers that support the clinical operation, supports the practitioner as presented in Table 8–4 and Figure 8–5.

As with all financial decisions, the lease/purchase should be considered with the assistance of the practice's accountant who appreciates the balance sheet implications of each option as well as the profitability of the procedure that will be conducted.

Capital Investment

In audiology there is often the need to open a new location to expand the practice into another lucrative market. As the expansion will not likely be funded internally, it is necessary to go to the bank for a loan to secure appropriate space, develop needed tenant improvements, and obtain requisite business and clinical equipment for the new office. Although this seems simple enough, the banker wants to know, "How long will it take you to 'break even' on this project" or, "Is the net present value on this project positive or negative?" The question the banker is really asking is, will it be profitable, and if not, how long until the project pays for itself.

The banker needs to make certain there is a high likelihood for success in this new venture. After all, they will be providing funding and the bank wants to insure they can receive consistent payments on the loan. In every business venture, there must be a solid plan that realistically forecasts profitability for a proposed expansion. As presented in Chapter 2, with a sound business plan and realistic financial projections in hand, the bank is more likely to loan the funds for the project at a favorable interest rate. There are a number of methods that can be used to figure the rate of return on your project, however, two methods commonly used: the breakeven analysis (BA) and/or the net present value (NPV).

Break-even Analysis (BA)

According to Kasewurm (2000), the break-even analysis provides a sales objective, expressed in either dollar or unit sales, at which the business will be breaking even (also discussed in Chapter 7). Described more technically by Brealey et al. (2010), the break-even analysis is the level of sales at which profits are zero or the point at which total revenues equal total costs. The calculation of a break-even analysis involves the use of the formula:

$$\text{Break-even (B)} = \frac{\text{Fixed}}{(\text{Gross Profit per Unit} - \text{Variable Costs})}$$

In the calculation of a break-even analysis, the fixed expenses are simply divided by the gross profit minus expenses to come up with the number of sales (or audiometric procedures or hearing aids) that it costs to break even. Of course, the practitioner is in business to make a profit and hopes to see many more procedures sold than to simply enough to break even (see Sidebar 8–10).

Sidebar 8–10
BREAKEVEN ANALYSIS

Described more technically by Brealey et al. (2002), the breakeven analysis is the level of sales at which profits are zero or the point at which total revenues equal total costs. The calculation of a breakeven analysis involves the use of the formula:

$$\text{Breakeven (B)} = \frac{\text{Fixed}}{\text{(Gross Profit per Unit} - \text{Variable Costs)}}$$

For example, Audiology Associates wants to open a new location for its diagnostic evaluations at the local hospital. At this alternative location, the practice will receive referrals from local physicians for routine audiometric evaluations, otoacoustic emission evaluations, videonystagmography, and auditory brainstem response evaluations. In the example offered below, the variable costs for items to conduct the tests, such as electrodes, forms, insurance discounts are an average of $78.00 per patient and the fixed costs for the new center are $4,500 per month to keep the clinic open. These fixed costs include an audiologist's salary, receptionist salary, rent, phone, and lease payments for equipment. For the full diagnostic services each patient is billed an average of $350.00.

Fixed Costs per month (Personnel, lease payments, space, phone, etc.)	$4,500
Variable Costs @100 Units (Insurance discount, forms, supplies, etc.)	$78
Average Fee (billed per patient)	$350

Therefore, the question to the practitioner that owns Audiology Associates is how many units of service must be provided each month to break even? Using the breakeven analysis calculation, simply take the fixed expenses of $4,500 divided by the gross profit per unit ($350) minus the variable costs ($78).

$$\text{Breakeven (B)} = \frac{\$4,500}{(\$350 - \$78)}$$

$$\text{Breakeven (B)} = \frac{\$4,500}{\$272} \quad BA = 16.54$$

From this analysis, the clinic must bill for 16.54 or 17 procedures each month to just break even. Of course, as this is only the point where the clinic breaks even, hopefully there will be substantially more than 17 units of service each month so that the new diagnostic center can stay in business.

Moser (2006) indicates that any expenditure made in the hope of generating more cash later can be called a capital investment project. For these large capital investment projects it is best to incorporate a calculation that considers the initial investment, everyday operation expenses, and the interest rate at which the funds for the project were borrowed. Although there are a number of financial calculations that attempt to predict the success of capital investment projects, a relatively simple calculation is the net present value (NPV); see Sidebar 8–11. The key to understanding the NPV calculation is, as indicated previously, the concept that the value of money is less tomorrow than it is today. This is why banks and other financial institutions charge interest. The value of the money may be less tomorrow but also the use of this money means that it cannot be used for another purpose if it is used in your particular project.

In capital investment projects it is often necessary to know if there is a possibility that the project will be successful while still in the planning stages. This allows the practitioner to choose the most successful project among a number of proposals based upon the calculated NPV. The chosen project is the one that has the highest return and a positive NPV value. Moser (2006) make a straightforward statement about negative NPV that all projects that carrying a negative NPV are losers and should not be attempted. The rules for the use of NPV indicate that the value of the practice will be increased by conducting those capital investment projects that are worth more than they cost—projects with a positive NPV.

Capital investment calculations, such as NPV and other project evaluations should be conducted with the assistance of the practice accountant to ensure accuracy of the cash flow predictions.

Sidebar 8–11
NET PRESENT VALUE (NPV) CALCULATION

Probably the most accurate technique to use in the estimation of the pay off for a remodeling or expansion project is one that actually considers the initial investment in addition to the everyday operation expenses and the interest rate at which the funds were borrowed. One method is to look at a calculation of the net present value or NPV often used by corporations to describe a number of project proposals allowing the manager to choose the project that will have the highest return and a positive NPV value. All projects, according to Brealey et al. (2002), that carry a negative NPV are losers and should not be attempted. A simple definition of the net present value (NPV) of a project or investment is that it presents the sum of the present values of the annual cash flows minus the initial investment. In a new clinic site, these annual cash flows are the net benefits (revenues minus costs) generated from new clinic site during its lifetime. In the NPV calculation these cash flows are discounted or adjusted by incorporating the uncertainty or risk of the success of the clinic and time value of money. In financial literature, the NPV offers the most robust financial evaluation to estimate the overall value of an investment.

Although there are Internet calculators for NPV, Odellion (2005) states that the calculation of NPV involves three simple yet nontrivial steps. The first step is to identify the size and timing of the expected future cash flows generated by the project or investment. The second step is to determine the discount rate or the estimated rate of return for the project. The third step is to calculate the NPV using the equations shown below:

$$NPV = Co + \frac{Cash\ Flow\ Year\ 1}{(1+r)} + \frac{Cash\ Flow\ Year\ 2}{(1+r)^2} + \frac{Cash\ Flow\ Year\ 3}{(1+r)^3}$$

Consider the following example, where the cost to remodel the space for the new diagnostic audiology center at the hospital is $27,000. The clinic can borrow the funds for this project at 6.5% for the project.

Initial Investment to remodel space (borrowed at 6.5% interest rate)	$27,000
Estimated Cash Flows	
Year 1	$25,000
Year 2	$40,000
Year 3	$75,000
Future Value of Practice if Successful	$75,000

This $27,000 includes items such as furniture, carpet, lighting, creating treatment rooms, reception area, wall coverings, art, and other appointments. The clinic also has some extra equipment that will be used in the new facility so there is not equipment cost. Cash flow estimates have been estimated by the accountant with input from the practitioner at $20,000 for year 1, $40,000 for year 3, and $75,000 at year 3. It is expected that after 3 years of operation; the new clinic could be worth $75,000.

$$NPV = -\$27,000 + \frac{\$25,000}{1.065} + \frac{\$40,000}{1.134} + \frac{\$75,000}{1.207}$$

$$NPV = -\$27,000 + \$23,474.17 + \$35,273.36 + \$62,137.53$$

$$NPV = \$93,885.06$$

As this is a highly positive NPV, the project should be conducted.

Epilogue

Fiscal management is fundamentally the practitioner's accountability for the practice. A fiscally responsible practitioner not only knows where the funds are, who needs payment, when they need to be paid, but also is current on everchanging costs and how to adjust to them. Reviewing financial statements and ratios regularly and tracking comparisons with other periods for monthly, quarterly or yearly comparisons, the changes in the landscape of the practice are evident. Knowledge of how to manage a fiscally responsible practice opens up many new horizons for the practitioner as to how to adjust to the external and internal changes in the environment.

Finance is an area in which most audiologists have no interest or background. A chief financial officer (CFO) is the chief financial policymaker in the company with duties often extending into many other areas including accounting, budgeting, and capital investment. Wise practice CFOs borrow smartly, expand cautiously, and invest in sound projects that will bring future success to the practice. Good financial investment may even counteract business problems, such as equipment breakdowns, slow business, or other unforeseen emergencies; providing a source of unencumbered cash to augment income as the situation changes. Since the audiologist is usually the CFO of their own practice, it is necessary to understand the accounting process, know how to review and track financial statements, prepare budgets to plan for the efficient use of funds, and calculate the benefits and realities of expenditure projects in our unrelenting quest for the unencumbered cash. Our goal with this chapter was to introduce the new practitioner to fiscal management, offer specific management points for increase efficiency to those that have been in practice for some time, and present the case that it is no longer safe and prudent to manage practices by the "seat of the pants." In today's competitive market, where most of us are doctors, these "seat of the pants" managers will fall by the wayside, victims of their own ignorance of the numbers and their valuable insight.

References

Accounting Coach. (2012a). Accounting principles: Basic accounting principles and guidelines. Accounting Coach.com. Retrieved June 28, 2012, from http://www.accountingcoach.com/online-accounting-course/09Xpg01.html

Accounting Coach. (2012b). Accounting principles: Basic accounting principles and guidelines. Accounting coach.com. Retrieved July 1, 2012, from http://www.accountingcoach.com/online-accounting-course/05Xpg01.html

Accounting Coach. (2012c). Multi step income statement. Accountingcoach.com. Retrieved July 1, 2012, from http://www.accountingcoach.com/online-accounting-course/04Xpg04.html#income-statement-multiple-step

Accounting for Management. (2012). Current ratio. Accounting4management.com. Retrieved July 1, 2012, from http://www.accounting4management.com/current_ratio.htm

ADP. (2012). ADP payroll services. Retrieved July 11, 2012, from http://www.adp.com/

American Institute of Certified Public Accountants. (2012). Retrieved June 28, 2012, from http://www.aicpa.org/Pages/Default.aspx

Answers.com. (2012). Defense interval ratio. Retrieved July 1, 2012, from http://www

.answers.com/topic/defensive-interval-ratio

Bankrate.com. (2012). Small business basics. Bankrate.com. Retrieved June 24, 2012, from http://www.bankrate.com/brm/news/biz/green/19990823c.asp

Brealey, R., Myers, S., & Allen F. (2010). *Fundamentals of corporate finance* (2nd ed.). New York, NY: McGraw-Hill.

Business Spreadsheets. (2007). *Lease Versus Purchase Decisions*. Business Spreadsheets. Retrieved April 6, 2007, from http://www.business-spreadsheets.com/solutions.asp?prod=91

Business Victoria. (2007). Types of leases. Business Victoria, Victoria, Australia. Retrieved April 6, 2007, from http://www.business.vic.gov.au/BUSVIC/STANDARD/1001/PC_50080.html

Edmonds, T., Edmonds, C., McNair, F., Olds, P., & Schneider, N. (2006). *Fundamental financial accounting concepts* (pp. 124–125). New York, NY: McGraw-Hill.

Freeman, B., Barimo, J., & Fox, G. (2000). Financial management of audiology practices and clinics. In H. Hosford-Dunn, R. Roeser, & M. Valente (Eds.), *Audiology practice management.* (pp. 351–362). New York, NY: Thieme.

Glaser, R. (2006). Point/counterpoint on issues in ethics. *Hearing Journal, 59*(10), 44.

Kasewurm, G. (2000). Business plan and practice accounting. In H. Hosford-Dunn, R. Roeser, & M. Valente, (Eds.), *Audiology practice management* (pp. 313–336). New York, NY: Thieme.

Lerner, J. & Gokarn, R. (2007). *Schaum's outlines of bookkeeping and accounting* (4th ed.). New York, NY: McGraw-Hill.

Marshall, D., McManus, W., & Viele, D. (2010). *Accounting: What the numbers mean* (9th ed.). New York, NY: McGraw-Hill.

McNamara, C. (2007). *Profit and loss statements.* Authenticity Consulting, LLC. Retrieved April 7, 2007, from http://www.managementhelp.org/finance/fp_fnce/fp_fnce.htm#anchor561785

Moser, K. (2006). *Lecture notes from Finance, 544.* Phoenix, AZ: University of Phoenix.

Newman, P. (2006). Eleven expectations to be set for your bookkeeper. Entrepreneur.com. Retrieved August 2, 2006, from http://smallbusiness.aol.com/manage/managing/article/_a/11-expectations-to-set-for-your/20060801161009990001

Odellion. (2005). NPV equation. Odellion.com. *Odellion Research Group.* Retrieved July 24, 2005, from http://www.odellion.com/pages/financial%20models/NPV/financialmodels_npv_equations.htm

Paycom. (2012). Online payroll services. Retrieved June 24, 2012, from http://www.paycomonline.com/landingb/?utm_source=google&utm_medium=ppc&utm_campaign=companies&keyword=Payroll-Companies-Paycom-Payroll-Company&gclid=COzJlpXNkbECFQZ5hwod-RHVdw

Quick MBA. (2012).Double entry bookkeeping. QuickMBA.com. Retrieved July 8, 2012, from http://www.quickmba.com/accounting/fin/double-entry/

Stratus.com. (2005). Advantages of leasing. *Stratus Technologies Bermuda, Ltd.* Retrieved July 27, 2005, from http://www.stratus.com/leasing/advant.htm

Tracy, J. (2008). *Accounting for dummies* (4th ed.). Hoboken, NJ: Wiley.

Tyson, E. (1996). *Personal finance for dummies* (2nd ed.). Foster City, CA: IDW Books.

Coding, Reimbursement, and Practice Management

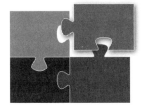

DEBRA ABEL, AuD

As audiologists, we have historically experienced road bumps and seemingly road blocks with coding, reimbursement, and the recognition by third-party payers for the services we provide. We have had a long, arduous road of educating third-party payers as to those services as well as defining "audiology" on a national as well as a grass roots level. Consequently, this education has also been conducted within the halls of the Centers for Medicare and Medicaid Services, otherwise known as CMS. Many third-party payers look to CMS, the Resource-Based Relative Value Scale (RBRVS), and the Medicare Physician Fee Schedule (MPFS) as the benchmark for establishing fee schedules, thereby perpetuating this flawed, inefficient system. The RBRVS and the MPFS is discussed next. Understanding the process of where we have been, and where we are going in terms of autonomy and professionalism, is essential to practicing within established federal and state regulations.

In addition to the reimbursement side, there are a plethora of issues and concerns to consider when contemplating the foray into independent practice, some legal and some practical, one hopes all touched upon here. This is not a limited list by any means. Federal, state, and local laws should be vetted prior to considering a private practice, with an attorney versed in health care law, offering legal guidance.

At the time of the publication of this book, CMS recognizes audiologists only as diagnosticians, and not as providers of treatment of hearing and balance disorders such as rehabilitation of hearing loss, tinnitus management, and management of the patient experiencing imbalance disorders. Many third-party payers with whom we interact establish their policies based on these Medicare imposed requirements. Although these restrictions fly in the face of our state licensure laws, which define our scope of practice, some payers do recognize and reimburse for all professional services that audiologists are licensed to provide.

With the movement to a doctoring profession, evolution has occurred with some third-party payers as well as with managed care and likely will continue. It is also incumbent upon us to educate these third-party payers as to who we are, what we do, and what the services are that we can provide to their subscribers. On a grass roots level, it is encouraged that you and a few of your local colleagues meet with the medical director of the insurance company who may not recognize audiologists. In your armament, you will want to have the American Academy of Audiology's scope of practice as well as redacted copies of several explanations of benefits (EOBs) from their competitors, illustrating how audiology services have been successfully reimbursed. The intent of this meeting is to educate that medical director about audiology as well as the cost-savings benefits we can provide.

To understand coding, one needs to know how a code is valued and the formula that determines Medicare reimbursement; Medicare bases payments on the Resource-Based Relative Value Scale (RBRVS). There are three components that compose the relative value unit (RVU). The first component is work or cognition and includes the time, physical effort, skill, and stress in providing the service. "Work" (RVUw) composes slightly over 50% of the total payment. The second component is the practice expense (RVUpe). This includes the overhead of operating and maintaining an office: the rent, the office's physical liability coverage, staff expenses, and the disposables needed for the equipment you have. Practice expense (PE) accounts for over 40% of the total payment of a CPT code. The final component is professional liability/malpractice (RVUpli), and accounts for the remaining 5% of the total payment. Each of these three components (work, PE, and PLI) is multiplied by the geographic price cost index (GPCI) to reflect practice costs that differ across the country. This takes into account the costs of maintaining a practice. For example, the costs of a metropolitan office will be higher in California than in a rural area in Arkansas. Finally, all components are then multiplied by the conversion factor (CF), which changes on an annual basis, as a result of congressional action. The final formula is:

$$\textbf{RVUw} \times \textbf{GPCIw} + \textbf{RVUpe} \times \textbf{GPCIpe}$$
$$+ \textbf{RVUpli} \times \textbf{GPCIpli} \times \textbf{CF}$$
$$= \textbf{Medicare payment}$$

What makes this situation more flawed is the process is budget neutral. To translate, that means if the cost of one procedure is increased, another will be decreased.

The Current Procedural Process (CPT) Code Evolution

As we open our new CPT manuals every fall to see if there are any new CPT codes that we may implement in our practices, it is helpful to know the process of how those codes appear. The American Medical Association (AMA) owns the 8,000 plus CPT codes and has since 1966, about the time of Medicare's genesis. The intent was to standardize codes for procedures performed for insurance submissions and for data collection. CPT codes comprise one of the components of the transaction and code sets of HIPAA which also includes the International Classification of Diseases-9-CM codes (ICD-9, the diagnoses codes), and the Healthcare Common Procedures Coding System (HCPCS), which includes supplies and ancillary services such as hearing aid related expenses not addressed by the CPT codes.

Utilization of CPT codes is tracked in the RUC (AMA's Specialty Society Relative Value Scale Update Committee) database. Prior to 2008, when the Centers for Medicare and Medicaid Services issued Transmittal 84, which specified that the services performed by an audiologist be billed with the national provider identifier (NPI) of that audiologist, many physicians billed audiologic services to Medicare beneficiaries as "incident to." "Incident to" services have requirements which did not include "other diagnostic tests," the category for audiologic tests. Therefore, the mistaken, pervasive practice of physicians filing claims for services performed by their audiologist-employee with the physician's NPI for the tests performed by that employee should not have been done and should have ceased in 2008.

A code request may be initiated by anyone. The majority of the code requests originate from interested parties such as professional organizations. When a potential code will be utilized by several organizations, often a code request is submitted by the organizations collaboratively. Several requirements need to be met: The equipment utilized must have the approval from the Food and Drug Administration (FDA), be performed in multiple locations by many other providers and that the procedure's clinical efficacy, and be well documented with peer-reviewed literature. A vignette, or scenario, that details the procedure for a "typical patient" also must accompany the request.

The CPT Editorial Panel is responsible for revising or updating the CPT codes. This 17-member panel is composed of 11 physicians representing the AMA, 1 each from Blue Cross and Blue Shield Association, America's Health Insurance Plans, the American Hospital Association, and the Centers for Medicare and Medicaid Services (CMS), and the co-chair and a representative of the Health Care Professionals Advisory Committee (HCPAC) (AMA, 2004).

There are two other groups who are involved in this process: the CPT HCPAC and the RUC HCPAC. The CPT HCPAC reviews the code requests that are brought forth through that process. The HCPAC is vital to audiology as this represents limited license practitioners and other allied health professionals (AMA, 2004) reviewing the two higher weighted components of the RVU: the work and practice expense components. The RUC HCPAC reviews recommendations on the RVU's for nonphysician specialties' work and practice expenses.

The CPT Editorial Panel meets three times per calendar year. It is at these meetings that new code requests are introduced or revised. Of course, the code request can be tabled or rejected. At this point if things go smoothly, a code will be accepted and will appear in the next published CPT manual, which may be a year or two later. There are three categories of codes that reflect usage, performance measurement(s), or emerging technology and the code request meets one of those category's descriptors. Contained in the request are four questions defining the impetus for the request: Is the suggestion a fragmentation of an existing procedure/service, can the suggested procedure/service be reported by using two or more existing codes, does the suggested procedure/service represent a distinct service, or is the suggested procedure/service merely a means to report extraordinary circumstances related to the performance of a procedure/service already included in CPT (AMA, 2004)? Category I codes are what audiology has utilized in the last several years to introduce a new code, meeting the requirements which addressed that it is a distinct service performed by many practitioners across the United States, that the clinical efficacy of the procedure is well established and documented in peer review literature, and that the procedure is not currently reportable by one or more existing codes (AMA, 2004). Category II codes track performance measures, such as those utilized for the Medicare Physician Quality Reporting System. Category III code are for emerging technologies and services.

This explanation may serve to help audiologists understand the process of a code becoming just that and the journey it takes. This may explain why we don't have codes for every service we do as the time and process may take 24 to 36 months to "bring them to market" once the request is filed. In addition, CPT codes are assigned a relative value unit, and in the recent past, the valuation process has not served the profession well.

Billing Practices

As with any professional organization by virtue of membership, we subscribe to the code of ethics of our professional home. The American Academy of Audiology (AAA), the Academy of Doctors of Audiology (ADA), and the American Speech-Language-Hearing Association (ASHA) all have codes of ethics that can be located on their respective Web sites. State licensure laws may also incorporate codes of ethics in either the statute or in the code. These codify acceptable practice for the profession. Not adhering to them may result in unethical and potentially illegal behaviors.

Audiologists and other health care providers utilize three coding structures: Current Procedural Terminology (CPT), International Compendium of Diseases 9th Revision Clinical Modification (ICD-9-CM), and the Healthcare Common Procedure Coding System (HCPCS). These manuals should be in each of our offices and ordered annually when they are published. The five-digit CPT codes are the procedures that we perform and are owned by the American Medical Association (AMA). The ICD-9 codes are the disease codes, with five-digit codes preferred for specificity, and the HCPCS codes are the supply codes that include codes for the specific styles of hearing aids, professional fees, and assistive listening devices codes. With all of these codes, they are utilized by other professionals, not just audiologists.

Any third-party payer has a specific contract between the patient and themselves as well as one between the provider and themselves. You may have a more general contract that applies to many of their subscribers and specifies the dos and don'ts of coverage. This may include discounts, the ability or inability to balance bill the patient for services above the cost of what they will reimbursed, and if you can, bill the patient or be forced to wait for their reimbursement. It is vital to remember that this is only a vehicle for reimbursement, not for payment.

There are many types of insurances: Medicare, Medicaid, Tricare, Health Maintenance Organizations (HMOs), Preferred Provider Organizations (PPOs), Point of Service (POS), Fee for Service (FFS), Worker's Compensation, and Disability, to name a few.

In order to bill a patient, most offices have an encounter form, routing slip, or superbill. This is a listing of the applicable and most widely utilized codes in that facility. The patient's name, date of service, and provider's name also need to be included on an encounter form. The appropriate CPT codes that were performed as well as the diagnosis or diagnoses need to be indicated and then submitted to the clearinghouse or insurance company that will be billing on your behalf for these codes on a CMS 1500 claim form. If hearing aids or supplies were billed, the HCPCS codes will also need to be itemized. Several ICD-9 codes per claim, if appropriate and applicable, may be indicated.

For example, you perform 92557, the comprehensive audiometry code that includes air, bone, speech reception thresholds, and word recognition that you perform on the patient who presents with a hearing loss after an airplane flight. An air-bone gap is the result and is then confirmed with tympanometry and acoustic reflex thresholds (92550). You may elect to utilize 389.03, conductive hearing loss, middle ear, for these procedures. Continuing with this example, if the patient also complained of tinnitus, you could choose 388.31, subjective tinnitus, as a secondary ICD-9 code for 92557 and 92550. You want all this documented in the chart along with the patient's history, assessment and recommendations. Documentation details are discussed later in this chapter. You will also need to have the patient's permission in order to bill their insurer on their behalf, which is often included on the facility's registration sheet. Also often included on the same sheet or a separate sheet, if allowed by the payer, is the patient's signature on an insurance waiver, the statement that if their insurer does not cover their services, they understand they then will be responsible for those service.

To ensure the highest level of accuracy and reimbursement, you need to utilize the five digit ICD-9 codes for specificity, but avoid those that end in zero. There is no ICD-9 code for normal hearing and "rule outs" are unacceptable submissions. As with any result, coding for the reason for the visit, for signs, symptoms, or the chief complaint the patient presented are acceptable coding strategies.

Medicare

Medicare, the largest insurer, has been in effect since the Lyndon Johnson years of the mid-1960s as a mechanism to supplement and provide health insurance for those aged 65 or older, blind individuals, individuals who have been on disability for at least two years, and those with end stage renal disease (ESRD). Medicare is usually the primary insurance, but with more people over age 65 and still in the workforce, Medicare may be secondary to their employers' health care benefit.

CMS Program Memorandum AB-02-080 heralds, "diagnostic testing, including hearing and balance assessment services, performed by a qualified audiologist is paid for as 'other diagnostic tests' under §1861 (s)(3) of the Social Security Act (the Act) when a physician orders testing to obtain information as part of his/her diagnostic evaluation or to determine the appropriate medical or surgical treatment of a hearing deficit or related medical problem" (CMS, 2002). It further states that, "services are excluded by virtue of §1862 (a)(7) of the Act when the diagnostic information is already known to the physician, or the diagnostic services are performed only to determine the need for or the appropriate type of hearing aid" (CMS, 2002, 2012).

Since 2005, Medicare beneficiaries who are new to Medicare (within the first twelve months of enrollment) are entitled to an initial physical examination. Hearing and balance disorders are addressed by screening questionnaires approved by a couple of professional organizations. This is a wonderful opportunity for audiologists to be the diagnostic professional to address either or both of these health issues and to educate the physicians on their importance by citing fall risk as well as the self-esteem and depression issues of the elderly hearing-impaired population.

At this point in time, CMS designed the Medicare Administrative Contractors

(MAC) jurisdictions to balance the allocation of workloads, account for integration of claims processing activities, and mitigate the risk to the Medicare program (http://www.cms.hhs.gov, 2007). The jurisdictions reasonably balance the number of fee-for-service beneficiaries and providers and are substantially more alike in size than the previous fiscal intermediary and carrier jurisdictions. This restructuring is to promote much greater efficiency in processing Medicare's billion plus claims a year (http://www.cms.hhs.gov, 2007).

The Centers for Medicare and Medicaid Services issue National Coverage Determination (NCD) policies. Each MAC may create Local Coverage Determination (LCD) policies which are specific to those designated states for which a MAC has jurisdiction. As each MAC has the authority to interpret the Medicare statute independently, Medicare regulations may not be the same from contractor to contractor. You will want to have the LCD policy for your contractor as well as the Medicare Physician Fee Schedule (MPFS), updated annually, for your area. There may not be an audiologic or vestibular procedure LCD for your area, but it is suggested that you review one from another MAC. LCDs describe in detail what is considered to be medical necessity, what CPT and ICD-9-CM or ICD-10-CM codes may be recognized for payment and other parameters that each Medicare provider needs to be familiar with. These can be obtained online at http://www.cms.hhs.gov. It may behoove you to have a contact person in provider relations at your Medicare contractor's office to consult for guidance. Contractors offer no-charge seminars periodically, which would be beneficial to keep abreast of changing information.

Medicare is composed of 4 parts: Part A (hospital based services), Part B (typically outpatient services), Part C (these are Medicare HMOs, with some having audiologic benefits for diagnosis, annual routine monitoring, and often a hearing aid benefit), and Part D (drugs). We discuss Parts A and B in greater detail and how they pertain to audiology.

Part A

The following components compose Medicare Part A: hospitalization, home health care, hospice care, and skilled nursing care after hospital discharge. Audiologists in hospital settings are Part A and those who bill independently will need to be contracted with the hospital who will then reimburse them for services provided. The Joint Commission for Accreditation of Healthcare Organizations (JCAHO) credentials hospitals and only accredited hospitals will be reimbursed by Medicare.

Medicare Part A is funded by payroll taxes, self-employed individual contributions, and contributions from railroad workers and their employers (Medicare New Provider Training, 2006). Payment to the hospital is via the patient's diagnostic related group (DRG), which is generally based on diagnosis, age, gender, and complications (Capturing Reimbursement, 2006). Beneficiaries can be enrolled in Medicare Part A and Part B.

Part B

Medicare Part B recipients have outpatient services as their Medicare benefit, including physician office visits. As audiologists, subscriber benefits would be exercised in the two most common outpatient settings: those in private practice who bill independently and those of our colleagues employed by otolaryngologists. Part B includes the following: medical expenses, home health care, laboratory services, ambulatory surgical services, and of course, outpatient medical services.

Part B Medicare is funded by premium payments, contribution from general revenues, and interest earned on Part B Trust Fund (Medicare New Provider Training, 2006). Part B providers have several categories in which to provide services: participating provider (par), nonparticipating provider (non-par), and limiting charge provider (LC).

Participating and nonparticipating providers have the choice of changing their status once a year. In an economically challenged area, it is usually more beneficial for the patients if you are a participating provider. Medicare will pay the provider 80% of the Medicare Physician Fee Schedule allowable amount for the procedures performed and the patient pays their 20% co-insurance or the claim is forwarded to their secondary, if one exists. That is the definition of a participating provider: accepting what is allowed via the MPFS. The co-payments (and unmet deductibles) must be paid at the time of service.

With a more affluent demographic, patients are often receptive and able to pay their share at the time of service. For nonparticipating or limiting charge enrolled providers, Medicare would reimburse the patient 80% of the allowable amount of Medicare Physician Fee Schedule, which yields better cash flow. Secondary insurances often will pay the co-insurance of 20%. A nonparticipating audiologist may not exceed the limiting charge. Nonparticipating providers receive 5% less than a participating provider. Limiting charge providers receive 10% more than someone who is participating.

For those who are Medicare providers, there is the opportunity to choose how one wishes to be paid by Medicare and/or the beneficiary. Regardless of the status, Medicare can only be billed for diagnostic audiologic services when there is a physician referral based on medical necessity.

Part C

Medicare Advantage Plans were created in the 1997 Balance Budget Act in order to afford Medicare beneficiaries choices with their health care. This is accomplished via a coverage plan which provides services not traditionally covered by Medicare. Annual audiograms and hearing aids which are statutorily excluded in the traditional Part B may be included in Part C when this Part C plan is in effect. It may take the form of a preferred provider organization (PPO), a health maintenance organization (HMO), a point of service (POS), or fee for service (FFS).

Part D

In effect since January 2006 as a component of the Medicare Modernization Act, beneficiaries may be eligible for a prescription drug plan. Monthly premiums and deductibles may apply (Medicare New Provider Training, 2006).

Advanced Beneficiary Notice

The alerting notice required for Medicare beneficiaries, the Advanced Benefi-

ciary Notice (ABN), is a component of the Beneficiary Notices Initiative (BNI). These statutory mandates are to ensure that the patient understands that all of their health care may not be a statutorily covered service, advises them of their expected out-of-pocket payment, and enables them to be more active participants in their health care decisions. They may choose not to pursue that service at that time. It is their option and they have the right to exercise it. The ABN informs the patient that their procedure(s) *may* be denied as, "Medicare does not pay for everything, even some care that you or your health care provider have good reason to think you need" (CMS, 2012). They are then expected to pay for those non-Medicare reimbursed services that are listed on the ABN. In other words, if there is doubt that the procedure will be paid, an Advanced Beneficiary Notice will need to be signed by the patient, dated with the procedure(s) to be performed, and a copy given to the patient. Also on the form is the reason the procedure may be denied or partially paid. In the event that Medicare does not pay, the patient may then be billed. A signature should be maintained on file and the modifier–GA appended to the claim so that Medicare is aware that the ABN was given to the patient. If an ABN is not issued to the patient and the service is denied, the provider is liable and cannot seek payment from the Medicare beneficiary. The ABN is not required to be issued for noncovered services, but is suggested so that the patient can understand their fiscal responsibility.

Although you may want to protect your patients and your practice, it is ill advised to have every patient complete the ABN. This is considered to be blanket utilization and is not a recommended policy.

If the patient's visit is due to annual routine audiologic monitoring for example, this is statutorily excluded and a voluntary ABN may be offered to the patient *before* any services are provided as it notifies them that Medicare will *not* pay for that particular service. A voluntary ABN could be given to the patient if the visit was due to anything related to hearing aids or vestibular rehabilitation, for example, because of statutory exclusion. Medicare is not billed for any of these services; therefore, the patient is financially responsible. If the patient has a secondary payer which requires a denial from Medicare, you can file the claim to Medicare to obtain the denial with the GY and GX modifiers (see Medicare modifiers listed in this chapter).

You will need to contact your Medicare carrier as local policies differ and therefore contractors may differ in their guidance. The ABN forms can be located on the CMS Web site (https://www.cms.gov/BNI/02_ABN.asp#TopOfPage), the American Academy of Audiology Web site (http://www.audiology.org), or in Appendix 9–A following this chapter. The ABN is form number CMS-R-131.

Medicare Participating Provider Status

This Medicare category is the most common among Medicare providers. It means that you accept Medicare assignment and agree to accept the assignment for the services that are covered for all patients. The assignment is 80% of the Medicare Physician Fee Schedule allowable amount for your region. This is paid to you on the patient's behalf. The patient then pays you their 20% co-insurance at the time of service. If they have a sec-ondary insurance, it is then automatically forwarded and submitted to that secondary by Medicare, if a coordination of benefits is in place. This category allows the patient to have a lesser expense at the time of service while the provider enjoys a 5% higher fee allowance than a nonparticipating provider, but 10% lower than a limiting charge provider. Medical necessity and a physician order are the two requirements in billing Medicare for diagnostic audiologic services at the time of the publication of this text.

If an overpayment occurs, when Medicare pays you more than the correct amount, you need to refund the overpayment as soon as it is discovered. If Medicare requests an overpayment, it must be refunded or notification served within 60 days, or it may be considered a false claim, carrying a stiff penalty. Of course, you have the right to appeal if in disagreement.

Medicare Nonparticipating Status

This category means that the provider does not accept assignment. Two subcategories are found here. The first is nonparticipating provider and is reimbursed at 5% less than a participating provider. The second category is limiting charge and allows 10% more than participating. This is the highest level of payment from Medicare to a provider. The benefit is that it is increases cash flow for the practice as the patient pays the provider and is then reimbursed by Medicare. Nonparticipating provider status is better received in a less economically challenged demographic. The limiting charge is the maximum amount a nonparticipating provider may charge a Medicare beneficiary on a non-par claim. Again, medical necessity and a physician order are the two requirements in billing Medicare for diagnostic audiologic services.

Opting Out—Not an Option for Audiologists

Audiologists are not one of the professions allowed to opt out of Medicare; therefore, audiologists must be enrolled in Medicare or provide diagnostic services at no charge. If a Medicare beneficiary requests their claim be filed to Medicare, the Social Security Act (Section 1848(g)(4) requires that claims be submitted for services rendered to Medicare beneficiaries on or after September 1, 1990 (CMS, 2011). The only way that can be accomplished is if you are enrolled in Medicare. Enrollment can be done online via Provider Enrollment, Chain, Ownership System (PECOS) at https://pecos.cms.hhs.gov/pecos/login.do or by filing the 855I enrollment form.

Medicare Compliance

Compliance with mandatory claim filing requirements is monitored by CMS, and violations of the requirement may be subject to a civil monetary penalty of up to $2,000 for each violation, a 10% reduction of a physician's/supplier's payment once the physician/supplier is eventually brought back into compliance, and/or Medicare program exclusion. Medicare beneficiaries may not be charged for preparing or filing a Medicare claim (CMS Medlearn Matters, 2011).

Medicare may require a medical review if there is concern about inappropriate billings, odd billing patterns, and over-utilization. This may be to confirm that services were rendered, to ensure that services were coded correctly as well as to confirm those services were medically necessary (Medicare New Provider Training, 2006). The reviewer/auditor may specify patient files for review. If there are issues, penalties may be assessed and an appeal may be instituted. Comprehensive Error Rate Testing (CERT) is another mechanism to identify potential problems via random claims review to determine potential billing issues and to address those issues.

There are five levels of appeal: redetermination, reconsideration, administrative law judge hearing, appeals council review, and judicial review in US District Court (CMS Medlearn, 2011).

"Incident to"

"Incident to" has been utilized for many years by physicians who billed Medicare for the services performed by audiology employees, not for services they personally performed. It does suggest that these are services that they did not personally perform, but supervised when performed by others. None of our CPT codes require physician supervision. Was the physician in the office? Out of the office performing surgery? "Incident to" supervision requires the physician to be in the facility and available for assistance (direct supervision) if a technician is performing the technical component of a CPT code that has the TC/PC split.

"Incident to" billing is not to be done when services are in the "other diagnostic services" category, which is where diagnostic audiology services reside. "Incident to" billing dilutes the work audiologists do within the RUC data bank, a proprietary repository of services performed on Medicare beneficiaries. In other words, our profession does not receive the credit for the numbers of audiologic procedures performed, when not filed directly by an audiologist. Audiologists have "qualified provider" status which allows us to bill for our services directly, with the caveat of having a physician order for a medically necessary reason.

CMS has established the following requirements in order to bill "incident to": a procedure or service must be furnished by a physician which initiates the course of treatment; the service is billed secondary to the medical visit, or "incident to'" that it is furnished in a non-institutional setting to noninstitutional patients; and finally, of a type commonly furnished in the office of a physician, furnished under the direct supervision of the physician, furnished by a physician, other practitioner, or auxiliary personnel and only for services that do not have their own benefit category. Again, this final point is the reason why this method of billing should not be done by way of the physician's NPI when performed by any licensed audiologist as we have our own provider category, "other diagnostic tests." In addition, as we do provide benefits that are statutorily covered, "incident to" should not be billed (Pessis, Williams, & Freint, 2006).

CPT Codes with Technical and Professional Components

Due to the technical component (TC)/professional component (PC) split, several families of CPT codes utilized by audiologists have three methods of payment. The codes that have the TC/PC split include the vestibular codes 92540–

92546, 92548; auditory evoked potentials for evoked response audiometry comprehensive (92585); and the limited and diagnostic otoacoustic emissions codes, respectively, 92587 and 92588. These codes have the TC or technical component and also the professional component indicated by modifier-26.

With the TC/PC split codes, if a professional only performs the procedure, then the technical component is billed. If another provider only does the interpretation and report, then the professional code is billed. If both are completed by the same audiologist, the procedure is then billed globally.

The technical component (TC) is to be utilized by the provider, likely a technician, who performed the test and per Medicare guidelines, the claim is filed by the physician who performed the direct supervision of that procedure. When the TC is billed by one professional, then the professional component (PC or -26), the interpretation of the test results and writing a report of the findings for the patient's health record, can be completed and billed directly by an audiologist, physician, or nonphysician provider (NPP), such as a nurse practitioner, physician's assistant, or certified nurse midwife.

Physician Quality Reporting System (PQRS)

CMS has stated in the last few years of this writing that they will be converting fee-for-service payment into "pay for performance" or "value-based purchasing." These methodologies are based on a merit system, to encourage excellence while trimming costs, and are likely to be based on successful outcome measure reporting and quality of care results. The Medicare Part B Physician Quality Reporting System (PQRS) is a likely step to this end.

The Physician Quality Reporting System (PQRS), a measures reporting system originally known as the Physician Quality Reporting Initiative (PQRI), is a voluntary program created to improve the quality of care to Medicare beneficiaries which offers a bonus based on all Medicare claims when successful reporting has been done by Medicare Part B eligible providers. Audiologists have been recognized since 2010 as an eligible provider for PQRS, which has resulted in recognition of the profession by CMS. Since 2010, the Audiology Quality Consortium (AQC), a coalition of 10 audiology organizations, has collaborated on the audiology quality measures.. When successful reporting on eligible measures is completed, all Medicare allowed charges will receive a 0.5% bonus until December 31, 2014. However, for those who did not report on a minimum of at least one PQRS measure in 2013 for 50% of eligible cases, effective beginning on January 1, 2015, a 1.5% disincentive on all Medicare claims will occur and for those who don't report in 2014, a 2% disincentive will be applied to all 2016 Medicare claims. As Medicare moves away from a fee-for-service methodology, outcome measure reporting may be one of the requirements for future payment. It's as easy as adding a G code to your Medicare Part B claims!

In 2013, audiologists have four measures on which to report:

■ *Measure #188:* Referral for Otologic Evaluation for Patients with Congenital or Traumatic Deformity of the Ear

■ *Measure #261:* Referral for Otologic Evaluation for Patients with Acute or Chronic Dizziness
■ *Measure #130:* Documentation of Current Medications in the Medical Record
■ *Measure #134:* Preventative Care and Screening: Screening for Clinical Depression and Follow-Up Plan.

For current information on PQRS and audiology measures, go to: http://www.audiology.org/practice/PQRI/Pages/default.aspx and for general information: https://www.cms.gov/PQRS/.

Other Third-Party Payers and Differences with Medicare

Although many third-party payers look to Medicare to set their policies and fee schedules, there are other entities that also need to be discussed when dealing with insurance companies as this is integral to our practices. This alphabet soup of HMO, PPO, FFS, and POS is overwhelming, but has been in existence for many years and is likely to continue. A short explanation of these follows.

Health Maintenance Organizations (HMO): The gatekeeper or primary care physician (PCP) is the conductor of health care for the patient. This may also be a pediatrician, an internal medicine physician, an obstetrician/gynecologist, as well as a family practitioner. Referrals to other health care providers are required and sanctioned by those listed above. Payment will not occur if a referral was not obtained.

This is designed to control health care costs.

Preferred Provider Organization (PPO): The patient's preferred choice as they do not need a referral, and in general may see the provider of their choice. Although it may be more of an out of pocket expense for an out-of-network provider and they may pay a higher co-pay for seeing that provider. An in-network provider is one who is contracted directly with the PPO. Out-of-network is therefore one who is not contracted with that third-party payer. Patient costs are minimized with an in-network provider as the co-pays are less and the reimbursement percentages (90% of the costs reimbursed for example, patient pays the remaining 10%) versus out-of-network that may have a higher co-pay as well as greater exposure (70% of the costs reimbursed for example, patient pays the remaining 30%).

Point of Service (POS): A step-down from an HMO, patients have more out-of-network options, but there are greater financial benefits for staying in-network as it the case for most of these health care structures. Higher co-pays or co-insurances are to be expected for utilizing a non-network provider as a disincentive.

Basic Coding Tidbits

When you perform a variety of audiologic procedures (CPT), these are often indicated on a superbill or encounter form, the mechanism for the staff/coders to know what you did in order for pay-

ment to occur. The next step in the process besides selecting that CPT code is to select a supportive ICD-9-CM code, the disease code. The reason the patient presented to your office is likely their chief complaint and "signs and symptoms" are often the mantra heard by many in completing this process. Patient symptoms and the outcome of the testing are also all legitimate reasons for specifying their diagnosis or diagnoses. For example, if a patient presents with bilateral tinnitus, ICD-9 code 388.31 can be utilized. If they also have a mild bilateral sensorineural hearing loss, 389.12 can then also be claimed. It is possible to have more than one ICD-9 code per patient encounter, depending on the reason for the visit or as a result of the outcome of the tests, but you will want to check with your payer's guidance to ensure the recognition of multiple ICD-9 codes when filing claims.

The most specific five-digit codes applicable for the ICD-9-CM's are the most advantageous and are less likely to result in a denial. That said, you also want to avoid those that end with a zero as they typically do not provide sufficient specificity. For example, 389.10 may not be the best choice for sensorineural hearing loss even though it is a five-digit code.

ICD-10 Codes

As of October 1, 2014, the ICD-10 coding system will be in effect for everyone covered by HIPAA, providers, and payers alike. This is the first coding change in the United States in 30 years, bringing the United States into the fold with nearly all non-third-world countries utilizing this coding system. Providers can look forward to greater coding specificity with the transition from a 17,000 code system to a 68,000 code system and to new codes not seen in the ICD-9 coding system, such as ototoxicity.

Co-Pays and Co-Insurances

Co-pays and co-insurances are likely a part of a patient's health care benefit. A co-pay is a specified amount that is indicated on their health insurance card which has to be collected from the patient at the time of service. A typical range is from $25.00 to $50.00. A co-insurance is a percentage of the visit that needs to be paid by the patient at the time of service, usually those who are insured by PPOs, fee for service, and also Medicare. Medicare Part B participating providers are required to collect the co-insurance and any unmet deductible.. As an example of co-insurance, if the total of the procedures performed was $250.00 for that date of service and the patient is to pay a 20% co-insurance, they would pay $50.00 to the provider. If the patient goes sees a non-network provider, they can expect to pay a higher co-insurance, for example 40% instead of their usual 20%.

Deductibles are another financial responsibility the patient needs to meet before their benefits "kick in." These amounts are paid annually and typically range from $500.00 to $5,000 per year for an individual. Family deductibles will be different if it is a family plan. If a patient comes in to see you in the early part of the year, barring any health care issues or visits, it is likely they have not met their deductible and they will need to pay the entire amount, which is then be applied to their deductible until it is paid.

"Balance billing" allows a patient to be billed for services that their insurance did not cover, for what was allowed, per that payer's specific fee schedule. For PPOs who often discount the patient's fees, this is disallowed as the provider has agreed to accept the discounted rate. If this is not specified in the contract, then the provider may balance bill the patient for services not covered. An example of balance billing would be if $425.00 was billed to the insurance company, they paid $399.00, then the patient can be billed the remaining $26.00, as long as this was not contractually disallowed.

You will want to trend and monitor the payments when the Explanation of Benefits (EOB) arrives in your office. This is a formal agreement of the covered and non-covered services for that date of service, the payment received or not, and, in addition, the patient's responsibility for payment. The patient is also likely to be the recipient of an EOB so they will also be notified as to what was paid and what is their responsibility, if any. You will want to have the payer's legend at hand to check what the abbreviations and their codes indicate as they may be specific for that payer. If you are just beginning a private practice, it would behoove you to set up a spreadsheet with each third-party payer you will be billing, what they reimburse for each code, and if you are permitted to bill the patient for unpaid services. This way you can observe trends, see if there's been a unilateral change to the reimbursements and also see if there is a trend in the appeals process. Write-offs will also be a component of the EOB and indicates the amount that is not billable to the patient and therefore must be written "off the books." For example, if services were billed to a PPO, the write-off amount would be what is contractually agreed upon by both parties and is then discounted and not billable to the patient.

You will need to establish a fee schedule for your practice of your usual and customary fees, based on your hourly rate and contact hours. Chapters 7 and 8 in this text will be resourceful in how to devise appropriate fees.

Evaluation and management codes (E & M) are not recognized by Medicare if billed by an audiologist. That does not eliminate other third-party payers from reimbursing for these codes, but there are several requirements to consider when billing E & M codes. The CPT manual is very specific in the requirements and includes the review of symptoms (ROS) for 18 body parts, some which have nothing to do with hearing or balance, but are required to be reviewed. The place and type of service, the content of the service such as history taking, detailed examination, medical decision making, the nature of the presenting problem, and the time element for face-to-face contact with the patient and/or family member is listed for each code as well as the history reported (AAA, Capturing Reimbursement, 2006). This is true for a new patient as well as an existing one to your practice. A new patient is considered one who you have never seen before or has not been seen 3 years previous to that date of service. An established patient is one who has been seen within that 3 year time frame. Level of complexity is also a consideration when choosing E & M codes, from Level 1 indicating the least involved level to a Level 5, the highest in complexity. It is recommended that private practice audiologists be conservative when selecting the appropriate level and

document the time you started and the time you completed the visit, if utilizing E & M codes. Documentation will be essential if the use of these codes prompts an audit. Audiologists should consult with individual payers about their specific guidance for E & M codes prior to filing claims for those services, to ensure that audiologists are recognized for payment for E & M codes.

It should prove to be quite beneficial to track all procedures and to whom they are being billed to see trends in payments, denials, and the time between billing and payment, as these can be addressed more expeditiously as well as correct internal billing problems within your facility.

Insurance or financial waivers are a mainstay of the patient registering in your office and should be offered at the time of service. By having the patient sign this document with the date of service and the procedures performed, they then become responsible for any payments not met by another party, if allowed by that party. This will allow you to bill them for that difference, as long as it is not contractually excluded. You will want to check with your specific payers to see if they offer their own waiver or if they will approve a generic waiver.

Although we don't like to consider that a patient may not pay the bill for our services, unfortunately, it does occur. Many practices send 3 notices to the nonpaying patient requesting payment. If nothing is received, the option of utilizing the services of a collection agency or an attorney in capturing this lost balance is urged. Generally if these mechanisms are utilized and if payment is then procured, only 50% of that amount collected is realized. This is why it is incumbent to collect at the time services are provided, if allowed by their third-party payer, and should include the required co-pays, co-insurances, or deductibles, especially for larger expense items such as hearing aids or extensive testing.

Bundling Versus Unbundling/Itemization of Hearing Aid Fees

For the last several years, the quandary of whether to bundle or itemize hearing aid fees, including professional fees, in the delivery of hearing aids has been a point of discussion. Bundling fees is best described as one fee for all hearing aid related services, including professional services. If you unbundle or itemize hearing aid related fees, you specify each of the incurred services or fees for the hearing aids; professional fees such as for dispensing, orientation, and verification; earmolds; earmold impressions; batteries; assistive listening devices; and follow-up visits. The Healthcare Common Procedure Coding System (HCPCS) codes provide the vehicle in which to itemize your fees in the provision of amplification devices and services. The hearing aid codes are listed as monaural versus binaural, by style (CIC, ITE, ITC, BTE, body), by technology (analog, programmable, and digital), and the combinations thereof.

By considering the itemization model, you demonstrate to the patient the "hardware" of the hearing aids/amplification system, as well as what it is "you," the software, and the services provided; these are value-added. This is one small aspect of autonomy that we seek and should be implemented, but may be payer specific. Patients should see the

value of the services they receive are by the one who is most qualified to provide those services: audiologists. Itemization sets the stage for patients to understand the breadth of audiologic services provided and for them to realize our worth. From a bottom line viewpoint, it helps increase cash flow so that you won't be spending many of your clinic days seeing no charge hearing aid rechecks all day. The American Academy of Audiology has created a step-by-step document to assist you in the itemization process: http://www.audiology.org/practice/reimbursement/Documents/20120110_AAA_Guide_Itemizing_Prof_Serv.pdf .

Modifiers

There are several modifiers commonly utilized by audiologists and can be located inside the front cover of the CPT manual. The first modifier, -22, increased procedural services, indicates that a procedure took a longer time than usual. An example of when to append this modifier would be applicable with a young child or a demented adult. If a comprehensive audiologic assessment was completed, the service would be appended as 92557-22. Documentation as to why this procedure took longer may need to accompany the claim when filed for payment.

Another common modifier for audiologists, -52, indicates reduced services. Often this is utilized when only one ear is tested since all of our diagnostic codes are binaural. If 92557, comprehensive audiometry, was performed for only one ear, the procedure would be appended as 92557-52.

The discontinued procedure modifier, -53, may be appended when the service is discontinued due to the patient becoming ill during the procedure and the provider chose to terminate it. In the same example, it would be appended as 92557-53. Although this has greater applicability with surgical procedures, you will want to consult with your payers for their guidance in using this modifier for audiologic procedures.

The -59 modifier is to be appended when indicating "distinct procedural service." In 2010, this became important to audiologists with the creation of a new bundled CPT code, 92540, Basic vestibular evaluation. This code includes 4 separate and distinct tests (CPT codes 92541, 92542, 92544, and 92545). When clinical decision making results in one to three of the four tests being performed, the -59 modifier indicates those tests are separate and distinct. If all four of the tests are completed, the bundled code is billed without a modifier.

Three families of codes, otoacoustic emissions (92587 and 92588), vestibular (92540–92546, 92548), and comprehensive auditory brainstem response (92585) have the ability to be billed globally or with the TC/PC split. Globally means the audiologist performed the procedure and did the interpretation and report. It would be billed as 92585 for the example of an ABR. With a few exceptions of a screening or limited code in the above families, if an audiologist performed only the test for CPT codes 92540–92546, 92548, 92585, 92587 and 92588, the TC or technical component would be appended. In the ABR example, it would be filed as 92585-TC and the provider who did the interpretation and report would append it with the professional modifier and bill it as 92585-26. The reimbursement of these two sub-fees per the Medicare Physician Fee Schedule, the

technical and professional components, equal the payment for the global fee. Although technicians are permitted to perform the technical component for Medicare beneficiaries, those services must be directly supervised and billed by a physician. Medicare-enrolled audiologists cannot bill for another provider's services, but you will need to consult with your commercial payers for their specific guidance pertaining to billing the services of technicians and audiology assistants.

Medicare Modifiers

Although the numeric modifiers described above apply to all services, although some are not recognized by all payers, there are alphabetic modifiers required by Medicare that pertain to medical necessity and the use of the ABN. Those modifiers are GY, GA, GX, and GZ. The Medicare beneficiary chooses one of three options on the ABN, directing how they want their claim to be filed (or not) to Medicare. The provider then appends the necessary modifier(s) to the claim.

GA, "Waiver of Liability Statement issued as Required by Payer Policy," is to be utilized when a required (mandatory) ABN is issued for a designated covered service. This indicates that the patient has a signature on file by way of their signed ABN, but the procedure may not be a covered service due to it not being medically reasonable and/or necessary. In the event it is not reimbursed, the patient can then be billed for that service since their signature is on file. This modifier is utilized when the provider expects Medicare to deny the service. Of the three Medicare modifiers, this is the least utilized by audiologists.

GY, "Item or service statutorily excluded or does not meet the definition of any Medicare benefit," is appended when the procedure is statutorily excluded and does not meet the definition of a Medicare benefit, such as hearing aids. Many third-party payers require a denial from Medicare in order for the patient to access the hearing aid benefit provided by that secondary payer. In this case, on line 19 of the CMS 1500 form, you would indicate that this is for denial by Medicare to initiate secondary payer coverage in order to generate that denial. This removes the onus of you billing fraudulently for a procedure that is statutorily excluded as the use of this modifier will result in an automatic denial. The GY modifier can be appended with the newest of the Medicare modifiers, the GX modifier.

The GX modifier, "Notice of Liability Issued, Voluntary Under Payer Policy," indicates a nonrequired or voluntary ABN, and would be issued for noncovered services such as routine evaluations not based on medical necessity, hearing aids, tinnitus treatment or aural rehabilitation. It is encouraged that patients be given the voluntary ABN, so their signature attests to their understanding of their fiscal responsibility, in case it is contested at a later date.

The GZ modifier, "Item or Service Expected To Be Denied As Not Reasonable and Necessary," is utilized when an ABN is not on file. When claims are submitted with this modifier, billing the patient for those services is disallowed.

Multiple modifiers could be listed as with this example: 92557-52GY if you performed comprehensive audiometry monaurally and you needed Medicare to deny this in order for the patient's secondary to pay for a hearing aid.

Collections

One of the potential problems of having a practice is having the patients pay their bills in a timely fashion. You may need to provide some type of payment plan or have a promissory note signed by the patient. Many offices avoid this problem with credit card payments that are confirmed in real time and there is no issue of nonpayment. There are several health care credit cards available so that the credit card company pays you and the patient in turn pays them. This eliminates your office having to bill the patient on a monthly basis, something that can only add to the cost of doing business.

Procedurally, many dispensing audiologists require half of the fee at the time of the hearing aid evaluation, the other half at the time the instruments are dispensed. One needs to be familiar with the device return policies of their state as they are quite variable and also specify the time frame in which the money has to be returned to the patient and how much has to be returned.

Audits

An audit may be triggered by several factors, but most often occurs when there is overutilization, especially in facilities where billed services are not typically performed on a regular basis, when processes are not followed, if there are direct patient complaints, or by a disgruntled employee or competitor. Third-party payers will perform random audits to ensure compliance to their regulations to ensure that procedures are followed within the confines of the parameters of appropriate billing practices.

One of the audit methodologies that Medicare utilizes is the Comprehensive Error Rate Testing (CERT). By randomly selecting a specific number of monthly claims, its goal is to educate the provider on appropriate and legitimate practices. Secondly, it is to ensure that Medicare is correctly processing claims. This is administered by an independent contractor, who will request records directly from the provider (Pessis, Williams, & Freint, 2006).

Another audit methodology Medicare has instituted as a result of the 2010 Affordable Care Act is data mining as well as categorizing levels of risk of providers who may commit fraud and abuse. Fortunately, audiologists are in the lowest level of risk. Medicaid is also required to perform audits and many commercial payers may also conduct audits.

To address Medicare audits, the Centers for Medicare and Medicaid (CMS) established a demonstration project in 2005 to 2007, with Recovery Audit Contractors (RACs) in Arizona, California, Florida, Massachusetts, New York, and South Carolina to identify and recover the monies from overpayments due them and to return the money to providers for underpayments, a less likely scenario. During these years, approximately $1.03 billion was recovered in improper payments. Now in all 50 states, RACs utilize proprietary software for outliers and violations, administered by incentivized contractors who receive a percentage of the money recouped. The OIG states that, "RACs are not responsible for reviewing claims for fraudulent activity," but are to refer potential fraud cases that are discovered in the RAC review process to CMS (CMS, 2010). Claims prior to October 1, 2007, will not be reviewed. CMS reported that in 2010, $75.4 million was recovered in overpayments; $16.9 million in underpayments. From January to September 2011, CMS reported $714.5 million in overpayments and $132.4 million in underpayments (DHHS, 2011).

In order to avoid an audit, you will want to have the most appropriate documentation in place as the chart for a specific patient likely will be reviewed by the auditors. One of the most common audit activities is to verify the completion of billed procedures for a specific date of service that is in the chart and noted. The diagnosis assigned to that date of service will also be verified with the report.

In the majority of cases, the auditors will assess a fee, possibly with a penalty to pay for any offenses. With the Centers for Medicare and Medicaid Services on their fraud and abuse campaign, this may proceed to the next level. You have the right to an appeal and it is recommended that you obtain legal counsel well versed in health care and Medicare/Medicaid/ thirty party doctrine. Utilization review will likely occur within a specific time frame post audit to ensure that specific procedures are being followed. Other consequences may ensue such as the payback of monies with a penalty and/ or interest fees, termination of the contract with that specific provider, and/or the potential for legal action.

Medicare Fraud and Abuse

Due to the 2010 Affordable Care Act, changes in fraud and abuse initiatives have resulted in improper payments being returned to Medicare; more than $4 billion dollars were recovered in 2010. In 2011, over $5.6 billion in fraudulent payments, a 167% increase from 2008, has been recovered. Consequently, fraud and abuse program integrity is a top priority with federal and state government agencies. Simply, it is defrauding the government, which results in unnecessary costs to the Medicare program.

Fraud is considered to include unnecessarily performed services, services not received, inappropriate documentation, and/or ineligible patients. Abuse may include misused codes, excessive charges for services/supplies, and billed services that were not medically necessary (CMS, 2011).

In order to combat fraud, one of Medicare's initiatives is to dispatch Senior Medicare Patrols (SMPs), trained seniors looking for violations performed in physician and health care provider offices. Medicare is also packing HEAT (Health Care Fraud Prevention and Enforcement Action Teams), a collaboration of the Department of Health and Human Services and the Department of Justice. At the time of this writing, nine major cities had infiltration of the HEAT, resulting in 270 convictions with over $240 million in fines, penalties, and paybacks within the first few years of the program.

In addition, Medicare has established practice patterns to predict fraud, based on overutilization in providers' offices. Three levels of risk screening, limited, moderate and high, establish the likelihood of fraud and abuse, based on setting and specialty. Licensure and background checks will be eventually investigated to ensure legitimacy, so that services are not provided to ineligible beneficiaries, such as those who are deceased, a common

fraudulent and abusive practice. It is suggested that audiologists conduct internal audits of billing practices and of their documentation to ensure compliance.

Contract Negotiations

Long ago we had the mentality of being grateful for any insurance company that would reimburse us for services. Since the health care landscape has changed substantially, this did also. Although the insurance company actually has the contract with the patient for the provision of health care, providers are also at their mercy. In pursuing contracts, a few choice questions for consideration may be in order:

■ Are patients allowed to share in the cost of upgraded technology?
■ If so, how will that be reflected on the EOB?
■ What is the fee schedule and how often is it revised?
■ Is balance billing allowed for services not reimbursed?
■ Is there a discount structure?
■ When can payment be expected?
■ What is the denial process?
■ How much liability do I need to carry?
■ What is the length of the contract?
■ How can the contract be terminated and by whom? What is the required time frame for advance notice?
■ Can the contract be changed unilaterally by the third-party such as with a unilateral change in the fee schedule?
■ Is there a credentialing fee? Withholds?

■ Will this secure patients in a designated demographic area?

■ Ease of verification of patient enrollment?

■ Are prior authorizations required?

The most critical component of any contract is the reimbursement you receive. Many plans devise their fee schedule according to the Medicare Physician Fee Schedule. Relying on this likely will not keep the doors open to your practice. You will need to know what your hourly rate is, what the contracted fees are (and re-negotiate if need dictates), and your expenses in order to maintain a healthy practice. Other chapters in this text can assist you in determining these rates.

Some commercial insurance plans continue to not include audiologists as providers, usually considering audiologists to be ancillary providers. If you want to exercise the "any willing provider" clause that your state has legislated, you will want to contact the provider relations department of that third-party payer in order to educate them about who audiologists are and by virtue of our qualifications, the services we provide. These services prove to be cost effective with audiologists being the first line of contact with the patient in their hearing and balance care.

In those situations of third-party payers not recognizing us for the work we do, it is suggested that several local colleagues arrange for an educational meeting with the payer's provider relations department as well as the medical director of that plan. It may be helpful to discuss with them our scope of practice, the services we provide, the outcomes and successes documented by patient testimonials and literature reviews as well as

redacted copies of several explanations of benefits (EOBs) issued by their competition, illustrating their competition's reimbursement for audiology services.

Often, discounts for services or giving away services in order to acquire more hearing aid patients as an example is illegal if you are offering the same service to Medicare patients since Medicare patients cannot be billed at a higher fee than another patient for the same procedure. In addition, Medicare contractors have guidance on solicitation of services. The cost of goods and the cost of maintaining an office at times can be greater than what appears to be an incentive to contract with that insurance carrier. I would refer you to another chapter in this book that can help you calculate the amount of funds needed to maintain your practice and overhead in order to make appropriate decisions for the financial health of your practice.

As with any third-party payer, there are many questions to be asked: what is the average reimbursement time frame, what is the denial process, what are the codes to be reimbursed and what is the fee schedule for those codes, can the patient be balanced billed for the difference in what is reimbursed by the insurance company and the fee billed, how often is the fee schedule updated, how much professional liability do I need to carry, are there administrative fees such as withholds and annual credentialing fees that are assessed, what is the contract termination policy, and what is the patient dismissal process, to name just a few. This certainly is not an exhaustive list.

In the case of hearing aid reimbursement, you need to know if there is a covered benefit, what it is, as well as if the patient can share in the cost for advanced technology, if an invoice is required, itemizing the hearing aid acquisition fee including batteries, earmold(s) and earmold impression(s) if applicable, the dispensing fee as well as the conformity evaluation, and other professional services. Also to consider is the expected payment time frame, the denial process, and the policy if a hearing aid(s) is returned. Again, this is not the entire list of potential questions, but ones to get you positioned for making the best decision with providing services to subscribers with audiology related insurance benefits.

For those who provide vestibular rehabilitation, you also want to know the nuances of billing as well as what codes are required and if they are reimbursed to audiologists.

Due to the changing health care landscape, it is no longer common for providers to "carve out" procedures that are more time consuming or expensive to provide. These would include amplification, central auditory processing, aural rehabilitation, and tinnitus treatment, to name a few.

You may recall the expression from your childhood, "safety in numbers," and it appears to be true in contract negotiating. Some audiologists have formed their own legal structure, an Independent Practice Association or IPA. This affords you the ability to contract with insurers that you may not be allowed to as a single practice yet allows you to maintain the autonomy of your own practice. This may afford you a larger geographic area and other economies of scale as well as sharing some expenses for a contract negotiator. There are several national audiology-related IPAs. There may be a sizable contribution at the front end per practice in order to hire an attorney to devise the corporate structure, an accountant to maintain the funds and

file the appropriate tax information to the required parties and a contract negotiator to obtain the necessary contracts, some of which may be exclusive to your particular IPA.

Managed care is a different entity and is much more restrictive and dogmatic: they will "allow" you to be on their panel of providers or network if they deem it so. The difficulty in penetrating this system is that often those panels are closed and no new providers are being accepted. This can potentially have great financial impact to your practice if many patients or potential patients have a contract with a payer that you cannot access.

Some states have "any willing providers," which means they have to accept anyone meeting their criteria. As plans often limit the number of providers and if they have reached that number, you will not be able to "get on" the plan. This is to their advantage as it allows them greater negotiating power in dealing with fewer providers within their network. Coupled with financial disincentives for patients to seek health care outside of their managed care plan, this will likely lead to greater benefits for that managed care plan, not necessarily for the patient. The patient may have the option of going "out-of- network," but it will come at a greater out-of-pocket expense if they opt to do so.

A member of this alphabet soup mix, preferred provider organizations (PPOs), is more flexible. Co-pays and out-of-pocket expenses may be slightly higher, but the patient does not require a referral and may see whomever they chose.

Health maintenance organizations (HMOs) require a referral from the gatekeeper, or primary care physician. Gatekeepers can be pediatricians, obstetrician/gynecologists, or internal medicine and family practitioners. You may not always be able to see your provider of choice and restrictions will likely apply.

Point of service plans (POS) combine the best of HMOs and PPOs: they are less restrictive than HMOs as the patient can chose to go out of the HMO network and utilize their out-of-network providers. This will come at a greater out-of-pocket expense by way of higher co-pays or co-insurances.

Documentation

Documentation details anything related to the patient's visit, provides the continuity of care between the professionals involved in that particular patient's care as well as providing a historical chronicle. It is required by third-party payers and as a legal document, it may be subpoenaed. In hospital settings, the chart may be reviewed for quality assurance (QA/CQI) issues.

The patient's chart needs to include that patient's demographics: name, date of birth, contact information, insurance information with a copy of both sides of their health care card, driver's license, the name of the referring professional, and the reason for their visit, case history including allergies, surgeries, hospitalizations, medications, and occupational and recreational noise exposure history. For the pediatric population, the prenatal, birth and postnatal histories should be included as well as familial history. For adults, all the above should be included as well as the age or time of onset of their hearing or balance disorder. All audiologic procedures are to be signed and dated. As Medicare and most commercial payers base payment on medical neces-

sity, this must clearly be documented in the chart.

The audiogram in isolation does not constitute a report. The interpretation of the performed procedures and recommendations for patient management are required in the chart notes, preferably on the audiogram, as well as an original signature and the date of service. A case history should also be included on the audiogram if space permits.

An emergency room physician once told this author, "If it isn't in the chart, it didn't happen." Those wise words are the basis of how we should document the course of the patient's visit for a particular date of service. When creating documentation, consider that the chart may be requested for an audit. It is imperative to include anything the patient describes to you during the history and physical intake, the tests you performed, and your findings and recommendations. In other words, these progress notes may follow the SOAP format:

Subjective is considered the description of the presenting problem as the patient relates it to you. This would also include the history, who if anyone referred the patient to you, and a review of the patient's medical history including medications, their occupational and recreational noise exposure history, and any other pertinent audiologic related information.

Objective should be the physical findings encountered upon the examination of the patient, including otoscopic findings.

Assessment includes the procedures performed and an interpretation of their results.

Plan includes your recommendations. This would include, but is not limited to, the treatment you recommend for the patient, further referrals, further procedures, as well as obtaining amplification, assistive listening devices, or undergoing tinnitus or vestibular treatment for example. Your signature should be on the audiogram as well as the chart progress note.

Electronic health care records (EHR) will require an encrypted signature and you may be unable to make changes to those specific progress notes once the signature is affixed and the chart note is saved for that time/date of service. Addenda may possibly be included. Paper/hard copy charts will soon be a fond memory as the electronic medical records transition marches on.

Notes need to be completed in a very timely manner and not left until later in the day when you have had several patients in between, possibly making facts blur. EHR will likely disallow this practice as one record will need to be completed before another record is opened in order to see the next patient. Templates can be created and the information adjusted for each patient as it pertains specifically to them. Letters to your referral sources need to be completed within 24 to 48 hours post visit. These should include a thank you for the referral as well as the name, date, findings, and recommendations for your mutual patient. This also solidifies the current physician referral requirement for Medicare and addresses the medical necessity requirement.

Documentation has six key elements: case history, procedures performed, findings and results, recommendations,

signature affixing, and the date of the evaluation and dictation.

If errors are made in the charting process, several guidelines need to be followed: Do not destroy what you have written. For a hard copy chart, correction fluid is not to be utilized; simply strike-out what you want to eliminate, initial it with your three initials, and place the date of action near those initials. Addendum notes may also possibly be attached, depending on the software of the electronic record. If using a hard copy, this will be sufficient with the date of the addendum added with your signature.

When charting, a guideline to follow is that the chart may be subpoenaed in a legal action or requested for a third-party payer audit. It needs to be legible, methodical and within the confines of what is considered minimum standard of care for audiology. To determine what constitutes standard of care, please consult *Audiology Clinical Practice Algorithms and Statements*. There are to be no sticky notes or other papers that are not affixed. Every visit, phone call, e-mail and any other patient contact needs to be noted, dated, and signed. For audiology practices falling under HIPAA regulations, legal authorities do not require consent (for treatment), but authorization for a single event, such as requesting a student's educational record, is likely to be required. The Notice of Privacy Practices (NPP) addresses how health care information is to be treated for that individual patient.

For those working in a hospital setting, there are guidelines to follow, courtesy of the Joint Commission in Accreditation of Healthcare Organization (JCAHO). In addition, there are other endorsing bodies that survey and accredit specific departments of a hospital or outpatient and/or rehabilitation facility.

Chart Composition

The following compose the necessary forms for chart composition:

- Patient registration form (needs to include the patient's demographic information (e.g., name, address, date of birth, phone number, insurance information, and referring physician)
- Copies of health care card (enrollment should be verified before they are seen), driver's license/photo identification
- Physician order if required by payer
- Adult or pediatric medical history form
- Insurance waiver
- Advance Beneficiary Notice if you are a Medicare provider and the service provided requires an ABN, or for a non-covered service, a voluntary ABN may be offered
- Medical waiver if required by state licensure
- Notice of Privacy Practices for HIPAA, signed by the patient
- Hearing aid related forms
  - Medical clearance by a physician if required by your state licensure
  - Hearing aid waiver if required by your state licensure
  - Contract/purchase agreement
  - Hearing aid checklist of covered points, signed by the patient
  - Earmold and/or cerumen waiver form, signed by the patient if either or both procedures were performed (sample form in Appendix 9–B)
  - Hearing aid warranty information
  - Post-warranty hearing aid service package document, indicating what the services are and the length of time they will be offered, if applicable

Records Retention

HIPAA requires that HIPAA related forms be retained for 6 years. It is suggested you contact your state's insurance commission for the state's record retention laws for the state(s) in which you practice. They may be listed on that state's website. If no specific guidance is offered, records of minors typically must be retained until 7 years after reaching the age of majority and for adults, records should typically be retained for 7 years after their last visit.

The patient does not own the chart although as a provision of HIPAA, they have the right to review their chart and amend anything with which they are not in agreement. The chart is to be maintained by the facility who "owns" it. If the chart is subpoenaed, the subpoena will specify if the original chart has to be submitted or whether a copy will suffice; preferred practice is to retain the original and offer a copy. Requested chart copies either by the patient, attorneys, or another third-party payer are to be issued in a timely manner. The patient may be charged for the copy of their chart and state insurance laws may dictate what that fee may be limited to on a fee per page basis.

Electronic Health Records (EHR)

In 2004, President George W. Bush envisioned electronic health records (EHR) being a reality by 2014 (CMS, 2007).

This will enable a paperless, computer-accessed health care record. The information listed above will still be a vital part of the EHR and signatures will be electronically encrypted for that date of service. In other words, the demographics, the progress notes, medications, history and physical will be a part of the EHR. Outcome measures reporting will also be a part of the EHR (CMS, 2007). The benefit of EHR is that in facilities such as a hospital, any health care information on a patient will be accessible by any provider in real-time who has the appropriate password to access their health care information. The provider is the one who maintains the EHR. Medicare Eligible Providers (EPs) were financially incentivized to include EHR in their offices, but at the time of publication, audiologists were not considered an EP, and therefore did not qualify for the incentive, or the disincentive, which will eventually result in a reduction in payments if EHR is not implemented.

Reports

The lifeline of an audiology practice is referrals. One way to ensure that the success of a practice continues is to inform the referral source via a well-written, succinct, and timely report as to the outcome of that patient's visit, preferably within a 24-hour time frame. This is an opportunity to have open communication regarding that patient, to demonstrate your expertise, and to make recommendations that are vital to patient care. From a marketing standpoint, it maintains your name and the work you perform on the radar of that referring professional.

Reports need to be well written and concise. The SOAP format is applicable to report writing. Many of the audiology specific software packages and EHR have report templates embedded in them. However you approach this aspect of the visit is critical to patient care and the health of your practice.

Referrals To and From an Audiologist's Office

Referrals to other specialties such as otolaryngology, neurology, primary care, internal medicine, pediatrics, speech-language pathology, and other audiologists are a vital aspect of the standard of care. You should expect a report from that provider. As we are experts in hearing and balance disorders, we can't always be everything to every one of our patients. Some of us are not comfortable with seeing a tinnitus or dizzy patient. If that is the case, it behooves you to refer to a colleague who is an expert in that particular area. That is responsible patient care and is addressed by some state licensure laws and professional organizations' codes of ethics.

Referrals will be forthcoming from other providers to your office. In order to keep the lines of communication open, report writing and appropriate thank you notes to that referral source in the way of a note and/or phone call is suggested.

The Laws That Bind: Anti-Kickback Statutes, Safe Harbors, Stark Laws, HIPAA, and State Licensure

As health care providers, we are required to follow the laws that apply to the provision of audiolgic and vestibular services, which include the Stark Laws, the Anti-

Kickback Statutes, Safe Harbors, False Claims Act, and Health Insurance Portability and Accountability Act (HIPAA). Each of these will be examined in detail individually and their applications to audiology specified. More detailed information can be found in Chapter 4 of this text.

Anti-Kickback Statute and Stark Laws

The Anti-Kickback Statute [42 U.S.C. §1320a-7b(b)] was promulgated to address the soliciting and receiving of kickbacks in return for referrals of patients whose items or services are reimbursable under federal health care programs. It prohibits any person from, "knowingly and willfully soliciting or receiving any remuneration (including any kickback, bribe, or rebate) directly or indirectly, overtly or covertly, in cash or in kind" to induce someone to refer an individual for, "any item or service for which payment may be made in whole or in part under a Federal health care program" (except the Federal Employees Health Benefits Program [FEHBP]) (Abel & Hahn, 2006). Lewis (2011) noted that the AKS was recently amended to include any activity, knowingly or unknowingly, thereby ensuring further transparency.

The AKS prohibits kickbacks because: (1) they create an incentive to overutilize reimbursable services, increasing costs to Medicare and other federal health care programs; (2) they distort medical decision making; and (3) they result in unfair competition by freezing out qualified providers who are unwilling to pay kickbacks (Abel & Hahn, 2006).

The AKS is a criminal statute. Violation of the AKS is a felony punishable by imprisonment (for not more than five years), heavy fines (up to $25,000), or

exclusion from federal health care program participation. "Civil Monetary Penalties may also be imposed up to $50,000 for each violation, plus the additional imposition of three times the amount of the remuneration offered, paid, solicited, or received, also known as treble damages" (Lewis, 2011). Unlike the Stark Law, which is a civil law, intent is a critical element that must be proved by the prosecutor. However, while intent to induce referrals or obtain money for referrals must be proven, it is not required to be the only purpose of the remuneration. The AKS is enforced by the Office of the Inspector General (OIG). Thus, the elements of an AKS violation are the following:

- Intent: acting knowingly and willfully
- Offering, giving, soliciting, or receiving remuneration
- Referral of patients to purchase, lease, order, or arrange for any item or service reimbursable under a federal health care program, except FEHBP.

The AKS is much broader than the Stark Law. Unlike Stark, it is not limited to particular designated health services. Instead, it applies to any item or service payable in whole or in part under any federal health care program other than FEHBP. A number of possible arrangements between audiologists and physicians may involve the AKS. Here are a few examples:

- An audiologist furnishes diagnostic tests to a physician's patients at no or reduced charge in return for hearing aid referrals, where hearing aids are covered by the state Medicaid plan. The audiologist is giving the physician remuneration (i.e., free or reduced price diagnostic tests) in return for referrals of hearing aid business reimbursable by Medicaid.

■ An audiologist rents office space from a physician and pays rental based on the number of referrals of Medicare/Medicaid patients received from the physician. The audiologist is giving the physician remuneration (i.e., above-market rent) in return for referrals of Medicare/Medicaid business.

■ An audiologist accepts remuneration (in the form of gifts, entertainment, loans, cooperative marketing funds, trips, or other benefits) from a hearing aid manufacturer in return for prescribing the manufacturer's hearing aids, where the hearing aids are covered by Medicaid or another federal program (other than Federal Employees Health Benefits Program). The audiologist is receiving remuneration in return for recommending purchase of hearing aids reimbursable by Medicaid (Abel & Hahn, 2006).

Safe Harbors

To avoid criminalizing innocent conduct, there are a number of "safe harbors" to the AKS. If a transaction meets all the requirements of a safe harbor, it is protected from prosecution. However, failure to qualify for a safe harbor does not automatically mean a transaction is not in violation of the AKS. The safe harbors include arm's-length agreements for the rental of office space or equipment, discounts, and bona fide employment relationships. While a complete discussion of the AKS safe harbors is beyond the

scope of this chapter, two of the harbors are worth mentioning because of their widespread use (Abel & Hahn, 2006).

To qualify for safe harbor protection, a discount must be "a reduction in the amount a buyer (who buys either directly or through a wholesaler or a group purchasing organization) is charged for an item or service based on an arms-length transaction" (42 C.F.R. § 1001.952[h][5]). The discount must be made at the time of sale (or, if a rebate, the terms of the rebate must be fixed and disclosed in writing to the buyer at the time of sale). The buyer receiving the discount must, upon request of the OIG or state regulators, provide certain information provided to it by the seller. In addition, the discount must be properly disclosed and reflected in the charges billed to the federal health care program paying for the item or service. Thus, the discount must inure to benefit of the Medicare or Medicaid program. The discount must be earned in the same fiscal year as the purchase of the applicable item or service. The safe harbor does not protect discounts in the form of cash payments (or cash equivalents) (Abel & Hahn, 2006).

The American Academy of Audiology Ethical Practice Guideline for Relationships with Industry for Audiologists Providing Clinical Care (2011), educates members about the ethics and legality of the acceptance of trips, cash, and other gifts in exchange for recommending items that may be paid for by a federal health care program. Abiding by these guidelines protects the audiologist from inadvertent violations of the Anti-Kickback Statute.

To qualify for the office rental safe harbor, an audiologist must ensure that rental payments are not disguised kickbacks to induce referrals by the physician-landlord. Specifically:

■ The rental agreement must be in writing and signed by the parties;

■ The rental agreement must cover all premises rented by the parties and specify the premises;

■ The term of the agreement must be at least one year;

■ If the audiologist is renting space for periodic intervals, the agreement must specify the exact schedule of usage;

■ The aggregate rental amount must be set in advance, consistent with fair market value, and may not take into account the volume or value of referrals; and

■ The aggregate space rented may not exceed what is reasonably necessary to accomplish a commercially reasonable business purpose.

For a more detailed discussion of this safe harbor, see OIG, Special Fraud Alert: Rental of Office Space in Physician Offices by Persons or Entities to Which Physicians Refer (February 2000).

Many states have their own anti-kickback and Stark laws, which may differ from the federal AKS. Whenever in doubt, consult with legal counsel well versed in both federal and state anti-kickback laws as it is beyond the purview of this chapter (Abel & Hahn, 2006).

Stark Laws

All audiologists should be aware of the federal antifraud laws (as well as any relevant state antifraud laws). Before embarking on a previously uncharted contractual arrangement with a physician or physician group, an audiologist should consult legal counsel familiar with health care fraud and abuse laws. The Stark Law and the Anti-Kickback Statute should be considered separately; activities or arrangements that are acceptable under one may violate the other (Abel & Hahn, 2006).

The Stark Law (42 U.S.C. § 1395nn) prohibits physician "self-referrals."[1] That is, it prohibits a physician (or a physician's immediate family member) from referring patients for designated health services to an entity in which the physician (or his or her immediate family member) has a financial relationship, unless a specific exception applies. The law also prohibits the entity receiving the prohibited referral from billing for those designated health services (Abel & Hahn, 2006).

The Stark Law is a civil, not a criminal, law. Violations may result in denial of reimbursement, mandatory refunds of federal payments, civil money penalties, and exclusion from federal and state health care programs. The Centers for Medicare and Medicaid Services (CMS) issued regulations (42 C.F.R. Part 411) implementing the Stark Law in two phases over a period of several years, with the third phase going into effect in 2007.

To violate Stark, there must be a *referral* by a physician (or his or her immediate family member) to an *entity* in which the physician (or his or her immediate family member) has a *financial interest* for the furnishing of *designated health services (DHS)*.

---

[1] The Stark Law is sometimes referred to as "Stark II." The statute originally only prohibited physician referrals to labs in which the referring physician has a financial interest ("Stark I"). When the statute was broadened to prohibit physician referrals to any entity in which the referring physician has a financial interest, it was designated "Stark II" (Abel & Hahn, 2006).

- A *referral* is any physician request, ordering of, or certifying, or recertifying of the need for a DHS for which payment may be made under Medicare. If the referring physician personally performs the service, there is no referral. A referral by an audiologist is not covered by Stark, unless the referral is directed or controlled by a physician.
- An *entity* is any person (including an individual, partnership, or corporation) that furnishes DHS. A person is considered to be furnishing DHS if it is the person to which CMS makes payment or to whom the right of payment has been reassigned. Thus, an audiologist may be an entity receiving a prohibited referral.
- A *financial interest* is broadly defined to include a direct or indirect ownership or investment interest or a direct or indirect compensation arrangement.
- *Designated health services (DHS)* are defined as the following items and services only:
  - Clinical lab services;
  - Physical therapy, occupational therapy, and speech-language pathology services;
  - Radiology and certain other imaging services;
  - Radiation therapy services and supplies;
  - Durable medical equipment and supplies;
  - Parenteral and enteral nutrients, equipment, and supplies;
  - Prosthetics, orthotics, and prosthetic devices and supplies;
  - Home health services;
  - Outpatient prescription drugs; and
  - Inpatient and outpatient hospital services.

Because of this narrow definition of DHS, the Stark Law has limited application to audiologists. The only audiology services that fall within the definition of DHS are audiology services furnished as hospital inpatient or outpatient services. However, as the entity furnishing DHS is the entity that receives payment from CMS, and as CMS reimburses the hospital for inpatient and outpatient services, it is the hospital (not the audiologist) that must comply with the Stark Law.

CMS considers the Current Procedural Terminology (CPT) codes 92507 and 92508 (evaluation/treatment of speech, language, voice, communication, or auditory processing; individual and group respectively) to be speech-language pathology services, and therefore DHS, lessening the applicability to audiologists. Audiology diagnostic tests, including cochlear implant mapping and reprogramming (CPT codes 92601 through 92604), are not DHS. In addition, CMS has clarified that hearing aids are not DHS.

The Stark Law and implementing CMS regulations provide a number of exceptions. These include bona fide employment relationships, arm's-length agreements for the rental of office space or equipment, and "in-office ancillary services." To qualify for an exception, a transaction or arrangement must meet specific requirements. For example, to qualify for the in-office ancillary services exception, the services must meet a supervision requirement (e.g., furnished by an individual under the supervision of the referring physician), a building requirement (e.g., furnished in the same building in which the referring physician normally furnishes services to patients), and a billing requirement (e.g., billed by the supervising physician, the group practice, an entity wholly owned by the physician or group practice, or an independent third-party billing company acting as agent of the physician, group practice, or entity). Because the Stark Law has limited impact on audiologists, the exceptions will not be discussed in detail in this chapter.

In essence, the Stark Law prohibits a physician (or his or her immediate family member) from referring a patient for the furnishing of DHS to an entity in which the physician (or his or her immediate family member) has a financial interest, unless an exception applies. Because the Stark Law only applies to referrals for the furnishing of DHS, and because the only audiology services that are DHS are inpatient and outpatient hospital services, the Stark Law has limited impact on audiologists. In the case of hospital services, CMS makes payment to the hospital, so the hospital is the entity that must comply with Stark.

Audiologists should be aware, however, that most states have their own Stark laws, and some of these may be broader than the federal Stark Law. Whenever in doubt, audiologists are advised to consult legal counsel well-versed in federal, state, and local laws (Abel & Hahn, 2006).

- Not billing with the appropriate provider number
- Billing for services known to be noncovered
- Falsifying a patient's diagnosis
- Upcoding or billing for the service at a higher rate
- Unbundling bundled codes (such as billing 92567 and 92568 individually when 92550 should have been billed).

Services that are determined to be fraudulent will result in the revocation of privileges in providing services to that insurer, potential legal action that may revoke state license(s), payback of funds with penalties and interest, and possible incarceration. There are potential criminal and civil penalties if found guilty.

Providers should bill only for services that are necessary when determining the patient's diagnosis. The Office of the Inspector General, in their pursuit of fraud and abuse, are on the lookout for false claims, especially submitting claims for services not rendered. In addition, as a result of the 2010 Affordable Care Act, any overpayment due a federal payer must be paid back within 60 days of discovery or it may be considered a false claim.

False Claims

The False Claims Act (31 U.S.C. §3729 et seq.) specifies these several ill-advised actions that would be considered fraudulent:

- Submitting claims for services that were not rendered
- Submitting claims for services not medically necessary

HIPAA

In 1996, the Health Insurance Portability and Accountability Act (HIPAA), Public Law 104-191, was promulgated by congress "to improve portability and continuity of health care when there was a change of jobs, to combat waste, fraud and abuse in health insurance and health care delivery to simplify the administration of health insurance, and for other purposes" (American Academy of Audiology, 2003). Because the deadline passed without congressional response to health care standards, the responsibility fell to the secretary of the Department of Health and Human Services (DHHS) and the Centers for Medicare and Medicaid Services (CMS) which has the responsibility of implementing them (AAA, Capturing Reimbursement, 2006). According to HIPAA privacy guidelines, when treatment, payment, or operational (TPO) information is involved, a medical release is not required. However, in a litigious society it may be prudent to obtain one for any exchange of information in order to protect your patients, your practice, and yourself. Consent according to HIPAA is optional, may be obtained once and can be revoked. After receiving the Notice of Privacy Practices (NPP), written consent is not required. The NPP should be updated annually with the patient's signature, attesting to how they want their Personal Health Information (PHI) handled. Authorization, typically for a one time occurrence, is required.

There are five titles that compose HIPAA with Title II, Administrative Simplification, being the most important in most of our practices, created in order to have PHI transmitted securely. Within this title are Transaction and Code Sets (effective date October 16, 2003), Privacy (April 14, 2003), and Security (April 21, 2005). The Unique Identifiers Rule, which includes the National Provider Identifier (NPI) for providers and the Tax Identification Number (TIN)/Employer Identification Number (EIN) for employers, became effective on May 23, 2007, and for small health plans, a year later to the day.

The Department of Health and Human Services (DHHS) oversees HIPAA. If any violations occur with the privacy aspect of HIPAA, the Office for Civil Rights at DHHS is responsible for the enforcement. Penalties may include criminal and civil penalties.

HIPAA has five titles, each of which addresses varied sections of this act. These are listed below.

- TITLE I: Portability and Renewability. Allows for the portability of health care for those who have changed or lost their jobs.
- TITLE II: Administrative Simplification. This section applies to any provider or facility that transmits health information and will affect nearly all health care providers as it addresses the standards of transmitting health care information via electronic methods. Due to concerns regarding the security of this information being processed electronically, Administrative Simplification was created. The following are also included with administrative simplification and are discussed in detail below:
  - Transaction and Code Sets (standardization of CPT, ICD-CM, and HCPCS codes, Unique Provider Identifiers). The transaction and code sets allows for all third-party payers to utilize uniform and standard sets of codes such as CPT, the ICD-CM's, and the HCPCS codes. However, worker's compensation in many states (and at least one state's Medicaid agency) has additional codes they may utilize, generally for hearing aid related procedures.
  - Privacy Rules. Protecting personal health information, Notice of Privacy Practices

- Security Rules. Safeguards to protect data, computers, and the information therein; disaster recovery
- TITLE III: Tax-Related Health Provisions
- TITLE IV: Application and Enforcement of Group Health Plan Requirements
- TITLE V: Revenue Offsets

A sample authorization release is included in Appendix 9–C or you may prefer to devise your own. It will need to include the name and address of your practice or facility, the patient's name, address, and birth date. In addition, the information that you need released or that will be released from you to a third-party with their identifying information should be included, as well as an expiration date for the authorization. The patient's right to revoke the authorization also needs to be addressed, as well as the notification that the information may be redisclosed by the recipient.

HIPAA addresses the importance of disseminating the minimum information necessary for treatment, payment, and operations (TPO) in dealing with patient care and privacy issues. We need to keep uppermost in our minds when speaking with colleagues that we do not reveal the name of the patient in the interesting clinical case we may be describing. This is not considered treatment, payment, or operations information. If recounting a case in a presentation or journal article, for example, names must be redacted and any identifying information deleted.

The privacy component of HIPAA addresses how personal health information is to be viewed, transmitted and stored. If you are a Covered Entity, a Notice of Privacy Practices (NPP) is given to the patient the first time they come into your facility. It addresses how any of their PHI will be treated, what is permissible for any contact with the patient and a family member. This aspect of HIPAA ensures that in the cases of treatment, payment, and/or operations, the consent is implied and information may flow among any of the covered entities involved in that patient's health care.

As audiologists, we may see evidence of abuse, domestic violence, and/or neglect. In cases such as this, privacy is "suspended" as these patients need to be reported to the appropriate authorities immediately, which may include and are not restricted to law enforcement, children's services and/or domestic violence shelters. This should be addressed in your NPP.

Incidental disclosures are addressed under HIPAA. This would be the inadvertent disclosure of PHI such as if a patient, lost in your office, happened to walk by as you were discussing something with another patient on the phone. You attempted to make it as private a conversation as possible, but an unforeseen circumstance transpired.

Anyone who provides health care services is considered a Covered Entity (CE) unless they do not transmit any health care information electronically. CEs include anyone who transmits PHI electronically, including health plans and clearinghouses. Electronic transmissions include Internet, dial-up, private networks, tapes, and CDs.

CEs need to have a business agreement (BA) in place when PHI is exchanged and it needs to be signed by both parties. Therefore, hearing aid manufacturers need to have BAs with your office since there is PHI exchanged on the patient's behalf when a hearing aid is ordered, for example. Of course, fictitious names could be substituted, but that is certainly more information to track. Other BAs that need to be in place is with anyone who processes your claims such as your insurance claims clearinghouse, those who do your billing, your accountant and attorney, and if you utilize transcription services, the transcriptionist. Due to the 2009 Health Information Technology for Economic and Clinical Health Act (HITECH), regulations were enacted so that BAs also have a contractual responsibility to the CE for providing services. HITECH also was enacted to address the processes and penalties when a data breach occurs. At the time this book went to print, a final rule for further HITECH requirements had just been released, including changes to BA agreements, so check with http://www.hhs.gov/ocr/privacy/hipaa/administrative/enforcementrule/hitechenforcementifr.html for further information.

Early in the HIPAA transition process, there were many myths about what was allowed, some of which have persisted. The patient may sign in on a sign-in sheet, but should not specify the reason for their visit. Many offices who utilize the sign-in process will have a line where the patient signs their name and it then can be pulled off after their visit is noted. Charts and computer monitors should not face the patient or be in a highly trafficked area, where they can be easily seen. Collection calls and informing patients of any test results should be completed in an area where one will not be overheard.

Reminder cards sent to the patient need to be in envelopes so that PHI cannot be viewed, such as the reason why the recipient will be seen in your office; any type of marketing requires authorization (Pessis & Williams, 2005). A newsletter that provides general information as long as it doesn't promote a specific product and/or brand and mass mailings that don't include PHI are permissible (Pessis, 2003).

Authorization in the form of written permission for a one time, date specific event or time frame is required. For example, audiologists need permission from parents to confer with school personnel regarding school-aged patients who wear amplification, such as the clinical audiologist and the educational audiologist exchanging information on a mutual patient, for example. The Family Educational Rights and Privacy Act (FERPA), the law for those in educational settings, was promulgated to protect student education records and is the educational setting's version of HIPAA.

The security side of HIPAA addresses administrative procedures, physical safeguards, technical data security services, and technical security mechanisms (Pessis & Williams, 2005). Administrative procedures cover documentation and formal procedures for selecting and executing information and how the staff will protect that data. All information security measures are to be reviewed (Pessis & Williams, 2005). Physical safeguards are necessary to protect the information within the walls of an office such as the actual computer system and the provision for fire, theft, and disaster recovery. The technical data security services safeguards the processes used to protect, control and monitor information access (Pessis & Williams, 2005). This includes any password application and may also include badge readers, smart cards, and biometrics (Pessis & Williams, 2005). Finally, technical security mechanisms address the utilization of unauthorized access to data transmitted over a communications network and may include a secure network, firewalls, as well as encryption (Pessis & Williams, 2005).

Every office providing health care in compliance with HIPAA has specified on their NPP the name of their privacy officer. This is to be used if a patient has a complaint which can then be addressed in-house. The patient has the right to review their chart and request a change in their record, an amendment. This change is then accepted or rejected by the provider and that decision is also documented in the chart. A complaint may also be registered by contacting the Office of Civil Rights. Fines for HIPAA violations can be substantial and may include exclusion from Medicare, civil monetary penalties from $100/violation to $50,000/violation, up to an annual maximum of $1.5 million. Criminal penalties range up to $50,000 and imprisonment up to one year. For offenses committed under false pretenses, the fine may be up to $100,000, with incarceration of up to 5 years.

Security

The intent of the security component of HIPAA is to protect data integrity, confidentiality and availability in safeguarding privacy. It was implemented on April 21, 2005 (Pessis, 2003).

The security section is composed of four categories: administrative procedures, physical safeguards, technical data security services, and technical security mechanisms (Pessis, 2003).

The administrative procedures discuss how staff protects the data as well

selecting and executing information on information security. Assessment and review of information security procedures, manuals, and records is required (Pessis, 2003).

Physical safeguards address the actual computer system from theft, fire, intrusion, and other environmental hazards. Technical data security services safeguards the processes used to protect, control and monitor information access (Pessis, 2003). Computer passwords are included in this component as well as biometrics, smart cards, and electronic signatures. It is recommended that passwords be changed periodically, a requirement in many facilities. Technical security mechanisms are geared to prevent the intrusion of an unauthorized, uninvited outside source into your data. Firewalls and encryption apply to this component.

Violations of the Administrative Simplification Regulations can result in civil monetary penalties of $100 per violation, up to $25,000 per year. In June 2005, the US Department of Justice (DOJ) clarified who can be held criminally liable under HIPAA. Covered entities and specified individuals, as explained below, whom "knowingly" obtain or disclose individually identifiable health information in violation of the Administrative Simplification Regulations face a fine of up to $50,000, as well as imprisonment up to one year. Offenses committed under false pretenses allow penalties to be increased to a $100,000 fine, with up to five years in prison. Finally, offenses committed with the intent to sell, transfer, or use individually identifiable health information for commercial advantage, personal gain, or malicious harm permit fines of $250,000, and imprisonment for up to 10 years (AMA, 2007).

National Provider Identifier

Effective on May 23, 2007, all health care providers and covered entities were required to have the 10 digit Unique Provider Identifier, the National Provider Identifier (NPI), one of the last vestiges of HIPAA's Administrative Simplification. Health care facilities must have the Tax Identification Number (TIN) or Employer Identification Number (EIN). HIPAA calls for a "standard unique health identifier for each individual, employer, health plan and health care provider for use in the healthcare system" (Federal Register, 2004). The NPI number is managed by CMS via the National Enumerator. This single provider number will replace all numbers assigned to you, is linked to your Medicare Provider Transaction Access Number (PTAN), and will be the only number you will use for your entire professional career for billing purposes. If you move to another state, you will utilize this same 10 digit number until the day you retire, but you may need to obtain a new Medicare Provider Transaction Number (PTAN). The NPI number carries no intelligence or mechanism to identify a provider or their specialty.

The NPI application process is quite simple and can be completed online in approximately 20 minutes at https://np pes.cms.hhs.gov/NPPES/StaticForward. do?forward=static.instructions. You will need to share your NPI with entities such as your employer, clearinghouses, third-party payers, or any others who would utilize it for billing purposes. Hospital employees have their services billed by way of the hospital's NPI.

The National Employer Identifier Number (EIN) became effective in 2007. This nine-digit number assigned by the Internal Revenue Service to all health care employers is required on all health care plan submissions and is required on the CMS 1500 billing form. Therefore, a private practice or a large medical center would need to have this number in place when billing for services.

HITECH

The HITECH (Health Information Technology for Economic and Clinical Health Act) was signed into law as part of the 2009 American Recovery and Reinvestment Act to promote the adoption of "meaningful use" of health information (not applicable to audiologists at the time of publication), to address privacy and security provisions concerning data breaches of PHI, and to define technologic specifications for secure nationwide electronic exchange of information. When a breach occurs, those affected by the breach as well as the Department of Health and Human Services must be informed within 60 days of discovery; if the breach affected 500 people or more, these entities must be informed as well as the local media outlets. Existing Business Agreements (BA) may need to be revised to be in compliance with HITECH, as BAs are now subject to part of HIPAA privacy and security rules, and subject to HIPAA civil and criminal penalties. Civil penalties range from $100 to $50,000/violation, with an annual maximum of $25,000 to $1,500,000 and the criminal penalty is up to $50,000 and imprisonment for up to one year. For those offenses committed under false pretenses, fines may be increased to $100,000 with up to five years imprisonment.

At the time this book went to print, a final rule for HITECH requirements had just been released, including changes to BA agreements, so check with http://www.hhs.gov/ocr/privacy/hipaa/administrative/enforcementrule/hitechenforcementifr.html for further information.

State Regulations/ Licensure

Currently audiologists are regulated by state licensure or registration in all 50 states. This is mandated and is the only requirement to practice, for the purpose of consumer protection. "Minimum necessary" in the standard of care is the only requirement. If one of our colleagues did not provide services under "the standard of care," liability issues will ensue when litigated.

It is incumbent upon every audiologist to know the state licensure laws in the state in which they practice or are licensed. Ignorance is not a defense when dealing with federal and state laws. Scope of practice for the profession is clearly delineated in position statements and documents on professional organization Web sites, but it is possible that a procedure that is in our scope of practice may not be delineated in the licensure law.

If you ever have any questions regarding the "dos and don'ts," it behooves you to vet those requirements. State licensure board offices will be happy to answer your questions. If they don't know the answer, they may poll that state's licensure board for an opinion.

Some states have also addressed codes of ethics and have included them as part of the revised code or law and they have to be abided as such. Something illegal may not be unethical and the reverse can also be true.

Certification

Although licensure is required to practice audiology, certification is not. Certification affirms your professionalism and is a mechanism of promoting the continuing education you have undertaken to hone your skill sets, to stay abreast of the rapid changes in our field. Currently there are two certifications for audiologists. One is voluntary, bestowed upon your meeting the requirements established by a free standing board whereas the other type of certification is a requirement of a professional organization. Continuing education is a requirement for licensure in most states as well as for certification.

Other Practice Issues for Consideration

The federal regulations above create the framework in which to be compliant. There are other issues to consider protecting yourself and your practice.

Liability

As audiologists, there are two types of liability to consider: malpractice and, for those who are in private practice, property liability. Malpractice is liability insurance that covers the provider in whole or in part if that provider errs by negligence or omission causing injury to the patient. Property liability covers the physical facility of the office for such things as fire, theft, and injuries that occur on the premises to name a few potential catastrophes or mishaps.

An umbrella policy that provides additional coverage if there is property damage or other potential calamities that exceed the limits of your current coverage is recommended. Your local insurance agent can be contacted for any of these insurance needs, but professional liability coverage is a benefit when a member of a national professional organization.

Informed Consent

We have all encountered the patient who does not seek audiologic treatment under their own volition, but by that of a well-meaning relative or friend. The patient has the ultimate right of determining treatment. When that patient is incapacitated and unable to make their own decisions, it is recommended that a power of attorney act on their behalf. It is suggested you include a place for the patient's signature on your practice registration form, indicating the patient is granting you permission to provide the necessary audiologic diagnosis and treatment options. HIPAA does not require consent for treatment. For those 18 years or younger, a note from the parent or guardian is necessary in order to provide audiologic services in that parent or guardian's absence (Abel & Hahn, 2006).

Impaired Practitioners

Rule 8b of the Code of Ethics of the American Academy of Audiology states, "individuals shall not engage in dishonesty or illegal conduct that adversely reflects on the profession." With the stressful lives we lead, there is the danger of being an impaired practitioner—drug or alcohol induced. If you are suffering from the

abuse of either, whether the drug is legal or not, you are placing yourself and your patients at risk. The personal and professional liability is not worth the cost. If you know of a colleague who is impaired, there are several options. Intervention strategies with friends and families can be of help if you are not comfortable discussing this with them on a one-on-one basis. Intervention is often used to confront the impaired practitioner and make him or her aware of their problem, the impact it has had on those that participate in that intervention, and their recommendations for seeking assistance in combating that problem. Audiologists have the ethical burden to report their colleague to the American Academy of Audiology's Ethical Practice Committee for review, and state licensure laws may compel you to report your suspicions about the licensee to that board as well (Abel & Hahn, 2006).

Incompetent Patients

A core professional rule of practice is cited as Principle 4 of the American Academy of Audiology's Code of Ethics and states, "Members shall provide only services and products that are in the best interest of those served." Rule 4a specifies that "individuals shall not exploit persons in the delivery of professional services." As audiologists serve the elderly, we often see confused or forgetful patients. In many instances, they are unaware they are experiencing these symptoms. Dementia may be accompanied with belligerence. These patients will require specialized care. If you cannot provide this care, refer to a colleague. Working closely with the family of this challenging patient may guide you to other avenues; for example, an assistive listening device may be recommended instead of a hearing aid (Abel & Hahn, 2006).

Dismissing a Patient

According to the American Medical Association, a physician is free to accept or decline an individual as a patient (Metz, 2006). There are many reasons as to why a patient may need to be dismissed from your service. Noncompliant patients, those who do not follow your recommendations, perpetual no shows, and those who don't pay their bills are patients whom you feel would be better served by another audiologist. This may also be due to personality traits or conflicts between the patient and the audiologist. Critical to making this decision, the patient needs to be notified in writing with 30 days advance notice providing a deadline of termination via certified mail with a signature request to verify their receipt of the letter. This then needs to be placed in their chart. These patients need to be offered the names of other audiologists whom they may contact for care. Document in the patient's chart the reason they are being terminated as well as provide them directly with copies of their records. As with providing any records to another health care professional or an attorney, you maintain the original chart and the patient receives the copy. Although our personal thoughts may color our thinking, we need to keep the patient's best interests tantamount to anything else. Clinical and life experiences often help circumvent potential conflicts before they become such.

You may be accused of abandonment if appropriate termination procedures do not occur. Abandonment generally means a unilateral severance of the professional relationship between a health care provider and a patient without reasonable notice at a time when there is still a need for continuing health care. Notification to the referring physician or health care provider is required (Gilliland Markette and Mulligan, LLP). As with many concerns discussed in this chapter, you will want to consult with legal counsel familiar with health care issues and federal, state, and local laws.

As you lay the groundwork to realize your professional home and ambitions, may the laws cited here guide you in providing the framework for your practice. The coding information may provide the mechanism for maintaining that framework.

As state and federal laws change in the health arena, it behooves every practitioner to know what those changes affect in order to effect compliance. In the next few years, we will be utilizing a new diagnosis coding system as well as likely seeing less reimbursement for services, and a change of core methodologies for how we are paid for our services. Additional bundled codes and the bundling of bundled codes may play a role in the evolution from defined moments such as the introduction of Medicare, regulations for compliance, and reduction in reimbursement paradigms, but the determination to continue to provide the utmost in care in even the most challenging situations will prevail for the benefit of those whom we serve.

References

Abel, D., & Hahn R. (2006). Ethical issues in practice management. In T. Hamill (Ed.), *Ethics in audiology: Guidelines for ethical conduct in clinical, educational, and research setting* (pp. 61–74). Reston, VA: American Academy of Audiology.

American Academy of Audiology. (2000). Audiology clinical practice algorithms and statements. *Audiology Today Special Issue,* August.

American Academy of Audiology. (2012). *Audiology superbill template.* Retrieved February 2, 2013, from http://www.audiology.org/resources/documentlibrary/Documents/2013_DiagnosticRehabSuperbill_tmp.pdf and http://www.audiology.org/resources/documentlibrary/Documents/2013_HCPCS_Superbill_tmp.pdf

American Academy of Audiology's Coding and Practice Management Committee. (2006). *Capturing reimbursement: A guide for audiologists.* Reston, VA: Author.

American Medical Association. (2004). *CPT process* (pp. 3–14). Chicago, IL: Author.

American Medical Association. (2005). *HIPAA violations and enforcement.* Retrieved March 29, 2007, from http://www.ama-assn.org/ama/pub/category/11805.html

American Medical Association. (2012). *HIPAA violations and enforcement.* Retrieved January 21, 2012, from http://www.ama-assn.org/ama/pub/physician-resources/solutions-managing-your-practice/coding-billing-insurance/hipaahealth-insurance-portability-accountability-act/hipaa-violations-enforcement.page

Centers for Medicare and Medicaid Services. (2001). *Program memorandum AB-02-080, Audiologists—payment for services furnished.* Retrieved June 3, 2002, from http://www.noridianmedicare.com/cgibin/coranto/viewnews.cgi?id

Centers for Medicare and Medicaid Services. (2008). *Transmittal 84.* Retrieved March 2, 2008, from https://www.cms.gov/transmittals/downloads/R84BP.pdf

Centers for Medicare and Medicaid Services. (2010). *Revisions and re-issuance of audiology policies-JA6447.* Retrieved September 4, 2010, from https://www.cms.gov/ContractorLearningResources/downloads/JA6447.pdf

Centers for Medicare and Medicaid Services. (2011). *Medicare benefit policy manual, chapter 15* (p. 98). Retrieved December 21, 2011, from https://www.cms.gov/manuals/Downloads/bp102c15.pdf

Centers for Medicare and Medicaid Services. (2011). *Medicare fee-for-service recovery audit program FY 2011.* Retrieved December 28, 2011, from https://www.cms.gov/Recovery-Audit-Program/Downloads/FY2011Corrections.pdf

Centers for Medicare and Medicaid Services. (2011). *MLN Matters Number: ICN_006562.* Retrieved December 15, 2011, from https://www.cms.gov/MLNProducts/downloads/MedicareAppealsprocess.pdf

Centers for Medicare and Medicaid Services. (2011). *MLN Matters Number: ICN 006827.* Retrieved on December 16, 2011, from https://www.cms.gov/MLNProducts/downloads/Fraud_and_Abuse.pdf

Centers for Medicare and Medicaid Services. (2011). *MLN Matters Number: SE0908.* Retrieved November 3, 2011, from http://www.cms.gov/MLNMattersArticles/downloads/SE0908.pdf

Centers for Medicare and Medicaid Services. (2012). *Medicare and you: 2012.* Retrieved January 18, 2012, from http://www.medicare.gov/publications/pubs/pdf/10050.pdf

Centers for Medicare and Medicaid Services. (2012). *Overview of electronic health care records.* Retrieved January 22, 2012, from https://www.cms.gov/EHealthRecords/

Centers for Medicare and Medicaid Services. (2013). *Advanced Beneficiary Notice.* Retrieved February 2, 2013, from http://www.cms.gov/Medicare/Medicare-General-Information/BNI/ABN.html

Department of Health and Human Services Office of the Inspector General. (2010). *Recovery audit contractors' fraud referrals.* Retrieved September 5, 2010, from http://oig.hhs.gov/oei/reports/oei-03-09-00130.pdf

Gilliland Markette and Milligan LLP. (2011). *Patient abandonment.* Retrieved November 14, 2011, from http://www.gillilandlaw

firm.com/Assets/Category/000010/0000/PatientAbandonmentwlogo2.pdf

Grider, D. J. (2004). *Coding with modifiers.* Chicago, IL: American Medical Association.

Hobart, R. (2006, April). *Medicare new provider training.* American Academy of Audiology. AudiologyNOW! 2006 Learning Module, Minneapolis, MN.

Lewis, D. (2011). Anti-kickback considerations for the Audiologist. *Audiology Today, 23*, 72–74.

Metz, M. (2006). Ethics of professional communication. In T. Hamill (Ed.), *Ethics in audiology: Guide for ethical conduct in clinical, educational, and research settings* (p. 45). Reston, VA: American Academy of Audiology.

Office of Inspector General. (2000). *Special fraud alert: Rental of space in physician offices by persons or entities to which physicians refer.* Retrieved May 28, 2006, from http://www.oig.hhs.gov/fraud/docsalertsandbulletins/office%20space.htm

Pessis, P. (2003, October). *Reimbursement: Am I playing by all of the rules?* Presentation at the Academy of Dispensing Audiologists Convention, Ft. Myers, FL.

Pessis, P., & Williams, K. (2005, March). *We're near the Capitol so let's increase YOUR capital!* American Academy of Audiology Annual Convention Pre-Convention Seminar. Washington DC.

Pessis, P., Williams K., & Freint, A. (2006, April). *Cracking the reimbursement code.* American Academy of Audiology NOW! 2006 Learning Lab, Minneapolis, MN.

Social Security Act. (2003). *Payment for physician's services.* Sec. 1848. [42 U.S.C. 1395w–4]. Retrieved April 4, 2010, from http://www.ssa.gov/OP_Home/ssact/title18/1848.htm

United States Federal Register. (2004). *NPI final rule.* Retrieved January 3, 2012, from http://www.cms.hhs.gov/NationalProvIdentStand/Downloads/NPIfinalrule.pdf

Appendix 9–A
Advanced Beneficiary Notice

A. Notifier:

B. Patient Name: C. Identification Number:

Advance Beneficiary Notice of Noncoverage (ABN)

<u>NOTE:</u> If Medicare doesn't pay for **D.** _____ below, you may have to pay.
Medicare does not pay for everything, even some care that you or your health care provider have good reason to think you need. We expect Medicare may not pay for the **D.** _____ below.

D.	E. Reason Medicare May Not Pay:	F. Estimated Cost

WHAT YOU NEED TO DO NOW:
- Read this notice, so you can make an informed decision about your care.
- Ask us any questions that you may have after you finish reading.
- Choose an option below about whether to receive the **D.** _____ listed above.
  Note: If you choose Option 1 or 2, we may help you to use any other insurance
    that you might have, but Medicare cannot require us to do this.

G. OPTIONS: Check only one box. We cannot choose a box for you.
☐ **OPTION 1.** I want the **D.** _____ listed above. You may ask to be paid now, but I also want Medicare billed for an official decision on payment, which is sent to me on a Medicare Summary Notice (MSN). I understand that if Medicare doesn't pay, I am responsible for payment, but **I can appeal to Medicare** by following the directions on the MSN. If Medicare does pay, you will refund any payments I made to you, less co-pays or deductibles.
☐ **OPTION 2.** I want the **D.** _____ listed above, but do not bill Medicare. You may ask to be paid now as I am responsible for payment. **I cannot appeal if Medicare is not billed**.
☐ **OPTION 3.** I don't want the **D.** _____ listed above. I understand with this choice I am **not** responsible for payment, and **I cannot appeal to see if Medicare would pay.**

H. Additional Information:

This notice gives our opinion, not an official Medicare decision. If you have other questions on this notice or Medicare billing, call **1-800-MEDICARE** (1-800-633-4227/**TTY:** 1-877-486-2048).
Signing below means that you have received and understand this notice. You also receive a copy.

I. Signature:	J. Date:

Form CMS-R-131 (03/11)   Form Approved OMB No. 0938-0566

Appendix 9–B
Cerumen/Earmold Impression Waiver Forms

CERUMEN REMOVAL WAIVER

I understand that I have impacted cerumen (wax) in one or both ears. I am therefore giving <u>(name of the audiologist who will be removing the cerumen)</u> the permission to remove it by way of the method best for me. I understand in the course of the cerumen removal I may incur a canal laceration, bleeding or the worst case and highly unlikely scenario, a tympanic membrane perforation.

I give my permission to have this procedure performed (please circle) in:

 Right ear   Left ear   **Both ears**

and understand that cerumen removal is in the scope of an audiologist's practice, for which they are licensed to perform.

_____

Patient Name

_____

Date

continues

EARMOLD IMPRESSION(S) WAIVER

In order to provide hearing aids, earmolds, swim plugs or custom hearing protectors, it will be necessary to obtain earmold impressions.

A block of cotton or foam with a string attached will be placed into your ear canal with an earlite. Impression material will then be injected into your ear canal. This will cure over a period of approximately 10 minutes. Your hearing may seem diminished during this time and is normal.

As with any procedure, there are rare risks. These risks can include a traumatic perforation of the eardrum, allergic reactions to the silicone impression material, cotton or foam; increased hearing loss; increased or change in tinnitus; laceration of the ear canal.

These risks have been reviewed with me, I understand them and give my permission to <u>(name of audiologist)</u> to have earmold impressions taken of (please circle):

Right ear   Left ear   Both ears

_____

Patient's sig **nature**

_____

Date

Appendix 9–C
Sample Authorization Form

SAMPLE RELEASE OF INFORMATION FORM

I, <u>(Name of patient), (Date of birth), (Address),</u> authorize and request <u>(name of facility)</u> to release my records to <u>(name of practice requesting information)</u> for dates of service from _____ to _____.

I understand that there may be a fee to copy such records.

I understand that this authorization will remain in effect from the date below until _____, and the information will be handled confidentially in compliance with all applicable federal and state laws.

_____

Printed name of Patient or Representative

_____

Signature of Patient or Representative (relationship if other than the patient)

_____

Date

_____

Witness

10

Policy and Procedures Manual

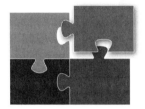

ROBERT G. GLASER, PhD

Introduction

Policy and Procedures Manual, Employee Handbook, and Employee Manual are titles for documents created to communicate the expectations of employers to their employees and what employees can expect from their employers. In some practice venues there may be two sets of documents that serve as operational guides.

The Policy and Procedures Manual (P&P Manual) may serve as the informational source developed for a spe-

cific individual or group of employees. Although the Policy and Procedures Manual serves as the basis for employee manuals or handbooks, it may also be reserved solely for the use of specific managers or directors within an organization. Employee Manuals or Handbooks may be developed from the P&P Manual for specific employees depending on their informational needs. An Employee Manual or Handbook for an audiologist may differ greatly from those generated for administrative staff despite the fact there will be operational issues common to all employees. No matter the title of the document, employee manuals or handbooks are critically important to optimize consistent operations in both small and large practices (Burrows, 2006).

Policies Versus Procedures

Policies establish the rules of the practice; procedures clarify operational issues. Policies provide the rules of engagement around which employees operate. They commonly include rules for paid time off (PTO), sick leave, jury duty, covered holidays, dress code, confidentiality, and a host of other parameters that sets forth the character and tone of the practice. For example, PTO must be readily delineated so that both new hires and long term employees understand the rules of computation and acquisition of time off, the nature and definition of various types of PTO (personal leave, military leave, sick leave), the process to request PTO, whether it is cumulative or needs to be used or lost, and so on.

Procedures prescribe and substantiate operational topics such as how the practice defines a comprehensive audiologic examination and delineating the acquisition of clinical information and data from the patient to come to an appropriate diagnosis. Although the procedure establishes the clinical components of what constitutes the examination in the practice, history, pure tone and speech threshold and recognition testing, otoacoustic emissions testing, and so forth, it should not be so detailed that it includes specific instructions of the technical components of the procedures. It is not so much how an audiologist gets to the data as much as the quality of the data gleaned from the clinical test battery

that has been chosen to constitute the comprehensive audiologic examination as a procedure for the practice. The decision to select a procedure for the comprehensive audiologic examination was determined based on the best methods to arrive at an accurate and valid diagnosis.

The Need for a Policy and Procedures Manual

The P&P Manual establishes operational and personnel characteristics necessary to provide professional services in accord with the Mission Statement or Practice Philosophy of the practice. It enables the practice owner or manager to establish these parameters in concert with his or her vision of how the practice is to operate and the manner and types of services to be provided.

Beyond systematizing administrative and operational aspects of the practice, the Policy and Procedures Manual provides rules and guidance for decision making and appropriate actions to be taken throughout the practice at every level of involvement: owner, director, department head, and clinical and administrative staff. It should be considered the ultimate resource document for an audiology practice whether the venue of service delivery is an autonomous audiology practice, a hospital department, an educational resource center, an ENT department in a medical school, or a private ENT/audiology practice.

Each employee must agree with and abide by these "rules of engagement" which clarify what the employer should expect from the employee and what the employee can expect from the employer. An employee's acceptance of these rules and procedural guidelines is critical to their becoming "stakeholders" in the practice. Additionally, employees who fail to comply with the tenets and principles in the P&P Manual do so under a stipulated understanding that they are jeopardizing their continued employment. That stipulation is completed by the employee signing and dating an acknowledgement form indicating his or her agreement to the tenets set forth in the P&P Manual as seen in Sidebar 10–1.

The P&P Manual can serve as a tutorial document for potential new hires and the basis for their orientation to the practice. Each person considered for employment must be able to follow the established rules and procedural guidelines. They should be encouraged to ask for clarification if they do not understand or have differing views on policies or procedures. If a potential employee is unable to agree with the tenets of the practice as set forth in the P&P Manual, they should seek employment elsewhere.

The P&P Manual sets the tone of the practice; how it feels and looks to patients and referral sources: employee dress and demeanor in the office or on the telephone; the structure, brevity, content, and turnaround time of reports; front office staff interactions with the referral source's office staff; and response to the number of rings on an incoming call. Many, if not all of the policies and procedures, are geared to developing patient

---

Sidebar 10–1
POLICY AND PROCEDURES MANUAL
ACKNOWLEDGMENT FORM

I have read the Policy and Procedures Manual for (*insert the practice or specific practice venue*). By acceptance of the Policy and Procedures Manual (P&P Manual), I acknowledge notice and agree to abide by and provide services or interact with patients, referral sources and others in accord with all policies and procedures set forth in the P&P Manual. I recognize the need and agree to maintain patient health information in a secure fashion such that each patient's health information is protected and secured in accord with current HIPAA regulations. I understand that changes may be made from time to time and that (*insert the practice or specific practice venue*) has the right and authority to make any representations contrary to the statements set forth in the P&P Manual. I also acknowledge that no one employed by, or acting on behalf of (*insert the practice or specific practice venue*), is authorized to make oral statements to change the at-will employment relationship between (*insert the practice or specific practice venue* and its employees. I understand that (*insert the practice or specific practice venue*) or I may terminate my employment at any time for any reason.

Signature _____ Date _____

satisfaction which has been identified as the critical element in securing the long term success of any practice.

Legal Considerations in Developing a Policy and Procedures Manual

As indicated in Chapter 3, a Policy and Procedures Manual is important no matter the number of employees. It establishes a basis for many otherwise unstated, ambiguous and/or misunderstood aspects of the employment relationship. Critically important to that relationship is the confirmation of the "at will" status of the employee and the right of the employer to terminate employment for any or no reason.

Some argue that a P&P Manual will not prevent an employee from filing a suit against the practice and its owner(s). Although it will not prevent a legal encounter by an employee, it may give them pause to do so. Having the rules of engagement set forth and the terms of employment stipulated by the employee may serve as an adequate defense against employee-related legal claims. A written document is the practice's best chance of not having a court case centering on the owner or manager's word against that of the employee. The remedy is to develop a well-written document that has been reviewed and approved by the attorney-of-record for the practice.

When preparing the P&P Manual it is best to assume that it may, right or wrong, be viewed as a legally binding contract. For that reason among many, the legal counsel for the practice must evaluate the entire document. He or she will ensure that appropriately worded disclaimers are in place and that the language in the document is in accord with the employer-employee relationship. Miller and Jentz (2006) aptly point out that employers have learned hard lessons from court decisions about what is said in P&P Manuals. They indicate that promises made in an employment manual may create an implied-in-fact contract. They suggest that employers make it clear to employees that the policies expressed in a P&P Manual must not be interpreted as a contractual promise and that the manual is not intended as a contract. They suggest the following disclaimer, appropriately adapted to the particular needs of the workplace venue, be set off and prominent from the surrounding text by the use of larger type, all capital letters or some other device that calls the reader's attention to it:

> **"This policy manual describes the basic personnel policies and practices of our Practice. You should understand that the manual does not modify our Company's 'at-will' employment doctrine or provide employees with any kind of contractual rights."**

An All-Encompassing Compliance Document

In the important arena of establishing the "rules of engagement" between an employer and an employee, consideration should be given to establishing a general compliance document. The employee signs the document upon employment. In this compliance document, the employee agrees to a variety of appropriate stipulations including records protection and confidentiality, information important to the practice, forms, electronic and hard copy files, and so forth. The employee, therefore, agrees to these stipulations on an a priori basis prior to his or her resignation or termination as an "at-will" employee.

Overview of a P&P Manual for an Audiology Practice

There is little uniformity across the tables of content for P&P Manuals, Employee Handbooks, and Manuals. Content varies with the practice venue, the practitioner/ owner and with the extent of clinical services offered in the practice. There is no set rule, order or list that might signal completeness of information. The spectrum of details in P&P Manuals ranges from minimalist statements to extensive descriptions of issues with definitions, footnotes and comprehensive legal precedents. It is important that the scope of issues in the P&P Manual be well met and adequately conveyed so that the document is clear and concise, leaving little question in the mind of the reader.

The best judge of completeness of information and topics covered relative to the venue of the practice is the attorney-of-record. He or she must review the document to ensure completeness, correctness and accuracy relative to current laws established both in the state in which the practice is located and according to federal guidelines. An attorney's view of the P&P Manual will be grounded in employment law and compliance as well as the best interests and protection of his or her client.

Each practice venue has different needs. If the practice is in a hospital department, most of the P&P Manual will likely have been completed at the corporate level. It may be left to you as the director or head of audiology to complete those sections pertaining specifically to the clinical services offered and the personnel delivering those services. The completed document will be reviewed by the hospital's legal staff as well as the administrator charged with oversight of your department or clinic. If you are in a university setting, clinical oversight as well as those with oversight of research activities will likely have to review the P&P Manual. As with corporate oversight in hospitals, universities may have even greater numbers of reviewers and personnel in oversight capacities with the final oversight commonly resting with the office of the provost.

The outline in Sidebar 10–2 may not appear logical to some, incomplete to others, and overextended by those who adhere to the "less is better" philosophy. It is offered as a guiding outline more than an all inclusive document. Each section should be given weight appropriate to your particular needs. Selected examples will be offered for your consideration. In some cases more than one option will be proffered with suggestions. Developing a comprehensive P&P Manual is beyond the scope of this text, however, this outline should enable you to get a good start and come up with a document that can be reviewed and edited by your attorney, accountant, and others with experience and knowledge in developing similar documents. The proposed text of the P&P Manual will appear in italics with commentary and suggestions, when issued, in regular font.

Sidebar 10–2
OUTLINE OF A POLICY AND PROCEDURES MANUAL

Policy and Procedure Manual
  Introduction to the Practice
  Manual as ultimate resource
    document; what it is and is
    not (disclaimers)
  The Mission of the Practice
  Practice Philosophy
  Management Rights
  Acknowledgment form(s)
    Acknowledges having read
    and willingness to abide by
    policies within P&P
    Compliance document
    regarding confidential and
    proprietary information
Policies
  Administrative Staff Priorities
  Billing-Collection Policy
  Certification vs Licenses
  Collection Policy
  Confidentiality
  Conflicts of Commitment:
    Conflicts of Interest
  Consent Forms for Procedures
    Audiology
  Consent to Perform EMI-
    Cerumen Removal
  Convention and Workshop Policy
  Customer Satisfaction and
    Complaint Resolution
  Disaster Policy
  Disciplinary Policy
  Discrimination and Harassment
    in the Workplace
  Drug and Alcohol Policy
  Equal Employment Opportunity
  Emergency Medical Assistance
    Protocol

Employee Access to Business
  Data
Employee Evaluation/
  Performance Review
Employee Standards of Conduct
  Dress
  Demeanor
  Collegiality
  Substance Abuse
  Smoking
  Harassment of Staff,
    Colleagues, and Patients
  Review P&P Manual Annually
Equipment Calibration and
  Replacement
Hearing Instrument Lost
Hearing Instrument Repair
Hearing Instrument Return
Incident Report
Infection Control
Internet Usage
Leave
Liability Insurance: Malpractice
  Insurance
Outside Employment
Patients with Prior Collection
  Action
Referring Patients to Other
  Practitioners
Release of Patient Information
Tuition Assistance
Weather
Clinical Procedures
Personnel: Position Descriptions
Documentation
Reimbursement Capture by Coding
  Optimization

Policy and Procedures Manual for Audiology Associates

Introduction

This Policy and Procedures Manual (P&P Manual) contains the policies, practices, and procedures of Audiology Associates. This P&P Manual is not intended to be all-inclusive. Audiology Associates reserves the right to make final decisions regarding the interpretation and application of its policies, practices, and procedures, whether or not identified in the P&P Manual, and to change or discontinue them at any time. The Manual also contains general information about the benefits that are available to you.

Audiology Associates is concerned not only with your job performance but also with you as an individual. If you have a question about work or any material in this Manual, contact the Practice Manager. Remember that a question can be answered only if it is raised, and conditions with which you are dissatisfied can be improved only if you bring the dilemma to management's attention.

Audiology Associates maintains an open, honest, and cooperative work environment. This work environment gives us an opportunity to get to know you and encourage you to understand and share the goals of Audiology Associates.

Please understand this manual is not intended to create nor constitute an employment contract between you and Audiology Associates. Because the P&P Manual is not contractually binding, you have the right to terminate our employment relationship at any time, with or without any notice or reason, and the Audiology Associates retains the same

right, unless specified differently by contract. Our employment relationship can be defined as employment "at will." Audiology Associates may have to make decisions without prior consultation with its employees. As such, Audiology Associates maintains exclusive discretion to select, hire, promote, suspend, dismiss, assign, supervise, and discipline employees; to establish, change, or abolish policies, procedures, rules, and regulations; to determine and modify job descriptions; and to assign duties to employees in accordance with the needs and requirements determined by Audiology Associates.

Purpose of the Policy and Procedures Manual

The P&P Manual was developed to provide you with guidelines and policies regarding your employment with Audiology Associates. This manual is an important guidebook to be used as a resource regarding policies, employee guidelines, and our practice standards. We hope that this manual will be beneficial in establishing the responsibilities of both the employer and employee to each other and eliminate any misunderstanding that may occur due to poor or misinterpreted communications. These policies have been developed to serve the current needs and may be adjusted periodically. Both Audiology Associates and the employees are encouraged to recommend revisions they feel are appropriate.

Practice Philosophy: A Mission of Commitment to Patients

■ *We pledge to always make decisions in favor of the patient and referral source at every opportunity knowing that we cannot be wrong if we are trying to be right for those whom we serve.*

■ *We are professionally, ethically, and personally committed to providing excellent care in a timely and caring manner to all members of the communities we serve.*

■ *Our Audiologists represent the finest professional resource for hearing and balance evaluations, tinnitus assessment and management, hearing instrument evaluation, fitting, and follow-up care in the communities we serve.*

■ *The entire staff of Audiology Associates recognizes and appreciates the importance of all health care providers and their staff who refer patients to us for our specialized care and consideration. We strive to maintain their trust by issuing timely, concise, and accurate reports and by maintaining an active liaison between our referral sources and their patients.*

■ *Each member of our practice subscribes to the following Patient's Bill of Rights:*

Patients in our practice should:

1. *Expect more from Audiology Associates than from any other provider in our community.*
2. *Know that each patient will be respected by everyone in our practice.*
3. *Expect us to answer your phone call in a timely, friendly, and welcoming manner.*
4. *Upon arrival, expect to be greeted in a friendly and appreciative manner by everyone in our practice.*

5. *Know that we recognize the importance of their time.*
6. *Expect a quick response and immediate action all the time by every member of our practice.*
7. *Require excellent communication from us.*
8. *Know that we will listen and understand their concerns.*
9. *Expect quick and accurate resolution of questions or concerns about your account.*
10. *Receive an apology if we are in error.*

Management Rights

It is important that any manual for employees has a clear statement of the rights of practice managers to conduct business in an appropriate and professional manner according to their terms. The statement need not be lengthy. It must clarify the roles, obligations, and expectations that management considers important to the continued operation of the practice as a business. Likewise, the employee should understand clearly where in the scheme of the practice he or she fits in relative to management. The wording is commonly straightforward and must leave little room for conjecture as to the roles of management and the intent to operate the practice as a business.

Rights of Management

Audiology Associates has and will always seek the opinions of every member of the practice about working conditions, ways, and means to accomplish all tasks important to the success of our practice and other matters that are of importance to the members of our team. From time to time, Audiology Associates must make decisions without the input from the members of the team. As such, Audiology Associates retains all managerial and administrative rights referred to inherently and by law. These rights include, but are not limited to, the right to exercise judgment in establishing and administering policies, practices, and procedures, and to make changes in them; the right to take whatever action is necessary, in management's judgment, to operate the practice; and the right to set standards of productivity and services to be rendered. The management of business and the direction of those working in the practice including, but not limited to, the responsibility to hire, promote, transfer, suspend, or discharge, and the responsibility to relieve employees from duty because of lack of work, or other reasons, are vested exclusively in the management of Audiology Associates. In addition, Audiology Associates has the right to amend, modify, or delete provisions of this manual with or without prior notice.

Acknowledgment Forms

Critically important to any P&P Manual is a statement signed and dated by the employee indicating that he or she has read the document and agrees with its content and implied or actual actions that may be put into effect by the owner or manager of the practice. Any document that stipulates specific compliance, duties, rules, or expected actions or response by an employee must be signed and dated during the earliest stages of employment. It is difficult to get docu-

ments signed immediately prior to or after an employee has been discharged.

Two examples follow. The first is an acknowledgment form that commits the signer to the tenets of the P&P Manual. It underscores the need for confidentiality and compliance with HIPAA regulations. The second is an equally important acknowledgment document specifying the proprietary rights of the practice. Although it will not prevent theft of documents, forms, and the like, the courts have taken a dim view of individuals leaving a business or practice with proprietary or trade information after they have affixed their signature to a compliance document describing specific proprietary items and information that must be left at the workplace. Of course, these documents can be combined; however, by having two separate forms, the underlying reasons and differing content are made clearer. Each should be signed in the early stages of employment, after the P&P Manual has been read and orientation to the practice has been completed. The second form lets the employee know that, in the event he or she decides to leave the practice or is terminated, there are specific rules regarding confidentiality, pirating forms, and removing items considered important to the practice is prohibited.

Acknowledgment Form

I have reviewed a current copy of Audiology Associates' Policy & Procedure Manual. By acceptance of the manual, I acknowledge notice of all policies contained therein. I agree to maintain patient information in a secure fashion such that each patient's health information is protected and secured, in accord with current HIPAA regulations. I understand that changes may be made from time to time and that Audiology Associates has authority to make any representations contrary to the statements set forth in the manual. I also acknowledge that no one employed by, or acting on behalf of Audiology Associates, is authorized to make oral statements which change the at-will employment relationship between Audiology Associates and its employees. I further understand that the Audiology Associates or I may terminate my employment at any time for any reason.

_____
Signature

_____
Date

General Compliance Document
Audiology Associates

In accord with my resignation or discharge as an at-will employee, I submit and agree to and with the following statements in compliance with office policies and HIPAA regulations:

- *Patient records, notes, and/or other information pertaining to the patients of Audiology Associates will remain confidential and will not be removed physically or electronically.*
- *Financial information about individual patients and/or any fiscal information pertaining to Audiology Associates will remain confidential and may not be removed physically or electronically.*
- *Information important to Audiology Associates including, but not limited to, personnel information, supplier information, and any/all statistics pertaining to the operations of Audiology Associates will remain confidential and will not be removed physically or electronically.*
- *Information about the current status, future plans, and other information deemed important to current and future operations of Audiology Associates will remain confidential and will not be removed physically or electronically.*
- *Forms, computer programs, equipment manuals, patient protocols, or other documents regarding operational and patient-related matters pertaining to Audiology Associates shall remain at the office in physical and electronic forms and information contained therein must remain confidential.*
- *Books, journals, and related materials not purchased by personal funds will remain the property of Audiology Associates.*
- *All forms developed for use at Audiology Associates are hereby copyrighted and remain the intellectual property of Audiology Associates. As such, none may be removed nor used in whole or in part for any reason except when permission has been granted in writing.*
- *All physical and electronic files used in the execution of duties as an employee of Audiology Associates remain the property of Audiology Associates and may not be removed in any form.*
- *In the interests of the patients served and the continuity of their care, all charts, and related correspondence will be completed by noon of the day immediately prior to the last day of employment.*

_____
Signature

_____
Date

Policies

Policies represent the rules of the practice. The following alphabetic list of policies with examples will not represent a comprehensive list for each and every practice. Each will provide a starting point to develop an appropriately written document for your particular practice venue. To enable both comments and instructions on the language to be considered in these policy sections, two different fonts will be used; italics for policy language and regular font for instructional comments.

Administrative Staff Priorities

1. *Booking patients into the office: We cannot help if they are not here.*
2. *Take care of referral sources: They and their support staff members are our partners in caring for THEIR patients: Courtesy, respect, and an abundance of assistance are critical to providing excellent service that will sustain referrals. If you take care of them, they assume their patients will be well cared for in our practice.*
3. *Smooth the process of every visit: Take the appointment from the hands of the referral source staff to our hands—let them get back to work while we book the appointment and get preliminary information from the patient.*
4. *Take great care of each phone call. Consider the caller your boss, as we all work for the patients coming to our practice. Always make decisions in favor of the patients and the referral sources.*

5. *To schedule follow up visits, call twice before leaving a voice message; if no response to voice message, send postcard asking them to call us.*
6. *Send handwritten thank you notes to those patients who have referred patients to our practice—they have entrusted their friend or relative to our care and they deserve our thanks and appreciation.*
7. *Call newly fitted patients or those with recently repaired instruments within 3 to 5 days of the (re)fitting to check their status <u>before</u> their return visit–if they are struggling, get them on the schedule PRIOR to their scheduled follow-up visit.*
8. *When a patient calls or presents a hearing instrument for repair, obtain their description of the problem, and when and how often the problem occurs. If the instrument is dead, check for occlusion and battery problems. Advise need to return for repair, turnaround time, and costs if applicable.*
9. *Hearing instrument repairs, accessories and batteries, out-of-warranty adjustments, or modifications are to be paid same day of service.*

Audiology Associates Financial Agreement

Payment is expected at the time of service unless other arrangements have been made. We accept cash, checks, Master-Card, Visa, and Discover Card.

■ *We will submit charges directly to your insurance carrier as a courtesy. Submitting the charges is no guarantee they will be paid.*

■ *Insurance policies may or may not pay for the services you receive in our office. Coverage varies with each insurance carrier; a few plans cover all charges, some cover 80% and others cover less than 50%. The amount your insurance company pays for the services you receive is between you and your insurance carrier.*

■ *YOU ARE RESPONSIBLE FOR PAYING ALL CHARGES INCLUDING DEDUCTIBLES, CO-INSURANCE AND SERVICES, DEVICES, AND RELATED ITEMS NOT COVERED BY INSURANCE. ACCOUNTS NOT PAID WITHIN 45 DAYS MAY GO TO A COLLECTION AGENT.*

■ *HEARING INSTRUMENTS ORDERED AND NOT PICKED UP WILL BE SUBJECT TO RESTOCKING AND HANDLING FEES WHEN RETURNED TO THE MANUFACTURER.*

■ *EARMOLDS AND/OR IMPRESSION COSTS ARE NON-REFUNDABLE AND MUST BE PAID IN FULL.*

I have read and understand the above and agree to pay all charges. I authorize my insurance company to make direct payment for all services rendered. Release is hereby granted to send records by any means appropriate to health care providers or others deemed necessary by Audiology Associates.

_____
Signature

_____
Date

_____
Witness

_____
Date

Billing and Collection Policy

Every patient in our practice has signed an agreement indicating they are responsible for paying any and all bills incurred during their care in our practice. The billing cycle for Audiology Associates is 45 days. Accounts with unpaid balances will be sent to collection if in that time period, payment in full or scheduled payment arrangements have not been established. There must be a written agreement on the method and dates of payment if balances are to be carried beyond the 45-day billing cycle.

Each patient must receive notification by phone or letter 15 days prior to our sending their account to collection. Once the account has been placed with the collection agent, all payments must be made to that agency. No attempt should be made to discuss accounts in collection since the account is no longer with our practice. They must be referred to the collection agency if they have questions or concerns.

Confidentiality

All information pertaining to the patients we serve must remain confidential. Conversations about patients entrusted to our care must be completed such that those in waiting or treatment rooms will not overhear the conversation. Patient charts and other information including the appointment book should be secured from view. At no time should a patient be discussed outside of the office with anyone including another staff member.

As all patient information obtained by Audiology Associates is confidential, it may not be released to an insurance company or any other party, without the patient's written permission on file.

Breach of confidentiality of patient information will result in immediate termination of employment.

Conflicts of Commitment and Conflicts of Interest

A conflict of commitment exists when an employee assumes obligations external to the practice which interferes with the employee's properly discharging his or her obligations and commitment to Audiology Associates. Full time employees must make full time commitments to Audiology Associates. Part-time employees with obligations external to the practice must ensure they are fully committed to Audiology Associates when discharging their duties on behalf of our practice. Full disclosure of any obligation external to Audiology Associates is expected regardless of the numbers of hours of employment.

Obligations external to Audiology Associates that represent direct competition for similar patients, referral sources or care contracts constitutes a conflict of interest. A conflict of interest must be disclosed by the employee and a determination made as to the course of action which will resolve the issue. Expeditious disclosure and resolution of such conflicts is in the interests of all involved. Failure to resolve conflicts may result in termination of employment.

Consent Forms for Specific Procedures

Consent forms will not prevent legal action. They exist as an acknowledgment that the procedure has been explained, risks have been discussed, and the patient

acknowledges having been advised of the risks.

Consent to Perform Cerumen Removal and/or Earmold Impression

Cerumen removal and/or earmold impression procedures involves the introduction of instruments and/or material into your ear canal(s). The audiologist will use accepted procedures to avoid adverse results. Cerumen removal and earmold impression involves the risks of discomfort, bleeding from the ear canal, puncture of or damage to the eardrum, and ear infection.

I, the undersigned patient, hereby acknowledge that I have read and understand the important notice printed above. I understand that no guarantee has been made to me as to the results. I recognize the risks of receiving the procedure(s) described. I hereby request and consent to the procedure(s).

_____
Patient Name

_____
Signature

_____
Audiologist Name

_____
Signature

_____
Date

Patient Satisfaction and Complaint Resolution

Every practice must ensure that the patient has a voice in his or her care. If the patient feels as though he or she has been treated inappropriately, unfairly, or has been otherwise ill treated, the patient should have a means to address the issues with the owner of the practice or the Practice Manager. The simpler the policy, the more expedient the result: complaint resolution is as much about the speed with which you reply as it is with the resolution of the complaint. The policy can be as simple as having all patients with unresolved complaints referred directly to the Practice Manager for resolution within 24 to 48 hours. He or she can deal with the situation directly after having discussed the situation with those members of the administrative and professional staffs directly involved in the patient's complaint. The goal is to resolve conflict in favor of the patient at every opportunity. That does not mean, however, that the Practice Manager needs to roll over every time a patient lodges a complaint. If the patient's complaint exceeds reasonable limits set forth in policies or guidelines and is beyond appropriate reasonability, resolution completely in favor of the patient might jeopardize the validity of the policies and procedures of the practice. Flexibility in favor of the patient is expected. Not responding favorably to a patient's unreasonable demand should not be construed as inflexibility. Every business has to draw the line somewhere and that includes businesses operating in the arena of health care.

Disciplinary Actions

Audiology Associates enjoys a fine reputation as a health care provider. That reputation in no small part is directly related to employees who take pride in the services they provide. Employees are expected to conduct themselves in a cour-

teous and professional manner towards patients, referral sources, and their fellow employees at all times. Policies and guidelines are to be followed to maintain the integrity of the practice and the standards of care we have established in the communities we serve. When difficulties affecting your performance or the performance of others dictate disciplinary considerations, the following disciplinary guideline represents the progressive steps that will be taken:

1. *A verbal warning*
2. *A written warning*
3. *Final warning*
4. *Termination.*

Management takes into account all the facts surrounding an employee's misconduct in determining appropriate discipline. Generally, however, a VERBAL warning may be given for initial minor violations of practice policies or procedures. The written warning is given for repeated violations or initial violations of a more serious nature. A final warning, which is always in writing, is given for the most serious offenses other than those calling for immediate discharge or for continued repetition of the type of violations for which one or more written warnings have been given.

Management reserves the right to bypass any of the progressive steps of discipline depending on the facts and severity of the offense. Management may give an employee a written or final warning as the first warning. Management can also terminate an employee without prior warning.

When misconduct is of a very serious nature, an employee may expect immediate discharge. The following acts are examples of serious misconduct, which may result in immediate discharge, and is not intended to be an all-inclusive list:

1. *Conviction of a felony.*
2. *Theft, misappropriation of funds.*
3. *Possession, use, or sale of an alcoholic beverage, non-prescribed drugs or illicit drugs while on Audiology Associates premises or while on duty at another practice site.*
4. *Reporting to work while under the influence of intoxicants, including alcohol, non-prescribed drugs, or illicit drugs.*
5. *Possession of firearms, knives, or other weapons while on practice premises or while on duty at another practice site.*
6. *Fighting or attempting to injure another person while on practice premises or while on duty at another practice site.*
7. *Engaging in horseplay or using abusive, threatening, or provocative language toward another person while on practice premises or while on duty at another practice site.*
8. *Engaging in sexual harassment.*
9. *Insubordination (e.g., refusal to promptly obey a work instruction or job assignment from a supervisor or the Practice Manager).*
10. *Dishonesty, including falsification of records (e.g., payroll, insurance, and personnel records).*
11. *Failure to report unexcused absences.*
12. *Immoral or indecent conduct on practice premises or while on duty at practice site.*
13. *Gambling on practice premises or while on duty at another site.*
14. *Willful destruction of practice property.*
15. *Unlawful possession, use, manufacture, distribution, or dispensing of illicit drugs, controlled substances or alcoholic beverages during the employee's work period, whether on the premises of Audiology Associates or at site(s) where the employee is carrying out assigned duties of Audiology Associates.*

Each employee is responsible for knowing the rules of expected conduct, as well as the procedures outlined in this manual. Should you have any questions about the application of any rule or any discipline you have received, discuss it with the Practice Manager.

Drug and Alcohol Policy

Audiology Associates maintains a safe and healthy environment for its employees and the patients and referring health care providers whom we serve. The use or trafficking of illicit drugs, on or off the job, has an adverse impact on our practice and will not be tolerated.

Possession of prescription drugs while on practice premises or representing Audiology Associates at a related site is permissible only if:

- *The drug is kept in the original container with both the employee's name and prescribing doctor's name on it.*
- *The drug was dispensed within 12 months.*
- *Written permission is submitted from the prescribing doctor who permits the employee to work while taking the indicated dosage.*

Even if the above conditions are met, Audiology Associates reserves the right to have a second physician determine whether the drug might adversely affect performance.

If an employee appears to be impaired or there is reason to believe that he or she may be in possession of alcohol or drugs, the employee may be ordered to undergo a drug and alcohol screen at the expense of Audiology Associates. Employees who are directed to undergo a drug or alcohol test will be suspended pending laboratory analysis of the sample. If the test is positive, the employee will be disciplined, up to and including termination of employment. If the test is negative, the employee will be paid for any lost work time. Employees are permitted to have the same sample re-tested at their own expense. If you are having a problem with drugs or alcohol, you can seek help. Our health insurance benefits provide for some treatment and counseling services. Please see the Practice Manager for any questions regarding the above.

Educational Allowances

Audiology Associates provides a minimum of three days for CEU eligible educational training at an approved meeting with approval of the practice manager. Registration, economy class airfare, accommodations, and reasonable expenses will be paid upon submission and approval of receipts. Additional funding for other CEU eligible educational meetings may be approved as needed by the Practice Manager.

Equal Employment Opportunity (EEO) Policy

In accordance with applicable local, state, and federal law, Audiology Associates is committed to a policy of non-discrimination and equal employment opportunity. All employment decisions will be made without regard to sex, sexual preference, race, color, religious creed, national origin, ancestry, age, non-job-related handicap, disability, HIV AIDS, or AIDS-related conditions.

Emergency Medical Assistance Protocol

Every practice must have a plan to respond to emergency situations. In the event that an individual in the practice becomes ill and requires emergency medical care, every member of the administrative and professional staffs must follow a set of steps to secure the situation and engage emergency personnel as soon as possible. The protocol should be practiced at least twice a year. Every telephone in the practice should have the office address and cross streets listed on the phone cradle—a handy reminder in the fast paced confusion of an emergency. The steps in the protocol will vary from setting-to-setting. At the minimum, a basic plan should include the following steps:

Emergency Medical Assistance Protocol

1. Upon determining a patient or guest is in distress, call out to other practice personnel for help.
2. Dial 911 and notify the operator of the situation and give the address of the practice.
3. Do not leave the individual; however, you must make sure that emergency personnel can access your location.
4. Another staff member should go outside to direct emergency personnel.

5. The Practice Manager should follow the individual to the hospital and make sure the family is contacted.
6. If the individual requiring removal from your practice has been referred by their physician, contact the referring physician immediately and apprise him or her of the situation.
7. Follow up with the patient or the family the next day.

Access to Operational Information of the Practice

Information in any form pertaining to the business operations of Audiology Associates is confidential. Daily business and professional operations such as, but not limited to, patient care visits, numbers of hearing instruments dispensed, billing and coding information, fiscal information, patient and referral source databases, and contracts to provide services and any similar information is considered confidential and access to these and other operational data is restricted to the Practice Manager and his or her designees on a need to know basis. Failure to comply with this policy will result in termination.

Performance Review

The first performance review for all personnel will be completed by the Practice Manager within the first 90 days of employment and at least annually thereafter.

The purpose of a review is to provide each employee with an opportunity to voice his or her concerns and to express thoughts about how their particular participation in the practice enhances patient care. He or she should take the opportunity to discuss items of interest or concern with the Practice Manager.

The Practice Manager will review the employee's performance and provide suggestions to improve specific areas. If significant resolution of deficiencies is considered necessary, additional training and re-assessment of performance may be established in a defined time period. The performance evaluation will be summarized by the Practice Manager in writing for the employee's personnel file and a copy will be provided the employee.

Professional Appearance and Dress Code

A professional image is important to our patients and helps solidify their positive attitudes about our professionalism and their perceptions of the quality of services we provide. Good grooming and a professional appearance are expected of all employees. Employees are required to wear white lab coats with their names embroidered or on a name tag. The practice will supply appropriate lab coats to all personnel. Dress shirts and ties with dress slacks or khakis and appropriate shoes and socks are expected for men. Skirts and slacks with appropriate blouses or sweaters and appropriate shoes are expected for women. Athletic shoes, jeans, sweatshirts, tank tops, and blouses displaying the midriff are prohibited. Additionally, professional attire is expected to be worn when attending professional meetings as a representative of Audiology Associates.

Replacement of Lost Hearing Instrument under Warranty

If a hearing instrument is lost while under warranty, a replacement instrument will be secured for the patient under the manufacturer's terms of replacement. There will be no charge for the replacement instrument. There will be an inclusive $350.00 fee for earmold impression, programming and placement of the replacement instrument including all adjustments necessary during three follow-up visits available for one year following the replacement.

Hearing Instrument Repairs

Hearing instrument repairs that are completed after the warranty period must be paid in full on the day the instrument is replaced. The cost of the repair may not include charges for reprogramming if the instrument has not been reprogrammed to the original settings.

Return of Hearing Instrument within Four Weeks Postfitting

In the event a patient returns a hearing instrument within the 4-week period following the initial fitting, the patient will be required to pay the restocking charge stipulated in the hearing instrument receipt booklet. Returns after the 4-week period following the fitting will be decided on a case-by-case basis.

Internet Usage

Information contained in Audiology Associate's computer and information systems (all of which shall be referred to as "information systems") are the property of the Audiology Associates.

E-mail Procedures

1. All e-mail correspondence is the property of Audiology Associ-

ates and is for business purposes only.

2. Employee e-mail communications are not considered private despite any such designation either by the sender or the recipient.

3. Messages sent to recipients outside of Audiology Associates, if sent over the Internet and not encrypted, are not secure. Encryption requires prior approval by Audiology Associates.

4. Audiology Associates will monitor its e-mail system, including an employee's mailbox, at its discretion in the ordinary course of business. Please note that in certain situations, Audiology Associates may access and disclose messages sent over its e-mail system.

5. The existence of passwords and "message delete" functions do not restrict or eliminate Audiology Associate's ability or right to access electronic communications. The delete function does not eliminate the message from the system.

6. Employees shall not share an e-mail password, provide e-mail access to an unauthorized user or access another user's e-mail box without authorization.

7. Offensive, demeaning, or disruptive messages are prohibited. This includes, but is not limited to, messages that are inconsistent with Audiology Associate's policies concerning "Equal Employment Opportunity" and "Sexual Harassment."

General Internet Procedures

1. Audiology Associate's network, including its connection to the Internet, is to be used for business-

related purposes only and not for personal use. Any unauthorized use of the Internet is strictly prohibited. Unauthorized use includes, accessing personal accounts or any form of social media, posting or downloading pornographic materials, engaging in computer "hacking," and other related activities attempting to disable or compromise the security of information contained on Audiology Associate's computers (or otherwise using Audiology Associate's computers for personal use).

2. *Because postings placed on the Internet may display Audiology Associate's address, make certain before posting information on the Internet that the information reflects the standard policies of our practice. Under no circumstances shall information of a confidential, sensitive or otherwise proprietary nature be placed on the Internet.*

3. *Subscriptions to news groups and mailing lists are permitted when the subscription is for a work-related purpose. Any other subscriptions are prohibited.*

4. *Unless the prior approval of management has been obtained, users may not establish Internet or other external network connections that could allow unauthorized persons to gain access to Audiology Associate's systems and information. These connections include the establishment of hosts with public modem dial-ins, World Wide Web home pages and File Transfer Protocol (FTP).*

5. *All files downloaded from the Internet must be checked for possible computer viruses.*

6. *Any data on any computer hard drives or electronic media (discs, etc.) which pertain to Audiology Associates, its patients or staff is considered the property of Audiology Associates and must be kept in confidence following the guidelines set forth in the Confidentiality Statement.*

7. *Upon termination of employment, all data must be returned to Audiology Associates intact and any copies must be deleted from hard drives and/or electronic media.*

8. *No software nor peripheral is to be installed on Audiology Associate's system without prior authorization.*

9. *Any employee who violates this policy shall be subject to disciplinary actions including termination of employment.*

Paid Time Off (PTO)

Employees are asked to schedule their vacation at least one or two months in advance of the time they desire to be away.

In the event that two employees ask for the same PTO dates and a conflict is deemed important and unavoidable, the individual who submitted his or her Request for Leave form first will be granted the PTO requested.

"Request for Leave" forms can be obtained from the Practice Manager.

All Requests for Leave forms must be competed and submitted to the Practice Manager. Emergency PTO will be considered accordingly, however, we expect a phone call regarding the situation and an estimate of time away from your responsibilities.

Paid Time Off Schedule

Full Time: (5 days a week; 32 to 40 hours and up; 50 consecutive weeks)

1st year	7 days
2nd & 3rd years	15 days
4th 5th & 6th years	20 days
7th 8th & 9th years	25 days
10th year and above	25 days

Part Time: (3 days per week; 30 hours and up; 50 consecutive weeks)

1st year	5 days
2nd & 3rd years	7 days
4th 5th & 6th years	10 days
7th 8th & 9th years	12 days
10th year and above	14 days

- *Above PTO must be used in one-hour increments.*
- *PTO earned but not taken during the calendar year is not cumulative from year-to-year and will be forfeited if not taken by December 31st (Use or lose policy).*
- *In the unfortunate event of a long-term illness, the employee will meet with the Practice Manager to discuss his or her PTO status.*

Patients with Prior Collection Actions

Individuals returning to our practice for re-assessment, hearing instrument repairs or follow-up visits with a history of having been placed in collections, must pay for all services on a cash or credit card basis only. Exceptions to this policy may be considered on a case-by-case basis.

Position Descriptions

Every position of employment within a practice requires a written description of general and specific duties, management responsibilities if appropriate, oversight and reporting responsibilities as well as specific areas of data handling and access. Qualifications for each position should be made clear including specific training requirements or degree requirements. Patient care responsibilities should be delineated relative to the expected clinical proficiencies necessary to provide specific services. An example of a position description for a receptionist follows:

Position Description for Receptionist

Reports To: Practice Manager

Managerial Responsibilities: None or as directed by the Practice Manager

Qualifications: Associates or Bachelor's Degree in business or related field preferred. Past work experience should include health care or related field as front office receptionist or position that included patient or practitioner interactions

Hours: 40 plus hours per week (flexible as needed)

Responsibilities:

1. Opening and closing the office
2. Confirming all appointments (Audiology and Speech patients) for the next business day and pulling charts

3. *Ordering supplies for the audiology department*
4. *Coordinates audiologists schedules*
5. *Schedules patient and vendor appointments*
6. *Greets patients and gathers billing information*
7. *Answers telephone, screens and directs calls, takes messages*
8. *Enters selected charges and payments in the computer*
9. *Prepares daily bank deposit*
10. *Organizes and files patients charts*
11. *Obtains medical concurrences*
12. *Performs receptionist duties at satellite offices*
13. *Researches and enters new patient data into the computer*
14. *Assists in the orientation and training of new employees as needed*
15. *Has joint responsibility for office maintenance*
16. *Faxing/mailing report results to primary care physicians and others.*
17. *Other responsibilities as directed by the Practice Manager.*

Referring Patients to Other Practitioners

Patients may be referred to other health care providers when needed, if he or she has come to our practice on a self-referred basis, independent of a physician or other health care provider's referral. If the patient has been referred to our practice by a primary care provider or other health care practitioner and there is a definitive need for referral to another specialist or health care entity for additional evaluation or treatment, the patient must be returned to the origi-nal referring source for disposition and management with suggestions.

Tuition Assistance

Tuition assistance may be provided for completion of an AuD or PhD in Audiol-ogy on a case-by-case basis. According to the Federal Tax Codes, up to $5,250.00 of payments received by an employee for tuition, fees, books, supplies, and so forth under an employer's educational assis-tance program may be excluded from gross income (Code Sec. 127; Reg. 1.127-1).

Inclement Weather

When forecasts indicate inclement weather that may result in school closings due to impassible road conditions, the Practice Manager (or designee) will take a copy of the schedule home (patient phone num-bers should be listed) the night before threatening weather. The Practice Owner and/or Practice Manager will decide on the following course(s) of action:

- *If conditions are obvious, scheduled patients may be cancelled and rescheduled the afternoon or evening prior to the anticipated weather situation.*
- *If severe, inclement conditions arise in the early morning, the patients may be cancelled and rescheduled before 8:30 am.*
- *The Practice Owner and/or Manager will contact each member of the staff to determine their ability to arrive at the office(s) or service sites. Depending on the response, patients may be cancelled and the workday may be considered cancelled.*

Clinical Procedures

Each clinical procedure offered in the practice should be delineated. Every CPT code employed in the practice constitutes a procedure; each should be well described with approximate times to complete the procedure with cooperative patients.

Summary

A P&P Manual is an essential part of communication within the practice. It stands as the rulebook, the reference book, and as a reminder of why patients and referral sources are the focus of the practice. Regardless of the number of people employed by the practice, a P&P Manual should be prepared and re-evaluated on an annual basis. There are no hard and fast rules about what should or should not be available to the readers of the manual. It can be easily adjusted to include speech-language pathologists, psychologists, physical therapists, or other health care providers and counselors with appropriate position descriptions and minor changes in language specific to each discipline included in the practice. Regardless of the numbers of employees and their relative contributions to the practice, the wise practice manager or owner will solicit as much input from every member of the practice team in the preparatory stages of the manual. After all, the P&P Manual is, at its basis, about the services and the contributions provided as members of the team that is the practice.

References

Burrows, D. L. (2006). Human resource issues: Managing, hiring, firing, and evaluating employees. In R. M. Traynor (Ed.), *Seminars in Hearing, 27*(1), 5–17.

Miller, R. L., & Jentz, G. A. (2006). *Business law today*. Mason, OH : Thomson Higher Education.

11

Patient Management

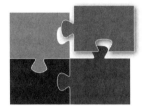

ROBERT G. GLASER, PhD

Beyond Clinical Service Delivery: Developing Patient Centric Practices

There was a time in health care when patient loyalty was not a noteworthy concern. People chose their practitioner and stayed with him or her throughout their lives. Commonly, the patient's children and grandchildren would be delivered and followed by the same practitioner throughout their lives. If a new associate entered the practice, the patients would rather see "Ol' Doc Jones" than the new practitioner unless there was absolutely no option beyond their perception of the urgency of their situation. Rarely did they consider leaving "Ol' Doc Jones," since he had been with the family for almost as long as anyone could remember: The only way out of the care and influence of the practitioner was when the patient or the practitioner died or otherwise moved elsewhere.

There was little or no concern about Doc Jones's academic or clinical training. Patients generally did not care what he knew; they appreciated that he not only cared for them but about them and their entire family as well. There was a reciprocal bond, a personal relationship between the caregiver and the patient that was inviolate. There was little-to-no

357

risk of legal action for mismanagement or malpractice in those times. Patients appreciated whatever attempt at resolution the practitioner could come up with as an honest, forthright endeavor. A documented standard of care was nonexistent nor considered necessary at that time.

The modern era of regulated practice in health care was introduced when Codes of Ethics were established by the respective health care professions and regulatory agencies were developed to set forth statutory descriptions of academic preparation and standards of care. With this new era came a different relationship between patients and all health care providers.

Successful patient management is not solely about assessment, therapeutic intervention, and clinical technique. There are a surprising number of patient centric activities that can significantly affect the continuum of a patient's care. This chapter explores how nonactivities affect your ability to provide quality care, increase patient satisfaction, and develop patient loyalty in your practice.

Developing Patient Loyalty

Patient care begins when a member of the front office staff schedules an appointment. The person on the other end of the line moves from caller to patient in a matter of minutes. The caller, now patient, will be arriving at your office expecting a high degree of professionalism, timely service, and attentive staff and caregivers sensitive to their particular needs. Every patient must experience seamless transitions from the waiting area to exam room, from exam room to payment window, and from departure to promised follow-up care. Seamless transitions in any health care setting depends on the synchrony of the front office and professional staff members and how well they take care of the patients at the center of their coordinated efforts.

Patient Loyalty Defined

Patient loyalty is the result of paying attention to what it takes to keep a patient and providing excellence in service on a consistent basis: Patient loyalty is important to your practice. Patient satisfaction is important to referral sources. Patient-centric care is sure to develop both loyalty and satisfaction. Patient-centric care creates a partnership across patients, their families, and the provider of the professional services to ensure that decisions respects patient's wants, needs, and preferences and that the patient receives the support and education they need to participate in their own care. Patient-centric care is, in its purest form, all about honoring the patent's perspective.

In their classic study of critical business relationships, Reinartz and Kumar (2002) establish several factual statements based on customer loyalty that are directly applicable to the services provided in everyday clinical practice. Their business relationship statement is followed by an interpretational statement appropriate for audiology practice in parentheses:

- Customer satisfaction is the key to customer loyalty. (Satisfied patients will likely return for repeat services.)
- Loyal customers expect tangible benefits for their loyalty. (Patients expect cost breaks on batteries, special "tune ups," etc.)

- Loyal customers become more price sensitive. (2nd or 3rd sets of hearing instruments expected to be "reasonably" more expensive than the last instruments.)
- Loyal customers may not be less expensive to maintain. (Consistent marketing efforts are necessary to retain patients—they are bombarded with opportunities to change providers)
- Loyal customers provide effective word-of-mouth marketing. (Satisfied patients will recommend your services to others.)

Building patient loyalty can be expensive in both time and capital. It is, however, a task that both front office and professional staff members must continuously and consistently strive to develop. Each patient encounter is an opportunity to foster patient loyalty: Developing patient loyalty must be considered in the diagnostic phase as much as the rehabilitative segment of a patient's journey through your practice. All forms of communication with your existing database of patients must focus on developing and maintaining patient loyalty; telephone conversations, newsletters, reminder letters, special offers, and other advertising media.

Research has demonstrated that effective communication between patients and providers increases the likelihood of: (1) positive patient outcomes, (2) accurate diagnoses and timely treatments, (3) patients and family members understanding and adhering to recommended treatment regimens, (4) greatly improved patient safety, and (5) patient and family satisfaction with the care they receive (Rao, 2011).

According to Wong et al. (2003), satisfaction ratings are likely influenced more by how well patients are treated than by the sound quality and improved speech intelligibility that their hearing aids provide. Satisfied patients are more likely to seek your guidance and care for the long term. If you are seeing the majority of your patient base annually, providing meaningful services delivered in a sincere and patient-centric manner, your patients will likely continue with your care and return to you for new hearing instruments when needed. It does not, however, take much to move a loyal patient in your database to one seeking an alternative location for their hearing care. The Research Institute of America reported on just how costly it is for businesses to be apathetic toward customer service. To underscore the point of importance to all in the business of providing professional services, I have inserted the word "patient" for "customer":

- The average practice will hear nothing from 96% of unhappy patients who receive rude or discourteous treatment.
- 90% of patients who are dissatisfied with the services they receive will not come back or buy again from the offending practice.
- Each unhappy patient tells his or her story to an average of nine other people.
- Only 4% of unhappy patients bother to complain to your office—they will complain to the referral source and will do so loudly and vociferously.
- Of those patients voicing a complaint, between 54% and 70% will do business again with the organization IF their complaint is resolved—that figure rises to 95% if the patient feels the complaint is resolved quickly.

■ 68% of patients who refuse to return to a practice do so because of the perception that the practice is "indifferent."

With conventional wisdom putting the average lifespan of contemporary hearing instruments at seven to eight years, it becomes crucial to the long-term success of your practice to have patients return consistently for their hearing care. Hopkins (2006), while highlighting the importance in developing close, clinical relationships with patients, points out another reason to maintain a loyal patient database: "Even if your product has a long life span and people shouldn't need to replace it for a long time, you still want to work on keeping those patients loyal to your practice. The reason: They will tell their friends, relatives and even strangers about what a great experience they had with you. They will be your biggest fans and provide free advertising for your services with their testimonials and referrals."

Marketers refer to three stages of the customer/patient life cycle, each with critical points of contact with the practice: First-time customers, repeat customers, and customer advocates (Marsh, 2005). Creating a group of customer advocates who voluntarily function as true "cheerleaders" is, without doubt, the greatest form of marketing and stands as a strong tribute to any professional practice.

Patient loyalty should be considered an outcome of the practice's dedication and diligence in developing and maintaining patient satisfaction. Long-term, loyal patients will be the desired outcome if they are well-satisfied, and treated with respect, dignity, and technical excellence by every member of the practice team. To maintain patient loyalty, each patient must be absolutely delighted with your services; being satisfied is no longer sufficient. Patients dissatisfied with your services for whatever reason, real or imagined, are likely to be lost forever.

Figure 11–1 depicts the interrelationship and importance of patients classified in one of three, distinct categories: **Dissatisfied**, **Simply Satisfied**, and **Absolutely Delighted**. Dissatisfied patients are in an area of discord. They are, for whatever reason, dissatisfied with all aspects of the practice, whether the front office staff, the professional staff, or their perception of the quality of the services received. When asked about their experiences in the practice they will quite likely issue strongly negative comments. Negative word-of-mouth comments are unequivocally damaging to the reputation of a practice.

To illustrate the impact of word-of-mouth comments, consider a restaurant you went to recently for the first time. Chances are high that you decided to try the restaurant based on a word-of-mouth recommendation by a family member, friend, or colleague. And if you valued the person's opinion because he or she is a good cook or an ardent gastronome that appreciates dining and knows his or her way around a wine list and a menu, the value of that recommendation will have added credibility and increase the likelihood of your acting on their recommendation. Consider the same scenario for negative word-of-mouth comments. If the comments about the restaurant were negative from these same, credible sources, chances are strong you would not even consider visiting the restaurant.

The same holds true for health care practices. Positive word-of-mouth testimonials may not ensure a new patient appointment in your practice, however,

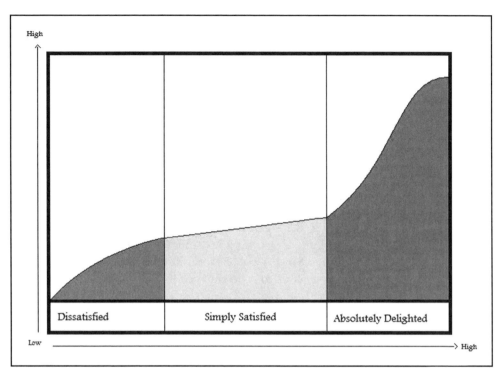

Figure 11–1. Levels of patient satisfaction and effect on loyalty to the practice.

negative word-of-mouth statements, will likely derail many more potential appointments than you can imagine.

Study after study in business journals and textbooks confirm that more people will be influenced by negative comments about a business or a practice than positive comments. The enduring folklore about the relative effectiveness of positive and negative word-of-mouth "reputations" suggests that a well-satisfied patient typically talks to three or five people whereas a disgruntled patient will replay a discordant event to as many as 10 or more individuals. Add to that the "word-of-mouse" world of Internet-bolstered communication and the potential numbers of contacts a determined, dissatisfied patient can reach in your local practice area expands at an alarming rate. Improving patient satisfaction

will decrease the likelihood of negative word-of-mouth comments about your practice. Nevertheless, it is best to always offer your patients the opportunity to communicate their dissatisfaction with any member of the practice team. Better those patients complain to personnel within the practice who can intervene and attempt to remedy a difficult situation than to have the patient issue complaints and indications of dissatisfaction to their family and friends.

Practices with even a few patients in the dreaded area of the **Dissatisfied** depicted in Figure 11–1 are operating suboptimally. Dissatisfied patients will leave the practice to reduce their stress (real or imagined) and to avoid conflict and uncomfortable interactions in the future. Retrieving these patients requires a frank assessment of their discord and an immediate, personal response to eliminate the source of the disharmony. Once the source of the discord is identified and an affirmative plan to resolve the situation is set into motion for the individual and his or her family, the patient may move into the area of the **Simply Satisfied**. It may not take much to achieve this shift: An acknowledgment of an error, an apology, an indication of your sincere appreciation of their being a patient in the practice, and perhaps a reasonable token of appreciation for their willingness to reconsider their position.

Patients in the area of the **Simply Satisfied** may not be the best asset to your practice since they are susceptible to competitor outreach in advertising or direct solicitation offering technical advances, simplicity of operation or compelling pricing strategies. As a group, these patients pay little attention to efforts to foster patient loyalty and many demonstrate the attitude of "what-have-you-done-for-me-lately?" at each visit to the practice. They are less concerned about the practice and more concerned about price than most patients. They rarely recommend the practice to others or comment on their experiences when visiting their primary care physician who referred the patient to your practice.

Practices dedicated to simply maintaining good, yet basic care; dwelling on avoiding mistakes; just meeting, not exceeding, patient needs; and retaining staff members with limited enthusiasm will have a large section of their patient database falling in the area of **Simply Satisfied**.

Patient-centric practices that value each patient as an engaged partner in their program of hearing or balance rehabilitation will generate a substantial number of patients in the area of the **Absolutely Delighted**. These patients frequently become cheerleaders for the practice, recommending your services to family, friends and strangers in casual conversations. They will thank the referral source for his or her wisdom in recommending your practice for their hearing care and will continue to sing your praises at every opportunity; bridge club, church group, or social gathering. These patients are worth far more to the practice than the revenue generated by their diagnostic studies, office visits and hearing instruments.

Several key elements, however, must be engaged in the practice from the onset of a patient's care to elevate a person to the ranks of the **Absolutely Delighted**. Those elements can be found in a comprehensive Patient's Bill of Rights, which sets forth what every patient should expect as a patient in the practice. There is a critically important stipulation that must be understood when a Patient's Bill of Rights is posted in the practice or written in documents the patient receives at their first visit. Everything listed in that document must be delivered on a consistent basis:

Patient's Bill of Rights

PATIENT'S BILL OF RIGHTS
Audiology Associates of Dayton, Inc.

- Know that quality care is our priority.
- Expect excellent service from Audiology & Speech Associates.
- Know that you will be respected by everyone in our practice.
- Expect us to answer your phone call in a timely and welcoming manner.

- You will be greeted in a friendly manner by every member of our practice.
- Know that we recognize the importance of your time.
- You can always expect excellent communication from us.
- We will listen to your concerns.
- We will deliver what we promise.
- To optimize your success, we will use state-of-the-art assessment and treatment procedures including the best hearing aids suited to your needs.
- We will provide prompt attention to all your service needs.
- Family and friends are welcome and encouraged to accompany you to appointments—everyone will benefit from their interest and presence.
- Questions about your hearing loss, your care plan, hearing instruments and billing information will be answered fully at any time.
- Expect quick and accurate resolution of questions about your account.
- If we make an error, you will receive an apology—we will make it right.

The Provider-Patient Relationship: Verbal and Nonverbal Communication

There is little doubt that negative word-of-mouth comments can destroy the reputation of a practice. Providing a patient with an avenue to express their dissatisfaction, gain resolution of their problem and an opportunity to stay in the practice that cares enough to resolve issues of discord will create increased patient satisfaction. Retrieving those patients lost to internal errors gives hope to all in the practice, patients and staff, that even the most egregious errors can be rectified to everyone's satisfaction and benefit.

The manner in which a clinician communicates information to a patient is as important as the information being communicated. Patients, who understand their care providers are more likely to acknowledge their health problems, understand their treatment options and modify their behavior accordingly (Travaline, Ruchinskas, & D'Alonzo, 2005).

Beck, Daughtridge, and Sloane (2002) reviewed an extensive body of published evidence linking specific verbal and nonverbal behaviors to short-, intermediate-, and long-term outcomes in interactions between primary care providers and their patients seen in their office practices. A total of 36 verbal and 16 nonverbal behaviors were considered from the 22 studies included in their meta-analysis. Despite the fact that these behaviors were included in controlled or descriptive studies involving Primary Care Providers, the consistency of impact noted throughout the studies between the provider and the patient enables an appropriate extrapolation to health care providers in general and audiologists specifically. Many of the behaviors fostering positive clinical outcomes (better patient compliance; improved response to various treatments; improved overall health status) describe a list of patient-centric behaviors necessary to develop patient comfort within the practice and to increase the likelihood of satisfaction with both professional and front office staffs. The list of behaviors linked to negative outcomes provides a guideline of behaviors to be avoided. Verbal behaviors associated with significant, positive patient outcomes are included in Figure 11–2.

VERBAL BEHAVIORS LINKED TO POSITIVE PATIENT OUTCOMES

- Empathy—intellectual appreciation of a patient's situation

- Provider statements of reassurance or support

- Encouraging patient questions

- Allowing the patient's point of view to guide the visit

- High proportion of objective statements by provider (explanation)

- Provider's expression of approval related to positive patient actions

- Laughing and joking from the provider's side (tension release)

- Provider addressing patient problems of daily living, relationships and emotions (psychosocial issues)

- Provider asking about and providing counseling for psychosocial issues

- Increased time spent on health education and sharing clinical data

- Provider fosters discussion of treatment parameters

- Friendliness and courtesy of the provider

- Receptivity to patient questions and statements (listening behaviors)

- Provider talking at the patient's level

- Provider ready to clarify and educate patient

- More time spent on history taking

- Increased encounter length

Figure 11-2. Verbal behaviors of health care providers linked to significant, positive patient outcomes.

Behaviors associated with significantly negative patient outcomes include those listed in Figure 11-3. These behaviors were found to consistently promote neg- ative feelings and disenfranchisement to the extent that patients did not return to the providers studied. Although not reported, the literature on the topic of

---

VERBAL BEHAVIORS LINKED TO NEGATIVE PATIENT OUTCOMES

- Negative social-emotional interactions

- Passive acceptance of information provided by patient to the provider

- Antagonism and passive rejection of the patient by the provider

- Formal, directive behaviors on the part of the provider

- High rates of biomedical questioning by the provider

- Interruptions issued by the provider

- One way information flow from patient to provider without response

- Lack of attentiveness on the part of the provider (disengaged listening)

- Provider directives issued with apparent irritation, nervousness or tension

- Dominance and verbal directness on the part of the provider

- Provider issuing opinions prior to completion of the evaluation

---

Figure 11–3. Verbal behaviors of health care providers linked to significant, negative patient outcomes.

verbal and nonverbal behaviors likely to develop negative attitudes, loss of confidence, and patient exits from practices appear to be those that can easily permeate the atmosphere of any practice. This is especially true of those practices that fail to focus on the patients, their integration into the practice and the levels of their satisfaction with all members of the practice staff.

Beck et al. (2002) describes 16 specific nonverbal behaviors found in one or more studies that were significantly associated with patient outcomes. Behaviors of interest to audiologists which were associated with positive clinical outcomes included: Less mutual gaze; positive head nodding of the provider; forward lean toward the patient; direct body orientation of the provider (shoulders squared to patient); and uncrossed arms and legs by the provider. Nonverbal behaviors that were associated with unfavorable clinical outcomes included: More patient gaze by the provider; provider body orientation 45 to 90 degrees away from the patient; backward lean away from the patient; crossed arms by the provider; frequent touch by the provider.

Selected Verbal Behaviors to Improve Patient Satisfaction

Professional and front office staff should be aware of both verbal and nonverbal statements and behaviors that can effect patient satisfaction and clinical outcomes. Beck et al. (2002) suggests that health care providers should focus on the following verbal behaviors linked statistically ($p < .05$) to patient satisfaction, compliance, comprehension, and positive perception of their provider: Empathy, courtesy, friendliness, reassurance, support, encouragement of patient's questions, explanation giving, and positive reinforcement or good feelings of positive patient actions or compliance in their treatment.

Many of the findings reported in their analysis were commonsense; for example, empathic patient-centered verbal styles were associated with high patient satisfaction. Participatory decision making was found to be a strong provider-partner interaction issuing significantly better clinical outcomes. Additionally, extensive sharing of clinical information and patient education about potential effects of treatment were found to consistently improve patient comprehension and satisfaction contributing to an overall improvement in clinical outcomes.

The extensive meta-analysis by Beck et al. (2002) indicates the strong impact of verbal and nonverbal behaviors in the development of the interrelationship between clinicians and their patients. Content, method of delivery, body positioning, as well as visual contact and other physical and nonverbal postures have been shown to significantly impact clinical outcomes. The importance and impact of these findings on daily clinical practice cannot be underestimated nor discounted. Practice owners and managers should include discussions and training about these opportunities for success as well as negative imagery and messaging to be avoided when interacting with patients in the practice.

Critical Points of Patient Contact: Office Staff

The first line of patient care begins with the front office staff. They may be called the office assistant, the receptionist, front office staff coordinator, or they might even be called a spouse or the owner of the practice (from this point forward in this text, we use the term "receptionist"). It all depends on who answers the phone.

The true value of the receptionist lies not solely in her abilities to organize and care for patients logistically and in a timely fashion but in her abilities to quickly and accurately assess patient distress and respond with a solution to their problem. An invaluable asset, the best receptionists are part mechanic, part counselor, part customer service specialist, part magician, always dressed appropriately, and, above all else, great listeners dedicated to the patient and their success in the practice.

They create the first and, often, most lasting impression on the patient. They are responsible for explaining financial policies, obtaining insurance information, and collecting co-pays. Not only must they be efficient in practice operations, they must also possess excellent interpersonal communication skills and a thorough knowledge of clinical procedures and treatment options available in the practice. Time spent instructing a receptionist to be a good listener, a good gatherer of information, an excellent communicator, and a host or hostess will contribute immensely to consistently high patient satisfaction ratings. Taylor (2006) reports that the interaction with the audiologist is the most important driver of patient satisfaction, the interaction with the receptionist had significant impact on overall patient satisfaction with the practice.

Fostering Patient Confidence

It is no easy task to have phones ringing, people at the payment window, and make a caller and prospective patient know that the office he or she has chosen or has been referred to will be a comfortable place to receive the type of care they need. The patient must know from the initial contact with your practice that the care they will receive will be comprehensive and excellent in every way. High patient confidence at the first patient visit is the responsibility of the receptionist. Confidence in the practice during and after the first visit is the responsibility of all members of the team; front office and professional staff alike.

The Receptionist as an Informational Source and Anxiety Reducer

The receptionist must be well trained and understand not only office procedures; specifics about billing, coding, and collection; and how to successfully guide a patient to the office from across town, he or she must also know and understand the clinical aspects of the office. A good way to train a receptionist about what goes on in the practice is to have them become a "patient." Undergoing a comprehensive hearing evaluation, a vestibular assessment with recording or watching a hearing instrument fitting provides lasting impressions and increases sensitivity to what patients experience during their visits.

The insight gained by the receptionist-as-patient will translate into valid experiential depictions of what to expect, how the patient might feel during the procedures, and what to expect on being fitted with hearing instruments for the first time. Patients respond favorably to having prior knowledge of the clinical situation. Reduced fears and increased confidence will set the stage for a comfortable visit and a far less anxious patient.

We learn well by what we experience. A receptionist who has undergone a vestibular study can immediately reduce a patient's anxiety about the procedure because she has "gone through it and lived to tell about it," With firsthand experience, the receptionist will be better able to answer patient questions and resolve concerns that might otherwise result in a missed or cancelled appointment. Receptionists are critical, front line members of the team and have as much duty to the patient on the front end of the appointment as does the professional involved in the clinical assessment, counseling, and rehabilitation on the back end of the appointment. The front line must be a strong line. Patient comfort and satisfaction is, after all, about outcomes and receptionists own a large part of setting the patient up for consistent, positive patient outcomes. Reduced fears and increased patient confidence sets the stage for a successful office visit for the patient and professional alike.

When the patient arrives for the appointment, the receptionist once again becomes the first point of contact. Her approach to each patient should vary with the patient's personal needs and anxiety level. Making the patients feel welcome and comfortable in the office should be a seamless transition from the booking conversation on the phone to the greeting at the reception room window. These patient interactions are crucial junctures prior to the actual patient-professional interaction. As a part of the team, the receptionist will develop observations and opinions on the patient's emotional status and perhaps a view of their expectations as well. By engaging the patient in conversation as they are about to fill out forms or as they are escorted to the examination room, the receptionist has the first opportunity to observe the patient's behaviors. Even with hearing instrument repairs, the receptionist should foster discussions about how the instrument is working, what the patient's observations have been, and when the problems began.

These informal discussions serve to cue the patient about questions to ask during the visit. They also provide the patient with an opportunity to vent frustrations about their particular situation or difficulties that have driven them back to the office. The more inquiries the patient hears about their particular situation, the more the patient develops a secure sense that everyone in the practice is interested in solving their problems. When every member of the practice team shows sincere interest and issues an empathetic response, a sincere smile or an encouraging statement, however brief, the probability of a positive outcome during the visit is enhanced.

The Patient's Perspective

The receptionist should be viewed as an interested, caring person, fully engaged in the best interests of the patient. The patient must have confidence that the receptionist will serve, at least to some extent, as an in-office advocate, who will get them to the appropriate member of the professional staff in a timely manner. In that sense, a receptionist is as much a care provider as any member of the clinical staff. No license is needed to be involved in fostering a patient's well being. The ultimate goal in all patient care is to have every member of the practice working toward a positive and comprehensive outcome for the patient. This goal is established on behalf of the patient as well as his or her family and the professional who referred the patient to the practice.

Long-term patients value the receptionist. They expect to hear his or her voice on the phone when they call with questions, to order hearing aid related items or to schedule a visit to the office. Relationship building is as important at the front desk as it is in the fitting room. The patient-receptionist relationship is important and should not be discounted in the continuum of care provided by the practice. Low turnover rate in the receptionist position is critical. Should the receptionist leave the practice, it is important to have her replacement spend adequate time integrating patient information and front office operations beyond the expected orientation with procedural and policy information contained in the receptionist's job description.

Aftercare Duties: Thank You Notes and Follow-Up Calls

The receptionist should be assigned the duty to contact patients after they have left the office. He or she should be responsible for sending each new patient an after-care thank you card in which he or she encourages the patient to call if there are questions about billing, setting up another appointment, or to review what the next step might be after the initial appointment. Patients remember these efforts and they are likely to tell their friends and families about the note and the excellent service they received in your practice. Building patient loyalty is critically important to the long-term health of the practice. Every member of the team must have a strong commitment to this effort and contribute to building patient loyalty on a daily basis.

Follow-up phone calls a few days after a hearing instrument fitting (preferably by the audiologist) or after replacing a repaired instrument are just as important as a thank you note to a new patient. Checking on their progress with their new or repaired instruments is an effective way to show interest in their response to your treatment regimen and to provide a spot check on the adequacy of the fitting and the stability of the repair. If the caller suspects the patient is struggling with adjusting to their new instruments or if the patient is concerned about the effectiveness of the repair, the patient should be scheduled for a return visit at the patient's earliest convenience. Waiting for their next scheduled visit simply prolongs the anxiety and promotes a loss of confidence in the fitting or repair replacement.

Occasionally, a patient may have a difficult time in response to segments of the vestibular evaluation. Patients who have a prolonged refractory period in response to caloric stimulation or who have a general weakness following the examination should be contacted by phone the same day of the test. Inquiring about their status and suggesting that they return to the referring physician as scheduled and reiterating the findings will go far in assuring them that their response to the test was nothing extraordinary. Of course, if their response was beyond that which is usually anticipated, the patient should be directed to consult with their physician immediately. The referring physician should be contacted and a course of action should be agreed upon.

Unfortunately, too few practices take the time to capitalize on easily managed opportunities like these to increase patient satisfaction and loyalty. Little time is involved in most patient management activities. Telephone calls can be completed during lulls in activities in the office or at the end of the day. If the caller (front office or professional staff) encounters the patient's voicemail, he or she should leave a message that imparts interest in their progress, reassuring them that all in the practice stand ready to resolve any particular issues that might have developed and issue an invitation to call back to let the practice know how they are doing.

Handling Challenges on the Phone or at the Window

Challenging interactions with patients occur on a regular basis. A variety of factors contribute to these, sometimes confrontational, episodes. Beyond instrument repair issues, errors on the part of the practice staff, and misinterpretation of information issued to the patient by the practitioner are two of the more common reasons for challenges by patients, their spouse, or other family members. Hearing loss, advancing cognitive deficits, medications, misinformation provided to family members by the patient, and confusion about the "next steps" to be taken in their care plan also contribute to challenges.

The first responder to problem situations is usually the receptionist. He or she must be empowered to resolve and manage as many challenges—usual and common; angry and outrageous. Receptionists must be great listeners and gatherers of information. Having a sense of humor is a definitive prerequisite for the position. They must have well-developed communication skills, patience, and commitment to patient satisfaction above all else. They must know when they cannot satisfy the caller or person at the window and how to deftly transfer the patient to the office manager or practice owner in a manner that appears to be part of the solution versus a means to get the patient out of his or her hair. Receptionists must be tactful, deft and sensitive to the patient's concerns and be fluidly willing to apologize for situations or circumstances over which they have neither control nor contribution to the difficulty at hand.

Every member of the practice team, however, must be able to identify patient concerns and immediately move to resolution (Figure 11–4). Prompt recovery when mistakes or misperceptions on the part of the patient occur, will make the difference between a satisfied patient and a "former patient" in the practice. The faster a situation is resolved, the better the likelihood the patient will be satisfied. All staff must remember one of the key elements in the rules for patient engagement: "Excellence at the speed of light." Patients, generally, are uninterested in who is to blame, nor should they be bothered with details of how an error or oversight occurred. If they are interested in an explanation, they should receive as detailed an account as seems appropriate for the particular situation.

RULES OF PATIENT ENGAGEMENT

- Patients are the priority
- We work for them
- Always with a smile
- Courtesy at all times
- Professional appearance is important
- Your boss is always on the phone
- Apologies are always appropriate
- Solutions not excuses
- Excellence at the speed of light

Figure 11–4. Rules of patient engagement.

The most common clinically relatable complaints include; repeat repairs (defined as a second repair within 45 to 90 days of the first repair), costs of the instruments, battery consumption, too many follow-up visits, time to adjust to instruments is too long, instruments are too conspicuous, noise reduction features fail to meet expectations and difficulty using instruments with telephone. Despite the fact that most of these issues are outside the purview of the receptionist, complaints must be addressed and the patient should be encouraged to realistically assess their complaints in view of their position in the continuum of the fitting process, the extent of their hearing loss and the goals set forth prior to and during the assessment and counseling period. Reassurance and a quick willingness to have the patient return prior to a scheduled visit is usually adequate in stemming the tide of anxiety in the early stages of adjustment to new or recently repaired instruments.

If the patient is concerned about an inordinate turnaround time for a repair or in establishing their appointment for their fitting, the receptionist should check the dates of the order or repair submission and advise the patient of the appropriateness of the time frame in question. If the repair or new order is outside the customary period from order to arrival, he or she should immediately call and check on the order, promptly contacting the patient the same day of their inquiry.

Patients deserve an acknowledgment of an error, an apology, and prompt resolution of their problem with the assurance that the error will not happen again. They expect the person to whom they are talking to be empowered to resolve the situation and they expect the staff person to be solution driven. Patient-centric practices embrace problem resolution without judgment and with one goal in mind: Total patient satisfaction. No blame, no excuse, no fault, just resolution to maintain long-term patient loyalty.

Challenges by Prospective Patients on the Phone or at the Window

One of the most common sources of confusion and error when talking with prospective patients on the phone rests with the unknown parameters of their hearing loss. Receptionists must be able to understand the reason for their call, make sure the patient has heard and integrated the appointment date and time and determine that the patient understands the services to be provided during their upcoming visit. Asking the patient to repeat the appointment date and time is one way to confirm their reception of the information. If the patient is obviously severely hampered on the telephone, the receptionist should ask to talk to another family member or friend. In some cases, having a "designated talker" for severely hearing impaired patients or those with known cognitive impairments will facilitate the process of issuing and confirming appointment dates and times. Family or friends are usually willing to call the office and exchange messages or confirm appointments for the patient.

Established Patients Who Develop Cognitive Difficulties

Long-standing, well-known patients in your practice with developing cognitive impairments present a unique challenge. The staff may not be privy to their decline and expect responses to questions, inquiries, or remembering appointment dates and times as had been successfully negotiated prior to the onset of their cognitive issues. Recognizing difficulties involving memory issues compared to the relatively consistent problems associated with the patient's hearing loss takes an attentive ear and a good sense of the clinical presentation of patients with memory-based difficulties. In this day of widely dispersed families, it is unwise to rely on family members to make a patient's developing cognitive issues known to the practice. By the same token, when cognitive decline is suspected, a call to the patient's physician may not only be informative to you and your office staff, it will likely be appreciated by the primary care provider and his or her staff as well.

When the appointment is made, the receptionist should advise each patient about items of importance to bring to their scheduled appointment: whether the initial visit or an annual hearing instrument inspection and cleaning. They should bring hearing instruments currently in use or any information describing the instrument; current instrument or repair warranties; information about their health care coverage; and if a hearing examination is needed, they should bring a medical concurrence form signed by their physician, depending on their particular insurance requirements.

New patients should be apprised of the extent of Medicare coverage or, if known, about their particular carrier's benefits for hearing assessment or, in some cases with private carriers, a hearing aid benefit. If your practice has specific policies about payment at the first visit or about missed appointments or other items of interest, that information should be issued on the phone or in writing to the patient prior to the first visit.

Critical Points of Patient Contact: Difficult Patients/Families

There are several chairs in each exam or fitting room. One chair is for the patient and the other chairs are for those interested in the outcome of your professional intervention and care. These chairs are filled with family members, friends, parents, children, sons and daughters-in-law, or girl or boyfriends. Each chair supports one person and each person is present at the visit because they are inexorably intertwined with the patient. As such,

they are as much a part of the diagnostic and rehabilitative process as is the patient. Each has a vested interest in the patient's success. After all, it would be nice to be able to talk to Aunt Edna without the conversation being heard above the blaring of the neighbor's television. Aunt Edna just wants everyone to stop shouting. The younger children in the family would be more likely to engage her in conversation if they did not have to talk so loud it hurt their ears. Each person has accompanied the patient for specific reasons: None should be ignored nor considered less important than the patient. They deserve to be included in the information processing, the fitting process and follow-up care. They will likely become care providers and will need assistance and guidance in proper insertion, cleaning and maintenance and battery replacement. These are the family and friends we like to see in our offices. Their involvement can only enhance the patient's experience and serve to develop realistic expectations in the circle of their family and friends.

Noncompliant Patient/Family/ Extended Care Facility

Individuals able to comply with a rehabilitative plan and choose not to follow the recommended plan must be considered non-compliant. Each takes a volitional step not to proceed as advised. Some will do so to gain a passive-aggressive advantage: Others because of depression or lack of interest in their living arrangements. Each will have a reason which, more times than not, is hidden from professional care providers, family, and friends. Noncompliant patients are not unique to the practice of audiology. Physicians, dentists, and other providers see them with surprising regularity.

Consider Mrs. Filbert, who is returning to her cardiologist following a three-month trial of a new medication for hypertension. During the office visit, the cardiologist notes that her blood pressure remains elevated and asks if she has been taking all of the five pills she is supposed to take each day. She replies that she decided it was too much trouble taking five pills so she cut it down to three a day. Concerned about the patient's obvious noncompliance, the cardiologist stresses the need to take all five pills as prescribed. Mrs. Filbert responds by saying that she can only take three pills a day, not five. The cardiologist must now decide to either discharge the patient or increase the strength of the medication so that three pills will work or find another medicine that does not require five tablets a day.

Audiologists are faced with similar difficulties. Many practices require their new patients to begin wearing their hearing instruments with daily regularity, morning until night. Others may create a schedule for the first and second weeks. When the patient returns to the first post-fitting visit and exclaims that he only needs to wear the hearing instruments when, "he thinks he needs them regardless of what his wife says," the audiologist must determine the best method to convince the patient that he will be less likely to adjust to his instruments if he fails to wear them as recommended, especially during the initial fitting period. If this noncompliance continues into the 2nd or 3rd postfitting visit, there is an increasing chance the patient will return the instruments or keep them and

become one of the dissatisfied patients who will complain how the practice and the professionals let him down and how hearing instruments simply do not work.

Much of the problem of noncompliance can be avoided by careful patient selection or at least having an idea of what a particular patient will be bringing to the overall clinical mix. Traynor (2003) suggests that although formal assessment with personality inventories like the Myers Briggs Type Indicator or the Kiersey Temperament Sorter would be an optimal approach to identifying difficult patients, this sort of assessment does not lend itself well to the rigors and time constraints of daily clinical practice. Informal assessment can be readily used to identify those patients in need of tailoring approaches to optimize outcomes. Observing and listening to how patients respond to questions or statements borrowed from these inventories will enable the clinician to localize each patient into one of four personality categories, each with its own characteristics to be addressed or considered during their assessment and treatment.

According to the characteristics outlined by Traynor (2003), noncompliant patients fall into the category of "Intuitive-Thinking Clients." Several of their characteristics outlined include:

- Can present as aloof, intimidating, argumentative, and arrogant
- Often impatient with the aural rehabilitation (fitting) process
- Complains about small problems
- When unsuccessful, may change recommended program on their own
- Skeptical and often require lots of references and rational for A/R process

■ Tend to overanalyze the problem and tries to fix it themselves.

Being able to identify a non-compliant patient early on in the clinical process can help in determining whether or not the difficulties the patient will likely bring to the practice will be more strain than benefit. If too many issue arise from his or her treatment and a point of decision is reached, prompted by patient or professional, to consider returning the hearing instruments, it may well be in the best interests of staff and patient alike to terminate the rehabilitative effort and issue a referral to another practice. As Traynor (2003) indicates so eloquently, "Clinicians should be grateful that (these patients) make up only 4 to 5% of the general clinical population."

Despite the best efforts at identifying problem patients, some will slip through even the most vigilant audiologist's sensors. The key question is what can be done to retrieve the situation and move the patient to a satisfied or delighted hearing instrument wearer? As a matter of the usual course in dealing with patients, there may not be any conceivable adjustment or tactic to take to alter the situation. There are a few measures that should be considered. The first includes evaluating the extremes by having the patient and family or friends assess his relative performance with and without the instruments. By recommending this assessment, a discussion will begin in the office and continue into their respective homes or workplaces about how much better the patient performs with the instruments in his or her ears than with them in a drawer or on the dresser.

Another approach is to have the patient return to the office for follow-up visits until he is wearing the instruments with acceptable consistency based on the observations of his or her family or friends. The goal of this approach is to assist the patient in appreciating the benefits of consistent instrument use. If you can move these patients to an acceptable schedule of consistent instrument use, he or she will develop increasingly greater satisfaction as the benefits of usage become readily apparent to both the patient and those around him.

Patients in extended care facilities (ECF) present a different issue concerning compliant use of hearing instruments. In many of these facilities, the patient may not be able to insert the instruments and must rely on the staff of the ECF to provide the necessary and appropriate assistance to do so. If the staff fails to appropriately place the hearing instruments in or on the patient's ear or places the instruments appropriately and fails to turn them on, change the batteries or clean the instruments, the ECF becomes the source of a noncompliance situation at the patient's expense. Finding an ECF that takes pride in the quality of care provided to their residents to the point that each patient wearing hearing instruments is functioning to their maximum hearing potential is a distinct rarity. Unfortunately, this seems to be the case no matter what the family is paying for their loved one's care in ECFs. Altering the course of this particular catastrophe will require intervention with the nursing supervisor and staff. Having the attending physician write specific orders of inserting, care, and cleaning might help. With orders written, oversight for appropriate hearing instrument placement and assessment of use becomes part of the medical record and is discussed during care conferences. The attending physician is now integrally linked to the quality of care provided under his or her medical management and adds a powerful ally to both the patient and family should disputes over the adequacy of care regarding hearing instrument usage develop in the care conferences. However, it is more likely that these simple but, time-consuming tasks will fall to the patient's family or friends. Following your patient to the ECF and providing instructional support to the staff will help. Nothing will supplant the watchful eye of demanding family members.

Angry or Disgruntled Patients

Anger fueled by declining health, frustrating encounters with insurance companies, and other health care providers or repeated yet needed follow-up visits or the out-of-pocket costs of hearing instruments can turn an otherwise kind, cooperative patient into a caustic, angry, and unsettled person bellowing at the receptionist's window.

Immediate steps must be taken to resolve his issues and to assure him or her that whatever it takes to reduce frustrations or change an irritating situation, will be done. Every member of the front office and professional staffs of the practice is responsible for patient satisfaction and patient loyalty. Recall that 68% of patients refusing to return to a practice do so because they felt the practice was "indifferent" to their concerns and needs. No one wants to think they are unimportant. Recall also that if the patient's issues are delineated, discussed, and resolved quickly, the patient will likely stay with the practice and develop an odd sense of

pride in generating what is perceived as much-needed change.

Service recovery is not just about fixing a particular patient's problem. It is about listening to the patient and recognizing their dissatisfaction. It should never take two members of a practice to resolve an issue for one patient nor should two people be required to foster patient satisfaction and loyalty. There are patients in every practice that are consistently cranky. It should be the goal of every staff person to make his or her visit the best, friendliest and pleasant visit on each and every visit to the practice. One patient who fit the bill for being consistently cranky had been coming to one of our offices (RGG) for many years. Every person in the office agreed to make his visits full of smiles and charm. One day the patient exclaimed, obviously peeved: "What is it with you people? I do nothing but moan and groan and you all stay so cheerful and upbeat no matter what!" The entire office staff celebrated this minor, yet important, team victory with a celebratory pizza lunch the next day. They were determined to charm his socks off and they had succeeded. In a patient-centric practice, every patient is treated in that manner, every day the office is open for business.

Conflict Resolution and Staff Safety

Every member of the practice staff must be trained to resolve patient issues and calm patients down when they are agitated or overly concerned. In addition, each staff member must be able to recognize when a situation has gotten out of control and what steps to follow to resolve the issue. Patients can, at times, become highly agitated and, in some cases, combative. Just as the practice should have an exit plan in the event of a fire and a plan for calling 911 in the event of a medical emergency, so too should there be a plan in place to protect the staff from a potentially dangerous patient. Just about the time the office staff begins to think they have seen everything or that " . . . our patients would never become physically abusive" a major eruption takes place at the payment window with the patient slamming his fist into the wall or tossing wall hangings on the floor in a frenzy.

In that event, an immediate 911 call summoning the police should be made. What about the time from the call to their arrival? What can be done to calm the situation and regain everyone's temperament and civility? Interventionists suggest that anything to defuse the situation should be done. Telling the patient not to worry about charges for the day and reassuring him that there has been no harm done as long as he begins to calm down will go far to lessen the tension of the situation. If the spouse or a friend is with him, ask for their intersession in the matter and have them help calm the situation. Conflict resolution needs calm more than focusing on immediate resolution in the early stages of an incident. Whatever it takes to calm the situation should be put into play. The goal is to have the patient leave the office without harming himself or others—or for the police to arrive and secure everyone's safety. Angry patient scenarios should be considered an important topic for discussion at staff meetings; just as important as fire safety or procedures for office closure for inclement weather.

Cool-down techniques to resolve conflict should be discussed and training should be completed at least annually. A procedural description of cool-down techniques to be used in the event of significant patient conflict should be developed with the help of mental health professionals. The basic components of cool down techniques geared to mollify patient anger includes: (1) engaging the assistance of the spouse or family member accompanying the patient to intervene; (2) if the interaction involves a member of the front office staff, immediately involve a member of the professional staff in the situation; (3) appropriate physical distance between the patient and staff members must be maintained; (4) immediate understanding and unequivocal agreement about the issue at the core of the disturbance should be exhibited on the part of the staff; (5) encourage the patient to talk about the problem without being patronizing: talk, talk, talk; (6) staff members should avoid any statement or behavioral posture that could escalate the situation—listen, listen, listen; (7) assure the patient that resolution of the circumstance will be in his or her favor; (8) resolution must be rapid, outcome(s) clear and assurance reiterated that all will be resolved to his or her satisfaction; (9) if the patient remains agitated despite best efforts to cool the situation to a tolerable level, the front office staff should be prepared to dial 911 Emergency to summon the police; (10) if there is no reduction in the intensity of the situation, the professional staff member must politely-yet-firmly ask the patient to leave the office; (11) if he or she refuses, advise the patient that you intend to call the authorities; and (12) if there is refusal to leave, 911 should be

Sidebar 11–1
BELLIGERENT PATIENT

Mr. H. came to the office on the referral of Dr. B., his primary care provider. During the history taking, Mr. H. became obviously agitated and angry in response to common questions about the development, severity and effects of his hearing loss in his daily living activities. His wife was in the exam room and noticed his agitation. At one point he stopped the questions and demanded to know why we needed to know so much about his hearing problems. He demanded that we "just get on with the testing" and that the "rest of this stuff is none of your business." It was obvious by his breathing and the extension of his neck vessels that he was markedly angry. His wife tearfully urged him to calm down. His response to her suggestion was to de-compensate into torrid remarks and movements that suggested he was about to escalate the situation into a physical confrontation. I stopped the conversation with an admonishment that he needed to "cool down," that we were trying to get information that would figure into a plan to help him and his family. I announced that I would give him five minutes to regain composure and that I would return to decide our next step in his visit.

The patient remained agitated and angry when I returned to the exam room. He announced that "you SOB's are only after the contents of my wallet so you might as well just open it up and take it now!" With that comment, he flung his wallet to the wall and his wife burst into tears. At that point, I asked him to leave the office. He refused and told me to "just go on with your damn tests and let's get this over with." I informed him that we were finished for the day and reiterated my request that he leave the office immediately. He said nothing yet stayed in the exam chair. His wife begged him to leave. I had alerted the front office to be prepared to call the police if needed. I informed the patient that if he did not leave immediately, that I was going to call the police and have him removed from the property. He muttered under his breath, told his wife to get the car and left the exam room. He left his wallet on the floor. I handed it to him before he left the office. It was empty. His insurance was billed for the visit and his primary care provider was called as soon as he exited the property.

The primary care provider indicated that the patient had a recent altercation with his billing staff, which he attributed to the patient's early stages of dementia. Organic brain syndromes including dementia do not lessen the dangers of physical confrontation with patients, indeed we should be aware of the possibilities of aggressive behaviors from even those patient known to have been mild mannered over the many years of care provided in the practice. In any event, aggressive or threatening behaviors toward professional or front office staff must not be tolerated. Staff should be well trained to identify and handle these situations. Annual reviews of emergency measures within the office should be part of a routine effort to reduce patient-related violence in your practice.

called—"This is Dr. _____'s office at XYZ address, we have a combative patient situation and we need help immediately—the patient's name is _____ he or she is a (description).

For the safety of all concerned, the practice staff must remain calm and in control of the situation. Physical contact with the patient must be avoided at all costs. Police response is usually quite rapid due to the explosive nature of these situations and the potential for physical altercations. Most municipal police departments have a community relations officer who will come to the office to discuss emergency notification and response times with specific instructions about reporting and responding to an incident involving an angry or agitated patient. Immediately following an incident, the referring physician should be contacted to explain the situation and circumstances under which the patient became agitated with a full disclosure of the resolution—no matter the outcome of the situation. A detailed, factual report of the incident from onset to final outcome should be prepared by each staff member involved. The comments should be signed by the staff member and each report should be reviewed by the attorney of record for the practice. A follow-up letter should be sent to the referring physician to confirm the telephone conversation and the resolution of the situation. The report should be part of the patient's continuing medical record. The

practice's attorney will advise how best to interact with the patient in the future. He may advise no further contact whatsoever or possibly sending a certified letter to the patient confirming the need for the patient to seek care elsewhere.

Statutory regulations governing the practice of medicine and dentistry commonly contain sections regarding patient abandonment. These sections usually stipulate the circumstances under which patients may be discharged from a practice and set forth guidelines or suggestions how best to advise a patient that he or she will no longer be seen for continuing care. Although required for physicians and dentists, it is not common to see these requirements in laws or other regulatory language governing the practice of Audiology. A thorough reading of your state licensing law and administrative rules should clarify whether or not there are specifically proscribed requirements or necessary means to inform a patient that he or she will no longer be seen as a patient in your practice. If in doubt, contact your state licensing board with a written request for clarification. When corresponding with your state licensing board or registration department, always send the correspondence, no matter the topic, via certified mail with a return receipt requested. This creates a documented record of your submission or inquiry. Should there be no response from the licensing board in a reasonable time period; a phone call to the Executive

Director of the board should be made to determine the status of your inquiry. If the Executive Director is unable to satisfy your request, contact the Chairman of the board or your elected state representative to make an inquiry on your behalf.

Baby Boomers: The Primary Population to Be Served

Maintaining customer/patient loyalty is becoming more difficult regardless of your profession. That may be especially true of the primary population to be served over the next 20 years. Primary care physicians, dentists, optometrists, and audiologists are becoming acutely aware of the markedly reduced tensile strength of the ties that bind baby boomers to their respective practitioners. As the baby boomer generation begins to access the health care system, new demands will be placed on the health care system in general and the hearing instrument delivery system specifically.

Boomers enjoy essentially unlimited ac-cess to medical and health care information through the World Wide Web. They are the best educated generation of Americans, 33% are college graduates, and those that did not finish college attended. Boomers are computer literate. For the most part, they are the generation responsible for incorporating computers and increasingly sophisticated technology into their existing workplaces. St. Clergy (2012) characterizes boomers and their use and acceptance of advancing technologies:

■ 90% use search engines
■ 78% use the Internet to find health information

■ 74% use the Internet as a news source
■ 70% search government sites for information
■ 91% use e-mail
■ The fastest growing group for social media is 55- to 65-year-old-females
■ 10% of boomers 55 to 64 have social media profiles, whereas 19% of those 45 to 54 have social media profiles.

According to Thornhill and Martin (2007), boomers think of themselves as 14 years younger than their years and generally do not consider themselves as "old." Boomers approach their health care like no other group. When they go to their providers for assessment or care, they are commonly well armed with an expansive knowledge of their particular health care issues. They seek the most qualified practitioners directly—*frequently without referral by their primary care physician*. They are more likely to schedule visits with practitioners having advanced degrees, specialty certification, or specific recognition as a specialist health care provider. They are abruptly critical of the quality of care provided and the surroundings in which the services are delivered. They are more likely to leave a health care provider to seek second opinions if they do not feel they are receiving accurate and appropriate information or care.

Boomers' trust and confidence in their health care providers develops from their perceptions of professionalism within the office, the efficiency and friendliness of the front office staff, and the important, yet ephemeral, doctor-to-patient relationship. They are less likely to accept mediocrity and less tolerant of problems arising from limited attention, common errors in billing and items, or issues in need of, what they consider to be, too much post-purchase attention.

Boomers are more likely to seek hearing care sooner than those in the previous generation and they readily accept well-credentialed, nonphysician practitioners as their health care provider for specific, well-defined health care needs (Traynor, 2011). As a group, they are more likely to seek alternative providers to their current providers based on price, time to schedule services, convenience of service locations, time spent in the office, and, most importantly, their perception of the quality and outcome of each professional/patient encounter.

In the final report in 2006 of the Clarity-Ear Foundation two-part survey that focused on the prevalence and impact of hearing loss in baby boomers, a number of interesting and important characteristics about this group came to light. This well-regarded and often quoted study began in 2004 with 437 randomly selected participants between 49 and 59 years of age. An initial online survey was completed followed by a telephone interview focusing on the prevalence of hearing loss. It focused on the how boomers felt their lives were impacted by their hearing loss. A group of 458 randomly selected participants 41 to 60 years of age completed an online survey which was also followed by telephone interviews.

These findings should be of special interest to audiologists since the first formal classes in audiology were begun in 1946 at Northwestern University; the same year the first batch of over 75 million boomers was born. The findings of the study confirmed many clinical observations and produced several interesting, and in some cases surprising findings selected below:

- About one-half (53%) of boomers have at least a "mild" hearing loss
- Men were significantly more likely to report a hearing loss than were women (62% to 38%)
- Three-fourths of those reporting a severe hearing loss were men
- 26% of those with hearing loss had their hearing loss formally diagnosed by a health care professional—37% had not had their hearing tested
- Only three out of four (73%) parents whose adult children say they have a hearing loss had their hearing tested
- One-fourth said their hearing loss affected their work; handling phone calls and conversations with co-workers were the areas most impacted
- One-fourth said their hearing loss had an impact on their earning potential
- 97% of participants stated they were aware of hearing aids
- 78% indicated they were aware of amplified telephones that could help individuals with hearing loss
- Among those with severe hearing loss, only 42% wore hearing aids.

A more contemporary view of the baby boomer group and how to approach them respectfully and with insight relative to established key descriptors of their interests, their need for control, and other important characteristics seen at both assessment and during the rehabilitation process was set forth in a set of 10 rules for working with baby boomers as patients by Traynor (2012):

- *Rule #1: Think Life Stage—Not Age.* In the past, people were mostly doing the same things at a certain age. Boomers have very diverse lives and do not do the same things at specific ages as the previous generation. Thus, there are boomers who have teenage children, college age children, have become empty nesters, grandparents, single, and caregivers. Basically, there can be a boomer in virtually any stage of life and we must respect this diversity and integrate it into the rehabilitative process.

■ *Rule #2: Diverse Clinical Needs.* As they come from many different stages of life, boomers have very different needs clinically. For example, boomers prefer 1 to 1 rehabilitative programs. They are not inclined to accept any form of group treatment programming.

■ *Rule #3: Emotionally Meaningful Treatment Programs.* Boomers do not respond to high pressure, they respond to emotional arguments and will purchase products if the situation "feels right." Clinicians need to talk about the future and how beneficial the advancements in hearing instruments will provide improved performance in real life situations. They readily accept sophisticated technology enabling them to hear better in difficult listening situations.

■ *Rule #4: Watch Out for Agism.* As they do not feel that they are old, baby boomers do not like things that make them feel old, such as bank accounts "for seniors," or senior citizen discounts. They respond well to sophisticated, progressive treatment programs and appreciate the attention counseling and being provided information on adaptive strategies to be used in situations of multiple talkers or noisy environments.

■ *Rule #5: More Information Is Better.* Gone are the days when a clinician selects a particular hearing instrument and informs the patient this is what you need—case closed. Boomers want as much information as possible about size, style, shape, adjustments, an explanation of the technology and why you, the clinician, has chosen the specific brand of instrument to be used. They often bring an internet file to the clinic with various types of products and information about care, cleaning, and postfitting follow-up. Internet files should be encouraged and appropriate discussion should focus on their questions and concerns. The discussions enhance their perception of you as a caring, professional willing to take the time they need to understand their loss and how they want to be involved in their hearing care.

■ *Rule #6: Tell a Story.* Boomers want to hear about other patient's success with the instruments being considered. Of equal importance, they appreciate the frankness about specific situations which may continue to present communication difficulties.

■ *Rule #7: Understand Changing Values.* Boomers had always focused on "becoming someone" and view themselves with their successes as "being someone." They value where they have been and what it has taken to get to this point. Despite the fact that hearing loss is more of a threat than the hearing instrument, counseling to realistically accept these changes can be difficult. Successful performance improvement with appropriately fitted hearing instruments will trump objections to the use of hearing instruments every time.

- *Rule #8: Make It Relevant to Me!* Boomers want to see themselves in your treatment program and it is necessary to paint a picture of how they will fit into the process. Describe the successes various patients have experienced in their everyday lives and in their efforts in the workplace. Discuss the impact on their interactions with family and friends.

- *Rule #9: Pay in the Gray.* This generation is tired of hearing things like the "Best of the Best" or "the finest available" relative to products and treatment programs. Just as "buy one get one free" is generally unappealing to boomers, absolute claims are equally unappealing. Better to present alternatives and give choices based on varied benefits from different circuit capabilities.

- *Rule #10: Learn Baby Learn.* This is a group that will continue to make Internet files of new technology, treatment techniques, implantable hearing instruments, and many other innovative products after they have been evaluated, fitted, and followed in your clinic. How they feel about you and your services will change over time as they view your efforts through the lens of the technology and the success or limitations it brings to their lives. These patients will expect you to stay on top of changing technology and to let them know what, if anything, has improved or is on the horizon when they are ready to consider changes in their hearing instruments

Follow-Up Care: Critical Element of Successful Long-Term Practices

Consistent follow-up care is a requirement in any health care practice. Follow-up care should be highly systematized and patient centric at the office staff level and engagingly personal at the provider-patient interface. Follow-up care is an operational method to increase patient satisfaction, foster patient loyalty, and an additional means to encourage patients to sing the praises of the practice not just to their family and friends but to the health care provider responsible for their referral to your practice.

The Art of Personalization

The era of "Sign in — Sit down — Shut up" health care is swiftly coming to a close. Baby boomers will be between 48 and 65 years old in 2012 and they will accept nothing less than active participation in their health care. The generation to follow them, Gen X, will be 34 and 48 and will be no less demanding as their older cohorts. Neither practice nor practitioner can prosper long term without creating a consistent atmosphere of patient involvement. Involving patients and those interested in their well-being, fosters high patient satisfaction and loyalty.

This is true for medical specialists and generalists, dentists, optometrists and audiologists as well.

It is important to personalize the patient's visit. As mentioned previously, sending a hand written note following the initial patient encounter thanking them for choosing the practice and encouraging their active participation in subsequent visits goes a long way in building a comfortable relationship. Consider creating a brochure informing the patient what to expect at the fitting and during subsequent follow-up visits. Underscore the importance of the follow-up visits as opportunities to "dial in" the instruments for use across a variety of listening conditions. Keep in mind that even the most seasoned hearing instrument wearer will admit to at least a bit of apprehension while waiting for their new hearing instruments. These efforts provide an appreciated informational bridge between visits.

Friends, Family, and Patient Referrals

Patients referring patients to your practice is the highest form of recognition for any health care practitioner. It sends a clear message to the incoming patient that the current patient has had a good experience with your practice, has been well served, and is confident enough to make a recommendation to a friend or another member of the immediate or extended family. The referring patient should be recognized in some way. A personal thank you note or a note

---

Sidebar 11–2
PATIENT BROCHURE: BEFORE HEARING INSTRUMENTS

Realistic Expectations

Hearing aids are just that, devices to aid your hearing. Hearing instruments will not return your hearing function to normal and they will not "cure" your hearing loss. If you use your hearing aids appropriately and wear them consistently, you can expect to hear better in almost all situations. There will be a few where you may experience difficulty, such as extremely noisy restaurants. But, for the most part, you and those around you can expect improved hearing and better communication.

Adjusting Takes Time

Realistic expectations are critically important. So too is the time it takes to get used to your new hearing instruments. Although periods of adjustment vary, many patients report continued hearing improvement and better speech understanding over a three to six month period. Since the auditory centers in the brain have not been subjected to these sounds, processing remembered sounds gets noticeably easier day by day.

Everyday Sounds

There is also an adjustment period to everyday sounds in our environment. Many patients report they forgot how annoying certain sounds can be and would just as well do without hearing them again. Clocks ticking, noisy refrigerators, and emergency sirens are examples of noises that may not seem important, but each contributes to your environment. Modern, digital circuitry has been designed to reduce the negative effects of noise in your listening environment.

Background sounds are no longer the greatest hurdle a hearing instrument wearer needs to overcome. Better technology coupled with better fitting techniques add up to a tremendous outlook for a successful outcome—even in areas with background noise, you will likely benefit from your hearing aids and hear those people seated at your table. It may not be perfect, but it will be far better than you can imagine with older hearing aids or by avoiding new instruments because you have heard they are so difficult to get accustomed to.

Keeping in touch with your environment is important. Enjoy all the sounds in your environment and recognize that even unwanted sounds have value. It's about taking a bit of the bad with all the good and staying in the everyday richness we call life. Welcome back to the world of all kinds of sounds!

Everyone Will Benefit From Your Hearing Instruments

Most of our patients come to us by referral from their family doctor. Others come to us by the "urgings" of their family or friends. They have a vested interest in your hearing. If you are hearing better, everyone benefits from easier and more accurate communication.

Good communication is a two-way street. If you persevere in wearing your hearing instruments, you and your family and friends will benefit from your willingness to improve your communication situation. Although it may be difficult at times, the more effort you put into adjusting to and wearing your hearing instruments, the more you will benefit from them.

Ultimately, better hearing is really up to you. You must wear your instruments consistently, maintain them well with regular cleaning and have an extra battery on hand at all times. Improved hearing takes but a few minutes of your time and attention daily. Our office is dedicated to your success and we are here to assist you in any way to make your journey to better hearing the best it can be. We will be available to you as long as you need us!

and a certificate for a free pack of batteries provide important recognition and appreciation. Although it is inappropriate and breaches a variety of organizational codes of ethics, actively seeking patient-generated referrals must not be considered a part of marketing or practice promotion. Accepting the recognition of a referral by a satisfied patient in the practice is appropriate: Actively seeking these referrals is, beyond the issues of ethics, simply unprofessional.

Notes in the Margins and Photo ID

A handy way to personalize your relationship with your patients is to jot notes in the margins of the chart so that you can recall events or circumstances important to the patient at the next visit. Birthdays, weddings, retirements, and funerals are items of great importance to your patients and if they feel comfortable sharing this information, you should take the time to listen and make an effort to inquire about it at subsequent patient visits. Staff should consistently peruse the obituaries and if it involves a current patient or one of their family members a note of condolence or sympathy card should be sent. When you work with a patient and their family for a number of years, you become important to them and as such, an appropriate response will be greatly appreciated and remembered for many years. Birthdays can be programmed to come up in most Management Information Systems and patient databases. Although some patients (and clinicians as well) have stopped counting birthdays, everyone likes to be recognized on their birthday.

Going beyond what is expected should be second nature when it comes to patient care. Extra effort cannot be taught, it comes not from a book but from the heart. Patients and their families appreciate extra effort. It bolsters confidence in the care they are receiving and reinforces their perception of your interest in their success.

Loyal patients are those with high comfort levels within the practice, both in the interest paid to them as a patient and in the quality of the professional care they have received. Loyalty is directly related to comfort and confidence and a sense of the staff having a genuine interest in the patient as an individual, not just as a person with hearing impairment seeking and receiving professional services to improve their hearing.

One of the most effective tools for front office and professional staffs to improve patient recognition is to keep a photo of the patient at the back of the chart for reference. Indeed, some third-party payers are requesting that patients be confirmed by reviewing an identifying photo on a driver's license or other form of identification bearing a photo of the patient. It is amazing how many times the practice staff will refer to a patient's photo to solidify their image with the name or to confirm they are dealing with a specific patient about a topic relevant to that particular patient's care or billing situation. Of course having access to these photos can also clarify the patient's identity in a rogue's gallery sort of way. Every practice has difficult patients and making sure who is who can serve as a means of alerting staff about particular problems, likes or dislikes, or patients with specific needs.

Newsletters

Practice newsletters are not only appreciated by your patients, they are anticipated and a welcome update about the goings-on in your office. Loyal patients feel a part of the practice and are interested in staff changes, training, and accomplishments. They want to know about attendance at seminars to improve technical and clinical skills. They like to read about new technology and will call and inquire about the need to consider "newer" technologies when discussed in the newsletter. There are services that provide practice newsletters. You send your database to them and they mail a newsletter at specified intervals. They are well written and contain a wealth of information. However, they lack the personal edge a practice-generated newsletter offers. Practice newsletters are time consuming. They should be formatted by a professional printing service, incurring both production and mailing costs. If you do not have the time, talent, and resources to develop and mail at least three newsletters per year, consider a commercial practice newsletter. Either way, practice newsletters provide an important opportunity to stay in the patient's view and to remain in the view of their significant others as well.

Summary

There is no substitute for well-developed patient management skills. Effective patient management skills are usually learned from the best teachers—the patients themselves. An ability to communicate and readily develop rapport and comfort in patients and those accompanying them to their office visits will set your practice above those merely interested in numbers of patients, procedures and instruments dispensed.

Whether in an independent private practice, an ENT-audiology practice, or a nonprofit community speech and hearing center, capable patient management must be the cornerstone of excellence in your daily clinical schedule. Patients referred to or seeking the professional care of an audiologist have come to expect clinical excellence and positive outcomes in their quality of life. Anything less and not only are patients and their referring health care providers poorly served, the whole of the profession of audiology loses important standing in the health care arena, one important patient at a time.

Every patient seen in your practice must know that their physician, friend, or relative issuing the referral to your practice has done so with great confidence in your patient management skills. They have made the referral knowing that audiologists are the professionals uniquely qualified to provide both diagnostic studies and appropriate treatment for patients with hearing and balance difficulties. They also refer knowing that after comprehensive assessment, patients will be appropriately referred for medical or surgical intervention when needed.

Each patient coming to the practice must expect professional, dedicated service from every member of the practice staff—at all times, every day the doors are open and telephones are being answered. Anything less than the items found in the Patient's Bill of Rights and the practice is not serving patients nor referral sources well.

References

Beck, R. S., Dautridge, R., & Sloane, P. D. (2002). Physician-patient communication in the primary care office: A systematic review. *Journal of the American Board of Family Practice, 15*(1), 25–38.

Hopkins, T. (2006). Do your customers feel ignored? Posting: February 06, 2006, *Entrepreneur.com*.

Marsh, D. (2005). Turning patients into patient advocates. *Hearing Journal, 58*(2), 48.

Rao, P. R. (2011 November). Our role in effective patient-provider communication. *ASHA Leader,* 17.

Reinartz, W., & Kumar, V. (2002 July). The mismanagement of customer loyalty. *Harvard Business Review,* 86–94.

St. Clergy, K. (2012). *Social media marketing to Baby Boomers.* Satellite presentation to the Business of Audiology Course, University of Colorado-Boulder.

Taylor, B. (2006). How quality of service affects patient satisfaction with hearing aids. *Hearing Journal, 59*(9), 25–34.

Thornhill, M., & Martin, J. (2007). *Boomer Consumer.* Great Falls, VA: LINX Corporation.

Travaline, J. M, Ruchinskas, R., & D'Alonzo, G. E. (2005, January). Patient-physician communication: Why and how. *Journal of the American Osteopathic Association, 105*(1), 13–17.

Traynor, R. M. (2003 August). Personal style and hearing aid fitting. *Hearing Review,* 16–22.

Traynor, R. (2011). Are Baby Boomer patients a worldwide phenomenon? *Hearing Health and Technology Matters.* Retrieved July 21, 2012, from http://hearinghealth matters.org/hearinginternational/2011/are-baby-boomer-patients-a-world-wide-phenomenon/

Traynor, R. (2012). *Baby Boomers: Our new patients.* Presentation to An Interactive Workshop in The Business of Audiology. Davenport, Iowa: Audiology Consultants, Inc.

Wong, L., Hickson, L., & McPherson, B. (2003). Hearing aid satisfaction: What does research from the past 20 years say? *Trends in Amplification, 7*(4), 117–161.

12

Supporting Practice Success: Counseling Considerations for Patient and Employee Management

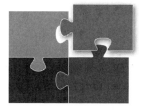

JOHN GREER CLARK, PhD

Introduction

Audiologists in management positions, whether practice owners or clinical service directors, are ultimately responsible for the success of the business enterprise. Those who are most successful clinically have developed a core set of attributes that they bring to their managerial roles that empower those they supervise thereby creating a team that builds the business from within.

To be most effective in serving patients and their families, audiologists must become adept not only in the diagnosis of auditory disorders and the treatment of these disorders, but also in the more elusive area of successful patient-professional relationships that may be built and maintained through the art of counseling (Clark & English, 2004, in press). Many of the same attributes that successful clinicians cultivate within themselves serve them well in both patient management and staff management. Routine information transfer (patient education, aka: content counseling) does not always address our patients' concerns or meet their counseling needs; nor does the simple provision of staff direction meet the professional growth needs of employees or build a cohesive team.

The majority of the patients and families we see for audiologic services are psychologically normal people. The emotional disruptions they may experience, that may block or seriously impede rehabilitative efforts, stem from the fact that they are currently confronting and trying to cope with one or more major disruptions in their lives. The counseling that we provide within our practices is a supportive counseling that may help patients to view their difficulties differently and then to build upon these renewed perceptions. The purpose of this chapter is not to present all of the approaches that strong counseling audiologists may bring to bear on the success of their patients. For full discussion of patient counseling for audiologists the reader is referred to other texts (e.g., Clark & English, 2004, in press; Lutterman, 2008). Rather, the purpose of this chapter is to review primary counseling attributes and motivation-building skills that need to be developed for successful patient and employee management—both of which are keys to a thriving business.

Counseling Attributes of Successful Practitioners

There are a variety of counseling attributes that successful practitioners may wish to develop within their interpersonal dynamic when working with both patients and employees. Carl Rogers's humanistic approach to patient management known as person-centered counseling (Rogers, 1959, 1979) embodies three personal attributes that we as audiologists may want to cultivate. Our embodiment of these attributes and two others reviewed here can enhance both our own counseling efforts with patients and our practice management success.

Congruence with Self

The first of Rogers's counselor attributes he referred to as congruence with self. Congruent clinicians, as well as congruent practice managers, are comfortable enough with their own strengths that they feel no need to continually place themselves above others. They do not portray themselves as one with all of the answers but one who continually seeks the greatest solutions. By decreasing patient or employee expectations that the clinician or practice manager has all of the answers, a self-sustaining partnership (whether between the audiologist and patient or the manager and employee) is fostered resulting in a symbiotic growth based on the empowerment of others that benefits all.

The attitudes and behaviors of the congruent audiologist/practice manager will help others find resources within themselves for growth. From an employee perspective, this growth may benefit employees directly as they expand on their skills and competencies and indirectly on the success of the practice. It is this trait of self-congruence that allows practice managers to maintain a relaxed and supportive manor that fosters a two-way exchange of constructive criticisms and suggestions from employees.

Unconditional Positive Regard

Rogers defines an unconditional positive regard as the professional's ability to accept patients as human beings of importance in their own right. The audiologist's code of ethics (AAA, 2011) requires that all patients be accepted for care and treated in accordance to the rights, dignities and privileges accorded to all humans regardless of their age, sex, ethnic origin, or religion whether they are a private, fee-paying patient of professional stature, or a welfare recipient whose bill is covered by a third party. Beyond what is dictated through professional ethics, unconditional positive regard dictates that we accept each patient's feelings as expressions of their current position within the rehabilitative journey. From a practice management perspective, unconditional positive regard dictates that we treat all employees with respect with an acceptance of conflicting viewpoints and varying opinion. An acceptance of statements made by others, be it parents or adult patients or employees, does not imply that we are in agreement with a given statement. It only means that we accept their right to express themselves and to hold the thoughts and beliefs that they may have. When we accept expressed attitudes or feelings, both positive and negative, we invite a more open dialogue and are afforded the greatest opportunities to provide guidance. Statements that may be intended to comfort, or that unintentionally pass judgment on what has been said, serve to give the impression that another should not feel as he or she does and stifles the desire to share further. When sharing stops, brakes are applied to collaboration: an outcome that is not conducive to patient management or practice operations. Certainly,

final practice decisions and ultimate responsibilities for the outcome of decisions rests with a practice owner/manager and this must be clearly conveyed to employees. But to foster collaboration and to empower employees to provide the best services to their patients and the practice as a whole, a sense of high positive regard should be mutually sensed by both employees and management.

Empathic Understanding

Rogers' third attribute for successful clinicians is an empathic, reflective understanding which requires a careful listening to others' explanations of their concerns and feelings thereby enhancing an appreciation of how they perceive specific problems. It is imperative that patients know their feelings have been heard even when not clearly expressed; and it is easy to see how empathic understanding is intimately intertwined with positive regard for another.

When we are unsure of the feelings or concerns that may lie beneath a statement, a reflection of our perception of the concern can quickly facilitate a more clear dialogue. Just as a facilitated understanding response is beneficial in clinical exchanges in patient management, so too is this beneficial in employee management.

The immediate gain from a reflective understanding response is that it reduces another's fear that we may pass judgment on what he or she may say, and thus opens opportunity for further discussion of topics needing exploration. This response can be developed only through practice and determined effort to combine the best aspects of active reflective listening, reassurance and probing with a sincere respect for the individuality and dignity of the other person.

Tied directly back to the first of the stated attributes, the success of the understanding response depends on an unconditional acceptance of other human beings as possessing importance in their own right. As Rogers (1961) has stated, this acceptance implies respect or regard for the patient's attitudes of the moment, regardless of how negative or positive these attitudes may be or how greatly they may vary from attitudes expressed in the past.

Active listening, as shown through one's ability to reflect the expressed feelings of the other person, is key to the understanding response. Reflection is an attempt to understand others' viewpoints and to communicate that understanding in a way that permits the examination of feelings or beliefs from different perspectives, thus allowing for a continued and perhaps broader consideration of the problems or concerns. A major pitfall of the reflective understanding response occurs when the content of the other person's statements is reflected rather than the feelings or underlying attitudes.

Reflections of feelings, although simple in principle, are often difficult in practice as they differ greatly from our long and more familiar experience of responding to content. When attempting to develop an understanding response through reflection of feelings with either patients or employees, the audiologist might try to select the one word that best describes the feelings underlying a given statement.

When patients or employees speak negatively of a situation they are in, such as a patient's perceived lack of progress in management or an employee's dissatisfaction with a change in procedure or policy, the audiologist/manager will make greater headway by openly recognizing this dissatisfaction than by becoming defensive. A reflection such as, "You don't feel the new compensation plan fully recognizes your contributions?" can help an employee view a supervising audiologist as more accepting and understanding, a perception that in turn may foster greater patience and cooperation from the employee. When another's negative feelings are consistently recognized and reflected, more positive feelings tend to follow.

In addition to statement reflection, the understanding response also may be conveyed through expressions of acceptance. Simply stating that we understand or appreciate a person's feelings may be especially useful when the patient or employee is disclosing information that might reveal feelings of shame or guilt (e.g., when discussions reveal a lack of follow through on recommendations, whether this be on the part of a patient or an employee). As stated earlier, acceptance should not be equated with either agreement or approval.

Moving Forward Through Silence

Employing the power of silence within clinical and managerial discussions is not one of Rogers's stated counselor attributes, although Rogers, like all good counselors, would attest to its value. In a social context, those brought up within Western cultures find silence to be awkward and uncomfortable. When a lull in conversation occurs we are quick to try to fill the void with a question or the introduction of a new topic.

In nonsocial contexts, such as clinical exchanges or business-related discussions, truncated silence can work against our progress or problem resolution. Silence, also known as "attentive waiting," serves as a response in itself, augmenting our empathic listening by allowing a temporal space for reflection and an opportunity for the other person to assume responsibility for his or her own progress or solutions. When we continually fill silent voids with questions or comments we run the risk of disrupting the other person's thought processes or sidetracking an issue that may need further exploration (Clark, 1994; Clark & English, 2004, in press; Luterman, 2008). By doing so we rob the other person of an opportunity for the empowering self-growth that comes when one's own solutions are put forth, discussed and possibly found of value.

Timing Is Critical

*Life is all about timing . . . the
unreachable becomes reachable,
the unavailable becomes available,
the unattainable . . . attainable.*

Stacey Charter

As with all in life, timing is ever important. A final counseling attribute that clinical and managing audiologists should embrace is recognition of information readiness. Whether we are working with patients or employees there are times when our listener's will be more prepared for both the reception and retention of information. Every audiologist has had the experience of a patient asking a question on a follow-up visit about something that was covered in detail at an earlier visit. Most have even had the experience of a patient who professed that the information was not provided before even though coverage of the infor-

mation is documented in the patient's record. How does this happen?

Neuroscientific research sheds light on this phenomenon (e.g., Cahill, Babinsky, Markowitsch, & McGauh, 1995; Canli, Zhao, Brewer, Gabrieli, & Cahill, 2000). When emotions are heightened the amygdala (the emotion center of the brain) is more highly activated. A highly active amygdala reduces the ability to process new information through the frontal cortex. Clinically, it is frequently at more emotionally charged times (immediately after sharing diagnostic findings) that we deliver critical information (details of test results, the need for medical follow-up, options for treatment) (Clark & Brueggeman, 2009). Practice managers should also keep in mind the research on patient information processing when managerial discussions bring forth strong employee opinions with heightened emotions.

Supportive Direction/ Collaboration

When practice growth opportunities arise, the managing audiologist frequently needs to provide supportive direction to help others achieve sustainable goals. In employee management, the key to the support we can give is exploration of possible barriers to success, which often relate to time management or a real or perceived need for additional training. The manager who works collaboratively will engage an employee through the attributes previously discussed as the managing audiologist and employee work together to find solutions. A counseling concept that works particularly well when providing supportive direction to or building greater collaboration with employees is one that capitalizes on the recognition of differing social style strengths and weakness that we all bring to both personal and vocational challenges. Social style recognition works equally well clinically when engaging with patients as they work toward greater success in the management of their own hearing difficulties.

Social Styles in Employee Management and Clinical Interactions

We all have our own social style that we bring to our interactions within both professional and nonprofessional settings. Others have previously noted the advantages of recognizing personality and social style differences in audiology practice (e.g., Clark, 1994; Clark & English, 2004, in press; Traynor, 1999; Traynor & Holmes, 2002). Our social styles develop as we learn to cope with life while simultaneously attempting to keep life's tensions at a manageable level (Wilson, 1978).

Our personal style of interacting with others can have a direct impact on how patients and employees receive the information we provide; how readily they may accept the recommendations, instruction, or guidance; and how comfortable they feel sharing their feelings and concerns with us. While a variety of personality descriptors exist, one view of social style provides a division of people's personalities into four basic styles of operation. Most of us have a dominant social style with a strong secondary social style and each of these can bring to an interpersonal dynamic both positive and negative contributions (Table 12–1; Wilson, 1978). Our primary style of interacting with oth-

ers is not necessarily constant and may vary within differing situations.

Assertion and Responsiveness

Social styles may be subdivided along the lines of an individual's degree of assertiveness and responsiveness. Those with higher assertion tend to step forward, take charge, and speak out. Those with lower assertion are viewed as more unassuming and cooperative tending to let others take charge. Like most personality traits, one's level of assertiveness falls on a continuum; each position on the assertiveness continuum has its own unique strengths and weaknesses.

Responsiveness is viewed as the effort, conscious or subconscious, that one may make to control emotions when interacting with others. As with assertiveness, responsiveness is placed on a continuum with different levels of responsiveness possessing different strengths and weaknesses. Those who are highly responsive may be viewed as enthusiastic, friendly, and informal whereas those who are less responsive may be viewed as more cool, unemotional, and businesslike.

Social Style Recognition

Knowing the characteristics of different social styles (see Table 12–1) can allow us to modify our own social style to facilitate interactions. From a patient management perspective, it is not practical to administer a social-style descriptor assessment or other measure of personality type, although such assessments can be beneficial in employee management. But even without formal assessment, our increased awareness of the different social styles can help us to recognize

Table 12–1. Four Basic Social Style Descriptors*

The Driving Style
Drivers are viewed as task-oriented individuals and may be described as people who give direction and whose emotions are more difficult to read. They appear to know what they want in life and where they are headed. They are highly assertive and self-controlled. From a positive view, drivers may be seen as thorough, decisive, and efficient, but can also be viewed as dominating, impersonal, and controlling.
The Expressive Style
Like drivers, expressives are also highly assertive people, yet they more openly display their feelings. Others may describe them as "people-people" placing more importance on relationships than on tasks. Expressives are said to be more intuitive and may rely on "gut" reactions more heavily than on objective data. Positively, the expressive may be viewed as personable, enthusiastic, and energizing, but may also be seen as opinionated and excitable.
The Amiable Style
Although amiables are less assertive than either the driver or expressive they share with the expressive a tendency for a more open display of their feelings. Others describe them as agreeable or as "peacemakers" who seem interested in establishing relationships. The amiable may be viewed positively as supportive, cooperative, and dependable, but they can also be viewed as conforming and noncommittal.
The Analytic Style
The analytics have a low level of assertion while possessing a high control of their emotions. These tend to ask questions and gather information so they may examine an issue from all sides. On the positive side, analytics may be seen as industrious and persistent whereas on the downside may be viewed as avoiding and impersonal.

*Most people operate within more than one social style with interplay of a primary and secondary style. No social style is superior to another and social styles may vary somewhat within different contexts (e.g., employment vs. social settings).

Source: Wilson Learning Company (1978); http://wilsonlearning.com .

behaviors that may guide us toward more meaningful interactions.

Modifications of our own social style to capitalize on our strengths and minimize our weaknesses can aid in the development of more comfortable, trusting and open relationships with employees and patients and can foster a better working relationship. Being able to recognize characteristics of our patients or employees that may indicate the social style from which they might operate can help us to mold our behaviors to be more conducive to theirs. For example, if an employer or manager is a driving/ analytic (primary and secondary social styles respectively) and is confronting an employee who is an amiable/expressive, the employer may want to tone down his or her businesslike persona, provide greater assurances and details than he or she might need in a similar discussion and strive to portray a more "friendly side." The benefits of a more open and productive exchange can make the conscious alterations worthwhile.

As stated earlier, the administration of a social or personality style assessment is not practical in the delivery of patient services; however, audiology managers can find this useful with staff or employee candidates. It would be a mistake to fail to hire a candidate simply because he or she operates differently than one's self. A staff with varying approaches to life's challenges can bring new and valuable insights for practice sustenance and growth. In addition, knowing the social style differences among employees can be useful when assigning employees to tasks or working groups. For example, if a supervisor is going to have one audiologist responsible primarily for hearing loss treatment and a second audiologist responsible for electrophysiologic assessments and one audiologist is an amiable/ expressive and the other more analytical in nature, social style awareness may make the choice more clear. This is not to say that an amiable/expressive will not work well in the provision of electrophysiologic assessment or that an analytical audiologist would not be a superb hearing aid audiologist. But playing toward an employee's natural strengths might be a consideration. Similarly, if pairing audiologists to work together on a project a mixture of social styles can often bring new insights to a task.

The relationship that evolves within our interactions with patients and employees develops over time and must be based on mutual respect and cooperation. An awareness of our own social style and that of others can foster enhanced collaboration and success when working with others. Readers wanting greater information on the implementation of social style recognition in clinical or managerial interactions are referred to Clark and English (2004, in press), or http://www.socialstyles.com.

Counseling Toward the Bottom Line

Audiology practitioners frequently see patients who are not yet ready to pursue amplification in spite of an apparent need to hear better. One might argue the audiologist has failed a patient and the patient's family when that patient is added to the pool of those we frequently call the "tested—not sold." When a patient who needs hearing assistance fails to attain that assistance, we have also failed the practice, as the financial bottom line, and ultimate success of the practice rests heavily on converting non-hearing aid users to successful hearing aid users. In this regard, successful patient counseling is intrinsically linked to the success of an audiology practice.

Self-assessment tools to help patients and their primary communication partners explore and discuss the impact of hearing loss have long been available for clinical use (e.g., HHIE, Ventry, & Weinstein, 1982; HHIA, Newman, Weinstein, Jacobson, & Hug, 1990; SAC/SOAC, Schow, & Nerbonne, 1982). Yet, in a large-scale survey of practicing audiologists across employment settings, Pietrzyk (2009) found less than 10% of audiologists routinely use self-assessment measures (Table 12–2). If audiologists hope to decrease the numbers of "tested—not sold" patients in their database, we must begin to more actively engage our patients in discussions of hearing loss impact within the various venues of their lives.

Health care providers have long acknowledged that change does not occur without motivation for change. This has been found to be true when working with patients on medication adherence, eating disorders, change in diet, substance abuse, smoking cessation, exercise improvement, or any host of areas (Tønnesen, 2012). Although audiologists have also long recognized that patient motivation is necessary for the acceptance of hearing care recommendations, patient motivation in audiology frequently relies on external motivators ranging from family persuasion and professional explanations of test results to marketing strategies that may rely on celebrity endorsements or financial incentives. However, time and again, life lessons have shown that motivation that arises from within one's self is not only more sustainable but ultimately leads to far greater success than any external motivators that are brought to bear, no matter how well intended.

The need for audiologists to successfully tap into patients' internal motivation has been addressed in the audiologic literature (Beck & Harvey, 2009; Beck, Harvey, & Schum, 2007; Harvey, 2003). A guided approach toward this end was first introduced to audiology through a series of interactive workshops for hearing health professionals (idainstitute.com) and subsequently through a series of publications (Clark, 2010; Clark & Weiser, in press; Clark, Maatman, & Gailey, 2012; Clark & Trychin, 2012).

Through motivational engagement, audiologists serve as a facilitative coach guiding patients as they reflect on the impact of hearing loss; their willingness to make the necessary changes in their lives to positively address this impact; and their perceived abilities to be successful in this endeavor. As audiologists help patients find an internal motivation for successful hearing loss treatment there is no better starting point than the

Table 12–2. Clinical Use of Self-Assessment Measures by Audiologists

- Master's Audiologists
  - Never use: 33%
  - Use less than 25% of the time: 34%
  - Use more than 75% of the time: 7%
- AuD Audiologists
  - Never use: 28%
  - Use less than 25% of the time: 31%
  - Use more than 75% of the time: 10%

Source: Pietrzyk (2009).

springboard provided by self-assessment measures.

Although the majority of patients who come to their initial audiology appointment are receptive to the audiologist's recommendations, there are those who only came to appease others not yet fully recognizing the impact of hearing loss, or who acknowledge the communication difficulties they are experiencing but have not fully taken ownership of those difficulties. Prochaska and DiClemente (1984) describe four stages leading to

successful change sometimes followed by a fifth stage in which an individual may relapse falling away from the change that had been made and returning to former behaviors (Table 12–3). Through our early discussions with patients and observation of their non-verbal behaviors, it is possible to ascertain how far patients may be on their own personal journey toward change.

Our perception of a patient's readiness for change is often based on what we know of the effects of diminished hear-

Table 12–3. Stages of Attitudinal and Behavioral Change in Hearing Loss Management

Contemplation	A patient may sense ambivalence toward change, possibly fearing what change may bring (e.g., not fully comfortable with the fact that hearing has changed and that a visible "prosthesis" may be needed to address the new deficiency).
Preparation	Ambivalence may continue but the patient is not fully sure how to proceed. This is an information gathering stage, often beginning with closer attention to marketing, information searches on the internet or discussions with friends who have obtained hearing aids.
Action	Patients are ready to follow the audiologist's recommendations at this stage. However, they may still need support and encouragement along the way as they may be unsure of their own ability to successfully adjust to amplification and follow through on recommendations.
Maintenance	Although normal ambivalence may still persist in this stage, patients are generally pleased with their forward movement to improve hearing. Support and encouragement are still needed to maintain the change they have made.
Relapse	Some patients go back to the psychological comfort experienced in the social isolation of hearing loss. Frequently, this reflects that the perceived benefit was insufficient to sustain the change. Support in the earlier stages along with a more comprehensive treatment that includes communication strategy training along with the "technological fix" helps to avoid potential relapse.

Source: Modified from idainstitute.com

ing, the test results in front of us and our assumptions of how the loss is impacting our patient. A full understanding of patient readiness is only possible when we attend to patients' stories, facilitated through discussions of reports on self-assessment measures. For some, it can be quite difficult to change a long-held view of "self" as one who is complete and whole and embrace a new self-image of one with a permanent disability requiring the use of a most-often visual prosthetic (Clark & English, 2004, in press). Although the majority of patients who seek our care arrive at the office ready to follow our recommendations, we must be prepared to assist those who have not yet reached a stage of readiness for the changes we are requesting of them.

Motivating Toward Action

When a patient is not ready to make the changes requisite to successfully follow our treatment recommendations (see contemplation and preparation stages in Table 12–3) and the audiologist proceeds, we may likely end with one of two outcomes, neither of which is good for the patient or the financial bottom line of the practice. One outcome may be that the patient gives any of a number of excuses to not proceed such as, "I can't afford it right now," "I need to discuss this with my spouse," or "I have a few more places to check before I make a decision." A second, and equally unsuccessful outcome, is a patient who acquiesces to the recommended plan, only to return the hearing instruments for a refund during the "trial period." Similar negative outcomes can be created with employees when management sees the need for changes in clinical policies or procedures but fails to ensure that the clinical team is all on board with the change.

When we sense reluctance toward change, it most often is not further information that is needed. When working with patients, a more proactive approach by the audiologist (and one that is more supportive of the patient's needs) simply would be to address their level of readiness by directly asking how important patients believe improving their hearing would be. The use of a visual prompt in making such rankings (Figure 12–1) is most useful. Frequently, audiologists fail to actively engage a patient's primary communication partner in these early discussions (Stika, Ross, & Cuevas, 2002). The importance of bringing this person into discussions is clearly evident when the importance of change is not judged highly by the patient.

If importance is ranked low, further exploration of hearing loss impact is necessary—possibly though a revisiting of responses on self-assessment measures.

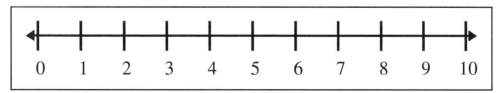

Figure 12–1. A visual prompt provided by a ranking line is useful in assessing perceived importance for making a change and one's self-perception of the ability to make change (Rollnick et al., 2008).

This should also include a weighing of the pros and cons of action versus inaction. Pros and cons should come from the patient and not be prompted by the audiologist as they carry far more weight when they come from within. The power of clinical silence cannot be underestimated here as the audiologist allows time for the patient to fill in the squares of a decisional box (Figure 12–2).

When a highly ranked importance for change has been acknowledged by all parties, successful change is not guaranteed. At this point, one should ask for a similar ranking on how strongly one believes in his or her ability to be successful in what is being asked. When working with patients, this self-efficacy question might be phrased as, "Looking at this scale again (see Figure 12–1), how strongly do you believe you can follow through with my recommendations, even if those recommendations include using hearing aids?" If the ranking is high on self-efficacy, successful intervention is highly likely. This is the time for patients in concert with their audiologist and an attending primary communication partner to begin setting the goals they want to achieve through the treatment process.

If the self-efficacy ranking is low, exploration can help ensure later success. Two questions may help with this exploration. Asking, "Why do you rank yourself as a three instead of a one?" gives patients the opportunity to reflect on possible strengths they may believe they have toward the task. Asking, "What is it that makes you unable to rank yourself, say, as an 8 on this scale?" opens discussion about the fears one may have regarding perceived abilities to follow though. With patients, these may be fears related to past failures when working

Benefits of Status Quo	Costs of Status Quo
Potential Costs of Change	Potential Benefits of Change

Figure 12–2. A decisional box (Janis & Mann, 1977) helps weigh the costs related to change versus the benefits derived when change is implemented.

with various technologies, fears that they will not be able to afford hearing aids, fears of how others will view them if they wear hearing aids, fears about how a boss may view their work capabilities if they show up at the job with hearing aids, or any host of concerns. The future success with any requested change is directly related to how adequately upfront fears or concerns are addressed with the audiologist.

The advantages of using tools of motivational engagement can be just as great when used in employee management as they can be within patient clinical interactions. For example, while an employee may agree to a change in clinical protocol as set by management, if done so reluctantly the effectiveness of implementation often suffers. Directly asking employees how important they view the change and their perceived self-efficacy for implementation can structure the dialogue that may be needed to uncover concerns and address them effectively. It is beneficial to use a decisional box to outline the benefits versus the costs (which are not always financial) of keeping a current protocol as opposed to implementing change. Assessing benefits and costs from both the perspective of the employee and how these impact the success of the practice can effectively move employees toward changes that may initially be feared to create more work, take more clinical time or have little beneficial outcome.

A more detailed discussion of the implementation of motivational tools in clinical practice with sample dialogues for each stage may be found in Clark and English (in press). An eTutorial on this topic is available for continuing education credit at http://www.idainstitute.com .

Summary

Audiologists frequently engage in both patient service delivery and employee management. There are a number of counselor attributes and counseling approaches that serve the audiologist well when working in either arena. Effective counseling, whether with patients or employees, enhances information comprehension and retention and success toward the implementation of needed changes in one's life or within a practice's established protocols. Readers interested in bolstering their counseling skills to enhance their clinical interactions and managerial style are encouraged to peruse the references cited in this chapter.

References

American Academy of Audiology. (2011). *Code of ethics*. Retrieved December 17, 2011, from http://www.audiology.org/resources/documentlibrary/Pages/codeofethics.aspx

Beck, D. L., & Harvey, M. A. (2009). Creating successful professional-patient relationships. *Audiology Today, 21*(5), 36–47.

Beck, D. L., Harvey, M. A., & Schum, D. J. (2007). Motivational interviewing and amplification. *Hearing Review*. Retrieved December 4, 2010, from http://www.hearingreview.com/issues/articles/2007-10_01.asp

Cahill, L., Babinsky, R., Markowitsch, H. J., & McGaugh, J. L. (1995). The amygdala and emotional memory. *Science, 377*, 295–296.

Canli, T., Zhao, Z., Brewer, J., Gabrieli, J. D., & Cahill, L. (2000). Event-related activation of the human amygdala associates with later memory for individual emotional experience. *Journal of Neuroscience, 20*, 1–5.

Clark, J. G. (2010). The geometry of patient motivation: Circles, lines and boxes. *Audiology Today, 22*(4), 32–40.

Clark, J. G. (1994). Understanding, building, and maintaining relationships with patients. In J. G. Clark & F. N. Martin (Eds.), *Effective counseling in audiology: Perspectives and practice* (pp. 18–37). Needham Heights, MA: Allyn & Bacon.

Clark, J. G., & Brueggeman, P. M. (2009). The Impact of grief on the delivery of information: Increasing student effectiveness. *Journal of the Academy of Rehabilitative Audiology, 42*, 1–12.

Clark, J. G., & English, K. (2004). *Counseling in audiologic practice: Helping patients and families adjust to hearing loss.* Boston, MA: Allyn & Bacon.

Clark, J. G., & English, K. (in press). *Counseling infused audiologic care.* Boston, MA: Allyn & Bacon.

Clark, J. G., & Weiser, C. (In press). Patient motivation in audiologic rehabilitation. In J. Montano & J. Spitzer (Eds.), *Adult audiologic rehabilitation* (2nd ed). San Diego, CA: Plural.

Clark, J. G., Maatman, C., & Gailey, L. (2012). Moving patients forward: Motivational engagement. *Seminars in Hearing, 33*(1), 35–44.

Clark, J. G., & Trychin, S. (2012). The operational model used by audiologists. In H. Tønnesen (Ed.), *Engage in the process of change—Facts and methods* (pp. 29–32). Bispebjerg, Denmark: WHO Collaborating Centre.

Harvey, M. A. (2003). *Audiology and motivational interviewing: A psychologist's perspective.* Retrieved December 4, 2010, from http://www.audiologyonline.com

Janis, I. L., & Mann, L. (1977). *Decision making: A psychological analysis of conflict, choice and commitment.* New York, NY: Free Press.

Luterman, D. (2008). *Counseling persons with communication disorders and their families.* Austin, TX: Pro-Ed.

Newman, C. W., Weinstein, B. E., Jacobson, G. P., & Hug, G. A. (1990). The Hearing Handicap Inventory for Adults: Psychometric adequacy and audiometric correlates. *Ear and Hearing, 11*, 430–433.

Pietrzyk, P. (2009). Counseling comfort levels of audiologists. University of Cincinnati, Unpublished Capstone.

Prochaska, J. O., & DiClemente, C. C. (1984). *The transtheoretical approach: Crossing traditional boundaries of therapy.* Homewood, IL: Dow/Jones Irwin.

Rogers, C. R. (1959). A theory of therapy personality and interpersonal relationships. In S. Koch (Ed.), *Psychology: A study of science* (Vol. 3, pp. 184–256). New York, NY: McGraw-Hill.

Rogers, C. R. (1961). *On becoming a person.* Boston, MA: Houghton Mifflin.

Rogers, C. R. (1979). Foundations of the person-centered approach. *Education, 100*(2), 98–107.

Rollnick, S., Miller, W. R., & Butler, C. C. (2008). *Motivational interviewing in health care.* New York, NY: Guilford Press.

Schow, R. L., & Nerbonne, M. A. (1982). Communication screening profile: Use with elderly clients. *Ear and Hearing, 3*(3), 133–147.

Stika, C. J., Ross, M., & Cuevas, C. (2002 May/June). Hearing aid services and satisfaction: The consumer viewpoint. *Hearing Loss (SHHH)*, pp. 25–31.

Tønnesen, H. (2012). *Engage in the process of change—Facts and methods.* Bispebjerg, DK: WHO Collaborating Centre.

Traynor, R. M. (1999). Relating to patients. In R. Sweetow (Ed.), *Counseling for hearing aid fittings* (pp. 55–80). San Diego, CA: Singular.

Traynor, R. M., & Holmes, A.E. (2002). Personal style and hearing aid fitting. *Trends in Amplification, 6*(1), 1–31.

Ventry, I., & Weinsitein, B. (1982). The hearing handicap inventory for the elderly: A new tool. *Ear and Hearing, 3*, 128–134.

Wilson Learning Corporation. (1978). *Managing interpersonal relationships.* Eden Prarie, MN: Author.

13

Referral Source Management

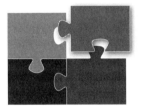

ROBERT G. GLASER, PhD

Referral Source Acquisition

A benchmark of the reputation of a practice within the professional community is the productivity of its referral base. It is an index of confidence and trust in the quality and consistency of services provided to their patients while in your practice. A productive referral base indicates confidence that your reports will contain important information that contributes to the overall care of the patient. A referral from the patient's primary care provider or other trusted, health care professional sets the stage for the initial patient encounter. It immediately develops a positive mindset about your services well

in advance of the patient's arrival at the receptionist's window. The patient recognizes that their physician has referred a portion of their care to you and your staff. It is an immediate vote of confidence and represents an assurance that you will have their interests as well as the reputation of the referral source in mind during your assessment and treatment.

Acquiring referral sources is important to ensure the long-term success of your practice. A creative blend of consistent, professional marketing strategies is necessary to populate the practice referral base. Besides satisfied patients, referral sources will include primary care and internal medicine physicians, pediatricians, neurologists, physiatrists, psychologists, optometrists, podiatrists, speech-language pathologists, nurses, a variety of other health care professionals, front office personnel, and practice administrators.

A Little Recognition Goes a Long Way

There is no harm in making the referring professional shine in the eyes of their patients. Recognizing the referral source for his or her insight into the patient's particular set of communication difficulties bolsters the patient's perception of the quality of care provided by the referring health care provider. Patients like to hear that those providing their health care are interested, insightful, and knowledgeable about when to refer to the proper professional to help with their hearing or balance difficulties. Just as the referral to your practice is a statement of your credibility as a provider, positive comments about the referring practitioner will boost their image in the patient's eyes. Consumer loyalty is as important to referring professionals as it is to the success of your practice. Physicians and other health care providers are interested in keeping their patients satisfied as much as keeping them healthy and functioning well in their daily life activities. Anything you do to bolster patient attitude and loyalty to the practitioner who referred them to your practice will help retain that provider as a productive member of your referral base.

Referral Source Retention

High patient satisfaction is elemental in retaining referral sources. It must be the foremost goal of every practice and a pervasive force that drives each member of the professional and support staffs. Patient satisfaction is not just about the patient. It includes encounters with family members, friends, and others interested in the patient's communication difficulties. Family and concerned friends will also provide impetus to those with hearing loss to come to your practice. They are interested in the outcome of your clinical intervention and have a vested interest in the patient's success as they also stand to benefit by the patient's improved communication capabilities; as such, family and friends should be included in the process at every opportunity.

Patients and a family member or friend should be invited into the examination or fitting room to observe. They should be included in the question and answer segments of the process and during counseling. Of course, this must be in compliance with the patient's wishes. With individuals other than the patient in the examination or fitting room, care must be taken to focus on the patient and his or her needs primarily. The patient must never be left out of the conversation nor become less than the center of attention of all involved. Having family or friends involved in the patient's evaluation and rehabilitation is a welcomed benefit for the clinician. They provide insight into the effects the patient's communication difficulties are having in their relationship and can serve as strong supporters for the patient after the fitting. Additionally, they may serve as keen observers of the patient's compliance, successes, and circumstances of poor performance. Most family and friends are pleased to be included in the process and have the patient's best interest at heart.

The practitioner will likely discuss the findings and recommendations in your report. That prompts the patient to share specific information about their visit to your office. If your practice has succeeded in its goal to develop high patient satisfaction, the patient will sing praises about the hospitality of the office staff from initial phone call and appointment making to their experience at checkout, and every step in between.

Satisfied patients will tell the referring practitioner exactly what he or she thought of your demeanor, your skills, and the completeness of your examination. Not much gets by patients and they readily advise their physicians (as well as their friends) about the positives and negatives of a practitioner. After all, your practice was entrusted to participate in a segment of their health care and as a result, your practice has become an integral link to both the referral source and their patient.

Patients trust their health care practitioner to refer them to another provider who is honest, fair, courteous, and above all, professional. This trust and anticipated confidence can unravel rapidly at the reception desk or if the patient is left waiting well beyond their scheduled appointment time. When a patient thinks the practitioner or his or her staff cares little about the importance of their time or if the receptionist meets them with a terse greeting, the likelihood of losing a referral source increases at an alarming rate.

There are other important ways to retain your referral sources. Any opportunity to fortify your service as a resource for referral sources will provide an enormous benefit to the numbers referred. Often times, the referral source may be unclear as to whether or not your services are the most appropriate for the patient's situation. If you have made it known to your referral sources that you stand ready to serve as a source of information readily available by phone or e-mail, they will appreciate that you recognize the immediacy of their needs and more referrals will likely follow. Other opportunities to retain referral sources include providing seminars in their office about how staff should approach those with hearing impairment, information about hearing aids and other communication difficulties and becoming a guest speaker at the referral source's civic group.

Patients without a primary care physician can be referred to one of your referral sources. Your office staff should contact their office to make sure they are taking new patients and that they know your practice is referring the patient to them. Consider the value a new referral is to your practice and the impact will be similar to the practitioner to whom you have made the referral.

Clinical excellence and high patient satisfaction are essential to retaining valued referral sources. On-time arrival for scheduled visits, having a sincere interest in their patient's well-being, and sending a reciprocal referral from time to time will go far to sustain the need for your referral sources to continue to send patients to your practice.

Communicating Findings and Recommendations

Report Turnaround Time

Though content may reign supreme when it comes to reporting clinical findings, report turnaround time from patient visit to the referring health care practitioner, will separate your practice from others. In this day of tomorrow-is-too-late information exchanges, consistently slow report turnaround time could result in your referral source searching for other providers to rely on for consistency and better accountability to their practice.

How slow is "too slow" depends on each referring practitioner's needs and practice pattern. Every setting providing clinical services should strive for 24- to 48-hour turnaround time on reports of findings and follow-up visits. Establishing a habit of writing your reports immediately following each patient encounter fosters a fresh perspective on important information obtained during the visit. Dictation used to be the method of choice to expedite documentation and create reports. With the advent of electronic medical records (EMR) and word processing programs loaded with pre written report segments, it is far more efficient to compile reports before the patient leaves the office, a lofty but readily attainable goal.

Referral sources and their office staff members take careful note of reports that are missing when the patient returns to their office. The worst-case scenario for the referral source is the patient in the exam room with the practitioner trying to explain why your report is not in their chart. The report may be languishing in the practitioner's to-be-filed basket (a common occurrence) and calls can be expected from the practitioner or a member of the practice's clerical staff for an immediate phone report, an admonishment, or both. Keeping records in your patient chart when the report was sent or confirmation sheets if sent via fax will enable you to advise that the report was sent and that you, of course, will gladly resubmit what is needed immediately.

An easy way around this dilemma is to develop an internal information routing sheet for the chart or use the left side of the chart jacket to record the date, time, description of the document, and where it was sent. Should the referring practitioner call your practice to inquire why they do not have a report in their file, your staff will have a complete record of report transmissions. If it was not sent, an apology and/or immediate fax or e-mail must be sent; if it was sent, the referring practitioner's staff "should" rummage through their piles of reports to be filed to locate the appropriate document. Your practice will, occasionally, be asked to resend a report because their staff person is too lazy or overworked to take the time to search through the pile for your report. If this becomes a consistent pattern, a call to their office manager must be considered to rectify the situation.

Report Format and Content

Good clinical reporting characterizes the symbiotic relationship of content and brevity. Content reigns supreme when it comes to reporting clinical findings; brevity is equally important. Health care practitioners sending patients to your practice do not have time to wade through three pages of discourse and data to get to the critical message that their patient has normal hearing. For the most part, they have no interest in looking at waveforms or output graphs. They may have such time constraints that they do not review the audiogram and go directly to the body of the report for your interpretation: they are interested in your findings and opinions about their patient's status and what you can do to help their particular difficulty.

The information provided by your practice will help solidify the diagnostic classification of their patient. Including a title or line segment in your report entitled "DIAGNOSIS" offers the reader an opportunity to move directly to the most important line in the report. An example of the written section of a brief format report is presented in Figure 13–1. The audiogram, speech threshold, and recognition score as well as other clinical information are immediately above the report language on the same page. Middle ear findings and otoacoustic emissions data are on the reverse side of the report.

In this recommended format, diagnostic classifications are listed followed by their respective ICD code numbers on the "DIAGNOSIS" line. The referring practitioner will use these codes to support their documentation about the patient's ongoing health care and diagnostic classification for a variety of reasons including reimbursement. An active medical record in a physician's office contains each patient's diagnostic codes. These codes are present whether specific treatment is underway even if they are not likely to change as in sensorineural hearing loss or diabetes mellitus.

When a patient has been referred to your practice or clinical area for an extensive evaluation, the reporting structure must be modified. The most efficient way to handle a great deal of information is to send relevant data along with a letter or cover sheet summarizing the results, diagnostic classifications, and listing recommendations.

The referring practitioner should be able to easily and quickly locate important diagnostic information and your recommendation(s) for treatment. A letter or cover sheet with a "quick-look" summary may increase efficiency for the referring physician and the likelihood

---

REFERRAL: Dr. Smith   **AUDIOLOGIST**: Robert G. Glaser, PhD

HISTORY: Pt. describes increasing difficulty understanding speech in a variety of communication settings. Wife & family concur. He reports non-disruptive, non-pulsatile, high-pitched tinnitus bilaterally for many years. He has worked as a toolmaker without hearing protection for >25 yrs.

HEARING: Severe, high frequency, sensory loss occurring symmetrically with distinctive "noise notch." Speech recognition is moderately reduced at each ear.

MIDDLE EAR FUNCTION: Normal middle ear function, bilaterally.

DIAGNOSIS: Noise-induced hearing loss 388.12
              Impaired auditory discrimination 388.43
              Tinnitus 388.31

PLAN/TREATMENT: Pt. and wife counseled with findings: Must use appropriate hearing protection consistently. Strategies to improve communication performance including hearing instruments were set discussed. Information was provided. He will contact our office to return for hearing instrument consultation. To return to Dr. Smith as planned.

Figure 13–1. Example of a brief format report.

of future referrals to your practice as well. Sending reports littered with multiple pages of information that the referring practitioner does not need nor may not understand, defeats the purpose of the summary page. For example, if the patient has undergone a tinnitus evaluation, the results of tinnitus mapping procedures, brainstem response data, and severity inventories will be meaningful to you as a clinician but not to the referring physician and should not be included. For fans of one of the earliest police procedurals on television (Dragnet), the term "just the facts" can never be understated when developing and delivering clinical information.

On the other hand, a patient who has been in an accident wherein he sustained a fracture of the temporal bone resulting in unilateral deafness, all clinical data obtained should be included with the summary since these data and informational points are important to the patient's ongoing and future care and may become critical in medicolegal documentation.

Recommendations

When a health care practitioner sends a patient to your practice for an evaluation, they do so because they are interested in your findings as well as your recommendations. They have invited you to become a participant in their patient's care and management. They expect recommendations; they do not have to agree with them nor act on them. If your findings support a high index of suspicion of a retrocochlear lesion, it is reasonable for you to suggest they consider further study such as an MRI of the posterior fossa. A recommendation couched as a suggestion gives the referring practitioner an option rather than an apparent order. Yet, should they disregard your statement and fail to identify a lesion in the posterior fossa, they may be subject to legal action. As such, it may be a better plan to state the findings without recommendations listed and to call the referral source to discuss the need for further, extensive studies based on your findings. Of course, the telephone call, date and time included, should be recorded in your chart notes. It is always better to offer suggestions that have ample room for the selection of medical diagnostic procedures by the patient's physician. It is not the audiologist's choice to make despite knowing that a specific medical diagnostic study has the necessary value in making the differential diagnosis.

When recommending treatment involving hearing instruments, do not overwhelm the referring physician with unnecessary information in an effort to demonstrate your knowledge or clinical prowess. State your suggestions with clarity: if the patient is a candidate for binaural placement, indicate that despite the fact that the patient has issued protests indicating his interest in a monaural placement. You must issue recommendations that will optimize your patient's outcome. If the patient chooses to wear only one hearing instrument, it becomes a choice beyond your clinical judgment and recommendation.

Indicate expected limitations and specific needs relative to the patient's hearing loss, speech recognition, and tolerance issues. If you foresee several options, or a lack of options, include that information in your recommendations. If you anticipate difficulties during the fitting and adjustment process, they should be stated in detail appropriate to the issue(s).

Reporting Interactions with Difficult Patients

Individuals with hearing impairment can, at times, become angry and explosive in the office. Diminished communication capabilities with attendant frustrations may cultivate inappropriate outbursts. The cost of the instruments and unrealistic expectations versus actual performance can set the stage for reduced patient satisfaction (Faiers & McCarthy, 2004). Anger is a common situational response during the assessment, fitting, and adjustment process. It is often displaced and the professional managing the patient's hearing care is a common target for the expression of anger (Hawkins, 2005). Despite appropriate strategies to provide evidence of value and effectiveness prior to and during the fitting process, anger and aggressive behaviors can sometimes escalate to a point where the patient may be asked to leave the office.

If the patient exhibits aggressive or threatening behaviors, they need to be documented in the record precisely as the events happened. Note who was an observer at the time and how staff reacted to the patient's behaviors. Immediately after the episode has been documented, the referring practitioner or the patient's primary care provider should be called and advised of the situation. That telephone conversation should be followed by written correspondence confirming the call and how you plan to address the situation with the patient in the long term. Depending on the extent of the outburst and the effects on you and your staff, you may be unwilling to see the patient again. If that is the decision, it must be so indicated in written correspondence to the referring practitioner. Additionally, a certified letter may be sent to the patient confirming that you will no longer participate in his or her care with an alphabetical listing of area providers. A copy of the letter should be sent to the referring primary care provider if seen on his or her referral. In any event, it is advisable to discuss this matter with your attorney prior to contacting the patient or referral source.

Practice-to-Practice Marketing to Retain Referral Sources

There is an old adage that is appropriate when considering your relationship with a referring practitioner and his or her office staff: "Nothing succeeds like success." Consistent and timely report turnaround, concise and accurate reporting of your findings, unequivocal diagnoses with associated ICD codes, and clear recommendations and suggestions for continued care or assessment characterize items and actions that should be in place on a routine basis. No gold stars should be issued for compliance with a practice standard of excellence. Adherence to clinical details, accurate results, and reporting enables a referring professional to rely on your participation in the care of their patients. And the successes you establish with the patients you serve as well as the response to the referring practitioners will likely enhance their level of care as well as their patient's loyalty.

In Chapter 6, a number of marketing strategies are set forth. Beyond those strategies, other opportunities arise to continue marketing on a different, more specific level. An often overlooked opportunity for marketing to referral sources within the practitioner's office includes their office staff—receptionist, billing and coding personnel, office managers, and the clinical staff—nurses, physician's assistants, and nursing assistants. When a patient calls the office to inquire about having their hearing evaluated, the front office staff might make the referral to your practice immediately by issuing your practice name, address, and phone number. If the call is passed on to the clinical staff, the nurse, for example, will likely triage the request to determine if the patient needs to come in or can be referred to your office for assessment. If you have developed a positive reputation with the front office and clinical staff in a referring provider's office, you will likely enjoy the luxury of direct referrals for your services. Some primary care physicians require seeing their patient before granting a referral to another health care provider's office for assessment or consultation. If that is the rule, and you have developed a positive reputation for consistent and reliable service provision with that physician, you will likely get a referral for that patient as quickly as you did from the front office or clinical staff in another office without a physician referral requirement: in fact, the former is occurring with much greater regularity.

Image Management

Image management is crucial to your success. It is most important that you foster and maintain a good, professional image within the medical community as well in the community at large. If you are viewed as a colleague in the give-and-take realm of professional referrals in health care, your future will be bright and your practice will be populated with a stream of patients. There are two simple ways to enhance your image by increasing your local professional visibility. One way is to provide lectures at professional functions such as meetings of departments of family practice and at the local medical school or during specialty group meetings of medical societies in your practice demographic. This will go far to establish your credentials and availability.

Another way to bolster your professional image in the health care arena is to advertise in the local medical society membership directory. These advertisements must maintain a minimalist attitude while establishing your office and location(s) as the best source of hearing (and balance) care available in the community. Call the local medical society to check out advertising possibilities and rates. They will be pleased to help you in your efforts to access their members.

Excellent services sell themselves. If you are receiving referrals from an individual health care practitioner within a practice group, that particular referring practitioner will likely inform the other practitioners or their respective clinical staff about the level of care and interest your practice has afforded his or her patients. These "internal referral systems" will, in effect, link your practice with theirs when it comes to the services available in your practice.

The more opportunities created to maintain good will and a good, professional image for you and your practice, the more patients you will see. Making it easy for the front office and clinical staffs of referring health care providers cannot be overstated. Taking over the appointment so that their office staff has less involvement in the booking is a small but important strategy. Get the patients off their plate and put them on yours. When your front office staff takes charge of the appointment, efficiency increases and the likelihood of booking errors that can result in patient frustrations are reduced: good for the patient and for both offices.

Image management also includes your reports of findings and informational and practice-related brochures. If your letterhead or reporting form has a list of services available on the left margin or elsewhere, all segments of the referring practitioner's office personnel will be reminded each time a letter or report is read or is to be filed or comes across the nurse's desk preparing the chart for the patient's visit. Helpful brochures about speech and language development, the damaging effects of excessive or unprotected noise exposure, and information about tinnitus are a few examples of informational brochures used by primary care physicians as waiting room items or when counseling their patients. It is best to tailor these brochures and have them printed locally. As for linking the brochures to your office, subtle listing on the reverse side of the brochure will increase the likelihood they will be accepted and used in their office. If it appears to be a commercial for your practice, it will limit use in medical practice offices.

Who Are Your Clients?

Your clients will vary depending on the professional circumstance. For a primary health care provider, patients may come from the entire population in a specific demographic area surrounding the office. The demographic area can be defined by drive times to the office, specific counties or municipalities, or by other markers of interest to that particular practice. As generalists in medicine see the young and the old, the urgent and the routine, their

potential client base is truly the entire population in a particular area (Rainer, 2004). For specialty care physicians, the population of patients narrows and dependency on referrals from primary care providers increases. Specialists, therefore, see those who refer patients to their practices as their clients.

Audiologists providing comprehensive diagnostic and rehabilitative care will have patients coming to their practice from their own advertising efforts, word-of-mouth referrals based on successful evaluation and treatment of other patients, and as walk-ins. Patients coming to the practice in this fashion become the clients of the audiologist. Those referred to the audiologist by another health care practitioner are certainly patients to be cared for in the practice; however, the client in this case is the referring health care practitioner.

Why does it matter how the patient arrives at your door? It is an axiom of good practice that every patient receive the same level of excellent care. When a patient comes to the practice without another health care provider's referral, their care from assessment to rehabilitative care is a matter of your management. That does not lessen the burden of communicating with their primary care provider as a matter of professional courtesy, a common occurrence in the medical community at large.

Medical Records and the Primary Care Provider

As the repository of medical records, primary care providers should receive reports of findings and recommendations as if they had referred the patient to your practice. If the patient has no primary care provider, recommend a provider or group that will most likely meet their needs within the community. Matching the patient to the right practice is important and the better you know your referral sources and their front office and clinical staffs, the better you can match the patient to the practice. Write a letter of introduction for the patient to the primary care provider after you have contacted their practice to ensure they are seeing new patients. It is best to make these connections prior to the patient leaving your office. Everyone wins when you match your patient with the right primary care provider. These referrals are appreciated and do not go unnoticed in the primary care practice. Think of the opportunity for both the patient and the physician to make a long-term commitment to a good patient-provider relationship. Not only is it a good fiscal benefit to the primary care provider, the patient will thank you for the referral for many years to come.

When another health care provider sends a patient to your practice for evaluation, you are bound to transmit your findings, diagnoses, and recommendations relative to your findings. As the referral came to your office, it is inappropriate for you to make referrals to other health care providers without involving the patient's physician directly. When asked to provide your diagnostic assessment and input, you are asked to do so with the unwritten knowledge that authority for referrals to other practitioners rests solely with the attending physician who sent the patient to your office.

For example, if your findings support the need for a referral to an ENT physician, a patient who walked into your office for an appointment on his own accord may be referred directly to the ENT physician. That same patient, when referred to your office by a primary care provider, should be returned to the primary care provider with your reasons and recommendations that he or she be referred to ENT. Referring a patient to another provider without notifying or consulting with the original health care practitioner who sent the patient to your office, is the fastest way to lose a valued, medical referral source.

Strategic Assessment of Referral Sources

Once your relationship with other health care providers in the community is established and referrals are coming in on a regular basis, you will want to learn how your practice can better facilitate their patient's care. Are you meeting their expectations for the patients referred to your practice? Knowing that each referring practice will have different needs and perceptions about how you are (or should be) servicing their patients, responses to these inquiries will vary greatly. Assessment can be as simple as a telephone call to the referring practitioner's office or clinical staff manager. Ask questions about their views on your practice's efficiency, turnaround time on reports, patient's perceptions of your services or office staff, whether your reports provide adequate information in a succinct fashion. The call need only take a few minutes to get to the heart of the questions. Expect truthful answers, and if they are negative, seek their input on a solution or ask if you might call back with a resolution based on a staff meeting or conversation with other members of your practice. If the negative response is coupled with a noted decline in referrals from their practice, it may be time to make an appointment to talk to their clinical staff or with the physician(s) in the practice to further explore the situation and to develop an equitable resolution. Another way to get feedback about the effectiveness of your practice and a referral source is to send a brief questionnaire about your services. It should contain no more than eight to ten items in a check-off format. A franked, return envelope addressed to your practice must be included. The idea is to make it as easy as possible to complete the task and put it in the outgoing mail basket. Address the envelope to specific individuals in the office. The office manager and members of the clinical staff are the most likely personnel to complete the task.

Evidence-Based Assessment of Referral Source Activity

Assessing the numbers of referrals made from specific health care providers can be a relatively simple matter. There must be a section on the patient information sheet to list the person who made the referral to your practice. Since that person may be different from their primary care physician, an additional line must be designated specifically for their primary care provider. These two opportunities will enable accurate tabulation of the referral source whether they are the primary care provider, another health care practitioner, or a friend or relative.

Numbers of patients referred to the practice should be tallied for each referral source. To consider referral patterns, these data can be listed monthly or by each quarter of the fiscal year to determine trends that may develop to guide your marketing efforts. If referrals for a particular provider decline in a certain period, marketing efforts should be directed immediately prior to that time period next year in an attempt at "smoothing" the referral pattern. If the referral source is a group of health care practitioners, it is best to tally the referrals by each practitioner within the group. Each practitioner may develop his or her own pattern depending on their level of participation within the group. Those practitioners who fall significantly behind in referrals in that group should receive more attention when marketing to the group at large.

Taking the pulse of your referral sources can lead to valuable introspective assessment of your practice and how it is interacting with a specific practice as well as the health care community at large. If a particular referring group or individual practitioner has fallen off their usual pace of referrals, it could signal dissatisfaction with your services or the availability of another provider in the area. A review of patient charts from that practice within the time period when referrals have declined might lend insight into the decline. One dissatisfied, vocal patient can affect the referral patterns of their physician or his or her clinical staff members who are also responsible for referring patients. Their response to the patient's complaints may seem punitive, and in some cases they are just that, but without your vigilance you may never have the opportunity of initiating a phone call to inquire about the decline in referrals. Straightforward inquiries usually get straightforward answers that can lead to dialogue and resolution of the problem, real or imagined. Taking the time to analyze drops in referral rates will provide information critical to both the short- and long-term success of your practice.

Once a collegial relationship has been developed with referring health care practitioners, you can expect direct communication when patients provide information (real or imagined) about a topic or situation that may have arisen from a recent trip to your office.

An example drawn from practice records describes a patient returning to the referring physician after a hearing assessment. He advised his physician that the practice no longer accepted Medicare patients. That was a surprise to the physician, who promptly called the office to validate their patient's claim. Medicare patients have always been welcomed in the practice despite the fact that coverage includes only the hearing examination without coverage of hearing instruments or related items or activities. In further discussions with the referring physician it became clear that the patient had confused statements regarding coverage by Medicaid versus Medicare. The physician was advised that the practice was unable to accept Medicaid patients in the practice unless the patients are enrolled in a Medicaid HMO system. This particular patient was covered by Medicaid but was not enrolled in the local HMO system. As such, the patient was not eligible for aural rehabilitation services through the practice. After the patient enrolled in the Medicaid HMO, the practice continued to provide services to that patient and many more referred by that physician, who took the time and trouble to get to the bottom of a dilemma that did not seem to agree with past actions of the practice. He cared not just about his patient but also about the practice in which his patients had received excellent care for many years.

References

Faiers, G., & McCarthy, P. (2004). Study explores how paying effects hearing aid users' satisfaction. *Hearing Journal, 57*(12), 25–32.

Hawkins, D. (2005). When you're attacked: Fight, flight, or what? *Hearing Journal, 58*(4), 76.

Rainer, C. (2004). *Practice management: A practical guide to running a medical office.* Lima, OH: Wyndham Hall Press.

14

Personnel Management

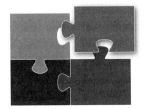

ROBERT G. GLASER, PhD

A conductor's baton is only so much. It is the rest of the orchestra that makes it happen.

Eric Kunzel, Conductor
Cincinnati Pops Orchestra

Introduction

Effective personnel management is the unifying force that establishes the tone and complexion of a practice. It begins when the practice owner hires an employee to complete specific tasks as directed. It is that "as directed" that forms the nucleus of personnel management. The owner/manager must be able to effectively impart what needs to be accomplished and how important that task is to the current and future status of the practice. He or she must make a commitment to the employee to establish what is expected in the position; to evaluate and provide regular feedback to the employee regarding their performance; to establish parameters of appropriate demeanor with patients and fellow employees; to clarify the need for teamwork focusing on the common goals of patient and referral source satisfaction; and to understand that failure to fulfill the duties and expectations in the job description may result in termination of employment.

Personnel management will vary as a function of style and experience. Some managers will rule in a top-down, do-as-I-say fashion. Others will state the objectives and desired outcomes and let the employees figure out the best way to accomplish the task to get to the defined outcomes. Savvy personnel managers will optimize productivity by recognizing that each employee responds differently—what motivates one employee may not motivate another.

Effective personnel management will develop a team pulling in the same direction with common goals where individuals step outside themselves to accomplish tasks in the best interests of the patients served in the practice.

Leadership and Personnel Management

Managing people requires leadership. The ability to lead is a collection of skills, nearly all of which can be learned and improved. Leadership has many facets; respect, experience, emotional strength, people skills, discipline, vision, momentum, and timing (Maxwell, 2002). It is about being the sort of person people will confidently follow and work diligently to gain your attention and approval. It is about becoming a person of influence and respect; each is earned by example and establishing model behaviors and developing an easily discerned attitude about the importance of patients and their success as a result of coming to the practice.

Leading a practice and managing a practice are different on several levels. Leadership is about influencing people

to follow; management focuses on maintaining systems and processes which may or may not be effective. There are fundamental differences in being the "boss" (manager) versus operating as the leader of a practice:

- The boss drives his workers; the leader coaches them.
- The boss depends on authority; the leader on goodwill.
- The boss inspires fear; the leader inspires enthusiasm.
- The boss says "I"; the leader, "we."
- The boss fixes blame for the breakdown; the leader fixes the breakdown.

From Employee to Associate

An effective leader recognizes those working in the practice as critically important assets necessary to achieve high patient and referral source satisfaction. The leader intuitively understands the role that selection, training, trust, respect, and empowerment play in the transformation of an employee to an associate. An associate shares the vision and goals of the practice and works as a partner and colleague in joint pursuit of patient and referral source satisfaction.

Practice leaders will doggedly pursue and find the most talented individual and provide the atmosphere for them to do their best work. No matter the position, a practice leader will find the person who best fulfills the preselection requirements based on the position description in the Policy and Procedures Manual. The process of selection may be time consuming and tedious; however, the more time spent, the more specific the preselection requirements and the greater the clarity of the position description, the better the outcome.

Be prepared for more than a few disappointments. Depending on the necessary skill level needed to fulfill the requirements of a position, the demographics of your area, and the competition offered by other positions available in your geographic location, you might become frustrated enough to take the next applicant walking through the door. That action may be costly in a variety of ways. A large group of mediocre candidates is not as valuable as a small group of good candidates with most or all of the characteristics and skills to fill the available position (Sidebar 14–1).

Sidebar 14–1
VALUABLE CHARACTER TRAITS IN POTENTIAL CANDIDATES

attentive	hard working	responsible
calm	honest	self-confident
cheerful	imaginative	self-motivated
common sense	independent	self-starter
conscientious	intelligent	sense of humor
courteous	interesting	sensitive
creative	kind	sincere
curious	likable	team player
dependable	likes challenge	tenacious
detail oriented	loyal	thorough
eager to learn	patient	tolerant
eager to please	perceptive	tolerates pressure
empathetic	persistent	understanding
energetic	personable	unflappable
enthusiastic	polite	vibrant
flexible	productive	warm
focused	punctual	willing to stay late
friendly	resourceful	work ethic
goal-oriented	respectful	zestful

Recruiting: Getting the Best Group of Candidates Through the Door

Whether adding a front office staff person to assist in scheduling, billing, and patient information management or searching for an audiologist as an employee or potential partner in the practice, recruiting talented candidates requires a great deal of planning and preparation. Once the decision to begin the search has been established, both administrative and professional associates should be involved in the process. Concerns about how the new person will fit in, what personal characteristics would add to the practice, what past experiences are considered most important for the position, and other issues will surface. Most of the concerns will boil down to one important factor: will the new person be a "good fit" for the existing team? The existing team, despite confidence in the practice leader's decision making, may be uncomfortable unless they have had a chance to participate in part or all of the selection process.

If your practice has a number of associates, you could select an independent team of associates to review resumes to arrive at a nucleus of candidates to consider for further evaluation. Deciding who to bring in for an interview is often adequate to fulfill an associate's need to participate in the process. Others may wish to become more involved in the process. Including staff members in this process is important not only for office morale, it provides the staff an opportunity to exert some level of control over the selection of the person who will be working with them. The goal is to develop a comfort level for both sides of the equation: when the selection has been made and the new hire walks into the practice on the first day of their employment, all members of the practice should be satisfied with their choice and provide an honest welcome to their new colleague. The newly hired associate should feel a part of the team on their first day of employment.

Establish a Recruiting Protocol and Stick to It—No Matter What

Developing a recruiting protocol to be followed consistently is important for a variety of reasons, not the least of which includes fairness and consistency in hiring practices. Though structured, the process need not discourage asking additional questions based on the applicant's responses. It is important to remain flexible in your line of inquiry, but be sure that all interviewees respond to an agreed upon set of specific questions so that direct comparisons can be made of each candidate on topics important to the practice.

Whether adding a new staff position or filling a vacancy, it must be recognized as an opportunity to improve the practice. Fresh looks, new ideas, and patient-centric operational strategies brought into the practice by new associates can provide new ways to address old issues. If nothing else, new personnel will provide thought-provoking conversations about a variety of operational and patient care issues that may have been brushed under the table until that important catalyst comes along as a potential agent of change.

The recruiting protocol (Sidebar 14–2) will differ from one practice to another. Each venue will need to consider specific items that may be part of a human resource department requirement or otherwise be important to the specifics of the respective practice.

Resume Review

The posting of the position should include specific directions to apply for the position. The candidate should submit a resume and follow the directions listed in the posting. If the applicant cannot follow these directions or submits a resume that is ill-prepared or other-

wise unacceptable, delete the application and continue the process. If the applicant does not convey the qualities deemed necessary for the position in their resume, eliminate the resume and seek those candidates with indications of achievements, complementary experiences, and education commensurate with the position. Select promising applicants for a telephone interview.

The Telephone Interview

The telephone interview is conducted to confirm the applicant's credentials, qualifications, assess their presence on the telephone, and gain additional, subjective

---

Sidebar 14–2
RECRUITING PROTOCOL

1. Post or advertise the position.

2. Issue explicit directions about how to apply for the position; request resume.

3. Resume screening develops pool of candidates.

4. Candidates sent position application with return-by date.

5. Schedule telephone interview based on qualifications listed in application.

6. Telephone interview to confirm candidate's qualifications; assess phone skills and demeanor and to verify prior work experiences.

7. Select candidates for face-to-face interview.

8. Develop structured questions tied to decision-making criteria.

9. Contact licensing board for confirmation of license and status.

10. Review background check by local or state police.

12. Complete face-to-face interviews.

13. Offer position to selected candidate.

impressions of the applicant: Did he or she return your call promptly or at the agreed on time? Was the applicant polite? Could this applicant interact well with the patient population in the practice? Based on the resume, the responses on the application, and a telephone interview, two or three candidates should be selected for face-to-face interviews.

The Face-to-Face Interview

Preparation for the face-to-face interviews should include contacting references by telephone to verify strengths and weaknesses and to get an idea of past performance. Past performance is a strong indicator of future performance. If the position involves a licensed professional an inquiry should be made at the licensing board to confirm their status and to ask if there have been complaints filed or adjudications levied. This information is a matter of public record. All applicants, regardless of the position they are applying for, should supply a copy of a current background check completed by state or local police. This is done for the protection of the practice and its staff as well as the patients to be served in the practice.

Questions should be prepared prior to the interview. The questions should be based on the job posting, tasks to be completed in the position, expected responsibilities, previous experiences, and accomplishments in prior employment. Ask the same questions of each candidate. "What if" questions or scenarios can be proposed to get an idea how each candidate would react or respond to specific situations that might arise in day-to-day operations of the practice. The interview should include those asso-

ciates in the practice with vested interest in hiring the applicant as well those who will be working directly with the applicant chosen for the position.

Tendering an Offer

When the decision to hire has been made, contact the applicant by phone with a verbal offer. If they accept the offer, a formal letter should follow confirming the salary structure, a tentative schedule for the first few weeks of their employment, documents or licensing information to bring to the practice on the first day, and other requirements relevant to the particular venue of the practice. If the candidate is considering several offers, set a time frame to respond to your available position. If the candidate is exceptional, there is no harm in asking where your offer stands on the pile and what conflicting issues are hindering their decision. If it is based on wages alone, you must decide whether this candidate is worth the difference in dollars and qualifications over the number two or three choice in your final pool of selected applicants. It is strictly a business decision. If they cannot make up there minds in a reasonable period of time (defined by your needs, not theirs), move to the next qualified applicant and wish your first choice well.

Orientation and Training

When going through the assessment process, candidates have an opportunity to evaluate the tenor of the practice. As representatives of the practice, those engaged in the interviewing process provide a snapshot of personnel attitude, dedication and interest the outcome of the hiring process. The staff wants to make sure they hire a "good fit" and the interviewee should be assessing their demeanor to add to his or her list of reasons to accept or reject an offer. If the interviewee feels as though the personnel doing the interview are arrogant or unfriendly, why would he or she accept a position working with a bunch of pretentious jerks? As such, an associate's orientation and training begins in the hiring process.

During orientation and training new employees should develop an understanding of the importance of patients and referral sources, practice operations, and the rules of the practice. Equally important is setting forth a clear picture of the culture of the practice, how everyone pulls together to complete the operational tasks that characterizes the reputation of the practice within the community of practitioners as well as the community at large.

The more time spent in high quality orientation and training, the greater the likelihood the new associate will be satisfied in his or her position, and will work diligently and consistently as a team member on behalf of the patient and the referral source. The well-trained associate will have the confidence to make mistakes in the beginning, develop the skill set to reduce errors over time, and understand the rationale behind the policies and procedures which guide the actions of all who participate in the practice.

On-Boarding

The concept of "on-boarding" an employee was developed by large corporations to efficiently integrate and improve retention of new employees in top management. It is a systematic method of introducing the newly hired individual to the people they will work with and report to during the initial stages of employment. First impressions are important and that is especially true in the first 30 days of a new position. New hires should feel welcome, valued, and well prepared for the demands of their position. Orientation and training should be personalized, simple, interesting, and focused. It should include information on both written and unwritten rules of operation, demeanor, dress code, and other obvious and not so obvious conventions that make up the "culture" of the practice.

All staff of the practice should be prepared to meet and greet their new coworker not as a set of job functions and duties but as a colleague and member of the team, regardless of the practice venue. An effective practice leader will guide and direct the on-boarding experience so that the new person in the practice is welcomed by the staff, well informed about their duties, and glad that they accepted the offer. Reviewing the position description, issuing keys and codes, orienting them to their work environment, and issuing a copy of the policies and procedures for the practice is a good list of first day accomplishments. Over the course of the first 90 days of employment, the new hire will continue his or her training. That training schedule should be prioritized based on input from incumbent members of the practice. Important tasks should be mastered first; those with less impact on patients, referral sources, and office operations should follow on the training schedule.

Health care systems such as HMOs and hospital-based audiology practices have human resources departments to issue information and details about health and disability insurance benefits, retirement plans, paid time off and leave of absence policies, dress code and demeanor expectations, parking, personal cell phone use, and other issues and rules. An independent audiology practice with three employees, now adding a fourth, will have no less need for completeness. The on-boarding process should be as systematic and complete as it is in larger health care facilities. The desired outcomes are the same, employee development, satisfaction with their position, and retention. On-boarding is designed to optimize an employee's knowledge and skill base through systematic training designed to develop necessary competencies in the first 90 to 120 days of employment. On-boarding in an audiology practice involves three distinct steps: meeting the players, teaching the tasks necessary to the job description, and evaluating performance.

Meeting the Players on the Team

Acceptance is important to all of us. That is never truer than on the first day of a new position. Meeting the other members of the team can be intimidating. A warm welcome issued by established members of the practice should be extended to every new hire. Those who lend support in the practice on a part-time basis should be included in the introductions and welcoming activities as well. Every member of the practice team is an important asset. Everyone contributes to the bottom line.

The attorney and accountant involved in the operational aspects of the practice as well as their staff who commonly interact with those in the practice should be encouraged to introduce themselves and clarify their respective roles in the practice. Introducing hearing instrument manufacturer's representatives and other vendors will underscore the importance and value of the newest member of the practice team.

Teaching the Tasks

Training is best accomplished by a knowledgeable person in the practice who has served as an audiology supervisor or in a related capacity. The trainer must have the necessary patience to serve as a guide to the nuances of each segment of the position. Certain competency levels should be achieved before the new hire is expected to function independently. He or she should not be placed at the front desk to answer phones, book patients, and record billings until such time that the tasks can be handled with at least a modicum of efficiency and accuracy. It is important to optimize the chances for early success by providing adequate training to master the daily operations of the practice.

Objectives to be achieved over the first 90 to 120 days should be outlined and the training should be achieved so that the new hire can meet their objectives. For example, it would be foolhardy to expect a new hire to complete the billings for services provided on the same day of service during the first few weeks of employment. A goal could be established, however, in which the new hire is expected to complete all billings for services rendered on the same day within 6 to 8 weeks of the first day of employment. When realistic expectations and goals are set and not achieved, training may need to be repeated or modified and another assessment time frame should be established.

Empowering Associates

As the leader in the practice it may fall to you to assist every associate in fulfilling the responsibilities in their respective job descriptions and to foster job satisfaction as they complete their tasks. Effective leaders develop a mutual respect; the associates respect the leader and the leader respects the associates. The practice leader must focus on the core of the practice, provide examples at every opportunity, and provide guidance, instruction, and praise to each associate pulling in the same direction. Everyone in the practice must hold high the importance of patient satisfaction and ensuring that referral sources remain satisfied with the outcomes of their referral to you as a participant in a segment of care of their patient.

The best way to make a commitment to an associate is to empower that person to make decisions based on the benefits to the patient, the referral source, and the practice. Their decisions should be made in that order. Empowerment is a strong drug. It implies trust and confidence. It provides validation. When the practice leader empowers an associate to make a decision, he or she is relying on the associate's assessment of the situation, their ability to come to a just and fair conclusion, and their confidence knowing that their decision will not be second-guessed nor otherwise undone. The practice leader, who enables his or her associates to make decisions about hearing instrument returns, repairs at no charge, or waiving charges for a situation that could use some salve on a wound caused by an error or misstep, demonstrates confidence and faith in their capabilities. Practice *owners or manag-*

ers readily delegate tasks to employees. Practice *leaders* empower others with decision-making capabilities to get things done. It takes a great deal of confidence, self-assurance, and security to transfer segments of authority to associates. By creating strong and effective associates who can work on behalf of the patient, the practice leader will have developed a group that can make the difference in the market place, a group that is known for competence and excellent care and patient satisfaction.

As you empower others, you will find that most aspects of your life will change for the better. Empowering others can free you personally to have more time for other matters in the practice, increase the effectiveness of your practice, and, best of all, and make an incredibly positive impact on the lives of the people you empower.

Performance Appraisal

McClain and Romaine (2007) state emphatically that despite the need for their existence, managers and employees inherently dislike evaluating performance. They contend that regular communication, daily or at least weekly, is the most effective way to both monitor and shape employee performance.

In practices with fewer than six to eight people involved in daily operations, there remains a need to complete formal evaluations although perhaps less critical than in larger practices. When an individual in a smaller practice fails to pull his or her weight, the work products of the entire team may suffer. Peer-generated appraisals are usually immediate and effective. In larger practices and those in corporate or health care settings, formal performance appraisals are necessary as a stipulation in hiring guidelines or for compliance with malpractice insurance coverage. The last thing a practice or a corporate entity wants to defend in a negligence case is why the individual involved had not had an appropriate performance appraisal in two or three years relative to the time the alleged incident was to have taken place.

There are as many ways to develop a performance appraisal as there are authors with opinions about the topic. It should be viewed as an opportunity for an associate's continued success and improvement. It should be tied to the associate's efforts to maintain and advance patient and referral source satisfaction and retention. Performance appraisals should be considered a formal part of a continuous program of assessment and quality improvement.

Probably the most unnerving and counterproductive aspect of formalized performance appraisal rests in the fact that financial parameters are commonly involved in the process. Burrows (2006), indicates that promotions, pay raises, bonuses, and job assignments should be made on the basis of a formal evaluation. No wonder people view performance appraisals with such overwhelming trepidation when so much of the outcome is clouded by the threat of loss of promotions and other financial matters. Performance appraisals and financial incentives are undeniably tied, however, by disengaging the appraisal meeting from the time when promotions, pay raises, and bonuses are granted (or denied), the appraisal meeting becomes less of a threatening circumstance and a greater opportunity to concentrate on performance assessment and strategies to improve. The focus of the performance appraisal moves from financial issues to performance issues which is exactly the core reason for the appraisal in the first place.

The key elements in a performance appraisal in an audiology practice should include at least the following:

- A review of the position description, related duties, and responsibilities as the basis for the performance review (clinical in the case of an audiologist; operational in the case of office staff);
- An assessment of the associate's contributions to patient and referral source satisfaction relative to their duties and responsibilities;
- An assessment of the associate's compliance with state licensing requirements for continuing education;
- An assessment of the associate's abilities to take direction, to work cooperatively, to follow policy and procedures, and to work independently;
- To establish recommendations to facilitate identified changes in the associate's work routines;
- To establish a time line for completion of change(s) in areas in need of improvement.

Employee Retention

Retaining associates is important for several distinct reasons: (1) it is expensive in time and capital to go through recruiting and evaluating potential candidates for the position; (2) there is a causal link between employee retention and high patient satisfaction; (3) continuity of care issue, even with the front office staff, patients like to see the same faces on a regular basis; and (4) the practice loses an associate with knowledge and skill sets specific to the position which will have to be re-established with the new hire for the position.

The goal of any employee retention program in health care is to keep those who add value to the practice. Competition for good people is intense and the practice leader must commit to the realities of their respective market. If he or she wants to hire good people who will become sources of patient satisfaction and continued revenue for the practice, it is essential to develop a compensation package that validates their worth.

The atmosphere that is the work environment contributes significantly to employee retention. Consistent interactions with members of the management team and access to the practice leader with liberty to discuss practice policies and procedures are also points of appreciation important to retention. An employer who will listen, cares about employee well-being and is sympathetic yet fair in the requirements of the position contributes greatly to retention. Well-trained, well-recognized, and empowered associates have pride in the practice and readily develop an allegiance that will likely transcend offers that might be attractive to those with less stature and unable to make decisions without permission. Trust is a critical element in retention. If an associate is trusted, they will work diligently to maintain that trust and the empowerment and positive self-image it brings.

Termination of Employment

Terminating an employment arrangement is never easy. It is probably one of the most difficult tasks a practice leader will face, regardless of the reason for the termination. In today's litigious society, justifiable terminations may be challenged by attorneys eager to gain a nuisance settlement in a wrongful termination suit. The advice of legal counsel to most health care practices is to reach a reasonable payout rather than incur a lengthy and expensive engagement. If supporting documentation is complete and the termination was appropriate relative to the Policy and Procedures Manual and discharge/termination documents, there is no reason (beyond the financial and time costs) to roll over and pay out excessive demands put on the table by your former associate's attorney. Indeed, if fewer practice owners or managers would roll over, perhaps there would be fewer incidences of wrongful termination lawsuits threatened or filed. Evaluate the potential costs realistically, remove your emotionality from the situation, and make a decision in the best interests of the practice in concert with the guidance of your attorney.

The Policy and Procedures Manual or employment contract should contain not only the associate's position description but clearly stated grounds for termination as well. In most instances of audiology practices, the employees are considered "at-will" employees and may be terminated at any time. Despite this status, it is good to document performance appraisals, specific situations that constitute non compliance in their position description or expected parameters of the workplace such as reporting on time, adhering to paid time-off policies, and other expectations that are required for continued employment in the practice. At every incidence of non compliance where the practice leader has had to discuss an issue or situation with the associate, it should be described in writing, with a plan to resolve the situation and/or a clear depiction of the consequences if the infringement occurs again. It should be dated and signed by the associate and the practice leader. In any event, never let an employee or associate dictate neither the terms of his or her employment nor hold your actions hostage by stated or implied threat of a wrongful discharge suit. The position would not be there if it were not for you starting the practice, managing the department, or otherwise serving as the employee's supervisor. If the employee or associate meets the criteria for dismissal, take decisive action on behalf of the practice, the patients, and the other members of the team who have been affected by the person's noncompliance as well.

Adding an Audiologist to the Professional Staff of the Practice

When adding a member to the professional staff of the practice, procedural contexts, diagnostic protocols specific to the practice, and a discussion of both philosophical and pragmatic approaches to patient evaluation, interpretation, and management must be considered. If the audiologist under consideration has been practicing for several years and carries the valuable mantel of experience, there will be little required of the practice leader save working with the new colleague on report formats, getting to know the ins and outs of all the referral sources, and filling in clinical vacuums such that they might exist. Perhaps the audiologist had been in a dispensing practice that did not offer vestibular evaluation. If so, the audiologist will need to re-establish a knowledge and skill set to participate in the clinical assessment, treatment or referral of patients with disequilibrium. The new audiologist may require course work or directed readings and clinical instruction in vestibular assessment techniques, interpretation of data, and report writing.

Fourth-Year AuD Externships

Adding a fourth-year AuD student to the practice does not constitute adding an audiologist to the professional staff of the practice. When the AuD degree was first considered and earnest discussions about curriculum and clinical training transpired, the fourth year was to stand as a beneficial circumstance for both extern and preceptor alike. The student was to enter the practice and "hit the ground running" compared to students in their clinical fellowship year (CFY) immediately following the master's degree. The fourth-year AuD student was to have had comprehensive academic and clinical training such that the preceptor would do little more than round off the rough edges. The culmination of that effort was to have produced a competent audiologist, able to work independently within a few months of arrival at their externship site.

Unfortunately, at the time of this writing, a number of practitioners serving as preceptors express concerns that contemporary fourth-year students fall markedly short of an ability to work independently and require as much time and attention as did the CFYs of yesteryear. This is to be expected to some limited extent as fourth-year externships remain in relative infancy in the developing continuum that is the AuD degree. One hopes the efforts of the Accreditation Commission for Audiology Education (ACAE) continues to develop and move forward credentialing methods such that both academic and clinical preparation will be stratified to the extent that fourth-year externs can indeed "hit the ground running" instead of needing to be brought up to speed to make up for limited clinical experience and, in some cases, less than stellar academic preparation.

These reports point to the need for an honest and open dialogue between universities and preceptors about the training program's strengths and weaknesses. Although the extern remains a tuition-paying student during their fourth-year rotation, the preceptor has, de facto, accepted the role of mentor and guide in an important, pragmatic phase of the clinician's development. It is not, however, the task of the preceptor to shore up an extern's academic and clinical preparation. The preceptor should focus on providing an opportunity for the extern to be intimately involved in patient management and exposed to the operational realities of independent practice. If the university fails to respond to the issues brought forth in discussions, the fourth-year externship will remain a catch-up time rather than the experiential opportunity it was intended to become.

This situation should not be taken lightly. The bedrock of any health care profession is the independent professional providing services and improving the quality of life for their patients. If we, as a profession, fail to produce practitioners able to hang a shingle and make a living by providing services as an audiologist, we have failed ourselves and future generations of audiologists who may be doomed to providing services directed by ENTs or working under the signature of a medical director in a corporate or hospital-based practice setting.

Summary

Successful personnel management requires strong leadership: an ability to lead and motivate and guide an individual's development from employee to associate. Every practice should develop uniform protocols for recruiting good people to provide the services described in a concise position description. Good people in the right positions will contribute significantly to the primary mission of any audiology practice, which must center around patient and referral source satisfaction.

Orientation and training formulates the substrate that is the culture of the practice. It is the process by which all associates in the practice pull together as a unified team to optimize positive outcomes for every patient referred for services. Retaining good personnel is critical to the long-term health of the practice. The practice leader must conscientiously strive to maintain employee satisfaction as diligently as maintaining patient and referral source satisfaction. The success of a practice hinges on the capabilities and dynamic involvement of the practice leader. It is his or her duty to hire the best, focus on the mission of the practice, and keep patient, referral sources, and associates secure in the knowledge that by selecting their practice, they have made the right choice.

References

Burrows, D. L. (2006). Human resource issues: Managing, hiring, firing and evaluating employees. *Seminars in Hearing, 27*(1), 5–17.

Maxwell, J. C. (2002). *Leadership 101: What every leader needs to know.* Nashville, TN: Thomas Nelson.

McClain, G. S., & Romaine, D. S. (2007). *The everything managing people book.* Avon, MA: Adams Media.

15

Career Management: What It Takes to Make It

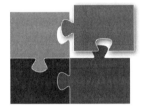

PATRICK N. MANGINO, AuD

Introduction

"Audiology is an expanding profession offering clinicians a variety of practice opportunities across a number of venues" (Traynor, 2008). Just as a business plan is essential to beginning a practice, planning your career path can significantly alter the success you experience during the course of your professional career. Regardless of your motivation, professional experiences and relationships play a vital role in a successful career. In the competitive environment that most health care professionals face

today, education and technical knowledge are not enough to assure success. Your success will also depend on characteristics such as, dedication, confidence, sincerity, attitude, and most of all, a passion for your profession.

As stated in a recruiting PowerPoint® developed by the American Academy of Audiology (2011), "The focus of the professional doctorate in audiology (AuD) is on the development of clinical proficiency" (slide 8). However, audiologists practice in many diverse settings:

■ Private practice
■ Community centers

- School systems
- Universities
- Hospitals
- Private clinics
- ENT/Otolaryngology offices
- Hearing aid manufacturing
- Federal and state governments
- General industries

As a result, audiologists frequently have had to learn business and management strategies. As the profession has evolved, a solid business and management foundation, business knowledge and acumen, and various personal skill sets are becoming increasingly important and essential. Without this type of knowledge and skill, the degree of success you experience as an audiologist can be severely limited. While your professional degrees provide the skill sets needed for clinical practice and prepare you with some basic business knowledge, the variety of settings within which audiologists practice require a broader bandwidth of skill sets and knowledge to be successful. Oftentimes, these skill sets are learned by trial and error.

Skill Sets

Character cannot be developed in ease and quiet. Only through experiences of trial and suffering can the soul be strengthened, vision cleared, ambition inspired and success achieved.

Helen Keller, Author, Activist, Presidential Medal of Freedom Recipient

Upon graduation, you will have the technical knowledge you need to start your career, but soon after, your professional experiences begin to require political,

business, and social knowledge in order to succeed within the many settings in which audiologists provide professional services. A plan for a patient may include diagnosis, treatment, therapy, counseling (e.g., family and significant others), prosthetic devices, training/teaching others (e.g., hearing aid orientation, listening skills), as well as administrative processes (recordkeeping, documentation), office/clinic management, financial management (financing services/products, payment plans, clinic operation budgets), and adherence to federal and state standards. Different skill sets will be required as you will have these varied work roles (e.g., financial management) and you will need key perspectives to be successful. You'll be applying unique strategies to the professional care of your patients and must be able to effectively communicate with others. You'll need team building skills and skills for developing professional relationships. Managerial and administrative skills will be required and keen decision-making will build and enhance your career. Since audiologists practice in so many different environments, to better serve patients, you may be called upon to coordinate care with medical, educational, industrial, social, psychological, manufacturing, and other business professionals.

Relationships

If your actions inspire others to dream more, learn more, do more, and become more, you are a leader.

John Quincy Adams, Statesman, 6th President of the United States

Much of your success will depend on several meaningful relationships. Core aspects of those relationships are patience and respect. If you take responsibility for those relationships, more often than not, at some point, the other person will also accept some responsibility for maintaining the relationship. With this sharing of responsibility positive things happen with individuals, organizations, teams, and so forth. Persistence in maintaining positive relationships and not giving up too soon when things get difficult will make a big difference in your level of professional success.

Relationships are an emotional or other connection among people: a connection, an association, or an involvement. The ability to develop and maintain relationships is often called "people skills." "People skills" are a primary skill required to successfully practice in almost any environment but development of these relationships is essential: (1) patient; (2) professional; and (3) staff and personnel.

A positive relationship with patients is critical to establishing your credibility and for gaining patient confidentiality in a clinical situation. Patients need to be convinced that you are not only an expert in your field, but that actions and strategies you conduct are done with the patient's best interest in mind. Patient relationships are critical to the establishment of a long-term plan for hearing health care, and positive relationships increase the likelihood of the patient's participation in the treatment plan presented. If a patient doesn't believe in you as a clinician, the benefit of the solution does not matter. He or she may not follow your recommendations or treatment plan to receive the benefit needed. To ensure that patients receive benefit from the clinical situation, a strong clinician-patient relationship must be built. Listening to patients engages communication strategies that serve to build strong relationships.

Relationships with other professionals can also serve to develop a patient base through referrals, assist with project developments, and provide opportunities to learn new or refined skills (e.g., administrative, managerial, networking). Positive professional relationships are longstanding and can have a positive influence throughout your entire career, helping to shape it, re-shape it, advance it, and validate your accomplishments. Many of these relationships are built by interactions with colleagues in your local community and by active participation in professional organizations.

Staff and personnel relationships are important to building an atmosphere of teamwork within your practice, clinic, or organization. In addition, they are a key factor within the organizational culture of your practice. Employee loyalty and involvement in your office or clinic is essential to your success. You must get personnel engaged in your business. You will need to earn their trust and instill values that everyone will respect. This builds a positive culture within your clinic, and will also contribute to professional relationships that may continue when a staff member relocates or accepts another position. These relationships can eventually assist in the future with recruiting new staff and sharing of professional knowledge in formulating treatment plans, and other interactions. Teamwork within your practice ensures a positive work environment and this adds to the quality of your professional services and builds a positive business and professional culture within your organization. In addition, this teamwork leads to the best hearing solutions for your patients and are the key to employee retention.

Within a private practice, business relationships are also important. To create a successful and efficient practice, a management team must include an attorney, an accountant, a manager, competent suppliers and a marketing specialist at the very least. Those involved in your business relationships need to share your perspective on your organizational goals, core values, and the nature of your business in order for their advice to be respected. Business relationships can also prove valuable in networking with other professionals care providers or product and service suppliers that have the same demographic target market. Opportunities for collegial cross-marketing and business development significantly improve the ability to grow and maintain your practice.

Success in any profession rests upon building relationships through confidence and trust. As an audiologist, you need to be confident in your ability to provide the best hearing health care solutions and convey them honesty and with sincerity to each patient. Similarly, the same confidence should be used with referral sources, business associates, staff members, and others to build trust and credibility and to ensure that your treatment plans will be successful. Getting others involved and engaged in your business culture does not require lighting a fire beneath people, but rather igniting the fire within to bring out your passion for the practice.

Communication

To effectively communicate, we must realize that we are all different in the way we perceive the world and use this understanding as a guide for our communication with others.

Anthony Robbins,
Leadership Psychologist,
Peak Performance Strategist

Communication can be defined as the imparting or interchange of thoughts, opinions, or information via speech, writing, or signs: an activity by one organism that changes or has the potential to change the behavior of other organisms. To express oneself properly and to get ideas across, communication must be effective and the message given from an expert, professional perspective. Expressing oneself clearly and effectively is required when communicating with patients about their treatment plans; with other professionals who are coordinating a treatment plan; with referral sources; with employees; and with superiors when presenting treatment options, procedures, unusual circumstances, or issues in the workplace. Effective communication involves not only delivering the message, but listening to and receiving the perspective of others. As an audiologist, you will encounter individuals with differing belief systems, value systems, needs, and perspectives. Understanding the perspectives of others, whether you agree with them or not, is a skill worth developing. The ability to understand the perspective of others is guided by listening and interpretive skills, along with a willingness for free exchange of ideas.

Communication begins with a measure of respect, an open mind, and an accepting attitude of another's point of view. An open mind sets aside biases and attempts to understand the other person's beliefs and value system. This requires withholding judgment and assumes approval; communications should encourage engagement in beliefs, perspectives, and values, as well as begin with an understanding of the other person's point of view. Beliefs and values are a matter of perception, and in most cases perception is reality. When understood through attentive listening, it is possible to understand a person's motivation, attitude, and reaction. This perspective taking can lead to consensus or, at least, to mutual agreement. The purpose or goal in most communications in your interaction with patients is to come to an agreement.

> Listening in dialogue is listening more to meaning than to words. In true listening, we reach behind the words and see through them, to find the person who is being revealed. Listening is a search to find the treasure of the true person as revealed verbally and nonverbally. There is the semantic problem, of course. The words bear a different connotation for you than they do for me. Consequently, I can never tell you what you said, but only what I heard. I will have to rephrase what you have said, and check it out with you to make sure that what left your mind and heart arrived in my mind and heart intact and without distortion. (Father John Powell, Professor of Theology Loyola University, Chicago)

For communication to be an effective process, the message sent has to be clear and concise, and simultaneously, the reception of the message has to be clearly understood. The content of a message and the choice of words can be the difference between success and failure in reaching a consensus on solutions. Much of the communication process is nonverbal; your body language (postures, facial expressions, gestures, eye contact), tone of voice, volume, and intonation, can make a significant difference in how effectively your communication is received. These nuances in the communication process set the tone and create the atmosphere for how a message is received and can often override the verbal message, affecting the whole conversation. Whether nonverbal or verbal, your communication skills will set the tone for

relationships, as one word, one phrase, one moment of poor body language can change the whole tone of a conversation. The main point in communication is to be consistent with what you say and how you say it. This avoids sending conflicting signals and eliminates any potential confusion about the message being delivered. Trusting relationships are built with consistent messages, even if they are not always agreeable. Consistency leads to sincere and trusting relationships. When the verbal and nonverbal parts of a communication are incongruent, the nonverbal influence is what people remember, and the nonverbal message becomes the primary message.

Negotiations

I've learned that people will forget what you said, people will forget what you did, but people will never forget how you made them feel.

> Dr. Maya Angelou,
> Author, Actor, Poet
> Presidential Medal of
> Arts Recipient

There are several skills sets needed to develop and maintain relationships requiring negotiations, including conducting or analyzing financial reports, understanding the process requiring negotiation, effective communication, and other components. Negotiation is a mutual discussion that usually consists of an arrangement of the terms of a transaction or agreement—the act or process of mutual agreement. The capacity to negotiate, formally or informally, is a valuable skill and crucial for reaching fair and mutually agreed upon settlement to issues. An ability to skillfully negotiate may be needed on several occasions during a successful professional career. In clinics, service and supply agreements, third-party pay agreements for products and services, community outreach programs, industrial hearing conservation programs, and satellite or remote facilities contracts are all instances requiring negotiation skills. In some instances, these negotiated programs can be the lifeblood of the financial basis for maintaining your ongoing business. Consequently, to maintain an ongoing relationship, it is important to begin with a fair and mutually beneficial agreement or contract. Another area where clinics may use negotiating skills is with work employee agreements or personnel contracts. Initial proposals should be put together with the assistance of attorneys, accountants, financial advisors, as there are many labor laws and other employee regulations that require consideration. Once negotiations begin, a clinic needs to comfortable with the fiscal feasibility of the agreement when viewed as part of the whole.

In audiology private practices, negotiations for agreements are also applicable. Certain components of the business, such as when renting/leasing office space is required, are negotiable and the end result can have a significant effect on the bottom line of your business. To negotiate successfully, an appropriate assessment of the value of the space for issues such as traffic flow, type of space (retail, medical), full-time or part-time location, amount of space required (square footage), what is included in the rent/lease (utilities, common area maintenance), maintenance costs, and the projected revenue for that location is critical. Once the value has been determined, negotiation from a position of strength can be accomplished.

Additionally, marketing agreements for television, yellow pages, newspapers, among others, offer standard proposals for various types and styles of media. Sales representatives rally for you to choose from one their standard marketing packages and may imply the fees are not negotiable; however, the fees are frequently negotiable. To determine the value of marketing options, the clinic or you in your private practice need to analyze and project the return on your investment and negotiate accordingly. Placements of ads, frequency, time slots, days of the week, and so forth all enter into valuing the importance of marketing arrangements.

When negotiating, initial proposals, are usually be skewed toward the party offering the proposal. Although it is reasonable to slant the initial offering, the initial offering cannot be so slanted that it is insulting. Since parties will be interested in getting the most they can out of an agreement process, "No" is a good place to start. During negotiations, realism and fairness for both parties may not become evident until a process of compromise brings the two sides together. For the negotiation process to be successful, there must be benefits for both sides.

Promotional/Public Relations Skills

Everything you do or say is public relations.

Anonymous

Promotion and public relations refer to the actions of a corporation, store, government, individual, or other entity in promoting goodwill among itself, the general public, the community, employees, customers, and all that interact with the practice. As part of developing a practice, promotion of your facility as expert in hearing health care is important. Taking advantage of public relations opportunities, using local media, is an effective and inexpensive means of presenting this message. By using public media, your message not only goes to consumers, but also to medical and other allied health care professionals, industries, and associations.

An element of public relations is educating consumers in your community about your products and services. This is a precursor to establishing meaningful relationships that will drive your practice or clinic's success. These marketing and educational communications reach the consumers and need to motivate them into taking action. Public relations strategies communicate important messages about the practice directly to consumers and influential associates. These strategies can put a particular practice "top of mind" when it comes to hearing healthcare services. Knowing your local media, their likes and dislikes, their scheduling, and their various formats for getting messages out (e.g., TV, newspaper, radio, Internet) is advantageous to getting your message heard and understood in the marketplace.

Public relations messages are frequently viewed as unbiased, sincere, informative, and less commercial. In addition, a public relations message frequently carries a human-interest theme. These human-interest stories can be informative and of interest to prospective patients, or of interest to those who may provide networking opportunities. They may be about you, a staff member, your facility, a patient, or work done within the community. In considering these messages, be confident, creative, and proactive. Use stories that fit into the bigger picture of hearing healthcare and emphasize the message of your practice. It helps for consumers to perceive you as an expert who is different and unique from the group of hearing health care professionals in your community.

Develop rapport with the reporter and other media professionals and attempt to become their go-to person for any questions they may have on hearing, tinnitus, or balance. Since these media professionals are looking for stories and repeat business, it is possible to become their initial and only contact for this type of information, giving you a big advantage in developing your business (Thomas, 2007).

Sales

If you work just for money, you'll never make it. But if you love what you are doing, and always put the customer first, success will be yours.

Ray Kroc, CEO, McDonalds

It's not the employer who pays the wages. Employers only handle the money. It's the customer who pays the wages.

Henry Ford, Founder, Ford Motor Company

"Sales" is operationally defined as transferring property for money, credit or other forms of recognition. In the not too distant past, the term "sales" had a markedly negative connotation in the audiology community. It was as if there was something inherently wrong with audiologists admitting they sold their services and attendant products: hearing instruments and related items. "Sales," however, is not a four-letter word.

The origins of these negative connotations began in many university programs as part of the educational process of audiologists. The concept was set forth under the guise of an "us" versus "them" debate based more in academic arrogance than any firm evidence beyond hearsay, as licensing boards were nonexistent or at best in their infancy at that time. Student audiologists were led to believe that there was an inherent conflict of interest wherein professionals would be sacrificing their integrity while pursuing revenue for services provided. A "true" professional could not be involved in "sales." This thinking persisted far too long in the face of other health care providers such as optometrists, dentists and physicians all of whom traded their particular expertise on a fee-for-service basis.

Wherever knowledgeable and credible resources for hearing health solutions are sought, selling our professionalism to a patient occurs. Selling takes place in any audiology practice venue: for-profit clinics, nonprofit community centers, private audiology practices, ENT offices, hospitals, and purely diagnostic settings.

Unless the patient believes in you as the professional to deliver his or her hearing health solution, he or she will not follow your prescribed treatment plan. When patients are in denial and need convincing, a selling proposition arises and how you set forth the options in your treatment plan will significantly affect the outcome of the journey about to unfold for the patient. The same is true in a research effort. The concept, the journey, and the benefits of the potential outcome(s) of the research must be sold well to secure funding and grants and other forms of support.

Sales skills are also valuable in the building of referral relationships, as you'll want to be perceived as ethical and credible as well as knowledgeable. In business relationships, it is essential to build a bond of trust. In personnel relationships, loyalty, sincerity, and honesty are important. In patient and professional relationships, credibility, knowledge, sincerity, integrity, loyalty, and commitment are all valuable assets and are personal characteristics you will need to "sell" about yourself.

In private practice, sales skills generally are important to all aspects of the business. Many functions within the office involve sales skills. Providing solutions for a patient involves the sale of varying levels of hearing instruments. Depending on your philosophy, there are many levels of technology at various price points. This complicates the process, as the consumer (and often other professionals) may be suspicious of anyone "selling" hardware (the product) versus someone selling his or her professional services (somehow that seems impartial to the patient). If the patient needs a more sophisticated instrument, with more features and incrementally more advanced technology, costs to procure and fit these technologies will increase the cost the patient will have to pay. Increased costs makes the patient hesitant, or at best, cautious. A more complex counseling and sales strategy is necessary in these situations. When it comes to a more costly purchase, confidence and trust in you and your skills are critically important.

Problem Solving/Analysis

What gets measured gets improved.
Peter Drucker,
Founder of Modern Management

To improve quality and promote growth, accurate tracking and analysis of treatment plans, business strategies, administrative processes, and management strategies is extremely important. Throughout the development of and, improvement in the efficacy of services, outcome measures must be calculated accurately and analyzed in such a way that areas of greatest need are emphasized. In any clinical practice, goals for treatment plans and for increasing the reach of your services are set. Goals can only be reached with consistent and periodic analyses of your services, processes, and strategies and any change that occurs is dependent on an appropriate set of performance metrics. This is the first step in an ongoing process of improving and building upon the hearing health care solutions you offer.

Many businesses have developed a set of key performance indicators that measure performance levels in several specific areas. Depending on the goals, the bandwidth of these metrics may yield important data about the efficacy of your marketing initiatives, your financial solvency (including pricing strategies and compensation strategies), performance comparisons year over year, your proximity to reaching goals set, training needs within your facility, staff motivation, market-shares, and/or staff performance. Once this information is gathered, analysis needs to be conducted in a logical, methodical manner to derive answers to the questions that allow you to focus resources and energy in the most appropriate areas. Analysis helps you maximize your efforts to achieve the desired change.

As an indicator of areas of greatest need, set benchmarks for each measure evaluated. These benchmarks will direct you or your manager to the areas that are in the most need, allowing prioritization of strategies for improvement. When measuring results that include several locations or care providers, the overall organization averages are the beginning benchmark. This allows focusing on those locations that are the most below the benchmark. At times, if the whole organization is underperforming, the average may not be your final goal, but it is a good starting point. As areas improve, the average will also improve, raising the bar and setting the goals closer to where you think is ideal.

The most important part of employing appropriate metrics is the ability to effectively analyze and interpret the results so solutions continuously improve the efficiency of the clinic. For example, if there is an unusually high cancellation rate or scheduled time is not utilized properly, it may be necessary to evaluate the effectiveness of your processes and/or protocols. Are appointments being confirmed in an appropriate manner? Is the right person doing the confirmations? Do they need to be scripted? Are appointments being scheduled too far out? Is there a need for training? Do you need to replace staff with insufficient skill sets? Is the staff used in a way that takes advantage of their strengths or weaknesses?

Not only have there been great changes in technology, but the marketplace has changed more in the past 5 years than it had ever in the previous 25 years.

Consumers, led by the baby boomers, are much more informed in their initial contact than ever before. These changes require continual evaluation of your clinic's performance and adjustment of processes, goals, and strategies in an ongoing manner. The only plausible method to make these adjustments is to use benchmarking, measurement, and analysis that facilitates the best, most cost-effective means for improvement.

Fiscal Responsibility

There is only one boss, the customer [patient]. And they can fire everybody in the company from the chairman on down, simply by spending their money somewhere else.

Sam Walton (1918–1992),
Founder of Walmart

In virtually any audiology setting, fiscal responsibility is required to ensure the continuance of services for an indefinite period of time. This assurance is provided through profitability and retained earnings, a natural result of accepting fiscal responsibility and the fiduciary duties of running a business. The first practitioner responsibility is to be profitable and stay in business to serve patients. Profitability cannot be viewed as a choice, but an obligation to patients. Continued and future earnings ensure that state of the art facilities and equipment are available for patient care.

The first step in accepting fiscal management responsibility of the clinic is the periodic review of financial statements, especially income statements (also called profit and loss statements) and balance sheets. Income statements are an indi-

cation of the practice's financial performance and assist in determining cash flow, pricing strategies, compensation strategies, operational costs, cost of goods, and other expenses. It shows how and where profit or loss was incurred during a specified assessment period. The balance sheet is a statement of a business's financial condition at any moment in time (as opposed to the income/profit and loss statement, which refers to a period of time). The balance sheet presents a summary of the business assets, liabilities, and equity, and is an indicator of liquidity and/or net worth. Although the income statements are a good indicator of profitability resulting from the effects of day-to-day operations, the balance sheet offers the overall results of a business's net worth, including the effects of loans, capital investment (equity), and any other liabilities. An informed, periodic, and methodical review of these statements is necessary to determine the effects of operational strategies on the solvency of the business. During hard economic times or unusual downturns in a business's profitability, financials can deteriorate fairly quickly. Knowing quick strategic reactions for maintaining solvency in a changing environment is critical. At times, small changes in pricing or compensation strategies can make the difference losing a business or making one profitable and self-sustaining.

The efficient use of financial statements requires setting up a financial plan with benchmarks to measure performance. This allows quick re-focus of efforts, should it be required, to appropriate areas. Setting benchmarks for the four or five most costly expenses that can be controlled is a part of a solid financial plan. For example, a hearing aid practice sets benchmarks or ratios for marketing, payroll expenses, the cost of goods, modified operating expenses, and net income. When a given measure falls outside the benchmark, an adjustment must be made in another area to stay profitable. The benchmarks may not totally define the issues, but they will point to the area where further due diligence is required to discover the problem and determine the solution. For instance, if cost of goods is outside the benchmark, negotiating a better price with a vendor or adjusting a pricing strategy may be required. If payroll costs are beyond the benchmark, revenue from sales may need to be increased or additional revenue-generating services/products added, or compensation strategies may need to be adjusted accordingly.

Benchmarking can also assist with budgeting for future performance and growth. In a mature business, a historical perspective provides a good basis for setting benchmarks and budgeting. In a new practice, industry averages or guidelines may be a starting point, but these data are difficult to find outside franchise operations or major buying group association. Even if the data are available, regional markets differ and the difference can affect the applicability of the figures to your particular market. Annual budgets set should be considered flexible and a budgeting a dynamic process. Budgets should be reviewed at least every quarter and adjustments made according to your business plan. (See Chapter 8, Fiscal Monitoring: Cash Flow Analysis).

Motivating Others

The rung of a ladder was never meant to rest upon, but only to hold a man's foot long enough to enable him to put the other somewhat higher.

Thomas Henry Huxley

As a manager and/or supervisor, the skill to effectively motivate staff, associates, and colleagues is very important. Mediocre results are easily achieved; obtaining various levels of excellence is more challenging. Motivating an individual to excel can require various forms of inducements or incentives. Depending on the values and personal style of the individual you are trying to motivate, the motivational tools used will vary. Motivation may be enticed using forms of verbal or intangible reinforcement on varying schedules. Some are motivated when they feel a sense of accomplishment, leading to satisfaction. Most people settle into their own personal comfort zones. An effective manager understands staff strengths and weaknesses. Placing individuals in positions where their strengths are maximized for benefit of the organization is crucial. Helping to set realistic, reachable goals and providing appropriate rewards for achievements will result in garnering efforts well beyond that which is simply required.

Incentives tend to motivate people to take action or make greater effort. Incentives, usually financial considerations given above the usual pay, can be offered as a reward for increased productivity. Financial incentives are often done in appreciation for work conducted, length of service, accumulated efforts, and are a premium paid for something extra or additional hard work given freely. As an audiologist, you may have been trained that receiving or providing financial incentives is an inherent breech of ethics, for there is an assumed conflict of interest. However, this ethical challenge can inhibit your pursuit of excellence. By motivating employees beyond their comfort levels, by motivating them to go from "good to great," from satisfactory to excellent, from achieving to overachieving, will ensure success in your business.

Ethics

Wisdom is to know the path to take, integrity is taking it.

Linda Lucas

Ethics is a set of principles that leads to a moral decision for justification of an action. They lead to rules of conduct that guide professionals through their careers. These rules are an internalized and personalized code of conduct based on an individual's moral principles and are difficult to apply to the general population. Rules of conduct guiding professional behavior vary from one profession to another and from one given situation to another. Most professional organizations set minimum standards that they believe define the minimum rules of conduct for ethical behavior. The varying nature and complexity of issues that professionals encounter and the unknown circumstances of practice cause quandaries in conduct and moral principles. Adherence to ethics must be considered paramount. No matter the personal benefit of a decision, it must be made in the best interest of the patient.

Ethical dilemmas often lead to a series of introspection and questions. For example, consider this dilemma: a patient purchased a hearing aid with a 2-year warranty from a competitor. The patient has never been satisfied with the device that is now 18 months old, but paid a lot of money for what could be considered an adequate hearing aid but not an optimal device. You could make adjustments to the device to address all of the patient's concerns, or you could recommend purchasing a higher-quality hearing instrument. Are both of these options legal? Are both of them ethical? Which one has more moral value? Most would consider them both legal, however, the ethical nature of the situation is a more personalized decision based on a set of internalized principles and values. The ethical question may be answered differently depending on your personal value system.

Developing a sense of ethical standards often depends on life experiences, morals, and internalized values. There may be times when colleagues do not agree on the ethical implications of a decision, but it may necessary to be consistent and true to your internalized values. Ethical decisions are always made in the patient's best interest but his or her best interest is not always obvious. Should patients be given all the information or is withholding some facts best to avoid undue stress to a patient? Should the audiologist only consider the product that is best for a patient or should the patient's financial status be considered? Or should the audiologist explain the value of best instrument and let the patient make the decision? Is it best to determine needs or to guide patients in making educated decisions? In making these decisions, ponder two questions: What and why is a particular course of action taken?

Summary

Although the above list of skills can be viewed as facilitators for a successful professional career, the list is not exhaustive.

Beyond formal education that prepares for "clinical proficiency," professional and life experiences will formulate your professional principles, ethical standards, personalized rules of conduct, and professional perspective that will shape your career. These principles, standards, rules, and perspective build long-standing professional relationships that will become crucial in establishing your professional and community credibility. Sales skills and appropriate analysis of fiscal measures will lead to the continuous development of your practice or clinic. These factors ultimately provide benefits to the patients you serve and ensure an indefinite continuance of professional service. As long as fiscal responsibility is maintained and ethical service providers are motivated, your clinic and the services it provides will benefit the patients.

There is a place within all of us which lies dormant until someone or something ignites the purest and most powerful source of energy known: passion. Passion drives the engine of greatness, leaving a wake of success behind. Draw yourself to those sparks that drive your passions: our world will change immensely.

References

American Academy of Audiology. (2011). *A career in audiology.*

Thomas, M. (2007). *Access Audiology*, *6*(2).

Traynor, R. (2008). Strategic business planning. In R. Glaser & R. Traynor (Eds.), *Strategic practice management: A patient-centric approach* (pp. 1–24). San Diego, CA: Plural.

16

Compensation Strategies

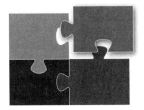

ROBERT M. TRAYNOR, EdD, MBA

Introduction

Probably the most difficult area of practice management is dealing with employees, also called human resources. Of course the goal is to be fair with employees, compensating them enough to be motivated and excited to go to work each day. Most practices, however, are small with no human resource department; usually the owner of the practice becomes the human resource director. Audiologists have generally maintained an anxious relationship with compensation since the 1970s when the profession first began dispensing hearing instruments. At that time, audiologists were compensated by a salary with a benefits package that sustained and motivated most professionals. These compensation packages, at the time, were, paid mostly by hospitals, physicians, universities, or government agencies. The profession typically provided services, evaluations, and other nonproduct related functions that, not only created difficulty making a decent living in the field, but was cumbersome clinically interacting with the hearing with the hearing impaired. Carrison and Walsh (1999) suggest that businesses, particularly human resources, should be maintained by the principles and techniques of the United States Marine Corps, building motivation for the mission and esprit de corps rather than merely a compensation package. They indicate that for all the differences between the military and the profit driven corporation, these enterprises share the same key goal: to create a high performance organization filled with committed, motivated personnel. Unfortunately, today's professionals are unlike the military and look to the compensation package first and motivation, esprit de corps, and the mission of the practice is usually secondary. The military takes each recruit and molds, shapes, trains, and educates to exacting standards for each and every job and at each base, the job will be essentially the same. Realistically, audiologists and our practices are very diverse and audiologists now toil for eight years in university program acquiring their clinical credentials. At the end of their study, they should feel well compensated for the time, energy, and effort spent in school and gaining experience to serve their patients.

This anxious relationship with compensation becomes complicated when there is a balancing act between fair compensation methods for clinicians, ethical standards created by the profession and fairness to patients. On the one hand, the profession and many clinicians are not comfortable with variable compensation methods, but typical salary compensation systems lead to less motivation, less overall compensation for professionals and, as a result, less efficiency in the revenue generation for the practice. Audiologist employees within a practice should be compensated to allow a good living commensurate with their credentials and experience and, possibly, an opportunity to buy into the practice over time. Clerical employees should receive salary, benefits, and other compensation based

upon their experience, longevity, and contributions to the practice.

Strategies for compensation are not straightforward; they are compounded not only by ethics and historical methods, but also by annual reviews, raise procedures, profit participation, incentives, rewards, new government regulations, and other frustrating but necessary complexities. Therefore, the purpose of this chapter is to present perspectives into various intangible and tangible components of compensation packages for an audiology practice with special emphasis on payment arrangements for practice owners, their professional audiologist employees, and clerical staff.

The Nature of Compensation

Atchison, Belcher, and Thomson (2010) presents that compensating people is a complex task requiring organizational systems and practices. In the discussion of the various compensation systems and practices and the influences on them both inside and outside the organization it should be noted that there are new outside influences on compensation expectations, such as Internet searches for differences in cities, components of the profession that offer more compensation for less work, and even chat rooms that discuss these issues. Atchison et al. (2010) also explain that compensation, like a coin, has two sides; it represents income to employees and cost to the employer. The term compensation is used to indicate the various forms of pay such as money, benefits, and nonfinancial rewards.

Compensation packages for any size business have two both intangible and tangible components and, according to

Elsdon (2003), the key to obtaining and keeping good employees, particularly professionals, is to create an environment in where employees want to stay and grow professionally with the practice. Although compensation packages in a small audiology practice are generally less than large firms, providing expertise and contributions to a small company has definite advantages for the employees. Shwiff (2007) indicates that these advantages include:

■ An opportunity to be more "hands on."
■ The need to wear multiple hats that result in a wider range of experiences and enhanced skills.
■ Greater chance for recognition for contributions.
■ The "big frog-small pond" factor that result in speedier promotions and greater personal benefits.
■ A stronger sense of ownership of work completed.
■ A culture more geared to fulfilling employee needs.
■ Job that better utilizes employee's aptitudes and interests.
■ Flextime and telecommuting.
■ A chance to buy stock options and possibly benefit financially from personal contributions to the practice.

Generally, there are three classes of individuals within an audiology practice each with different compensation packages; the owner, employee audiologists and the clerical staff. Audiology practice owners are entrepreneurs, investing in a business to offer private clinical services to the public. For the practice owner, their monthly salary is sustenance. The perquisites (perks) of ownership can provide special benefits; the hope to sell the practice for a retirement income, independence, and, one hopes, the sat-

isfaction of watching their small business grow into a thriving practice. Mathis and Jackson (2004) present three common elements of employment compensation packages; the psychological contract, job satisfaction, and loyalty and commitment. A portion of the package offered by the employee and paid for by the employer includes these factors that may be an exceptional value or a substantial problem, depending on the practice situation and the employee.

The Psychological Contract

Lavelle (2003) defines a psychological contract as an unwritten expectation between employees and employers regarding the nature of their work relationship that is, to some degree, based upon past experiences of both parties. This psychological contract is a direct result of the downsizing of companies over the past few years and the resulting "free agent" nature of employees. In the past, employees may have given their loyalty and commitment to a company and been disappointed as the company had minimal commitment to them, cutting their pay, or involuntarily modifying their work relationship. When a company (or a practice) has a minimal commitment to their employees, they often become free agents offering their services to the highest bidder with no particular commitments beyond the contract dates.

Although, recently employees have questioned if a company (or a practice) is worth their loyalty and commitment, Lee (2001) offers that when individuals feel they have some control and perceived rights in the organization, they are more likely to be committed to the organization. Thompson and Bunderson (2003) have also indicated that psychological contracts are strengthened and enhanced when an organization (such as an audiology practice) is involved in a cause that the employee values highly. Audiology practices working toward a better quality of life for their patients are very likely to obtain a psychological commitment from both the employer and the employee since they both firmly believe in the cause. Clerical employees also feel a sense of belonging to the process and usually become psychologically involved, working toward the common goal of better hearing for the patients.

Job Satisfaction

Mathis and Jackson (2004) broadly define job satisfaction as a positive emotional state resulting from evaluating one's job experience. Conversely, job dissatisfaction occurs when expectations are not met for either the employee or the employer. Figure 16–1 offers factors that affect job satisfaction. For an audiology practice the satisfaction of the employees with their position is very important to success since often it is the employees that represent the practitioner to the patients.

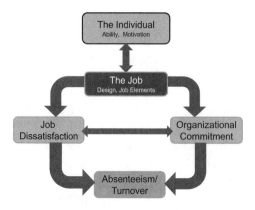

Figure 16–1. Factors affecting job satisfaction and organizational commitment (Mathis & Jackson, 2004).

Performance should never be of concern if the employee is a fully educated, licensed audiologist or an experienced clerical employee. Although an employee may have the training and the experience, sometimes motivation to provide the evaluations, products or support services may be lacking. Motivational difficulties may include, but are not limited to:

- Illness.
- A fight with a wife or husband that morning.
- A bad day.
- Low or reduced respect for the boss.
- Disagreement with the policies and procedures of the practice.
- General laziness.

Whatever the motivational problem, it is essential that these difficulties be rectified as soon as possible as they will only get worse, creating even more concern for the practice owner, the other employees, and, ultimately, the patients.

Job satisfaction also is part of the job itself. Although employees expect to be able to perform in the position for which they are hired, a clerical employee may not expect to clean hearing aids as part of their position or an employee audiologist may not expect that they will need to answer the phone, as these activities may have not been part of their former positions. Part of creating satisfaction is the explanation of the position so the employee knows, up front, the practice owner's expectations. Job satisfaction is greatly enhanced by openness in the job interview and is greatly assisted by the use of job descriptions presenting the specifics of each position in the practice along with expected extra duties. This "up front" presentation of expectations leads to high overall job satisfaction, which results in the employee's commitment to the organization. Motivated, committed employees have less absenteeism and are less likely to be looking elsewhere for employment. In tight labor markets or where audiologists are not readily available, job satisfaction and loyalty to the organization are clear factors in turnover (BNA.com, 2007).

Organizational Commitment

According to Mathis and Jackson (2004), organizational commitment is the degree to which the employees believe in and accept the organizational goals and desire to remain with the organization. Their data suggest that employees with a minimal commitment to the organization are not as satisfied with their jobs and are more likely to withdraw from the organization. Wasti (2003) offers that the relationship between job satisfaction and commitment with absenteeism and turnover has been affirmed across cultures, full and part time work, genders, and occupations. Findings demonstrate that absenteeism and turnover are related as both involve withdrawal from the organization, absenteeism being a temporary withdrawal from the organization whereas turnover is permanent.

Types and Philosophies of Compensation

In a comparison of the human resource literature, philosophical differences exist in terminology for various types of reward systems but, in general, compensation may be either intrinsic or extrinsic (Hay Group, 2002; Mathis & Jackson, 2004).

Intrinsic or Intangible Compensation

Intrinsic rewards are intangible and may include praise or expressions of appreciation for a job well done or meeting performance objectives. Other psychological and social forms of compensation, such as paid time off, social status, travel opportunities, and retirement plans are also intrinsic forms of employee rewards.

For many employees, the most valuable part of a compensation package is the intangible benefits offered by the position. Randolph (2005) in a study of 500 allied professional subjects found that intrinsic factors such as professional growth and having a work environment in line with personal values are more significant in predicting career satisfaction than extrinsic factors such as pay and continuing education. Obringer (2007) indicates that balancing lives has become more important than ever making flexible schedules, relaxed atmospheres, child care and other lifestyle benefits almost as important as salaries. In a poll of 10,300 employees, Levey and Levey (2000) found five important qualities most desired by employees in the United States, Europe, Russia, and Japan:

1. The ability to balance work and personal life.
2. Work that is truly enjoyable.
3. Security for the future.
4. Good pay or salary.
5. Enjoyable coworkers.

Tangible compensation appeared as a distant fourth on their list of reasons for quitting positions, suggesting the importance of intangible benefits. More than two thirds indicated that they would be willing to leave their company for such opportunities. Obringer (2007) also indicated that 90% of 1,000 workers felt work/life balance was as important as health insurance and more than one-fourth of those surveyed considered the balance of work and family was more important than a competitive salary, job security, or support for an advanced degree.

In a study supporting the importance of indirect or intangible benefits of employment, Anderson and Zhu (2002) found that 30% of all employees planned to quit their jobs in the next two years. Their survey indicated that it was not necessarily due to their cash compensation package but rather a function of the following reasons presented here in their order of importance.

1. Dissatisfaction with the manager.
2. Lack of career opportunities.
3. Job not "stretching" enough.
4. Personal reasons (spouse, partner moving on, maternity, etc.).
5. Cash compensation.

Note that cash compensation, at least in this study, was the last reason people

were quitting their jobs, suggesting intangibles are substantially more important than actual cash. Thus, the literature indicates that it is usually the intrinsic compensation not salary dissatisfaction that leads employees to explore alternative job prospects (Anderson & Zhu, 2002).

Extrinsic or Tangible Compensation

Extrinsic rewards are tangible and may be both monetary and nonmonetary. Tangible rewards are of two types:

- Direct compensation
- Indirect compensation.

Direct compensation is the money that changes hands in the form of base pay and variable pay, offered by the employer to the employee in exchange for the work performed. Indirect compensation usually refers to the employee benefits, such as health insurance offered to all employees as part of employment in the organization. Figure 16–2 clarifies direct

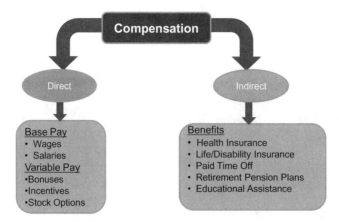

Figure 16–2. Components of a compensation system (Mathis & Jackson, 2004).

and indirect compensation for employees and represents the system by which most practice employees are compensated.

Compensation Philosophies

Professional employees can be compensated in a variety of arrangements. Shwiff (2007) offers some business models for paying professional employees that are not unlike those offered to employee physicians, dentists, chiropractors, and other health care professionals.

Entitlement-Based Programs

Entitlement programs are those that assume all employees who have worked another year are entitled to pay increases with little or no regard for performance. Organizations that use an entitlement philosophy will commonly refer to these yearly increases as "cost of living" increases and they may or may not be tied to actual economic indicators. The net result of using an entitlement philosophy is that the employer will pay more for their employees each year, no matter what the performance of the business, since raises and bonuses become income to which employees feel entitled. Characteristics of entitlement compensation programs are as follows:

- Seniority bases.
- Across the board raises.
- Pay scales raised annually.
- "Santa Claus" bonuses.

Performance-Based Programs

Lawler (2003) indicates that there is a trend to offer pay for performance among Fortune 1000 companies. In a performance-based compensation philosophy, pay changes reflect the true differences among employees. Employees that perform satisfactorily or better advance in their positions, whereas those who are poor or marginal performers fall behind in the pay scale. These performance-based systems award bonuses and incentives according to the performance of an individual, the team, or the organization. Characteristics of performance based compensation systems typically are:

- No raises for length of service.
- No raises for longer service poor performers.
- Job market adjusted pay structures.
- Broader compensation comparisons across the industry.
- Bonuses tied to performance results.

Audiology practices need to decide what type of a compensation system they want to offer. The particulars of the system offered will be based on the philosophy of the practice owner, the job market, economic conditions and the competitive compensation packages available within the region.

Straight Salary

According to Shwiff (2007), employees often prefer the straight approach, whereas more companies and professional practices are moving toward the alternative methods of compensation to get more out of their employees and spread their human resource costs across good and bad business seasons (Table 16–1).

Straight salary compensation systems are the traditional method of payment where the professional audiologist works in the clinic for a certain number of hours per week and are compensated with

Table 16–1. Compensation Philosophies

	Straight Salary	Variable Pay	Skill Based
Advantages	1. Easy 2. Dependable for employees	1. Incentives 2. Rewards 3. Motivating 4. Variable cost	1. Incentive to learn new skills 2. Training for the employee 3. Higher trained staff
Disadvantages	1. No incentive 2. No rewards 3. Fixed cost	1. Ethical concern 2. Pay varies	1. Base pay begins lower 2. Must build skills to advance base pay 3. Training costs

a salary. In this model, the employee obtains the same amount of salary each month for the work provided if the clinic is active or slow. The individual will actually be contracted for all the work they can possibly do within the confines of the practice schedule. These systems usually offer no rewards for extra effort, hard work, cross-training, and/or overtime, and there is usually none exerted. Although experience suggests that straight salaries work relatively well for clerical individuals and part timers, this system usually fails to provide sufficient motivation for a full time audiologist. A straight salary compensation method does not consider:

- The practice cash flow situations.
- Incentives for the employee.
- Rewards for extra work or creativity.

Practices generally are susceptible to seasonal highs and lows. Many patients return to spend the summer in climates they have left due to the cold in winter months. In extremely slow periods, it would not be beneficial for the employer to pay a salary when the opportunity to produce revenue is at low ebb. Conversely, when these "snow birds" return the audiologist employee will be working extremely hard.

Variable Compensation Model

The variable compensation model, sometimes referred to as "pay at risk," places a portion of the compensation contingent upon performance. This model provides incentives for employees by allowing them to share the profit that is generated by their increased contributions to the productivity of the practice. Meek (2007) indicates that most compensation systems are boring, do not pay for performance, or encourage commitment to the organization. In many fields, surveys point out that employees are not motivated by their current compensation system and in fact, do not even believe their performance has any influence on compensation. She suggests that, among others, a variable compensation program should include the following components:

- *Profit Sharing.* Profit sharing programs are employee incentives wherein a portion of the practice's profits will be set aside at year end and distributed to the employees.
- *Group Incentive.* Group incentives are given for participation in a group project or an overall goal of the practice.
- *Recognition, individual incentive, or key contributor awards.* These awards are for the individual achievement by a particular employee, such as the completion of an AuD, obtaining skills that will be useful to the practice, high sales, or other individual contribution to the practice that results in benefit to the practice. These awards may take the form of a lump sum bonus, awards of stock or equity in the practice, or simply a restaurant coupon or a plaque, but are to recognize their individual contribution.
- *Project/Team Incentive.* Group awards that involve a team of individuals that work together to further the goals of the practice. These awards are for group efforts that contribute to the success of the practice, such as a busy month, learning a new office management system, or other group effort that makes the practice more efficient.
- *Participative Peer Award.* Nominations of an employee by another employee for a job well done that may not be obvious to the practice owner. These are also individual awards that may take most any form, but are usually reserved for small rewards such as lunch or dinner, plaques, or some other simple recognition.

Designing a variable compensation program is no small task. An incentive program that rewards employee for diligent, hard work and providing excellent patient centric care will go a long way employee motivation. McNamara (2007) indicates that special care should be taken by the practitioner in the design of a variable pay program offering the following:

- A program that links variable pay to the practice business philosophy, preferably patient-centric practices.
- A program based on long-term objectives possibly geared to partnership or practice ownership, not just short term results.
- Deferred compensation opportunities, such as sharing the profit of the practice to attract and retain good professional employees.
- Well-understood details by every employee through education and regular scheduled face-to-face meetings about practice success or challenges.
- Sets realistic goals within the reach and control of the professional employees.
- Rewards team accomplishments, such as the clerical and professional teams as well as individual goals.

Skill-Based Compensation

Murphy (2004) defines a skill-based compensation program as a nontraditional pay system that ties base wages of the employee to knowledge and skills obtained rather than simply the job to which they are assigned. Shwiff (2007) explains that these skill-based programs reward individuals for acquiring certain work related skills or for being able to perform additional technical tasks. For example, if the practice conducts intraoperative monitoring, and an employee audiologist acquires the knowledge and skill sets necessary to provide monitoring services, that audiologist should be appropriately compensated for learning and using the new skill. Compensation should be issued as a raise in base pay or in the form of a pay differential when providing services in the operating room. Skill-based compensation could be applied to audiologists who seek and attain specialty certification in cochlear implants or pediatrics or advanced training that would enable the practice to expand or add new diagnostic or treatment protocols. Furthermore, practices often hire new audiologists directly out of school and these individuals are not initially able to conduct all evaluations on all populations in a timely manner or working with their own patients immediately. Skill-based compensation works well for these new clinicians as they will get used to the equipment, specifics of the practice's procedures in a short time. Thus, the base starting pay for a new clinician may need to be lower and increased as the skills and the capability to work independently increases. Lawson (2006) presents that skill based compensation programs are developed to:

- Encourage skill development.
- Reward learning.
- Increase individual productivity.
- Encourage more flexible staffing.

Computing a Tangible Base Salary and Salary Range For Employees

An important step in compensation for a practice is setting the base pay and salary ranges for all employees. This should be part of every position job description.

Obringer (2007) describes the procedure for establishing a standard base pay program. She offers fixed salary ranges for employees performing the standard duties of their jobs. In her system, an audiologist that has only conducted diagnostics for five years or a new audiologist directly out of school might be on the lower end of the scale, whereas veteran clinician able to see a full range of patients for services would be a the top of the compensation range. Although setting a base pay structure can be confusing, the following points should be considered:

- Determine where your practice falls relative to competitive compensation packages within the region.
- Set up your base pay levels to be competitive with other practices in the area or else you risk losing good employees.
- Use the Internet to review salaries, nationally, and regionally. A good starting place for these salary reviews is the American Academy of Audiology (http://www.audiology.org) or Audiology Online (http://www.audiologyonline.com).

Market Banding

Mathis and Jackson (2004) offer a method called "market banding" used by human resource professionals to establish base pay and salary ranges. Market banding is used for smaller groups and classifications of employees and is ideal for use by audiology practice owners to compute base salary and salary ranges. The easy steps to tangible salary and salary ranges using the market banding approach are outlined below:

Step 1—Job Families

The first step in this process is to set job families. In most audiology practices three distinct job families will surface, the practice owner, audiologist employees, and the clerical assistants.

Step 2—Salary Review Surveys

The second step is to launch a regional survey that reviews salaries the various job families, noting median salaries and the range in percentage from the highest and lowest salaries from the median in percentage. For example, if the median base salary for an employee audiologist with 10 years experience is $60,000 and a 13% adjustment up and down is noted between the highest and lowest salary surveys, then the raw survey result would be $60,000 ± 13%.

Step 3—Adjustment for Practice Personnel Expenditure

Once obtained, the median salary ($60,000) must be adjusted according to the practice budget for overall personnel expenditure. This adjustment amount is found a result of calculations on the personnel budget by the practice owner and the accountant. The median salary amount may be either adjusted up or down depending on the practice owner's philosophy, the accountant's input and/or the revenue of the practice relative to the overall expenditure for personnel. From the $60,000 figure (obtained from survey information) a negative personnel expenditure adjustment of $4,500 (suggested by the practice accountant) is made to adjust the median base salary to $55,500.

Step 4—Figuring the Salary Range

In the example presented here, $55,500 would be the median salary adjusted for practice personnel budget limitations. The survey also indicated that there was a 13% salary range from the adjusted medial salary. Thus, the base salary range for an audiologist employee in this practice would be ±$7,215 or a salary range of $48,285 to $62,715. Audiologists looking at this position would be able to plan as to how their experience and expertise fits into the organization and the practice owner then has the latitude to adjust the salary slightly up or down according to the quality of the application.

Step 5—Figuring the Hourly Rates for Clerical Employees

The same "market banding" procedure can be applied to hourly employees by the use of a survey to determine median hourly rates for clerical employees. For example, if the survey indicated that medial salary for qualified receptionist with 5 years experience and computer skills was $12.00 per hour and a negative adjustment according to practice owner's philosophy and the accountant's personnel budget recommendations of $1.00 per hour would bring the hourly employee to $11.00. If the survey indicated an hourly wage variation of ±10% for employees with these qualifications then the hourly wage for the practice clerical staff would be $9.90 to $12.10 per hour.

Another method to compute salaries and salary ranges is to use a Web site such as Salary Source.com (http://www.salarysource.com). At this site, for a fee, average salaries for audiology employees and clerical assistants are readily available. Although often not as regionally accurate as market banding, these sites can be valuable in the determination of salaries and salary ranges when it is difficult to obtain information from surveys and local sources.

Benefits for Employees

Audiologist employees and clerical staff may be offered a number of other tangible benefits that all add up into a package. The practice owner may decide to include all of those listed here or work out another list with their accountant and/or human resource consultant. This list of benefits for employees is modified from that offered by Jensen, McMullen, and Stark (2007) in Figure 16–3:

■ *Bonus or spot rewards.* These are bonuses offered for an individual's job well done, teamwork on a specific project, or simply meeting the goals of the practice. Specifically, these rewards could be for meeting a sales goal for a particular number of ABRs, VNGs or hearing instruments for a particular month and might take the form of a restaurant certificate, lunch, expenses to a meeting, or just plain cash, but usually a small amount that simply serves to acknowledge the extra effort and encourage it in other employees.

■ *Performance shares in the company.* As an incentive or reward, the practice owner may choose to offer shares in the company for a job well done. As the extra effort to meet a goal demonstrates interest in the success of the practice, shares in the company can be a method to reward

loyalty and/or the beginning of a transition process.

■ *Annual employee incentive or bonus program.* These programs reward the employee for meeting sales and/or marketing goals over the year. Usually, they are based on targets for the year and, if the practice meets these targets the bonus is offered. Annual bonuses can be given during the holidays, the anniversary of employment, or at the discretion of the practice owner. Khera (2004) indicates that annual incentives and bonuses should be rewards for a job "well done" and not given all the time and in the same amounts. If awarded incorrectly, these incentives will be perceived by the employees not as a bonus but as part of their usual and customary compensation, defeating the purpose of the bonus program.

■ *Income replacement (disability insurance).* Short-term disabilities, such as broken ankles, or hospital stays can be outlined as part of the overall employment package or simply handled internally by the practice owner according to the policies and procedures manual. Income replacement or long-term disability insurance is not a common benefit of employment but may be offered by some practices to employees for long term disabilities as part of the overall insurance package. Long-term disabilities are considered serious injuries that cause major life changes, such as confinement to a wheelchair, brain injuries or other physical modifications that affect the employee's capability to be productive. Long-term disability insurance

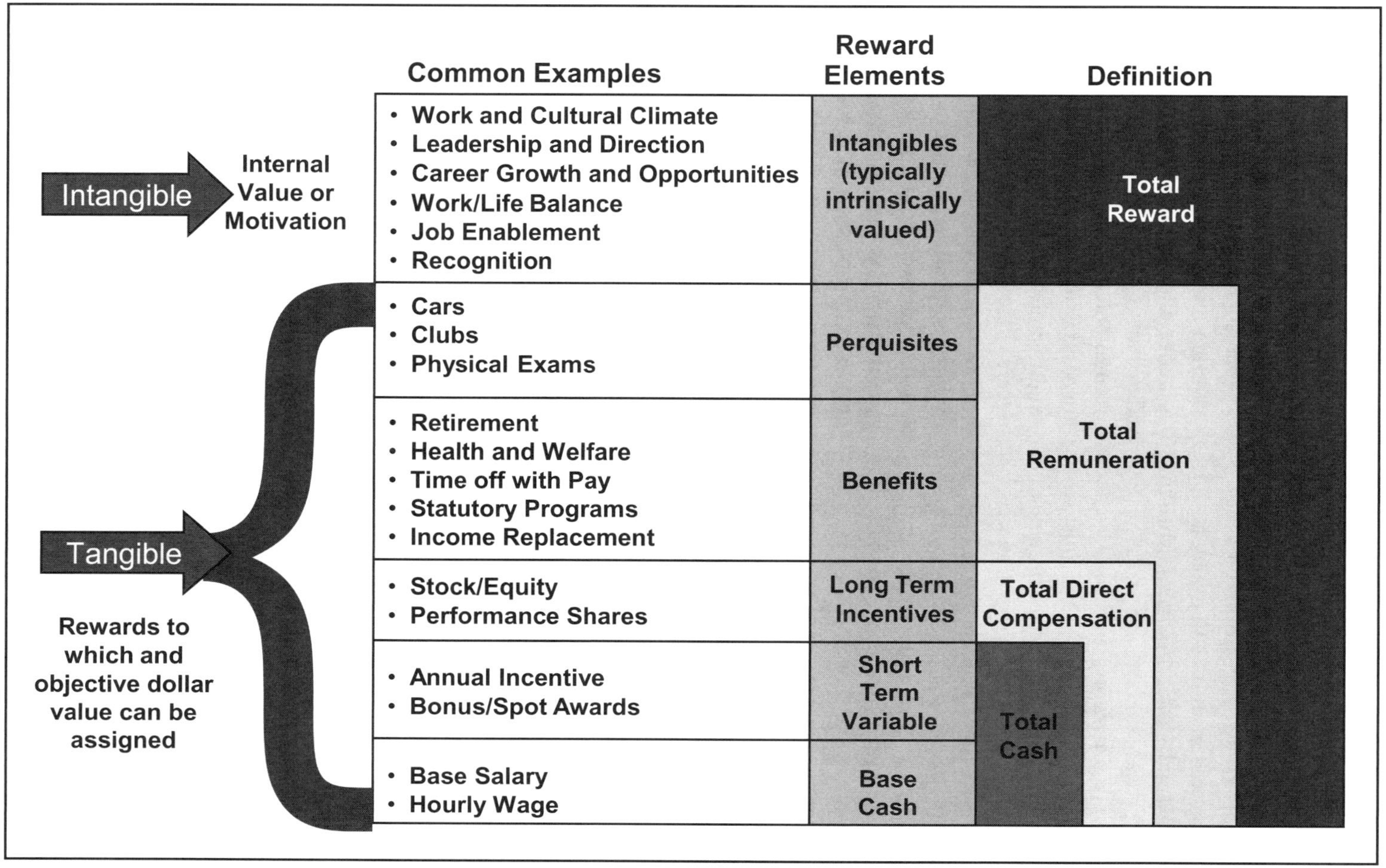

Figure 16–3. Model of employee reward program (Hay Group, 2002).

is a must for the audiology practice owner, but usually not part of the employee's package. When offered as a benefit to the employees these benefits are usually presented as an optional insurance that may be purchased by the employees through their private funds.

- *Statutory programs (workers' compensation).* In all states, it is mandatory that employers purchase workers' compensation insurance. Employees are never required to pay any part of the premium for this coverage since it is the employer that is covered by these policies. The purpose of these policies is to protect the practice and the practice owner from damages that could be awarded in lawsuits that could conceivably put them out of business. For example, a faulty infection control program in an audiology clinic could be grounds for a workers' compensation claim.

- *Paid time off.* Specific types of time off are usually presented in the policies and procedures manual (see Chapter 10), but special time off with pay can be awarded to employees as an incentive or reward for extra work on a specific project or reaching a goal.

- *Health and welfare insurance.* At this writing, health insurance benefits are in a state of flux. Due to the passage of the Affordable Care Act in 2010, businesses are hesitant to hire and offer health and welfare insurance, whereas in the past this benefit was essential to obtaining and maintaining quality employees. These benefits provide security for the employee and their family and insure that health difficulties can

be taken care of expeditiously at reasonable cost. Health insurance, discussed in detail later, is usually available through insurance brokers, specialists in the insurance business offering a variety of policies to the practice and its employees.

- *Retirement program.* Programs for retirement, though beneficial and necessary for employees, have been significantly reduced in the past few years. Practice managers may choose to offer these programs, offer them with modifications, or not to offer them at all. When offered, retirement programs can take on many different forms, such as stock option programs, 401(k) plans, simple savings plans, and other retirement packages. As the practice owner providing benefits to the employees, it is best to discuss these programs with financial advisors, the practice accountant, and the practice attorney as regulations for these programs can be quite complicated and vary from state to state.

- *Physical Exams.* Some practices offer wellness exams in their clinic or at an outside office. These wellness exams are considered a nice benefit, but are usually outside of the usual benefit package offered by audiology practices.

- *Clubs.* Dues to a country club, social club, golf club or other activity are usually reserved for the practice owner. Occasionally, the employee audiologist may be invited to become a member as part of an incentive or a benefits package. When offered to employees, there is usually a particular marketing reason to provide such a benefit. For example, a club where referral sources gather, or a country club to gather contacts where the owner may not care to attend.

- *Automobiles.* Transportation benefits are not part of the usual tangible package for an employee audiologist or clerical personnel. There may be, however, special situations where travel is required that makes this benefit necessary for employees. Rather than supplying a vehicle for employees, it makes more sense to provide transportation or pay mileage and expenses according to procedures outlined in the policies and procedures manual (see Chapter 10) if the employees are required to travel distances to maintain clinics in other cities.

- *Education benefits for employees.* Fenton (2004) indicates that most practice owners consider their employees an important investment both to accomplish the practice's current goals and to have the right people in place for the future. Practices want to hire the best and the brightest and then give them the experience and education they need to advance to the doctoral level. For the past few years, continuing education benefits have been a major issue for young master's degree audiologists eager to obtain an AuD. As part of their benefit package, the employer may choose to offer an education benefit to enhance the package. According to IRS 15B (2007), up to $5,250 of payments received by an employee for tuition, fees, books, supplies, and so forth under an employer's educational assistance program may be excluded from gross income. This employer tax incentive to provide education

was extended until the end of the 2012 tax year by the Tax Relief Act of 2010 (Minnesota Office of Higher Education, 2012). This act allows the employer to pay tuition but cannot cover tools or supplies that the employee retains after the completion of the course and the cost of meals, lodging, or transportation. Thus, the practice owner can offer an education package for an AuD program and deduct up to $5,250 per year for an employee's AuD program as long the costs covered by the employer do not cover meals, lodging, or transportation. An agreement with the employee, drawn by the practice attorney, is highly recommended, as many employees do not honor verbal agreements. The agreement should specify the amounts to be paid back, any work commitment necessary, and a specific repayment program for the educational experience. These commitments vary from 1 year to 3 years depending on the length of time required to complete the program. As with other employee benefits a discussion with the practice's accountant and attorney as to how to structure the employee education benefit before it is offered. After the tax year 2012, audiologists who are employers should discuss offering this benefit with their accountant to ensure that the tax incentives are still available.

After the base salary, the tangible benefits of the position are incentives to provide a comfortable situation for the employee so that they will be able to concentrate on their work each day as well as feel well rewarded for their labor and expertise.

Insurance Benefits

Insurance benefits are essential to any business operation and the audiology practice is no exception. To attract and retain high quality employees the practice must offer competitive insurance benefit programs. The specific programs offered are determined by the regional employment market, the needs of the employees, and the companies that offer policies in the area.

Health Insurance

Health insurance is an important benefit for every employee, including the practice owner. There are several questions a practice owner must ask when considering healthcare insurance for the practice employees:

■ What coverage plans are available in the area?
■ Does my insurance broker carry health insurance?
■ Should I use an HMO or a PPO to save costs?
■ Should I pay all of the policy for the employee or only a portion of the premium?
■ What other ancillary services, such as vision and dental care should I offer in addition to standard health insurance?
■ How will government regulation of the provision of health insurance change what the practice needs to do for their employees in the next 5 years?

The above questions and others are answered by health insurance brokers that have studied all of the various policies and providers in the area. Insurance is their business and they are eager to present a proposal to the practice considering a number of companies with the costs versus benefits presented. The broker typically has analyzed these programs and makes recommendations depending upon needs of the practice. It is recommended to invite the health insurance broker to the practice discuss insurance options at least once a year with the entire staff. All employees should participate in the discussion of this important benefit as it facilitates an understanding the advantages and disadvantages of the various health insurance options and the rationale for the choice of a particular program.

Since the passage of the Affordable Health Care Act in March 2010, the health care industry has been in a state of flux. Thus, the provision of health insurance will be precarious for quite some time. If the act remains intact, there will be implications for audiology practices. Some of the specific implications overviewed by Health Care.Gov (2012):

■ If the practice has fewer than 25 employees and pays average annual wages below $50,000, while providing health insurance, it may qualify for a small business tax credit of up to 35% (up to 25% for nonprofits) to offset the cost of providing health insurance.
■ Starting in 2014, the small business tax credit goes up to 50% (up to 35% for nonprofits) for qualifying businesses.
■ In 2014, small businesses with fewer than 100 employees can shop in an Affordable Insurance Exchange, which a small audiology clinic can

have power similar to large businesses to obtain better choices and lower prices. The exchange is a new marketplace where individuals and small businesses can buy affordable health benefit plans. Exchanges will offer a choice of plans that meet certain benefits and cost standards.

■ Employers with fewer than 50 employees are exempt from new employer responsibility policies. They don't have to pay an assessment if their employees get tax credits through an exchange.

Since health insurance rates have been rising at alarming rates and benefits have been drastically reduced over the past 10 years, it makes good sense to review the system. Whether or not the Affordable Health Care Act is successful, practitioners should seek professional advice about essential health insurance programs.

Disability and Life Insurance

The offering of disability insurances and life insurances to the employees may be a simple matter of another program offered by the insurance broker that the practice owner can either subsidize or simply have available for those employees that need these policies. This coverage is not normally part of a regular compensation package for employees of a small audiology practice but are, as presented earlier, essential for the practice owner.

Depending on the size of the practice group life insurance can be offered to employees for as little as 5 cents per $1,000 worth of coverage. The practice employees and prospective employees

appreciate this benefit as they do not usually need a physical before they are covered by the policy, and they can often convert the plan to an individual life insurance plan, if they when they leave the practice. The actual amount of this policy should be discussed and decided by the practice owner and their accountant. Additionally, if the practice pays for the benefit, it is considered taxable income whereas if the employee pays for the benefit, it is considered insurance and is nontaxable.

Vacations, Holidays, and Personal Time Off

Generally, practitioners will spend about 10% of their payroll on paid time off for their employees, but it is a highly rated employee benefit as people attempt to balance work, family time, and life experiences. An established policy for paid time off (PTO) should be written and included in the policies and procedures manual (see Chapter 10). It should include the number of days granted relative to years of service, specifying lunch and break times as well as holidays paid and unpaid.

Practices usually provide paid holidays for their employees. Although the specific holidays offered to the employees vary according to the individual practice owner by philosophy, religion, region, and state. Typical holidays offered include:

■ New Year's Day
■ President's Day
■ Memorial Day
■ Independence Day

- Labor Day
- Thanksgiving Day and the day after
- Christmas Eve and Christmas Day.

In addition to standard holidays, the practice may also choose to provide one to two floating holidays or personal days. These days can be used whenever the employee would like to use them and often make up for religious holidays that are not part of the practice's standard paid holiday schedule.

Obringer (2007) indicates that the average number of vacation days provided by businesses for new employees are 10 per year, with increases to 15 after five years and 20 after 10 to 15 years. Vacation time is usually accrued on a monthly or quarterly basis, and most practices use a calendar year to make their recordkeeping easier. She indicates that the business standard for a practice is to provide 6 to 9 sick days per year. Unlike vacation time, the number of sick days offered typically does not increase with increasing years of service and do not carry over unused sick leave to the following year. Another necessary decision for the practice owner is if employees will be allowed to use their paid sick days to take care of the illnesses of family members. Most audiology practices have less than 75 people and do not fall under the Family Medical Leave requirement, thus the practice owner is not generally required to provide for the employees families (Burrows, 2006; Ellison, 1999).

Stock Options

Sometimes used as a tool to retain employees, a stock options benefit has some appeal in today's job market. As Glaser (2006) suggests, doctors of audiology are not necessarily looking for a job, but a position within a practice. Stock options represent an attractive incentive in the hiring and retention of quality professional and administrative personnel. These programs are under the control of the US Securities and Exchange Commission. Consultation with the practice's accountant and a licensed securities broker is imperative before stock options are offered. The plan must also be viewed by the attorney of record for the practice.

Retirement Programs

Retirement may seem like a long way off, but it is an important item to consider in attracting and retaining employees. There are several types of plans to choose from for retirement programs the questions and specific needs of your practice should be considered by the accountant, financial advisor, and the practice's attorney for specific advantages and disadvantages of each type.

General, Cash, and Deferred Profit Sharing Plans

Although not always a retirement program, some companies offer profit sharing programs. Profit sharing programs require establishing a formula for distribution of the company profits. These plans are usually based on a distribution percentage of the employee's salary, but require the employee to be in their position for a specified period of time before the profit sharing programs available to them. This vesting period makes profit-sharing programs primarily an incentive to retain employees.

Cash and Deferred Profit Sharing Plans

Cash profit sharing plans pay benefits directly to the employees in cash, check or stock as soon as profits are determined. Profit sharing allows the practice owner to decide if a contribution will be affordable and, if affordable, how much the company will contribute to the plan. Learner (2012) indicates that a designated profit level should be established as a goal to achieve allowing the program to automatically go into effect when profits of a certain amount are achieved for the year. The percentage of profits or the arbitrary level at which the program initiates is usually shared with the employees and is normally established and articulated in advance. For example, the practice owner may say that 10% of all profits over $50,000 will be set aside for the profit sharing program.

In corporations, profit sharing contributions are usually made by a fixed formula or an amount decided by the board of directors (BOD) (often the BOD is simply the practice owner). In high profit years, contributions are made; during less profitable years contributions can be deferred. Profit sharing plans also allow the practice owner to control how the money is invested and is not as expensive to administer as other plans that require expensive administrative professionals for management. The major drawback to a cash profit sharing programs is these programs do not qualify as a retirement plan since they are difficult to predict contribution schedules and at the discretion of the practice owner (Armstrong, 2007).

Deferred profit sharing plans are profit sharing plans designed to provide benefits upon retirement. The benefits at retirement are based on the total of the contributions and the results of the investments made over time. The difference between cash and deferred plans is that a deferred plan must provide a definite predetermined formula. The benefits at retirement are based strictly upon the sum total of the contributions made according to the formula and the quality of the resulting investments.

401(k) Programs

US Legal (2012) defines a 401(k) program as a contribution plan that enables employees to choose between receiving current compensation and making pre-tax contributions to an account through a salary-reduction agreement. Employers may, but are not required to, make contributions to employees' accounts. These plans defer federal income taxes and, in most cases, state income taxes as 401(k) contributions are made before payroll tax deductions. This is conducted to effectively reduce the employee's income before the taxes are figured allowing them to invest with before tax dollars and pay taxes on the income later when their incomes are lower during retirement. As part of the process, the employee receives an investment return on their money, often with the practice matching their contributions. This use of "before tax dollars" to defer taxes allows the employee to simplify their investment decision and contribute through a payroll deduction. The US Department of Labor (2007) states that when the practice owner establishes a 401(k) plan there are certain basic preparations that must be conducted:

- Find an administrator or service provider for the plan.
- Decide if the practice will make contribution to the plan.

- Inform the employees that there is a 401(k) plan.
- Arrange for a trust fund or other account to receive the proceeds of the 401(k) program.
- Submit a written plan to the IRS that describes the type of 401(k) plan, how it operates. Most of the administrators, such as banks, or mutual funds can assist with this requirement.
- Learn about the fiduciary responsibility, reporting, and disclosure requirements that are a part of managing a 401(k) plan.

The 401(k) plan is a major commitment to employees. Although there may be years when there are no contributions, the employees still have their own contributions and they are making money with before tax dollars that allow them to benefit greatly from the program. For the practice owner, there is a significant amount of paper work and administrative monitoring that goes along with these programs but, once organized, the day to day operation of the plan will be handled by the administrator who the works out the payroll deductions and makes the appropriate deposits of practice profits to the appropriate accounts.

Base Salary, Benefits, and Perquisites for the Practice Owner

There must be tangible and generous monetary rewards for the practice owner to offset the risk assumed in the initial and continuous investment in the practice. Market banding works very well to figure base salaries and salary ranges for employees, but not for practice own-

ers. Most practice owners do not readily offer their salary and benefits to others in a survey and, therefore, these market banding ranges are difficult to obtain for practice owners. A good "rule of thumb" here is for the practice owner to set their salary about the same or slightly above the employee audiologists and then use the perks and management skills to offset the difference.

In close consultation with the practice accountant the perks of practice ownership can be used to glean other forms of direct and indirect compensation that generally goes along with business ownership or executive level employment. Increased perks will sometimes work to the practice's advantage as they are often partially or fully deductible.

Virtually all tangible and intangible rewards presented in Figure 16–4 from Jensen et al. (2007), as well as others not listed, may be available as compensation to the practice owner. Compensating the owner of the practice, who is often the chairperson of the board of directors for the practice's the corporation, may require a formal discussion and a resolution at a corporate board meeting to allow the practice owner certain perks. The board of directors of these small corporations usually consist of the owner's accountant, attorney, and relatives, so they will likely vote for a liberal salary and benefits. Most states allow the practice owner, that is, the chairperson of the board of directors, to have compensation for their service on the board that may consist of extra perks or actual tangible salary. Although the practitioner may choose a salary that is virtually unlimited; as presented above, their base salary should follow some logical compensation sequence similar to the other audiologist employees of the practice.

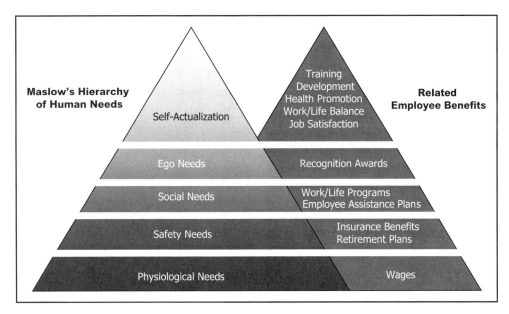

Figure 16–4. Comparison of employee compensation to Maslow's hierarchy of human needs (Jensen et al., 2007).

Benefits and rewards of being in business or perks belong to the practice owner. Bank prizes for depositing money, benefits from suppliers (if the ethical choice is to accept them), and other incentives normally available to business owners are a tangible benefit of entrepreneurship. Other tangible rewards include other short and long-term monetary compensation that make practice ownership worth the investment and more comfortable as the practice develops over time. For example, it is quite common for audiology practices to pay many of their supplier accounts payables on credit cards. The benefits of the credit cards, such as airline miles, cash rebates, points for merchandise, and other benefits are usually a tangible reward for the owner of the practice.

When business is good, the practice owner can present themselves a handsome bonus, a reward, an incentive, extra retirement contributions, time off, or other benefit, provided that all legal, corporate and tax regulations are observed. Benefits such as travel to meetings, books, continuing education, country club memberships for themselves and their families may be also written off as legitimate business expenses.

Disability and Life Insurance

Insure.com (2005) indicates that nearly one-third of all Americans will suffer a serious disability between the ages of 35 and 65. Practice owners need to weigh these statistics and consider disability and life insurance as an essential part of their compensation package. Disability and life insurance policies on the practice owner allow an income cushion to continue practice operations in the event of the disability or death of the owner. These benefits are not necessarily just for the practice owner, but also for the good of the employees, the owner's family, and the patients.

Short- and Long-Term Disability Insurance

Short-term disability, in the United States, is not provided by many employers, and certainly not by most private practices, even for owners. Short-term disability insurance, however, is designed to replace an employee's income on a short-term basis as a result of a disability. Short-term disability (STD) would pay a percentage of the practice owner's salary if they are temporarily disabled. Temporarily disabled is defined by Insure.com (2005) as not able to work for a short period of time due to sickness or injury (excluding on-the-job injuries, which are covered by workers compensation insurance). Short-term disability policies typically provide a weekly portion of the practice owner's salary, usually 50, 60, or 66 percent for 13 to 26 weeks, depending on the program selected. If the practice owner has enough in savings to meet personal and practice needs for a 3-month period without working, then short-term disability insurance is not necessary. However, if there is not much in savings or the practice is a solo operation, a short-term disability policy is essential.

Long-term disability is not required by law, but it should be considered as an essential benefit for the practice owner. Long-term disability insurance helps recover about 60% of the insured income for an extended period of time, usually ending after five years or when the disabled person turns 65, when Social Security benefits usually replace the disability benefit. There is usually a period of time before the long-term disability policy will pay benefits, usually 30 to 180 days or when the short-term disability policies end. The economic security of the practice and, therefore, the practitioner, all the employees, and their families are at risk when illness or injury strikes the practice owner. Although some degree of protection is secured automatically from Social Security Disability through FICA deductions, Social Security only guards against catastrophic loss of all work capability. When dealing with the government, there are specific rules and regulations that must be adhered to by these agencies. Qualification for Social Security disability requires that a claimant must be unable to perform any gainful work at all; there is no partial or percentage disability under the Social Security Act (DeBofsky, 2006). Private insurers, however, offer income protection in the event of a disability over a wide range disability types and levels, including temporary disruption of capability (short-term disability) to perform in your profession, permanent or long-term disability and partial disability coverage. Qualifying for private disability benefits is not as demanding, and in some cases as not as demeaning, as meeting the requirements of Social Security. Less demanding qualification does not mean that an assessment of your ability to perform your duties will not be evaluated. Private insurers will assess the capabilities of the insured and cover needs relative to that assessment.

In any event, disability income insurance is an important benefit that should be paid for with after-tax dollars, especially for the practice owner. As there are many variables in the selection these policies, it makes sense to use an insurance broker to assist in their selection. These policies are often handled by the same broker as the practice's health insurance and their job is to present an insurance package that includes the state minimums as well as some optional program that meet the needs of the practice. Some of the variables of these policies include everything from the exclusion period, which can be based on different time periods if it's an injury or illness, to pre-existing condition limitations, self-reported claim limitations, own-occupation protection, and rate guarantee. The specifics of the amount of income replacement and the benefits to the practice should be discussed in detail with the practice accountant to insure that cash flow to the practice as well as cash flow to the practice owner will replace their income.

As with disability insurance, life insurance for the practice owner is essential. Proceeds of the policy should insure the survival of the practice in the event of the death of the owner. Although the proceeds of the policy will pay necessary practice expenses until arrangements for its disposition are finalized, the actual amount of life insurance should be discussed with the practice accountant.

Automobiles

The practice may lease or purchase a vehicle for use by the practice owner. This vehicle is technically to make deliveries, provide transportation to peripheral clinics during the day, and other places required for business. Any other use of the vehicle is considered to be personal use and is usually taxable to the practice owner. Thus, most practices provide the practice owner with a company vehicle (either leased or purchased) and declare a percentage (85 to 95%) to be used for business purposes and another percent-age (5 to 15%) to be used for personal purposes. Of course, the practice owner gets to choose the car, drive it most of the time, and deduct all of the acquisition costs and maintenance expenses.

Country Club Dues

Along with practice ownership goes the ability to become a member of the exclusive clubs in the area as a marketing expense. Similar to other incentives such as automobiles, the wise practitioner pays a portion of the dues themselves. This allows most of the expense to be considered as a business deduction, but also a portion is paid by the owner with his taxable income to ensure there are no questions about the personal or business use of the club.

Summary: The Road to Self-Actualization

As a summary of compensation for a practice, an analogy that is offered by Jensen et al. (2007) draws a parallel between employment compensation and the hierarchy of needs theory (Maslow, 1943). According to Maslow's theory, once a person has satisfied their basic physiological and safety needs, attention is then focused on social and ego needs with self-actualization being the pinnacle of achievement. Figure 16–4 offers a correlation between components of compensation packages and Maslow's theory, suggesting that self-actualization or job satisfaction will only exist if there is a fair salary that meets physiological needs; health benefits, for ensuring safety needs; work/life programs, for the social needs; recognition to feed the ego;

and training and employee development. The road to self-actualization, or job satisfaction, seems to follow a clear progression from tangible compensation components to the intangible and, once the tangible needs are met, it appears that intangibles become extremely important to job satisfaction and ultimately retention of good employees.

As practice owners, consideration of the self-actualization theory as to how and why we compensate employees and ourselves offers perspective to an otherwise complex issue. This concept simplifies the compensation issue into certain specifics that can be considered in light of the practice, its revenue, and the owner's philosophy.

References

Anderson, K., & Zhu, G. (2002). *Organizational climate technical manual.* Chicago, IL: Hay Group.

Armstrong, F. (2007). Profit sharing and 401(k) plans. *Investor Solutions.com.* Retrieved July 21, 2007, from http://www.investor solutions.com/v2content/Profit%20Sharing%20and%20401K%20Plans.pdf

Atchison, T., Belcher, D., & Thomson, D. (2010). Online compensation and benefits education. *Distance Learning Center.* Retrieved June 19, 2012, from http://www.eridlc.com/index.cfm?fuseaction=textbook.chpt01

BNA.com. (2007). Study says 30% of workers are loyal. *Bulletin to Management.* Retrieved June 28, 2007, from http://www.bna.com/products/hr/btmn.htm

Burrows, D. (2006). Human resource issues: Managing, hiring, firing, and evaluating employees. In R. M. Traynor (Ed.), *Seminars in Hearing, 27*(1), 5–17.

Carrison, D., & Walsh, R. (1999). *Semper Fi: Business leadership the Marine Corps Way.*

New York, NY: American Management Association.

DeBofsky, M. (2006). What every physician needs to know about disability insurance. *Journal Medical Practice Management, 22*(2), 113–118.

Ellison, K. (1999). *Managing employees.* Lectures for CAS 7803, Business and Professional Issues, University of Florida Working Professional Doctor of Audiology Program, University of Florida, Gainesville, FL.

Elsdon, R. (2003). *Affiliation in the workplace: Value creation in the new organization.* Westport, CT: Praeger.

Fenton, E. (2004). Employer provided education benefits. *Journal of Accounting.* Online issues. Retrieved July 18, 2007, from http://www.aicpa.org/PUBS/JOFA/sep2004/fenton.htm

Glaser, R. (2006). *Strategic Practice Management Seminar.* Los Angeles, CA: Sonic Innovations.

Hay Group. (2002). *Ensuring culture change at Arbella: A case study in the effectiveness of rewards.* Presentation at the World at Work Conference, May 13, 2002.

Health Care.Gov. (2012). *Small business and the Affordable Health Care Act.* Retrieved June 23, 2012, from http://www.health care.gov/news/factsheets/2011/08/sm-bus-aff-care-act.pdf

Insure.com. (2005). The basics of short-term disability insurance. *Insure.com.* Retrieved July 20, 2007, from http://info.insure.com/disability/shorttermdisability.html

IRS Publication 15B. (2007). *Employers guide to employee benefits.* Retrieved July 18, 2007, from http://www.saonm.org/pdf/additional-employers-tax-guide.pdf

Jensen, D., McMullen, T., & Stark, M. (2007). *The manager's guide to rewards.* New York, NY: American Management Association.

Khera, D. (2004). Establishing an incentive compensation program. *The Profit Advisors.* Retrieved May 13, 2007, from http://www.morebusiness.com/running_your_business/profitability/tip16.brc

Lavelle, L. (September 29, 2003). Coming next: A war for talent. *Business Week,* p 1.

Lawler III, E. (2003). Pay practices in Fortune 1000 companies. *World at Work Journal, 4*, 45–54.

Lawson, F. (2006). Skill-based pay: Results of a national survey. *Fox Lawson and Associates.* Retrieved May 13, 2007, from http://www.foxlawson.com/newsletter/newsletters/v3n1.cfm

Learner, D. (2012). Profit sharing plans: One way to share the pie. *David Learner and Associates, Inc.* Retrieved June 24, 2012 from, http://news.davidlerner.com/financial.php?include=143511

Lee, G. (2001). Towards a contingent model of key staff retention: The new psychological contract reconsidered. *South African Journal of Business Management, 32*, 1–9.

Levey, J., & Levey, M. (2000). Reflections for leaders. *Journal of the EAPA Exchange*, Employee Assistance Professionals Association, Florida State University, Tallahassee, FL.

Maslow, A. (1943). A theory of human motivation. *Psychological Review, 50*, 370–396.

Mathis, R., & Jackson, J. (2004). *Human resource management* (11th ed.). Mason, OH: Thomson Learning.

McNamara, C. (2007). The basics of employee motivation (the steps you can take). *Free Management Library.* Retrieved July 19, 2007, from http://www.managementhelp.org/guiding/motivate/basics.htm

Meek, C. (2007). Variable pay. *Meek and Associates.* Retrieved May 12, 2007, from http://www.meekassoc.com/opinion/variable_pay.htm

Minnesota Office of Higher Education. (2012). *Get ready for college.* Retrieved June 24, 2012, from http://www.getreadyforcollege.org/gPg.cfm?pageID=116

Murphy, S. (2004). *Design and implementation of a skill-based compensation program in a physician group practice.* University of Kentucky Capstone Project. Retrieved May 13, 2007, from http://www.martin.uky.edu/~web/programs/mha/2004mha_capstones/murphy.pdf

Obringer, L. (2007). How employee compensation works. *How Stuff Works.* Retrieved May 14, 2007, from http://money.howstuffworks.com/benefits1.htm

Randolph, D. (2005). Predicting the effect of extrinsic and intrinsic satisfaction factors on recruitment and retention of rehabilitation professionals. *Journal of Healthcare Management, 50*, 49–60. Retrieved June 21, 2012 from http://ukpmc.ac.uk/abstract/MED/15729907/reload=0;jsessionid=oUPXQS05Wbq1i9DzwSUz.2

Salary source.com. (2007). *Salarysource.com.* Retrieved July 10, 2007, from http://www.salarysource.com/articles.cfm

Shwiff, K. (2007). *Best practices: Hiring people.* Irvington, NY: Hylas.

Thompson, J., & Bunderson, J. (2003). Violations of principle: Ideological currency in the psychological contract. *Academy of Management Review, 28*, 571–586.

US Department of Labor. (2007). *401(k) business plans for small business.* Employee Benefits and Security Administration. Retrieved May 17, 2007, from http://www.dol.gov/ebsa/publications/401kplans.html

US Legal. (2012). 401(k) Law and legal definitions. *USlegal.com.* Retrieved from http://definitions.uslegal.com/4/401-k-plans/

Wasti, S. (2003). Organizational commitment, turnover, intentions, and the influence of cultural values. *Journal of Occupational and Organizational Psychology, 76*, 303–321.

17

Hearing Instrument Manufacturers and Suppliers

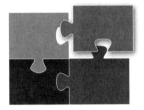

ROBERT G. GLASER, PhD

Introduction

Hearing instruments and those who develop and manufacture them, differ in many and varied ways. In the last several years, cutbacks have occurred in research and development (R&D) departments in many instrument manufacturers. R&D is expensive. Without it, however, there will be a diminution in advances in circuitry design and chip technologies, which will impair necessary advances to improve the lives of those with hearing loss. The advances in chip technology over the last five years have resulted in significant improvement in reducing difficulties in varied backgrounds of noise. Patients are enjoying success with these technological advances in noticeable numbers; not only in my offices, but in offices across the country. Both patients and the audiologists fitting and following them are noting significant differences in acceptance and improved communication performance in a variety of settings.

It has never been more important to know how to select a manufacturing group and their line of hearing instruments and, equally important, when to move on to another manufacturer. How to select and when to depart manufacturers are two very different decisions. Each impacts the quality of services provided in your practice as well as the bottom line. This chapter sets forth methodology to develop ideas and metrics for decision making in selecting and maintaining hearing instrument manufacturers and associated vendors important to a practice. Evaluating various software packages is also critically important and suggestions here will enable practitioners to select and purchase the most appropriate system for their particular needs.

Consider the Following Worst-Case Scenario

Patients and their family members are, generally, a forgiving lot. However, that is true only up to a critical point of intolerance that is consistent in today's health care consumer and particularly so with baby boomers.

How many times has this happened in your practice? A patient returns to pick up his repaired hearing instrument, wife waiting patiently in the room with him. You enter the room with appropriate greetings, perhaps a comment on the weather and full confidence that the hearing instrument about to be replaced in the patient's ear is in full working order with the same programming, the same shell, all ready to go when you notice the serial number does not match the patient's records or the instrument fails to ignite despite a new battery. Or you have a left instrument in your hand when you sent a right one in for repair; or the patient says the hearing aid sounds terrible in his ear and objective mea-

sures confirm there is a gross mismatch between need and output.

As beads of sweat develop on your forehead, the patient and his wife look at you like this is some sort of cruel joke since you are responsible for all things that make up the total picture of hearing care including the repair, the replacement, and successful rededication of patient and instrument. It matters not to the patient that the audiologist-case manager could not open the instrument and replace a chip or a microphone assembly if his or her life depended on it: It is the audiologist's responsibility, not the repair team at the manufacturing facility. Because the audiologist will bear the brunt of patient and family dissatisfaction, it is up to you as the care provider to step up to the plate and swing away as the patient's advocate. That duty is unequivocal and clearly defined no matter the venue of your practice.

"I Am Only as Good as You Will Permit Me to Be"

The line above should be repeated to every repair manager and inside sales representative until such time that each finally begins to see the big picture of having patients in your office appropriately disgusted by the fact that their hearing instrument needs to be sent to the manufacturing facility for its third repair in as many months. They sit at their desk on the phone while you are facing down an angry patient who is convinced the hearing instrument you placed in their ear will never work despite extensive diagnostic testing, counseling, and emotional preparation to the contrary.

Repair managers do not have to figure out a reasonable apology scheme for disgruntled patients and family members. It is true, as the audiologist, you are only as good as the repair team or manufacturer (new instruments DOA) will permit you to be. As clinicians, each of us have experienced this type of disappointment such that we sometimes fantasize about how it would feel to be able to jam our hands through the telephone and around the neck of the repair manager or inside sales representative each of whom promised the world and delivered more problems.

Hearing Instrument Manufacturer and Audiologist: A Symbiotic Relationship

Audiologists and hearing instrument manufacturers alike have contributions to make and responsibilities to assume in a patient's journey from diagnostic assessment to wearing hearing instruments with a high degree of satisfaction. It is the responsibility of the audiologist to blend the needs of the patient with the manufacturer offering the most appropriate technology. It is the audiologist's critical contribution of assessment, instrument selection, and application/adjustment that is the continuum of successful aural rehabilitation.

The hearing instrument manufacturer has the responsibility to provide sophisticated instruments and support systems such that audiologists can readily apply these technologies within the continuum of aural rehabilitation. A symbiotic relationship exists when reliance becomes mutually beneficial so that the patient is the direct recipient of the interdependent function of each group.

Instrument manufacturers have tremendous responsibilities in the relationship. It is their responsibility to provide audiologists with innovative solutions to hearing loss including improved chip technology and transducers, better clarity in noise, improved reliability of operation, user-friendly fitting software, ease of modifiability, and excellent in-house service. The instrument manufacturer logically and for obvious, intrinsic reasons accepts the burden of educating audiologists about the options and instrument-specific advantages available to maximize the benefits available in their product lines. Whether the training is delivered in the audiologist's office by a manufacturer's field representative, provided at their facility, or in a Continuing Education Unit (CEU) event, the manufacturer must have a readily available, systematic training program to ensure that audiologists are maximizing the potential of their technologies. If the instruments and their particular technological advantages are not applied effectively in the patient's ear, the expense of extensive research and development is lost.

It is also the responsibility of instrument manufacturers to produce evidence that all claims made about their products are valid, unequivocal, and, most importantly, readily noticed by the patients wearing the instruments. The ultimate metrics of success of the relationship between manufacturers and clinicians is the level of patient satisfaction and the observations of those communicating with the patient wearing the hearing instruments.

Patient Satisfaction and Digital Technology

Patient satisfaction with their hearing instruments has been steadily improving over the last several years and it appears to be directly related to increasing numbers of fittings of hearing instruments with digital signal processing (DSP). In a study at the early stages of widespread use of digital technologies, Kirkwood (2001) surveyed audiologists and commercial hearing aid dealers regarding their patient's satisfaction with DSP hearing instruments. They rated overall patient satisfaction to be 78% better with DSP instruments, 89% better in sound quality, 82% in listening comfort, 77% better in speech recognition in noisy areas, and 70% better in feedback reduction or suppression.

From 2000 to 2005, DSP hearing instruments as a percent of fittings grew from 5 to 90%. The use of digital hearing instruments is associated with significantly higher ratings of overall user satisfaction and benefit, improved sound quality, reduction in feedback, improved performance in noisy situations, and greater utility in a number of important listening situations (Kochkin, 2005).

Groth and Mecklenburger (2011) point out that the growth in behind-the-ear instrument usage has increased from 20% in 2000 to over 60% use in 2011 due primarily to advances in open-fit and feedback suppression technology. As advances in technology continue, improvements in patient satisfaction and consistent use of hearing instruments in all communication settings is expected.

With the advent of improvements in verification techniques coupled with advances in hearing instrument technologies, patients are enjoying increased success in their process of aural rehabilitation. And it usually begins when the hearing-impaired person begins to accept the fact that his or her hearing loss is causing difficulties for themselves and others in their communication sphere.

Then, and perhaps for some, only then will they begin to consider hearing instruments as an opportunity to improve their difficulties (Kochkin, 2012).

Technology

Audiologists should choose a hearing instrument manufacturer based on much more than "the best technology choice for my patient, and how I can keep my costs as low as possible" (Smriga, 2004). Technological and connectivity considerations, instrument costs, warranties, financial operations, repair resolution, and educational opportunities are but a few important items to consider when choosing a hearing instrument manufacturer for your particular practice venue. "In the United States, roughly 90% of all hearing aids dispensed in 2007 were digital, offering improved fitting flexibility, feedback reduction, and multichannel compression strategies to ensure audibility for soft, moderate, and loud sounds. Open-fitting platforms have regained in popularity due to improved fitting flexibility in combination with feedback phase inversion systems that may be used to dynamically cancel feedback" (Fabry et al., 2007).

There is little question that advances over the last ten years in hearing instrument technology and the ear-instrument interface can appropriately be viewed on a logarithmic scale in comparison to the advances noted since the first vacuum tube hearing aid was invented by Hanson in 1920. The Vactuphone was made-to-order for the Globe Ear-Phone Company by the Western Electric company and was commercially distributed in 1921 (Berger, 1984).

When evaluating a manufacturer's line up of available hearing instruments, a number of characteristics should be considered. The most logical starting point in the evaluation should be the needs of the patients seen in your practice. What are the general characteristics and range of hearing levels commonly seen in your practice? For example, if your practice is in a highly industrialized area, there will be a higher percentage of noise induced hearing loss with attendant high-frequency "noise notch" configurations. The manufacturer's line up should, therefore, include high frequency emphasis offerings with open fitting platforms. If you are practicing in a pediatric hospital seeing youngsters with moderate-to-severe losses, your fitting needs will differ and the manufacturer should have a well-developed series of pediatric-focused instruments with adequate power and processing capabilities linkable to FM systems. A manufacturer should have sufficient breadth of offerings to cover at least 85% of the hearing loss parameters seen in your particular practice venue.

If you are an independent practitioner seeing children and adults in a community with a broad base of employment opportunities including noise exposure possibilities, the same 85% criteria should hold comfortably true. Most major manufacturers offer realistic technological opportunities from open fitting platforms for steeply sloping sensorineural hearing loss to powerful behind the ear instruments with appropriate compression and feedback management systems for moderate-to-severe sensorineural hearing loss. Of course, there is no rule that you have to maintain allegiance to only one or two manufacturers. However, the ease of knowing one line of instruments thoroughly and maximizing the utility in one

programming system are only two reasons to seek a single manufacturer as the primary source of your hearing instrument needs. If a single lineup of instruments covers only 85% of your patients needs, there will always be room to seek solutions elsewhere for the remaining 15% of your clinical population.

Assistive Technologies and Compatibility

There are a host of adjuvant devices to improve hearing and listening in specific conditions that are coupled to hearing instruments via direct audio input, infrared and Bluetooth integration, and by electromagnetic inductance. Both assistive listening systems (ALS) and assistive listening devices (ALDs) require specific interfacing technologies from tele-loop compatibility to inductor coils specifically designed to enhance cell phone use. Compatibility with an ever expanding group of devices developed to improve the signal-to-noise ratio and enhance speech recognition in difficult listening situations must be considered an important part of every aural rehabilitation effort. A manufacturer should have a well-developed grouping of ALS or ALDs or have easy access or modification routines so that their hearing instruments can interface readily with systems available elsewhere in the market. Whether it be something as simple as enjoying a sermon at church or hearing well at a meeting in a hard walled, highly reverberant conference room, these new technologies are critically important to the patient and to their families as well. They lend a level of communication integration in difficult listening situations and

Sidebar 17–1
EVALUATING SUPPLIERS

Audiologists rely on noninstrument suppliers for equipment, tools, supplies, and resale accessories used in their daily practice. The following factors should be considered when selecting a supplier:

Price. Pricing is an important factor in selecting a supplier. However, given the instability of product pricing in the hearing health care industry, price may not be the most critical element in choosing a supplier. Occasionally, suppliers offer lower prices on a particular product as a limited, promotional effort. Suppliers with greater sales volumes may pass their price breaks, and lower prices, on to their customers—but don't hold your breath waiting.

Breadth of Product Line. Breadth of product line refers to the number and variety of products offered by a supplier. The more products offered by a supplier, the less likely a practice will have to divert staff effort engaging multiple suppliers. If you find a good supplier, support them.

Resource Capability. Suppliers committed to and effective in serving as a resource to their customers offer invaluable advantages. Those willing and able to research alternative products when items are discontinued provide an important service to busy practitioners.

Ease of Doing Business. Suppliers who forgo complicated credit applications and minimum purchase requirements should be considered over those with rigid requirements. Suppliers should offer a variety of opportunities to order products (i.e., phone orders, fax, Web site, e-mail) with varied payment methods and straightforward payment terms.

Return Policies. It is important to establish a relationship with a supplier offering reasonable return policies. Suppliers with limited opportunity for customers to return defective items or items that did not meet expectations may not be acting in the best interest of the audiologist nor the patients served. Return policies should be unencumbered and without significant delay in issuing credits or refunds for returned products.

Product Availability/Backorder Policy. Suppliers should provide products in a timely fashion. Avoid those who are routinely out of stock or need to consistently back-order items. In the event of a back-order situation, use those suppliers willing to deliver back-ordered items without additional shipping charges.

Supplier Independence. Independent distributors, not owned nor financially affiliated with product manufacturer(s), are in the best position to offer customers an unbiased, objective perspective about products.

(Special Thanks to Dr. A.U. Bankaitis, Vice President, Oaktree Products) reduce the numbers of environments or communication situations that may have been avoided altogether.

Connectivity: Ease of Connecting to the Instrument

With the advent of programmable hearing instruments a dilemma developed for both instrument development engineers and for audiologists fitting the hearing instruments: How best to connect the instrument with the programming system. This dilemma seemingly went from bad to worst in a brief period. Initially, most of the connectivity was completed with cumbersome yet easy to connect plugs to fit into capped receptacles on the instrument. Once connected, they remained connected and data transfer was relatively easily completed. Pull the connector, replace the cap to the programming port and the commands or data were transferred and the session was done. The ports were large and the economy of space issue inherent in the miniaturization process of hearing instruments began to win out as programming ribbons and other smaller connection systems were developed.

These attempts at size reduction created, in some instances, an entirely new set of problems for the end user. The manufacturing community could have come together and agreed on consistent usage of size and shape of connectors but that would have been too easy. As it stands, every audiologist must have an ugly array of connecting gear and ribbons and "whatnot" to access the hearing instrument for programming or adjustment of the instrument. There are problems within a single manufacturer's lines where ribbons must be changed for this or that reason or another cable must be used here or there. And none of the software appears to be sensitive to this dilemma, save one that gives a description and number of the cable and ribbon to be used for the instrument specified in the fitting software. It is truly a puzzle as to why hearing instrument manufacturers seemingly have to compete right down to the connectivity of their instruments to a universal linking system. It does, however, give the audiologist a reason to evaluate a manufacturer on the basis of ease and speed of connectivity. If a hearing instrument cannot be connected with data on screen within two minutes, serious consideration must be given to looking for another manufacturer with better connectivity throughout their product line. Time is money no matter the venue of your practice and connectivity problems are not a good sign to a patient awaiting his new instruments or the replacement of a repaired instrument that has to be reprogrammed. Connectivity should not be an issue; connecting hearing instruments to a programming system should be essentially instantaneous.

User-Friendly Software

There are great differences in the usability, effectiveness and simplicity of hearing instrument manufacturers' programming software systems. Some require wading through two or three screens before approaching the initial programming screen. Other programming software has little or no navigation indicators to advise the user as to exactly where he or she is in the programming sequence.

This can create a sense of being lost within the program and often results in having to restart the programming sequence. Time and confidence in the programming system are lost as the patient perceives palpable frustration. No matter the intent of the software developers, programming protocols that require disproportionate amounts of time and effort will subject the manufacturer to the financial risk of losing valuable dispensers.

Evaluating the usability of programming software systems does not require the skills or knowledge of a software developer. The audiologist working with patients every day quickly develops a sense of usability and inherent time constraints a poorly designed program brings to the patient's visit. There are several, basic aspects of software programs that can be used to evaluate hearing instrument programming software. Although not a set of absolute rules, these recommended actions, programming transformations, screen prompts and messages adapted from Hedge (2007), provide guidelines to be used in comparing software program offerings of hearing instrument manufacturers:

1. A time-focused hearing instrument software system should permit initial programming within four keystrokes after auditory data describing the patient's hearing loss are entered in the program.
2. The software should provide an instant reading of the instruments being programmed and display the serial number and specific model details upon initial connection to the software.
3. Software users (hereafter, audiologists will be considered the "users") must be able to accomplish their task in a naturally occurring order of events: the programming task must be in an order that makes sense to the user so that he or she does not have to change screens or otherwise search for solutions in other levels of the software.
4. Wording in on-screen messages and instructions should be easily understood, concise, and unambiguous.
5. All recent actions or commands completed by the user should be easily reversible by "undo" commands that would allow escape routines from specific operations in motion.
6. The programming software should be solution driven with "go to" symptom and solution selection lists to logically help the patient with their various performance complaints. The more automatic the resolution of definable problems, the faster the instruments are programmed or reprogrammed and the quicker the patient can begin to adjust to their new instruments.
7. The software must permit access to all definable parameters of the hearing instrument. Compression ratios, output by channels or frequency bands, processing speed and integration of attack and release times, and similar modifiable functions should be accessible to the audiologist programming the instrument for the patient.
8. The software must provide pull-down lists and reminders to foster recall by the clinician. With so many opportunities for optimizing the instrument fitting, it is difficult to commit to memory various routines and subroutines that may be important for the unique needs of individual patients.
9. The software must be configured to provide a printout or easily retrievable electronic record of actions

by dates for each instrument programmed or adjusted after the initial programming. This record is important as it is not uncommon to have to undo programming that failed to improve a patient's particular situation. If a record is retained, the original programming configuration can be reinstated in the hearing instruments. This is an important feature since many patients unsure of the adjustments made following the initial fitting will want to return to the initial settings to compare their performance in varied environments.

10. Photos of the hearing instruments in situ and patient-friendly lists of features along with audiologic findings superimposed on the effective fitting range of the instruments should be readily available to the audiologist and patients in the initial phases of counseling and preparation for the fitting.

Additional information, readily visible on screen or in a print out for the patient, should include the battery size, estimates of battery life, and information about compatibility with assistive technologies including cell phones and land-line telephones.

Costs and Financial Operations

Hearing Instrument Acquisition Costs

One of the most important determinants in selecting a hearing instrument manufacturer is instrument acquisition cost. More than just the cost of the instrument should be included in the assessment. Some of these issues may not seem relatable to costs and they will impact your practice and how it is viewed as a participant in the health care arena at large. A good example of an important, yet nonmonetary cost factor involves the time span from placing an order to the arrival of the new or repaired hearing instrument. If Manufacturer A takes 10 days to two weeks to deliver a new or repaired instrument and Manufacturer B delivers in seven days, these different schedules can be critical to patient satisfaction and therefore the long-term success of your practice. A few days to a week from order to arrival is often a critical time frame for a patient and family waiting for a new or repaired hearing instrument. There are other determinants involving costs and financial operations to consider in choosing a hearing instrument manufacturer.

Range of Instrument Costs Across the Product Line

Most major instrument manufacturers develop a wide-ranging lineup of circuitry and instrument types within their product line. Manufacturers strive to provide a comprehensive array of offerings so that an audiologist will be able to select an instrument appropriate to a broad base of patient needs. In essence, each line should be able to cover 85% of the fitting needs seen in most clinical venue. That is important to instrument manufacturers for a variety of reasons not the least of which is developing brand loyalty in the ranks of audiologists using their products.

Paying the Bills

Instrument manufacturers generally function on a 30- to 45-day payment policy. You are expected to pay the bill for the instrument completely (net) within the specified payment period. The longer the payment cycle, the greater the time the manufacturer has granted to pay the bill in full. In effect, the manufacturer is providing you with a loan for the period of the defined payment cycle. There might be penalties or interest charges if the bill is not paid within a specific time period. Depending on your status as a customer, you might be able to get an extended payment time period. The terms of payment should be taken into consideration when choosing a manufacturer. The longer the payment cycle, even by as little as 15 days, the longer you keep your operating funds remain intact. Penalties for overextending the payment deadlines should be clearly stated, and if not, contact the accounting department and have someone clarify the situation, preferably in writing. An additional measure of a good manufacturer is a readily available accounting department focused on account resolution and most are quite happy to review your statement and assist you in resolving any confusions or correcting wrongs.

The statement of your account should be easy to read and it should balance relative to known orders, payments and credits for returns. The accounting department must produce a readable and logical account statement. If your office personnel or your accountant has trouble making sense of the format of the account, ask to have the format changed. Should the accounting department fail to consistently provide an accurate state-

ment, a true accounting of the orders, payments, and credits, do not stop at the head of the accounting department to resolve the problem. Statements should be carefully confirmed upon receipt and errors resolved swiftly. If they cannot figure whether you have appropriately scheduled payments to your account or if the accounting department is calling to request payments when your records indicate payments have been made in full and on time, consider another manufacturer. Resolving errors on your statement is time consuming and frustrating for you and your office personnel and your part of the bargain in the business transaction is paying their bills on time. Their part is to provide an accurate accounting of transactions in your statement and that is not an inordinate expectation.

Repair Resolution and Warranties

Hearing instrument repairs are perplexing to the wearer and to the audiologist managing the patient's aural rehabilitation. Despite the improvement in patient satisfaction with digital hearing instruments, there remains the ever present issue with hearing instrument repairs. Clinically, it matters little to the patient and their family whether the repair was necessitated by their actions. They are more interested in how long the repair will take and why their instrument cannot be repaired in the office. In an odd sense, their concern is less an unrealistic expectation as it is a tribute to the effectiveness of the instrument in need of repair. They want their hearing aid back as soon as possible. Their response is coincidental to the observations reported by Kochkin (2005) in which 93% of digital hearing instrument wearers noted a significant improvement in the quality of life.

Rates of Repairs

It is difficult to determine the rates at which hearing instruments require out-of-office repairs. Although statistics on hearing instrument repairs are kept by manufacturers, neither the consuming public nor the audiology community is commonly privy to these data. Conventional wisdom (largely based on the experiences of clinicians) suggests rates of repairs on most instruments in the first year post fitting ranging from 10% to as much as 18% of instruments dispensed. The second and third year rates of repairs flatten to approximately 20 to 25%. By the fifth year post fitting, 30 to 40% of instruments likely will undergo an out-of-office repair.

Almost all instruments dispensed today are fully digital. Repairs on these instruments in their first year post fitting appear to have decreased significantly. Glaser (2012) has monitored the incidence of repairs and post fitting rates of occurrence in his practice for over 25 years across several manufacturers, instrument styles and various levels of circuitry. The data indicate there has been 18% fewer returns to manufacturers for repairs within the first postfitting year from 2008 to 2011. Additionally, the rate of re-repairs (defined as a repaired instrument returned to the manufacturer within 45 days of the original repair date) has declined at a similar rate within the same period. The reasons for the improvements most likely include improvements

in the stability of transducers and chip technology to better preventive measures to reduce repairs related to cerumen. There remains no substitute for training the patient and at least one other family member how to clean the hearing instruments and to do so at least three or four times per week. With the advent of electronic drying systems and better instruction in instrument care, cleaning and maintenance, less returns for repairs should continue to improve.

Establishing a Benchmark for Instrument Repairs in Your Practice

It is difficult to establish a benchmark for an "expected" number of hearing instrument repairs. From the patient's viewpoint there should be zero tolerance for repairs. Audiologists agree there should be zero tolerance for repairs. The reality of the situation, however, dictates reasonable acceptance of some repairs since electronic equipment in general and hearing instruments specifically are inherently prone to failure from time-to-time. It is unreasonable to assume that hearing instruments can be developed that are not subject to the need for out-of-office repairs. It is also difficult to develop a benchmark on repairs without an accurate accounting of numbers of repairs occurring as a function of the date of the instrument being fitted. Knowing the pattern of repairs as a function of the fitting date provides an opportunity to develop a prospective guide of what to expect of a specific model within an instrument line.

Based on well-kept anecdotal records of a single practice (Glaser, 2012) described above, the following represents an example of an anticipated repair rate that has been generated on the basis of previous data for an approximated volume of 250 instruments per year:

■ Fewer than 18% of instruments fit within the first year require out-of-office repair.

■ Fewer than 15% of instruments in the second and third years post fitting required out-of-office repairs.

■ Fewer than 15% of instruments in the fourth and fifth years post fitting required out-of-office repairs.

Considering the numbers of repairs that will require a return trip to the manufacturer for repair, it becomes readily apparent that out-of-office repairs cost a great deal of time and money as well as increased levels of patient dissatisfaction and discord. However, by reducing repair rates not only will the practice have more time to schedule new patients, there will be a concurrent increase in patient satisfaction. No matter how fast you return the repaired instrument nor how many warranty extensions the manufacturer is willing to issue, repairs are unacceptable to patients and family members who have come to appreciate the benefits of appropriately fitted hearing instruments.

Counseling Patients About Hearing Instrument Repairs

Beyond counseling and advising the rates of repairs known to your practice, there are few methods to assist patients in developing realistic expectations about hearing instrument repairs. As with counseling the patient and family about the importance of developing realistic expectations of improved communication performance, counseling about the incidence of hearing instrument repairs should be equally realistic. Zero percent repairs is an unrealistic expectation despite remarkable advances in contemporary hearing instrument technology. Warranty periods are made available to the patient for a reason. They stand as indicators of likelihood that instrument repairs will be needed within a two or three year period after the fitting. Why else would a manufacturer build the cost of anticipated repairs into the single unit price of their hearing instruments with additional years of coverage available at an additional cost? The fact remains that hearing instruments are subject to a variety of external and internal forces that work against developing a performance history without repairs.

Patients and family must be given appropriate training on maintenance and the importance of consistent instrument care and cleaning. They must be given every opportunity to develop good maintenance habits. At the fitting and during the immediate follow-up visits, care and maintenance routines should be assessed, restated, and all involved must demonstrate competencies in care and cleaning, proper insertion and removal of the battery and use of dehumidifying equipment. To reduce instrument loss, advise patients and family members to place the instruments in their case whenever they need to remove them. Putting their instruments in a pocket or purse is inviting loss and damage. The more the family is involved in the care and maintenance of the patient's hearing instruments, the less likely they will be lost or require an out-of-office repair.

> ### *Sidebar 17–2*
> ### THE IMPORTANCE OF MANUFACTURER
> ### FIELD REPRESENTATIVES
>
> Manufacturer field representatives provide a great service to practitioners and patients alike. They offer quick, pragmatic information not readily available in printed bulletins or product descriptions issued by the manufacturer. Their information is gleaned from their customer base and, therefore, represents real world information. Some of the services they provide include:
>
> - Training regarding products, software, and specific technical information
> - Establishing which patients are best suited for specific instruments
> - Offers circuit-by-circuit comparisons of products offered by others
> - Training to maximize fitting utility of fitting software and instruments
> - Sharing tricks, gimmicks, insights gleaned from other users of the product
> - Solving specific patient difficulties common to an instrument line
> - Assisting in developing realistic pricing for the practice's demographic
> - Advise in-house contacts to resolve billing difficulties, repair problems, and so forth
> - Assistance in resolving billing errors
> - Stands as the practice's in-house liaison to the manufacturer
> - Assist in marketing strategies and co-operative marketing opportunities.

Return of Repaired Instruments by the Manufacturer/Repair Facility

Repairs should be returned to the practice by the manufacturer/repair facility within 7 to 10 working days. Most repairs require a 2- or 3-day in-house period. Shipping to and from manufacturers and repair facilities is commonly facilitated by retail shippers (e.g., FedEx, UPS). Pick-up and delivery at the practice door reduces critical out-of-ear time and reduces the risk of loss and damage in transit. With improvements in shipping, the onus to improve the time it takes to repair and return the repair rests with the repair manager and the productivity and accuracy of his or her staff of repair technicians. And then there is the extra cost of an expedited repair. Does it really warrant the extra cost? Does the repair turnaround in-house faster with the extra fee? The answer, of course, depends on the manufacturer or repair facility but there is usually a savings of one or two days at the most, perhaps worth it to the executive who has an important board meeting or to a mother who must hear her children in the middle of the night. If repair facilities can improve turnaround time to your practice for an additional charge, it seems reasonable to expect that same repair department to improve their turnaround time without an additional charge levied for expected work.

Repair turnaround time should be monitored consistently and reviewed regularly. If the data indicate turnaround time is increasing, it must be considered a critical measure in deciding whether to seek another manufacturer or repair facility. Repairs are always a rough spot for our patients. The longer it takes to return the instrument to the patient's ear, the greater the probability of reduced patient satisfaction and a loss of confidence in both the hearing instrument and the practitioner.

Re-Repairs

If the patient experiences greater than three repairs in an 18- to 24-month period postfitting, manufacturers commonly replace or replate (replace all major components within the shell) the instrument at no charge to the patient. If they do not consider this an option, they should be urged to do so on behalf of your patient and your practice. This replacement scheme covers the patient's needs, however, it does not account for diminishing profits in the practice when greater time is spent in repeated visits, reprogramming efforts, refitting, and recounseling the patient and family to regain at least a bit of confidence lost in the instrument and the practice. Too many unplanned "re-'s" result in lost revenue and respect that will not be replaced by an instrument manufacturer or repair facility.

Beyond Improving Rates of Repair: What Manufacturers Can Do

As manufacturers generally do not reimburse practitioners for lost time and revenue due to multiple repairs, there are a few items or issues manufacturers could incorporate to lessen the burden of audiologists responsible for fitting their products.

Return Repairs with Programming Intact

Repaired instruments returned without the original programming is irritating, time consuming and an unnecessary addition to the mayhem. Granted, it may take as little as 15 minutes to re-establish patient specific programming data to re-repair status: it also includes the fact that a significant number of patients perceive differences in performance with the repaired instrument. No matter the programs nor manufacturer nor whether or not have we informed them of the need for the reprogramming. Even if the chip must be replaced it is best for all concerned when the repair technician spends the time transferring the programming information rather than having to repeat the programming in the office with patients and family members overseeing every move the audiologist makes. Retrieving and reprogramming the instrument at the repair facility must become an institutional priority and duty of repair technicians and every instrument manufacturer or repair facility. If you ask any audiologist fitting hearing instruments, each will tell you that they would happily pay a bit more for repairs if those completing the repairs would at least try to replace the programming. And if it is a matter of laziness, then repair facilities managers should find individuals eager to work hard and do the job right!

Software Upgrades for Chips in Use

When chip technology and accessibility becomes readily available to clinicians, upgrades can and will be provided to the practice patient base. Upgrades could be purchased from or provided by the instrument manufacturer. Patients with accessible chip technology could be called in for an upgrade at no cost or at a nominal fee relative to what the manufacturer charges to download the upgrade. *Upgrade availability would go far in reducing the concerns of purchasing a sophisticated hearing instrument that is subject to technological obsolescence.* Unlike a safety recall common to the automobile industry, upgrades will be viewed as a positive opportunity for a practice to offer additional opportunities for improved hearing with their instruments. It affords the audiologist another, positive opportunity to preserve the patient's confidence in both instrument and practitioner alike.

Liberal Warranty Extensions on Re-Repairs

Re-repairs are poison to a patient and to a practice as well. Re-repairs provide the greatest source of broken confidence in both the hearing instrument and the practice. As one irate patient said recently: "What is it with you people? You can't even get a broken instrument repaired correctly at the manufacturing plant? That damn thing hasn't worked right from day

one and here I am a year and a half later and it still doesn't work right and you can't get it right even with two tries."

Little will satisfy a frustrated patient after having had his instrument repaired only to have it fail a second time within a month or two. Re-repairs should be discussed at the initial fitting but few practitioners dwell on the topic for obvious reasons. A realistic expectation about a repair is one thing; there is no reality to the patient when it comes to multiple repairs in a brief time period. Re-repairs should not happen in this modern era of digital technology and improved transducers and improvements in the manufacturing process.

Unfortunately, re-repairs do happen and the manufacturer should provide a liberal warranty extension after the fact. Issuing an additional 6 to 12 months of warranty on a four-year-old instrument may represent a formula for loss for a manufacturer but it should be the minimum consideration given the patient for no other reason than to stand as an indication of confidence by the manufacturer that another "re-repair" will not be an issue. Simply put, the repair facility should have enough confidence in their capabilities to extend warranted repairs at no charge or with attenuating costs with each successive repair.

Manufacturer's In-House Staff Dedicated to Rapid Resolutions

Members of a call staff in a manufacturer's repair section are the first responders in the calamity that is a hearing instrument repair. They must be well trained in complaint resolution, knowledgeable about the product line in general and specific idiosyncrasies of each particular circuit and they must know the internal tracks to resolution. They must be as efficient and accommodating as your front office associates and just as available for consultation and inquiry. They represent the human touch of a system that can quickly become impersonal and inattentive. And if they cannot solve the problem over the phone or by quickly consulting with the repair section, they should request the instrument be sent to their desk for personalized attention. Each member of this important team must be dedicated to complaint resolution and acknowledging the caller's problem as unique to his or her practice deserving an equally unique response and prompt resolution.

Monitoring Performance: Products and Providers

Part of maintaining a practice as a center of excellence requires evaluating the performance of others as they integrate their products or services into your practice. The practice, after all, is only as good as the sum of its parts. Each part must be consistently monitored with expectations defined in the parameters of participation that affects the overall performance of the practice. Just as administrative and professional staff members should undergo performance evaluations on a regular schedule, so too should hearing instrument manufacturers and other suppliers to the practice undergo consistent performance assessment.

Standards have been set by two governmental agencies have administrative oversight regarding hearing instruments: the Food and Drug Administration (FDA) and the Federal Trade Commission (FTC).

The FDA has regulatory authority over the manufacturing and sale of hearing instruments. The FTC regulates sales activity, including fraudulent and deceptive claims and assesses the appropriateness and accuracy of promotional efforts.

The FDA requires that the audiologist obtain a written statement by the referring physician indicating the need for the hearing evaluation. If the patient is 18 years of age or older, he or she may waive the medical evaluation by signing a form contained in the Code of Federal Regulations, Title 21, Volume 8, Revised April 1, 2012 (21CFR801.420):

Warning to Hearing Aid Dispensers

A hearing aid dispenser should advise a prospective hearing aid user to consult promptly with a licensed physician (preferably an ear specialist) before dispensing a hearing aid if the hearing aid dispenser determines through inquiry, actual observation, or review of any other available information concerning the prospective user, that the prospective user has any of the following conditions:

(i) *Visible congenital or traumatic deformity of the ear.*

(ii) *History of active drainage from the ear within the previous 90 days.*

(iii) *History of sudden or rapidly progressive hearing loss within the previous 90 days.*

(iv) *Acute or chronic dizziness.*

(v) *Unilateral hearing loss of sudden or recent onset within the previous 90 days.*

(vi) *Audiometric air-bone gap equal to or greater than 15 decibels at 500 hertz (Hz), 1000 Hz, and 2000 Hz.*

(vii) Visible evidence of significant cerumen accumulation or a foreign body in the ear canal.
(viii) Pain or discomfort in the ear.

Special care should be exercised in selecting and fitting a hearing aid whose maximum sound pressure level exceeds 132 decibels because there may be risk of impairing the remaining hearing of the hearing aid user. (This provision is required only for those hearing aids with a maximum sound pressure capability greater than 132 decibels [dB].)

In the provision for waiving the medical examination, the following precedes the signature line:

Federal law restricts the sale of hearing aids to those individuals who have obtained a medical evaluation from a licensed physician. Federal law permits a fully informed adult to sign a waiver statement declining the medical evaluation for religious or personal beliefs that preclude consultation with a physician. The exercise of such a waiver is not in your best health interest and its use is strongly discouraged.

DiSogra (2012) provides an excellent summary of the provisions and regulatory constraints set forth by the FDA, the FTC, and the National Center for Complementary and Alternative Medicine (CAM). This is a must read for all clinicians, students and their professors. An extensive reference for relevant Web sites offers an expansive opportunity to assess supplements and medications and their positive and negative impact on patient care: "Audiologists must continuously ask new questions during the case history review that include the use of FDA-approved drugs, herbal medicines, and nutritional supplements whose side effects could impact on subjective and objective data interpretation."

Evidence-Based Decision Making

Evidence-based practice in health care requires explicit and judicious use of information in making decisions about matters that directly influence the quality of care provided to patients. In health care, it covers the gamut from counting numbers of visits to a patient's bedside by nursing personnel during hospitalization to counting the numbers of repairs sustained within a specific hearing instrument model or, more generally, by a specific manufacturer.

Incidence of Repairs

The incidence of hearing instrument repairs by manufacturers must be monitored regularly. When repaired instruments are sent or received, a few minutes spent logging information about the repair provides compelling information about the manufacturer, instrument model and repair history of the instrument. It takes little effort to gain additional important information beyond counting the number of repairs. By documenting repairs by circuit class or model, the practice will get a failure rate for each class of instrument dispensed (Figure 17–1). Should a spike in the incidence data occur, an analysis will be at hand and a call to the manufacturer to discuss the dilemma must be made immediately. If the particular circuit class or model of interest continues to fail, it would be appropriate to stop fitting that particular instrument class or model. It

Records of Repairs by Manufacturer												
	Jan	Feb	Mar	Apr	May	Jun	Jul	Aug	Sep	Oct	Nov	Dec
Model #												
<1 yr												
1–2 yrs												
2–3 yrs												
3–5 yrs												
Re-Rep												
Cost												
Turnaround												

Figure 17–1. Repair records.

would also be appropriate to reassess the past records of repairs and determine whether it is time to consider finding another source for hearing instruments.

How much data should be required to contact the manufacturer? That depends on several factors. Certainly volume should be a factor: If the practice is dispensing a significant number of a specific model, the data will dictate the need quite readily if there is an inherent problem within the circuit class or model. If the data signals a developing panel of evidence that one in five instruments requires a return for repair, the manufacturer should be contacted immediately. Advise the manufacturer of the findings and ask if they have noted similar difficulties with that particular model. They may have a fitting or modification suggestion that will resolve the repair issue completely. If the repair manager replies they have not seen a pattern in that particular instrument model, advise them that, in your hands, the instrument is failing. After you have stated your case with the data, make it clear that if these failures continue, there will be no more orders forthcoming from the practice for this particular instrument model.

Confirm the telephone conversation with the repair manager via e-mail and include copies to the inside sales staff member assigned to your account and

to the president of the company. Presidents of hearing instrument manufacturing companies are sometimes the last to know there is a flaw in a specific model or circuit class. They understand you must act as your patient's advocate in these matters. They also understand that you will cease to dispense their products if situations such as repeated failures continue. Consistent problems in your practice should become known to every level within the product side of the instrument manufacturer's hierarchy.

Changing Manufacturers: When It's Time to Go

Patient satisfaction is tied to a variety of factors. When managing patients, audiologists must recognize and accept the fact that patient satisfaction is tied directly to the hearing instrument and to the services provided by the audiologist directing the patient's hearing care in about the same measure.

Factors to Consider in the Decision

Hearing instrument manufacturers must share in the responsibility for declining

---

Sidebar 17–3
**TO CEO OF XXXXX HEARING INSTRUMENTS:
UNRESOLVED PROBLEMS**

8-13-2012
Mr. XXXX, CEO:

We are seeing wax springs in both new instruments and repaired instruments. We have made it known on MULTIPLE occasions that we do not want wax springs in new and repaired instruments. If you are unable to comply with our request we will simply stop using your products. There is no excuse for this.

We have requested that tubing on RIC instruments include appropriately colored tubing for our patients of color. The first discussion and request was issued 12/16/2011. We have had 5 subsequent complaints from our patients and I agree with their complaints completely. We have tried coloring the tubing; however, no matter what we use, the coloring wears off. I should not have to do this sort of cover-up for an issue you fail to recognize as important. There is absolutely no reason why XXXXX Hearing Instruments cannot avoid this obvious discriminatory practice.

We are experiencing a marked increase in repairs on instruments less than a year old. Several of the instruments were returned with no changes nor adjustments. It is obvious that no repair was completed. Re-repairs within 45 days are unacceptable. Too many repairs produce too many patients dissatisfied with your products. This makes XXXXX Hearing Instruments look bad and makes the level of our care decline in the eyes of our patients. This is unacceptable and another reason to cease using your products.

I have been a user of XXXXX Hearing Instruments products for many years. Of course there have been bumps along the way but nothing like the issues we are seeing currently. Something is seriously wrong. I have discussed this with a number of colleagues across the country and it appears difficulties (well above the usual grumblings) are not isolated to my region of the country. If these issues are not resolved, we will find another source for our hearing instruments.

Robert G. Glaser, PhD
XxXxXx

---

patient satisfaction when directly relatable to the hearing instrument. Lack of or lethargic responses to inquiries in the face of well-documented evidence that a segment of their product line is consis-tently failing should be a strong factor in the decision to seek another source for hearing instruments. In some cases, it may be the most important or singular reason to move to another instrument manufacturer. If the incidence of repairs exceeds established practice benchmarks; if turnaround time on repairs is excessive; if the incidence of re-repairs is increasing and re-repairs are on the rise, the need to move to another instrument manufacturer becomes undeniably evident—a "no-brainer." The bottom line of the practice requires optimum product reliability and fast and reliable resolution of product line difficulties.

Establishing Perspective: Continuous Monitoring of Acquisition Costs

Practice owners and managers tend to overlook the amount of money spent in the purchase of hearing instruments. It is as if they get lulled to sleep by the fact that instrument costs never decline and always increase so why worry about that which you cannot control. Changes in costs of instruments seem to be coming more frequently than ever before. As such there is an ever stronger need to consistently monitor acquisition costs. It takes little time to read the invoice and do the addition and it clarifies the amount of money the practice sends to each manufacturer. It will put each manufacturer into a financial perspective and appropriately embolden the practice owner or manager to become more assertive in their advocacy efforts for their patients. If an instrument cost

has increased a substantial amount, contact your representative and find out why the spike in cost and ask about alternative pricing or suggestions about other items in their lineup that might serve as a viable alternatives. Of course if the alternatives offer little or no benefit, it is a valid signal to seek options available from other manufacturers. The previous year's total amount spent should be in the heading of the column to further recognize the level of participation with each manufacturer. A running tabulation of acquisition costs is a simple statistic to maintain relative to the perspective it provides (Figure 17–2).

Factors to Consider Other Than Product Lines and Repair Parameters

An interesting revolution in the profession of audiology began in the late 1990s. It began when major hearing instrument manufacturers decided to solidify distribution outlets for their products. In essence, manufacturers determined the need to secure and manage clinical outlets that would dedicate dispensing efforts specifically within their respective product lines. These efforts paralleled ongoing activity in "managed care," where health care services are delivered to member-patients of health maintenance organizations (HMO) or networks at specified locations by a panel of partic-

Records of Instruments Ordered and Received				
Patient Name	Instrument Make/Model	Acquisition Cost	Running Total Manufacturer	Dates Ordered/Received
	/	/	/	/

Figure 17–2. Record of instruments ordered/received.

ipating providers or employee-providers of the HMO or network. In managed care organizations, medical care, therapies, and hospitalization are controlled by corporate entities. Managers assign patients to participating providers or employee-practitioners for general or specific health care. Medication regimen, surgical intervention, selection of specialists, specific testing protocols, and other utilization activities are carefully controlled with strict guidelines and utilization reviews. Participating providers may suggest particular therapies or medications; however, these suggestions are subject to review and approval by corporate managers.

Similar efforts have been ongoing within the hearing care industry in the form of corporate and practice consolidations. Soaring operating costs including research and development, production, facilities, personnel and a host of other costs have contributed to this trend. So too has the opportunity for greater control and profitability within the marketplace in the United States and throughout the world. On the positive side, greater application of resources will continue to foster improvements in technologies and, therefore, greater opportunities for success for those patients described as nonadopters (Kochkin, 2012). The forms of these consolidation efforts fall primarily into three categories: company owned outlets, manufacturer branded distribution, and manufacturer affiliated provider practices:

■ *Company owned outlets* are retail outlets purchased and owned by the consolidating instrument manufacturer. Both administrative and clinical staff members are employees of the manufacturer and overhead considerations such as rent, utilities, office outfitting, and leasehold improvements are the responsibility of the manufacturer.

■ *Manufacturer branded distribution* facilities are recognizable members of a chain of retail outlets exclusively dispensing the retail brand of the instrument manufacturer. The manufacturer covers expenses for advertising and promotion and supplies leads to the chain's participating providers. Overhead costs remain the responsibility of the owner of the distribution outlet.

■ *Affiliated provider practices* are independent practices with a contract to purchase instruments and related products from a distributor-consolidator. The practice agrees to buy instruments from the same corporation that owns retail outlets and manufacturer branded distribution chain locations. The corporation sets the prices the practice pays for the instruments. Overhead costs including administrative and professional staff are the responsibility of the owner.

The Final Note: Patient Advocacy

Patient advocacy is a time-honored tradition of all health care practitioners: whatever it takes to guarantee the quality of patient care, dedicated health care practitioners work diligently on behalf of their patients. Whether it is establishing or improving licensing and regulatory issues for audiologists or whether it is the concerted efforts of an entire profession actively advancing providers to doctoral level training and expectations, patient welfare, and quality of care are at the core of professional health care providers.

Audiologists are advocates in the relationship between hearing instrument manufacturers and the end-users of their products. It is the audiologist's job to work diligently on behalf of the patient to ensure appropriate instrumentation is placed and applied relative the patient's need. No matter the situation or circumstance, the audiologist as health care provider must first and foremost put the interests of his or her patients before those of the practice and the hearing instrument manufacturer. The audiologist must function as the patient's intercessor in matters of conflict that may arise from time-to-time with hearing instrument manufacturers and suppliers. The practice must insist that instrument manufacturers, suppliers, and related vendors participate as actively as any member of the practice in placing the patient at the forefront of interest in all deliberations and resolution of conflict.

In contemporary hearing health care, adhering to the concept of patient centric care is as much the responsibility of the audiologist managing the patient's aural rehabilitation as it is the responsibility of instrument manufacturers and suppliers. In the final analysis, we are all in this together with the success of those whom we serve at the core of all we do.

References

Berger, K. W. (1984). *The hearing aid: Its operation and development* (3rd ed.). Livonia, MI: National Hearing Aid Society.

DiSogra, R. M. (2012). Adverse herbal and nutritional/dietary supplement side effects. *Audiology Today, 24*(6), 40–48.

Fabry, D. A., Launer, S., & Derleth, P. (2007). Hearing aid technology vs. steeply sloping sensorineural hearing loss. *Hearing Review, 14*(1), 18–24.

Glaser, R. G. (2012). Unpublished data on rates of hearing aid repairs.

Groth, J., & Mecklenburger, J. (2011). Do's and don't's of open fittings. *Hearing Review, 18*(5), 12–18.

Hedge, A. (2007). Ergonomic guidelines for user-interface design. *CU Ergo.* Retrieved January 28, 2007, from http://ergo.human.cornell.edu/ahtutorials/interface.html

Kirkwood, D. H. (2001). Most dispensers in Journal's survey report greater patient satisfaction with digitals. *Hearing Journal, 54*(3), 21–32.

Kochkin, S. (2005). MarkeTrak VII: Satisfaction with hearing instruments in the digital age. *Hearing Journal, 58*(9), 30–37.

Kochkin, S. (2012). MarkeTrak VIII: The key influencing factors in hearing aid purchase intent. *Hearing Review, 19*(5), 12–31.

Smiriga, D.J. (2004). Are we asleep at the wheel? The delicate future of audiology private practice in America. *ADA Feedback, 15*(4), 7–15.

18

Practice Management Considerations in a University Audiology Clinic

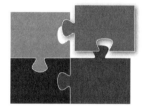

GAIL M. WHITELAW, PhD, MHA

Introduction

It may seem unusual to find a chapter on the management of a university-based audiology clinic in a text on strategic practice management targeting profit-based practice models. Historically, university clinics have been based on a model in which they are viewed as a "teaching laboratory." In this lab model, services were provided at no charge or at a significantly reduced fee and often only during periods that coincided with the university calendar. The focus in this model was assuring that students in audiology programs had subjects on whom to "practice" their clinical skills.

However, transitions in both the profession of audiology and of higher education have resulted in an evolution from this "lab model" to a model that recognizes the university clinic as a business. The demands of doctor of audiology (AuD) programs require that university audiology clinics provide breadth and depth of clinical experiences delivered in an environment that prepares the AuD student to enter the profession of audiology. A not-for-profit mantra of "no margin, no mission" must be the guiding principle for university audiology clinics, both to provide a clinical model appropriate to support AuD education and to survive in the changing University environment. This principle supports a strong clinical education model with the clinic being a critical entry point to prepare students for the demands of the profession of audiology both now and into the future. As suggested by Novak (2004), it is imperative that there is consistency of clinical preparation for students entering the profession, so that the transition from university audiology clinic to clinical sites that partner with the university support the development of professional knowledge and skills. As noted by Newman, Sandridge, and Lesner (2011), the best clinical education models incorporate direct patient care, which extends beyond a traditional classroom model and supports using the "clinic as a classroom." Therefore, the university audiology clinic must be an environment that sets the standard to nurture the entry of young audiologists into their profession.

The challenge facing the university audiology clinic is the need to "serve many masters," although often simplified into a dichotomy of clinical education and patient care. On the one hand, as already described, the mission of the university clinic is indeed, to create the "clinic as classroom" environment for AuD students, as previously suggested. On the other hand, exceptional patient care must be a mission of the clinic. An example of this split is reflected in the leadership role of the university audiology clinic director; as Bartlett, McNamara, and Peaper (2006a) note, the director's skills must

be broad based and "are bifurcated and continuously being diverted into separate but equal, intersecting, and interdependent lines of responsibility (p. 1)."

One could make the point that "if you've seen one university audiology clinic, you've seen one university audiology clinic"; although this point could likely be made regarding any audiology practice setting, it may ring particularly true for university audiology clinics, due to the variations in higher education (e.g., public, private, associated with a medical school, etc.). A unique challenge may be considered to be the longevity of many audiology programs that house university audiology programs. University speech and hearing clinics, where many of these audiology clinics are housed, are among the oldest clinical service providers in the United States, with clinics like those at the University of Iowa or the Ohio State University, founded in the 1930s, and those at Washington University in St. Louis and the University of Texas-Austin, operating since the 1940s. Clinics with this type of history have many benefits, such as that of name recognition and university reputation. This type of tradition, however, may result in either a real or perceived lack of flexibility and responsiveness required to meet the needs of patients and to provide clinical education. The traditional university audiology clinic is in a period of transition, even with the development of more flexible models that do not rely on the "brick and mortar," such as consortia arrangements and distance learning options.

Along with the benefits of association with a university, the audiology clinic may have the limitations of more constraints and less autonomy than for a community based or independent audiology practice. The benefits of being able to access support and services from the university, such as cleaning, risk management, or legal, are offset by needing to use a monopoly and the need to pay for these services, which may be priced at a rate higher than if the clinic were able to seek independent estimates. This defies the myth that clinics housed at public universities have the unfair advantage of receiving free "taxpayer subsidized" services and clinics housed at private universities are offered tax breaks over their community "competitors." The fact is that taxpayer support of universities continues to decline (Meister, 2011). The current demands on the university audiology clinic is to be more self-sustaining than in the past and is certainly an impetus in managing the practice in a strategic manner.

Funding and Support

As the landscape in higher education funding continues to change, the impact on university-based audiology clinics is evident. Universities are viewed as businesses and administrators are charged to be fiscally responsible. The model followed in many universities requires cost shifting so that costs incurred by an individual unit (e.g., department or clinic) are assigned to that unit. In the past, the cost of "education" was typically borne by the university, usually in a centralized model. The university, as an entity, received tuition revenues from students; in turn, the full cost of the education of the student was covered. In the current model, the differential cost of education, such as additional costs incurred in a clinical education program, is assigned to the individual "unit" providing the education, such as the department or the clinic. In this decentralized model, the audiology clinic may be responsible for

covering costs associated with its operation and, presumably, the revenue generated by the audiology clinic is "earned" by the clinic and can be assigned to the costs of running the business. Any revenue that exceeds cost, or profit, should be available for the clinic to expand programs and services, provide care for the indigent, or purchase equipment, among other activities related to the mission of the clinic. However, it may be difficult to generate a profit in this environment due to the demands and expectations of the University. Costs allocated to the clinic may be similar to those of practices in the private sector; leasehold and other space-related costs, insurance costs, specific facility charges, and other overhead costs. In addition, audiology clinics housed within Universities are often viewed as "earnings units," with the expectation that the clinic has both the ability and responsibility to generate revenue to the point of being self-sustaining. In many University settings, this business model for the audiology clinic is a paradigm shift from the past. It is, however, clearly a trend that will continue into the foreseeable future (Lundy, 2006). This shift coincides with changes in professional preparation in audiology that support the need for the University clinic to be based on a business model, as a foundation for professional preparation.

The Changing Landscape for Service Provision in the University Setting

The strategic management tenets identified in this text certainly apply to the management of a university audiology clinic. Effective management is a critical topic; however, a review of the literature suggests a dearth of information specific to this practice setting. A chapter on administration of speech-language-hearing programs within the university setting by Hardick and Oyer (1987) highlighted some of the same issues that will be identified in this chapter. However, review of the Hardick and Oyer chapter demonstrates both the evolution and revolution in the delivery of audiology services that have occurred in the past few decades. The challenges facing audiology, including implementing a clinic technology platform, the everchanging human resource environment, use of electronic health records, and enhanced government regulation, as mandated in the privacy and security components of the Health Insurance Portability and Accountability Act (HIPAA), could not have been anticipated 25 years ago. Developing a university clinic model that emulates other practice settings is crucial, as the issues facing the university clinic are more similar to those in other practice settings than in the past, a trend that will certainly continue.

The Council of Academic Programs in Communication Sciences and Disorders (CAPCSD) is an organization with a mission to support undergraduate and graduate programs in communication sciences and disorders. CAPCSD has as one of its goals to support the clinical education process, thus the organization has an interest in both the university-based audiology clinic and the "town-grown" partnership between the university program and the community preceptors. A review of the proceedings of the annual meeting of Council of Academic Programs in Communication Sciences and Disorders (CAPCSD) for the past 10 years reveals many presentations on the topic of university clinics; however, the vast majority focuses on the broader perspective of clinical education. These topics

include changes in certification requirements, approaches to clinical supervision, or the focus of preparing future personnel to meet general requirements in the workplace (ASHA, 2000; CAPCSD, 2011). In addition, only five articles that deal exclusively with issues related to university clinic administration have been published among the more than two hundred fifty articles that have appeared in *Perspectives in Administration and Supervision,* the journal of ASHA's Special Interest Group (SIG) Eleven since its inception (Special Interest Group 11: Administration and Supervision, 2011).

The purpose of this chapter is to focus on the unique challenges and opportunities of running a practice within the university environment. This chapter will focus on a number of areas, including physical facilities, personnel, pricing of goods and services, and marketing.

Physical Facilities and the Practice of Audiology

The university setting provides a unique environment in which to develop and maintain an audiology practice. In addition to the number of audiologists employed, number of patients served, and other services, such as speech-language pathology or physical therapy, available in the practice, a number of issues are distinctive in the university environment. The type of university, whether state funded or privately funded, can have a significant impact on the federal and/or state rules that govern the function of the clinic and types of funding support that may be available to support the clinic's mission. The college or "unit" in which the clinic is housed can also guide the practice. University clinics are located in a wide variety of units, including colleges of allied medicine, education, social and behavioral sciences, arts and sciences, optometry, and medicine. In many cases, the audiology clinic may be the only clinical education program within the college, a lone "earnings unit" and/or facility providing patient care within the college. Deans of colleges with backgrounds not related to audiology may comment on the expense of clinical education, often without recognizing the benefits of the clinic to the department, college, or community.

As noted previously, university audiology clinics may receive significant benefits from being housed within the university. These benefits may include access to legal services, assistance with purchasing, fiscal management services, and marketing consultation. The clinic may benefit from the economy of scale available based on the size of university and also the specialized knowledge and skills of those employed by the university. Specific benefits may include access to services that facilitate contract negotiation with knowledge specific to this setting, an understanding of target marketing within the university community, and access to discounts on office equipment and supplies based on the purchasing power of the University. In addition, the reputation of the university may provide a "halo" effect for the clinic, in which patients choose to seek their hearing care at the clinic due to positive regard for the University or one of its sports teams.

Challenges of Operating in the University Environment

The university environment can provide unique challenges to effectively operating an audiology practice. Choices that are available in other practice settings, such as location, signage, or décor of the office may not exist in the university setting. University clinics may be required to pay physical facilities assessment, similar to rent, however may have little ability to make decisions about the space and literally no ability to negotiate the amount charged for the space assigned. This also applies to the overhead rate charged by the university. Assuming the university audiology clinic operates on a business model, the clinic should expect to pay for the resources utilized. However, there must be a vehicle to negotiate. Information is power and the clinic director must know the cost per square foot for the "rent" charged and how these decisions are made by the university. The clinic director should carefully analyze the space needs for the clinic and assure that the clinic is not paying for more space than is actually needed. In addition, space needs should be analyzed in terms of purpose of the space. If the space is used primarily for research or shared with department administration, only the actual space utilized for clinical activities should be counted in this process. This also requires that the department chair and/or college dean understand the use of space and advocates for the clinic in the space allocation process. In addition, the clinic may receive benefits from developing a coalition with other clinical education programs providing services on campus. This type of coalition may be either formal or informal and may include clinics such as those housed in optometry, psychology, and/or education. Such a partnership can provide leverage in discussions with the university related to rates or overhead and opportunities to educate university administrators about the breadth of clinical education on their campus.

As mentioned previously, the university clinic location may be fixed. Most clinics are housed within their department, which limits choices of location on campus. Decisions are not likely to be based on patient need, but rather on where space is available, the location of the college in relation to the department, and other factors which do not address the needs of clinical service provision nor the population being served. In an era of privatization in higher education, some university clinics may be able to take advantage of opportunities to rent space off campus or generally think outside of the proverbial clinic location "box." An example of this would be the model at the University of Pittsburgh, which does not have a traditional "in-house" university audiology clinic, but utilizes partnerships throughout the Pittsburgh community to support the majority of the clinical education model. AuD students are placed in these sites and supervised by university-employed preceptors, who fulfill the roles of clinical supervisors for the university and of clinical service provision for the sites.

In addition, a program may raise funds through university development to build their own clinical facility or share with similar programs within a college. An example of this is the Bill Wilkerson Center for Otolaryngology and Communication Sciences at Vanderbilt University, designed to encourage interdisciplinary collaboration and research in all of the speech, language and hearing sciences, and otolaryngology specialties. The amount of funds required to build a facility along with space being at a premium are factors that would limit the feasibility of this model in many universities. In addition, most audiology programs in universities cannot easily move locations.

Patient Care Considerations in the University Audiology Clinic

Assuming that the clinic location is generally a nonnegotiable, a number of factors that impact patient care must be considered. On most university campuses, parking is a valuable commodity. Parking generally reflects a delicate balance of supply and demand and the supply of available parking is often a significant distance from the location of the clinic. Universities have historically been designed to meet the needs of young adults for whom parking a distance from academic or recreational facilities may be less of a physical challenge than for clinic patients and their families. However, with changes in the demographics of higher education, demands for accessibility on campus, and an increased focus on consumerism on campuses, improvements in parking services with an eye toward accessibility are likely to occur. In addition, increases in online education and virtual classrooms even on traditional campuses suggest changes in demand for parking in the future. The current situation is generally the same on most college campuses: although physical access to the clinical facility may be appropriate, the distance from the parking area may be significant, parking options may be limited, or the parking area may present challenges in terms of related factors, including grading of walkway that take into account the clinical population served or signage that clearly identifies the clinic. Parking may require that creative solutions, such as valet or dedicated parking options available only to audiology clinic patients, be implemented. These types of solutions can facilitate access to a clinic, but often come at a cost higher than would be negotiated in a private practice setting. In addition, if the clinic building is "landlocked" within a university campus, limited options may be available. In this case, the growth of the clinic may be constrained by how many patients may park to access the building at any given time. Obviously, it is critical to educate those in both administration and customer service at the university's department of transportation or parking regarding the missions and functions of the clinic and the special needs of those seeking hearing and balance services at the clinic. Utilizing specially designated clinic spaces or spaces designated for those with disabilities can provide options that increase both access to the clinic and number of patients that can be accommodated. Patients may be able to access special parking permits or tokens to park in restricted areas or be able to access parking meters located close to the clinic. Patients, however, may be sensitive to the additional cost of parking, a factor that may be viewed as a negative in utilizing services at the university audiology clinic. Paying a parking meter in order to access services is consistently cited as the most frequent complaint on patient satisfaction surveys over the past 10 years in the author's clinic setting. This issue virtually disappeared when Transportation and Parking Services changed access to a lot adjacent to the clinic and patients were able to obtain permits allowing them to park in that lot at no charge. Of course, the university passed the cost of "renting" these spaces on to the clinic; however, the improved access to parking has been worth the additional cost incurred.

Other types of overhead assigned from the university may include building services, such as housekeeping/cleaning. As discussed earlier in this chapter,

communication regarding the mission of the clinic, the patient population served, and consumer expectations are critical to successful management of a patient-centered practice within the structure of the university. University services, such as cleaning, are often hired as subcontractors based on a bidding process. The bidding criteria should include specifications for the specialized needs of the audiology clinic population, such as vacuuming after hours to minimize noise interference during audiometric testing or additional cleaning needs when serving young children. The audiology clinic director should participate in developing the bid criteria or communicate specific needs in working with janitorial subcontractors. In addition, the clinic director should participate in the evaluation of services provided as a criterion of the contract between the service provider and the university. This participation allows for clear communication regarding expectations of cleaning, providing a vehicle to document these expectations, and the ability to develop corrective actions if the criteria are not met. These corrective actions may include the ability to modify the contract or to be granted the flexibility to hire a cleaning service independent of that provided by the university.

The advent of telepractice in audiology, or "teleaudiology," may provide increased opportunities for both the University clinic and for patients and may help to minimize clinical space and physical facility concerns. Telepractice may be defined as "the application of telecommunications technology to deliver professional services at a distance . . . for assessment, intervention, and/or consultation" (Romanow & Brannon, 2010). As noted previously, distance education options are common on university campuses and telemedicine options available through medical schools, establishing a precedent on university campuses. Thus, the university audiology clinic may be well positioned to establish services through a telehealth practice model. This model may address patient care needs, along with concerns about access to audiology services, both in terms of increasing demand and ongoing issues in rural and underserved areas. (Donahue, Dubno, & Beck, 2010). University clinics often have a increased supply of available "hands," with AuD students able to provide teleaudiology services under the direction of a preceptor. The clinic may be able to provide much needed outreach and the AuD students will gain exposure to a different model of service delivery, perhaps for a population that will diversity their clinical experience or opportunity. Clinical education is no longer constrained by geography or facility and access to clinical service is clearly a benefit to the patient. However, to date, teleaudiology services are not covered by Medicare and are generally restricted by third-party payers (Romanow & Brannon, 2010). Thus, the benefits of access and quality of service provision and opportunity for clinical education may be offset by limited opportunity to charge for these services. From a revenue perspective, there may be other opportunities available to the university clinic, including grants or interdisciplinary partnerships that will help to offset the cost of providing these services.

Personnel in the University Audiology Clinic

There are a number of personnel challenges that are unique to the university setting. First, the person that oversees the clinic may be a skilled clinical supervisor, researcher, or teacher, but may have little preparation for administrative and management demands of an audiology practice. This person may be selected based on seniority or as part of their "service load" within the Department and have little knowledge, skill, or interest in running a business. A clinic director dedicated to managing a business helps to ensure both the fiscal success of the clinic and its strength in the clinical education process. It is important that both the personnel in department and college understand the demands of running a practice and the unique skills and knowledge required to effectively administer this practice.

Administration of the Clinic

The university clinic director must have many of the same skills as an audiologist in private practice, incorporating functional areas such as marketing, finance, and human resource management. However, the clinic director may be constrained from making independent decisions available to those in private practice due to restrictions inherent in the university setting. Based on the university model, the clinic director may be forced to utilize the skills and knowledge of others within the department, such as a fiscal officer, or employees within another unit, such as purchasing or business and finance. These employees may have little knowledge or interest in issues related to practice management, and the tasks required for clinical management may differ significantly from the skills required in a traditional university department. Bartlett, McNamara, and Peaper (2006) describe the balancing act of clinical education demands with clinic operations demands in an era of shrinking resources in higher education. Their survey of clinic directors in university settings described personnel challenges including an inadequate number of clinical supervisors and inadequate or nonexistent clerical staff that are critical for managing a successful clinical practice.

In addition to the clinic director, audiologists are employed in university-based clinical settings. These audiologists may have a role either as a clinical supervisor or preceptor, as a direct service provider, or as a hybrid of the two. Historically, services were only provided in the university audiology clinic when students were available and audiologists employed in this type of setting usually did not provide direct service. This trend has changed with consumer demand and the fact that problems with hearing aids do not happen only on the university schedule. This requires that audiologists employed in university settings are not only knowledgeable in the process of clinical supervisor and clinical education, but also in the current practices of the profession. In many university medical center settings, a marketing slogan is related to the concept of "we practice what we teach," which characterizes the current trend in the university audiology clinic. Just as in other practice settings, audiologists in the university setting must consider how their time is spent and the value of that time in the overall profitability of the practice (Kasewurm, 2011a.) Not only is this important in order to meet financial targets for the clinic but also to provide a model of professional behavior for future audiologists. Another issue is how to provide continuity in patient care, so that patients both understand that services are provided in a clinical education environment yet have their needs effectively and efficiently met. The scheduling of appointments must be as realistic as possible in order to strike a balance of providing the opportunity for learning yet to ensure that the patient's time is valued. These are challenges in the clinical education process and the audiology preceptor has to balance the importance of patient care with the demands of clinical education. Patients should be given the opportunity to request an audiologist that will provide their clinical services and ever effort should be made to assure that the patient will be followed by that individual. Although it is generally the audiology supervisor with whom the relationship will be established, it is also not unusual for a patient to request a particular AuD student with whom they have developed a relationship to provide continuity of care. The limitations of this type of schedule may discourage some patients from seeking services in the university clinic; however, others will see that participating in a clinical education model as having significant benefit. Just as with any practice setting, it is impossible to be all things to all patients and audiologists employed in this setting must capitalize on the strengths available.

Guidelines for clinical supervision and mentoring are evolving with changes in accreditation and certification guidelines. These changes require new approaches to mentoring and innovative methods of assessing student performance, often developed by the audiologists employed as supervisors. Audiologists employed in the university may also be responsible for developing and nurturing partnerships with audiologists in the community. In addition to their clinical responsibilities, university-based audiologists are often engaged in planning the fourth year preceptorship for AuD students, thus strengthening the "town-grown" partnership that is critical in preparing students for independent practice of the profession of audiology and directing clinical education. The critical nature of this relationship cannot be underestimated and the importance of developing and maintaining strong relationships with community practitioners to participate in the educational process is key to the future of the profession. As clinical education in audiology has transitioned from a master's degree with a separate clinical fellowship year or professional experience year model to the current model with fourth years as an educational experience, the university has the significant role in developing a comprehensive clinical education program. This model must incorporate a plan where the university and preceptor enter into a relationship that is mutually beneficial and contributes positively to the student's educational program. To that end, the university-based audiologists must make the professional contacts with preceptors and not rely on students to contact preceptors independently. In addition, preceptors must understand the mission and vision of the clinical education program and that they will participate in an educational partnership with student. Several programs have been developed that address these partnerships by integrating academic and clinical education across settings and providing training in being a mentor. These programs include Mentoring AuDs (MAuDs), a program sponsored by the Illinois Academy of Audiology, and the preceptor education model developed by the Northern Ohio Audiology Coalition (NOAC), the joint partnership between the University of Akron, Kent State University, and the Cleveland Clinic.

Clinical Faculty Rank

Many universities have a clinical faculty rank that provides an appropriate framework for hiring, retaining, and promoting those employed in clinical education. This classification differentiates from the traditional faculty ranks in the university, for which the requirements may have little flexibility to recognize the clinical education component of these position and recognize teaching and research as the primary criteria for evaluation. Other universities have administrative and professional (A&P) classifications for those employed in the clinic. Although the A&P model may provide a mechanism that reflects the types of skills required for service provision, it can fail to recognize the critical role that these professionals have in the student's education. An important consideration in this discussion is whether the audiologist is on a traditional university 9-month or 10-month contract, or on an annual contract. Obviously, the need for year-round employment of audiologists in a university setting is critical, as most practices cannot be successful if they cannot meet the patient's needs. Most AuD programs are full-year programs based on a professional school education model and not the undergraduate educational model constrained by an academic calendar.

In addition to audiologists/clinical supervisors, appropriate support personnel are as critical in the university setting as they are in the private practice setting. These may include a clinic business/financial manager, billing personnel, clinic secretary, and/or office manager. In some university settings, these roles may be filled by one person, and in some cases, a person who has other job responsibilities within the department and the clinic responsibilities are "add-ons." Every effort should be made to assure that the clinic has dedicated personnel with knowledge and skill sets appropriate to advance the mission of the clinic. Just as in the private practice setting, training of front office personnel is critical. The number of support personnel, and therefore the need for a generalist and/or specialists, is driven by a number of factors, including the number of patients served, the amount of revenue generated, and the size of the program. All personnel should have appropriate training in both their functional areas, such as accounts payable or receivables, and in university procedures specific to these areas. A cost-effective approach for expanding support personnel may be hiring graduate assistants from among students enrolled in the AuD program. These graduate student assignments may include checking in hearing aids, scheduling appointments, or assisting with insurance claims. The employees, because of their status as students, may bring skills and ideas to the work setting, such as technology savvy or knowledge of social networking to promote the clinic, that others in the clinic do not possess. In addition, they have knowledge of audiology. The benefit to the clinic is obvious; however, the student also obtains a more intimate understanding of business-related functions of audiology and an appreciation of attention to detail required in these functions. Hiring graduate assistants may be a cost allocated to the clinic budget or may be an option for the department to provide as a benefit to the clinic in partnering in the clinical education function.

Another option may be to hire audiology assistants, who can provide assistance with hearing aid management,

particularly during times that students may be unavailable, such as when they are in class or on university-designated breaks. The added benefit of employing an audiology assistant in the university clinic is for students to have exposure to a clinical model using a clinical care extender. However, an added demand of supervision of an assistant is placed on the audiologists employed in the university clinic who already may have significant demands on their time.

Salary and benefits are structured and lack flexibility in most universities. Some university employees, depending on their classification, may be members of unions and benefits and working conditions are prescribed with minimal options. The clinic director may need to actively develop mechanisms that recognize audiologists and support staff for their productivity and service, which may include paying for continuing education opportunities, licensure and certification, and liability insurance. The challenge in the university audiology clinic is to elicit "buy in" from audiologists and support staff when the opportunities for "reward" are limited by the constraints of university policies that emphasize a didactic education model. As professional education models in audiology evolve, it is important for the audiology clinic director and the administration of the department and college to advocate models that recognize the contributions of the clinical staff for productivity in the university clinic environment (e.g., patient satisfaction, revenue generation, and student outcomes are some possible measures that may reflect the staff contribution).

The option of housing a clinic that is established like a private practice or a faculty practice model is available in some university settings although prohibited in others (Windmill, Cunningham, & Preminger, 2004). A faculty practice is arguably a more effective clinical education model that emphasizes business management, due to increased autonomy afforded to the partners in the practice. Regardless of the relationship between the university and the practice, all university employees are required to sign conflict of interest statements. These statements should be reviewed carefully so that audiologists affiliated with the university understand the opportunities and limitations of their specific employment setting.

Issues Related to Clinical Education Activities in the University Clinic

A critical component of clinical education and personnel development in the university audiology clinic is the AuD student. Historically, the "corporate culture" of the university audiology clinic reflected the "teaching lab environment" referred to earlier in this chapter. Students may have had a relaxed approach to clinical service provision, assuming that they were "students who were learning in this process" and someone else, usually the audiology clinical supervisor, was the one responsible for ensuring that the patient (often referred to as "clients" in University clinics, particularly in the past) was well served, that the paperwork was filed appropriately, and that the clinical areas were clean and organized. As noted by McCarthy (2006), the doctor of audiology degree was developed in response to external factors including evolution in health care, advances in information and technology,

and the changing demographics of those requiring hearing and balance services. The master of arts degree was inadequate at preparing students academically or clinically to meet the escalating demands of the workplace, thus the knowledge and skill sets were expanded to meet the needs of professional preparation (McCarthy, 2006).

It is imperative that university clinics challenge AuD students by defining clinical service broadly and by setting the expectation of professional behavior that is also modeled by the clinical staff. Generally not paid employees (although a fourth year placement, if in the university clinic, may be a paid), every effort should be made for students to understand that they are to view their role in the university clinic as that of an employee. Students must understand that placement in the university audiology clinic is a critically important segment of their professional preparation. This may require a number of paradigm shifts including those issues related to dress and behavior. The dress code must be clearly communicated and enforced for clinic-employees and AuD students alike. Students may be required to wear a lab coat and must wear a name tag clearly identifying their affiliation with the university audiology program and their role in the clinic as an AuD student. AuD students should have a firm understanding of how to greet patients in an appropriate, professional manner. Students should have the opportunity to observe, develop, and execute skills related to conflict resolution with patients, counseling patients regarding the need for and acceptance of hearing aids and assistive technology, and providing timely, effective, and efficient clinical services. Although this may be critical in all practice settings, word of mouth marketing may be the primary method of marketing the university clinic. As discussed by Kasewurm (2011b), positive word of mouth marketing is critical since satisfied patients pay less attention to the competition, are less price sensitive and cost less to serve than patients who are dissatisfied. In addition, flexibility is certainly a cornerstone in the profession of audiology and should be an expectation that is nurtured in the university clinic.

As noted earlier in the chapter, continuity of patient care should be a focus for the audiology student placed in the university audiology clinic. In some university audiology clinics, student assignments are based on their level in the program or clinical experience in a specific area, such as diagnostics or hearing instruments. In these cases, the student is assigned to a "diagnostic only" clinic during a semester or quarter. Although this may have good face validity as a clinical teaching model, there is no empirical evidence to support that this is the most effective model. From a patient centric approach, a model that provides a broader training experience will yield better continuity of care. This provides a more realistic clinical education model and requires that the audiology supervisor/preceptor and student clinician work together as a team to meet the patient's needs.

The university clinic setting should allow students to develop the knowledge, skills, and values that will transfer to other clinical placements and to the practice of audiology. AuD students should understand their role on the "team" in the clinic by showing respect to the clinic staff and their colleagues. Students must see the clinic as their own and should treat the patients, staff, equipment, and facility with the same respect as if it were their own business. They should have a clear

understanding of the policies and procedures of the clinic, as outlined in clinic manual or handbook. This handbook should be viewed as similar employee policy and procedures manual in a private practice setting and should outline expectations, policies, and protocols that apply to the AuD student. This handbook or manual should be reviewed by the university attorney to ensure it is consistent with university policy. A mechanism for documentation of clinic requirements outlined in the handbook, such as criminal background check, immunizations, training in HIPAA and/or universal precautions procedures, and annual liability insurance update, is necessary, along with a protocol to update this information on a regular basis. This documentation should be provided by the student and kept in a secured area.

The university clinic provides an excellent opportunity for students to learn about issues related to human resource management, even if discussed through hypothetical scenarios. At this point, most university clinics do not employ audiology assistants; however, it is likely that during their careers, audiologists who are currently being educated will be responsible for hiring, supervising, promoting, and terminating employees, including assistants. Peer supervision may provide an excellent mentoring opportunity and enhance patient care, as is implemented in clinical education in other fields (Williams, 1996). These areas of personnel management and supervision are appropriate topics for clinical seminars, courses within the program, or as part of a specialization that a student may choose to take as part of their degree. In addition to providing supervised clinical services within the university clinic environment, students may be given other assignments or projects related to their clinical education. Such projects may include developing and publishing brochures and patient newsletters, participating in community education events, creating marketing plans and activities, and maintaining a hearing instrument loaner stock and hearing-related informational materials. These types of projects may result in materials that can be utilized immediately by the student, provide templates for future reference, and represent a set of transferable skills that will be desirable to employers. However, the unique mission and vision for the clinic, in keeping with the strategic plan, should guide all materials and products so that students develop an appreciation of branding and image in marketing activities (Foltner & Mansfield, 2006).

Just as students have a responsibility to the clinic, they have a right to expect certain types of support within the university clinic. Students must have access to equipment that provides the opportunity both to serve the patient population of the clinic and to learn new procedures and techniques. The number of individuals and relative inexperience of these individuals using clinical equipment should be considerations when purchasing equipment and budgeting for repair. The replacement cycle for equipment may differ from that in other practice settings due to these factors. The clinic and department should work together to allocate equipment costs associated with patient care and those cost associated with clinical education so that an equitable plan for equipment calibration, repair, and replacement is developed. This also applies to associated materials and disposable accessories, such as electrodes.

If the expectation of the student is to view their position as an employee of the clinic, resources must be provided to support this approach. In the past, audiology students performed clinical responsibilities only related to direct patient care.

Currently, the expectation is that student should perform all aspects of professional care, including ordering hearing aids and providing patient follow-up with appropriate supervision and direction. Due to confidentiality issues, the student should have telephone access in a private office area adjacent to relevant patient charts. Private areas should also be available to complete chart notes, write reports, contact manufacturers, and return patient phone calls, as requested by their clinical supervisor. Computer database access with appropriate software programs including access via personal digital assistant technology must also be available.

Although it may be easy to rationalize that current computer scheduling and billing methods are difficult to implement in a University clinic due to planned turnover in students, the number of "hands" on the system (presumably increasing possibilities for errors), and need for ongoing training, both online scheduling systems and electronic medical/health records must be considered as part of the clinical education process therefore integrated into the university clinic. An online booking system has been found to result in a lower "no show" rate in the university clinic setting, despite the patients using this system being significantly older in age than those scheduling by traditional means (e.g., calling to schedule/cancel an appointment) (Parmer, Lange, Madden, & Das, 2009). Jurgens (2008) suggested that an integrated data-management system enhances accuracy of record keeping and allows more time to provide quality care, among other benefits. Clearly, health care has moved to the electronic medical record (EMR), a standard for patient care and a growing necessity for third party reimbursement. This type of technology defines the profession that students educated in the university clinic are entering and support for developing these types of options, from both a clinical education and patient care perspective must be considered.

Cost of Services and Reimbursement Issues

A confusion held by many involved in clinical education in universities and by potential patients of university clinics is that services should be provided at no charge. These attitudes are based on a number of misconceptions including that patients are somehow "guinea pigs" in the education process or that taxpayer dollars cover the operation of the clinic. The mission and vision of the clinic should certainly drive decision making regarding patient care and service provision. Establishing fees for the services rendered should also be in line with the mission of the audiology clinic as well as the university's policy on fee-for-service charges for student provided, faculty supervised service provision. In addition, a patient centric approach to clinical education is critical. Students should be supervised appropriately so that patients receive professional care and do not perceive that they are participating in an "audiology experiment." Participation in research studies associated with the clinic may be an added opportunity and benefit to the patient. However, such participation must be clearly differentiated

from the clinical services provided. In this era of strict regulation and protection of human subjects participating in research, the rules established for subject participation established and enforced by the Institutional Review Board (IRB) differ greatly in need and scope in comparison to patients receiving clinical services.

As noted earlier in the chapter, most university clinics are viewed as earnings units which are expected to cover some or all of the cost of operation. University audiology clinics face the same issues as the universities in which they may be housed: decreased state and federal support, increased regulation, and economic uncertainties, as noted earlier in this chapter. The university clinic cannot count on long-term support from the university to survive or thrive. States continue to reduce taxpayer support for public, higher education, offsetting those reductions with higher tuition to the students (Fish, 2003). A model may exist in which the audiology clinic can access some portion of the tuition paid for the clinical education courses to support the clinic operation. In addition, many professional education programs in universities assess students a lab or clinic fee that is designed to acknowledge the added cost of clinical education, such as the need for additional equipment or materials over and above those necessary for clinical service provision. The university clinic may be able to access a portion of this fee if it currently exists, or to advocate for the development of such a fee if it does not.

A brief discussion on the nonprofit status of the clinic is included in order to address some possible misconceptions about the implications of this classification. Nonprofit organizations are incorporated and exist for education and/

or charitable reasons and from which trustees or shareholders cannot benefit financially. One of the cornerstones of nonprofit organizations has been to build capacity (e.g., financial resources, facilities, personnel) in which to meet their mission. These capacity building activities are generally based on money, and may be based on private contributions, grants, or other sources, viewed as "indirect customers" that are able to support the mission of the organization (Foster & Bradach, 2005). Receiving revenue from goods and services provided to "direct customers" is another method for nonprofit organizations to build this capacity. There is a national trend toward nonprofit organizations engaging in earned-income ventures as they become "more businesslike" and attempt to reduce their reliance on other sources of funds, such as grants or development gifts, which may be less stable sources of income in the current economic and higher education environments (Foster & Bradach, 2005). However, it is noted that these organizations are often poorly prepared to meet the demands of running a successful business. Foster and Bradach (2005) point out that those running nonprofit organizations must have knowledge of issues related to pricing and generating revenue in order to be successful and meet their missions. This principle should guide decisions made related to pricing products and services in the university environment.

An informal survey of a number of university clinics revealed that at least some of these clinics provide services "for free," no fee is associated with the provision of services at the clinic. This may reflect a historic model for a university clinic in the past; however, the transition to the AuD requires students entering the profession to understand the value of the services they provide. As noted earlier in the chapter, the mantra of "no margin, no mission" is a critical one for young professional to integrate into their practice of audiology. Students must understand the "value" of what they provide. As noted by Pessis (2006), "professionalism is not easy to teach, but it is essential to convey by the modeling we provide." A fee-for-service clinic establishes a professional and realistic practice model.

Determining pricing of services and products is covered in other chapters in this book and will not be reviewed here. However, the university clinic director must have a strong knowledge of the cost of providing services within the university environment. Concerns regarding the university "undercutting" cost of products, such as hearing aids, are often noted by audiologists in the community who may also participate as critical partners in the clinical education of students. The university clinic must price products and services in the same manner as every other business: pricing should be based on the actual cost to provide the services or products with an appropriate profit margin based on the mission of the clinic. Just as each audiology practice sets their prices based on their cost of doing business, so should be true in the university setting. Prices of goods and services in the clinic should reflect a business model that incorporates the cost of doing business in this environment. This model should be carefully reviewed by the university administration to assure that pricing of services is also consistent with University policy.

A current topic in the profession is that of bundling versus unbundling hearing aid pricing, with the thought that the unbundled model may be perceived to provide greater transparency to the patient and better addresses patient value-based needs (Amlani, Taylor, & Tara, 2011). On the bundling/unbundling continuum, the university clinic may appear to have a greater degree of flexibility in this decision than other practices, due to what may be perceived as "more hands on deck" that can provide support and counsel to patients fit with hearing aids; what has been described as "cheap labor" by some practices. It is imperative that regardless of whether services are bundled or unbundled, AuD students understand the value add of the services they provide and the role of the quality of the services in dispensing a product.

The mission of the university clinic may allow for provision of services and products not readily available or feasible in other practice settings. University programs may find benefit, for example, in providing education opportunities in adult group aural rehabilitation or educational audiology services. The clinic may develop a contractual relationship with a nursing home or school district for provision of services to meet the educational mission but is also mutually beneficial to the facility receiving the services and the clinic. These contractual relationships should be billed on a fee-for-service basis as suggested above. The benefit to the clinic is that these types of contractual relationships follow a fee-for-service model and are not subject to the types of "discounting" commonplace with third-party payers. These contracts provide an important platform to teach the economics of engaging in fee-for-service health care delivery. As noted in the bundling/unbundling discussion they also provide an opportunity for the student to develop

awareness that the service he or she provides has economic value. Their services are meaningful both clinically and fiscally. In addition, university clinics may have the opportunity to provide outreach using a student-initiated clinic model for providing direct service to those who are under- or uninsured or to increase access through telehealth provision of services (Meah, Smith, & Thomas, 2009).

Another unique aspect of the University clinic is the "bench to bedside" application of research available to enhance patient care. Students should have the opportunity to apply the research results obtained in their labs and discussed in courses and integrate evidence-based practice into patient care. An example of this is the University of Western Ontario Pediatric Audiologic Monitoring Protocol (UWO PedAMP), a tool developed at University of Western Ontario and integrated into their clinical protocol for addressing amplification outcomes as part of a comprehensive hearing aid fitting in children (Goldstein, 2008).

In the current environment, it is likely that university clinics will have relationships with third-party payers, including private health insurance companies, Medicaid, and Medicare. It is critical that students understand the requirements of dealing with third party payers in terms of coding, supervision, and accurate attention to detail related to paperwork. If the clinic accepts third-party payment, an employee who is knowledgeable in this area must be on the clinic staff or hired as a consultant. The clinic should have someone who is knowledgeable about Medicare regulations, specifically as they apply to student supervision and the university setting. As in every other practice setting, audiologists who are preceptors must have a National Provider Identifier

(NPI) and the clinic may also need to apply for a group NPI (Kander, 2010). As with any practice setting, third-party billing is complex and constantly changing and requires the attention of dedicated personnel. Many universities are self-insured and this fact may drive decision making regarding provider status with third-party payers. It may be most efficient and effective to focus efforts in the university insurance plan, as there is consistency in the plan, presumably ease of access to those developing and administering the plan, and a build in marketing benefit, due to the ability for the clinic to participate in university health fairs and plan sponsored wellness events.

Regardless of the source of reimbursement, the university audiology clinic must have an effective billing system in place to track payables and receivables and a mechanism for assuring that bills are paid in a timely manner and that receivables are collected effectively. Students should be exposed to this aspect of practice management by becoming directly involved in these critically important efforts. As noted previously, the audiology clinic should integrate effective software that tracks patient visits, services provided, procedural and diagnostic codes, and charges, among other information. Software programs should be carefully evaluated and matched to the needs of each clinical venue. Those designed for a small private practice or for use within the framework of a hospital setting may be inappropriate for the university audiology clinic. Clinic directors should consult with others in university audiology and or speech/language/hearing clinics to determine options and to obtain feedback about the benefits and glitches of particular clinic management software currently available. Just as with any business, a certain percentage of patients will not pay for services or products they receive. A plan to address collections must be in place in order to recover as many of these funds as possible, along with write-off criteria. The university setting may limit the types of collections options available to the clinic, and may include a collections department within the university or the state attorney general's office. The clinic director and/or business manager must clearly understand the university policies for collection.

The university will have specific rules related to purchasing and accounts payable that are likely to limit some decisions available to the clinic. Vendors may be required to participate in a "competitive bid" procedure, the clinic may have to select from "university-approved vendors," or there may be categories in which minority vendors must be considered. Based on the nature of the hearing instrument industry, the clinic staff will need to educate those in procurement regarding options for selecting hearing instrument manufacturers. The audiologists involved in hearing instrument dispensing should be able to put their specifications and criteria in writing. Universities have protocols that provide multiple cross checks related to purchasing, based on concerns related to ethics, conflict of interest, and prudent use of taxpayer funds. The challenge for the university audiology clinic is to implement these protocols without collapsing under the weight of the bureaucracy. This will take communication with those in purchasing regarding the mission and function of the audiology clinic along with the desire to operate as a business within the constraints of these protocols. A relationship with accounts payable is of particular importance due to the fact that hearing aids will not be received by the clinic if payables do not take into account the patient service mission of the clinic and the need to pay invoices in a timely manner. There may also be more than one clinic on a campus that provides hearing and balance care services and procedures must be in place to assure that charges and refunds are assigned to the appropriate clinic.

Other Considerations

As in all practice settings, the university clinic should have a marketing plan, even if it is very basic. The clinic may have a plan designed by the staff, or may consider other options. Participating in a buying group, like Sonus or American Hearing Aid Associates (AHAA), could provide marketing support to the clinic, along with other benefits. The clinic director may be able to take advantage of marketing or communications resources within the university that will capitalize on a consistent marketing message or program that promotes the clinic utilizing the university's slogans and materials. In addition, the clinic may benefit as a volunteer as a "case study" with a marketing or business class which can provide a market analysis and recommendations at no charge, with the side benefit of educating future marketing professionals about the profession of audiology. The cost of marketing must be included in the clinic budget and should include current needs and methods to address the future, such as an enhanced Web site or resources to support social networking.

Referrals to the university clinic may come from a variety of sources, including university faculty and staff, physicians and health care providers within the community, and self-referrals. The marketing adage of "perception is reality" may apply to the university clinic more than to any other practice setting in audiology. On the one hand, there may be a perception that services and products provided in the university setting are the most up-to-date and cutting edge due to the educational mission of the clinic. On the other hand, there may be a perception that services are provided by students with little experience making decisions independently. Marketing programs should target referral sources and the community and address these perceptions. Certainly, the name of the university provides a competitive advantage in certain markets. However, marketing should also highlight the clinical education mission of the clinic and the implications of this mission.

Clinic staff and students should be involved in all marketing activities, including activities that recognize and thank referral sources, promote services in wellness events, and provide community presentations. Understanding patient expectations, perceptions, and responses is enhanced by participation in these types of activities and is critical in the clinical education process. These experiences also reinforce clinical education activities and expectations, such as the importance of delivering services in a timely and efficient manner, a frequent criticism of university audiology clinics. Conversely, everyone involved in marketing of the clinic must understand the mission and vision of the clinic and communicate the message that the model utilized in the university audiology clinic may not be one that meets the needs of a specific patient. If all services are provided by students supervised by a licensed audiologist, the patient should understand that the supervising audiologist may not be providing direct or exclusive services to the patient. As stated previously in this chapter, this falls in the category that the university audiology clinic cannot or should not try to be "all things to all people" and understanding the target market helps to utilize time and resources most effectively.

As noted earlier in this chapter, it may be a paradigm shift for a university to have a patient centric service focus, since historically clinics housed in universities have been set up to primarily address the educational needs of students. This trend is certainly changing in universities and it is the responsibility of all associated with the clinic to promote the "patient centric" focus described in this text both within the clinic and in the larger environment of the university. This focus is the right one if optimal patient care is to be provided. It builds a clinical education model that will guide students effectively, and may have unintended benefits to the university community. A satisfied patient may be a significant factor in the marketing plan, since, as mentioned earlier; word of mouth is often a strong marketing component in the university setting. This may generalize to other clinical settings within the university, making this patient a "loyal customer" of other service providers available within the university. In addition, patients who are satisfied with the services they receive at the clinic may donate to a clinic development fund, which can support the missions of the clinic such as new equipment or a loaner hearing aid bank, which enhance both patient care and clinical education.

In the current era of higher education financing, it is clear that there is increased pressure for clinical programs and university-based clinics to be self-sufficient; however, these clinics may be constrained by regulations and policies that impact autonomy in options and decision making. Despite all of these considerations, the transition to the AuD has provided both an opportunity and imperative to transform the university audiology clinic to an efficient and effective nonprofit business. The tenets set forth in this book should help guide that plan, along with specifics addressed in this chapter. The university audiology clinic has a critical role in meeting patient needs, providing clinical education, and facilitating clinically relevant research. This role will increase with demands for services, changes in the model for AuD education, and with greater emphasis on evidence-based practice. This is framed by continued issues in funding of higher education and reimbursement for hearing and balance services. In order to be successful, the university clinic will need to transition to a nonprofit business for the new millennium. The clinic may benefit from the development of an advisory board made up of community partners, patients, families of patients, and other health care providers that may provide insight into issues facing the clinic, such as marketing and development fundraising. New collaborations will be developed with community partners to meet patient needs while expanding on clinical education opportunities (Doran, Solomon, & Brasseur, 1997; McCready, 2000; Solomon-Rice, 2004). Most importantly, the concepts that drive successful practices in the "real world" must be those that guide university clinic: provision of high quality, cost-effective, time-efficient, and patient-centric services.

References

American Speech-Language-Hearing Association. (2000, March). *Responding to the changing needs of speech-language pathology and audiology students in the 21st century* (A briefing paper for academicians, practitioners, employers, and students). Retrieved from http://www.asha.org/ students/changing.htm

Amlani, A., Taylor, B., & Tara, W. (2011). Increasing hearing aid adoption rates through value-based advertising and price unbundling. *Hearing Review, 18*(13), 10–17.

Bartlett, S., McNamara, K., & Peaper, R. (2006a). *New and used clinic directors: Dwindling resources.* 2006 Annual CAPCSD Conference Proceedings.

Bartlett, S., McNamara, K., & Peaper, R. (2006b). *Factors influencing the activities of clinic directors in university settings.* Presentation at the Annual Convention of the American Speech-Language-Hearing Association.

Council of Academic Programs in Communication Sciences and Disorders. (2011). Retrieved from http://www.capcsd.org/ proceedings.html

Donahue, A., Dubno, J. R., & Beck, L. (2010). Accessible & Affordable hearing health care for adults with mild and moderate hearing loss. *Ear and Hearing, 31*(1), 2–6.

Doran, M. C., Solomon, B. S. W., & Brasseur, J. A. (1997). Partners in professional preparation: Collaboration between universities and off-site settings. *Administration and Supervision Newsletter, c5,* 17–21.

Fish, S. (2003). Give us liberty or give us revenue. *The Chronicle of Higher Education,* p. 4.

Foltner, K., & Mansfield, B. (2006). Branding audiology: It's a budding opportunity. *Hearing Journal, 59*(5), 41–44.

Foster, W., & Bradach, J. (2005). Should nonprofits seek profit? *Harvard Business Review, 83*(2), 92–100.

Goldstein, B. A. (2008). Integration of evidence-based practice into the university clinic. *Topics in Language Disorders, 28*(3), 200–201.

Hardick, E. J., & Oyer, H. J. (1987). Administration of speech-language-hearing programs within the university setting. In H. J. Oyer (Ed.), *Administration of programs in speech-language pathology and audiology.* Englewood Cliffs, NJ: Prentice-Hall.

Jurgens, M. K. (2008). An integrated data-management system saves time, leaving more for patient care. *Hearing Journal, 61*(3), 48–51.

Kander, M. (2010, August 31). Medicare rules and university clinics. *ASHA Leader.*

Kasewurm, G. A. (2011a). Are you too busy? *Hearing Journal, 64*(11), 40–42.

Kasewurm, G. A. (2011b). Patient satisfaction surveys: A key to word-of-mouth referrals. *Audiology Practices, 3*(3), 34–39.

Lundy, E. (2006). University facilities respond to the changing landscape of higher education. *APPA Thought Leaders Series 2006.* Alexandria, VA: APPA.

McCarthy, P. (2006). Clinical education in audiology: The challenge of change. *Seminars in Hearing, 27*(2), 79–85.

McCready, V. (2000). The changing face of the university clinic: Reaching out to the community. *Proceedings of the Council of Academic Programs in Communication Sciences and Disorders.*

Meah, Y. S., Smith, E. L., & Thomas, D. C. (2009). Student-run health clinic: Novel arena to educate medical students on systems-based practice. *Mount Sinai Journal of Medicine, 76,* 344–356.

Meister, B. (2011). Debt and taxes: Can the financial industry save public universities? *Representations, 116*(1), 128–155.

Newman, C. W., Sandridge, S. A., & Lesner, S. A. (2011). Becoming a better preceptor: The clinic as classroom. *Hearing Journal, 64*(7), 10–18.

Novak, R. (2004). Thought on the development of our audiology profession. *Audiology Today, 16*(4), 18–19.

Parmar, V., Lange, A., Madden, C., & Das, V. (2009). The online outpatient booking system "Choose and Book" improves attendance rates at an audiology clinic: A comparative audit. *Informatics in Primary Care, 17*(3), 183–186.

Pessis, P. M. (2006). *Creating a culture of professionalism in audiology.* 2006 Proceedings of the CAPCSD Conference.

Romanow, K., & Brannon, J. A. (2010). Telepractice reimbursement is still limited. *ASHA Leader.* Retrieved November 14, 2011, from http://develop.asha.org/Publications/leader/2010/101102/Bottom-Line-101102.htm.

Solomon-Rice, P. (2004). *Enhancing university clinical programs through collaborations with nonprofit organizations.* ASHA convention, Philadelphia, PA.

Special Interest Group Eleven: Administration and supervision. (2011). Retrieved December 20, 2011, from http://div11perspectives.asha.org/content/by/year

Williams, A. L. (1996). Modified teaching clinic peer group supervision in clinical training and professional development. *American Journal of Speech-Language Pathology, 4*(3), 29–38.

Windmill, I. M., Cunningham, D. R., & Preminger, J. E. (2004). The University of Louisville: The AuD in a medical and business environment. *American Journal of Audiology, 13*(2), 110–117.

19

Transitions: Optimizing Entry and Exit Strategies

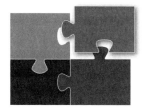

GAIL M. WHITELAW, PhD, MHA

Introduction

In recent years, the profession of audiology has undergone a significant transition that includes increased professional autonomy. From an autonomy perspective, many assert that audiology as a profession is best served when audiologists are self-employed and own their own practices. Engelmann and his colleagues (2008) contend:

> The future of the audiology profession and the provision of comprehensive and effective patient care will be best served by audiologists securing ownership of the audiology profession. This will be best accomplished by strategically ensuring that practice ownership is the predominant practice model for audiologists, consistent with the recognized character and success of other traditional doctoring healthcare professions. (p. 3)

Additionally, Smriga (2011) suggests that although all forms of audiology practice are essential to the survival of the profession "independent, autonomous practice is particularly critical" (p. 1). Although the exact number of audiologists who own their own practices is uncertain, it has been suggested that 15 to 20% of audiology services provided in the United States are owned and controlled by audiologists (Englemann et al., 2008). Fourteen percent of audiologists report being a private practice, according to the 2011 Compensation and Benefits report (American Academy of Audiology, 2011). Of 693 audiologists who listed employment in a private practice setting on the 2010 Audiology Survey, 44% reported being practice owners (American Speech-Language-Hearing Association, 2010). In addition, responses on the 2010 Audiology Survey indicated that 47% were self-employed in a private practice, 33% reported being employed in a private practice owned by nonaudiologists, and 19% were employed in a private practice owned by other audiologists.

A number of factors in the current practice environment frame transition issues related to practice ownership. Although health care may be less affected by fluctuation in the economy than many other professions or industries, it is not totally immune in a slowing economy (Mabry & Ollapally, 2009). The current demographic of aging of baby boomers thought to fuel the potential growth of audiology is also likely to be a factor, with audiologists of the same baby boom generation making plans to sell their practices in anticipation of retirement (Nemes, 2009). However, as with other professions, despite the "boomer" practice influx, linking young professionals seeking to buy a practice with those audiologists looking to sell a practice requires considerable attention to the transition, which may include the need for creative options, such as "work-to-buy" agreements (Silverman & Mohon, 2008). Even when the situation is right,

education debt may present a perceived barrier for young audiologists interested in owning their own practices (Foltner, 2008; Ousborne, 2007). The trend toward corporate ownership and franchising of audiology practices may also be a factor that impact decisions in purchase and sale. In addition, financial demands of being a small business owner, constant changes in the regulatory landscape, and maintaining audiology and staff "talent" are considerations in this transition process (Mabry & Ollapally, 2009).

Despite challenges related to independent practice in audiology, the current opportunities are unparalleled. Over 80% of AuD students and audiologists surveyed by the Academy of Doctors of Audiology (ADA) either agreed or strongly agreed that audiology should move from a "wage-employment" model to primarily an "ownership" practice model (Engelmann et al., 2009). As with other doctoring professions, audiologists enter the profession both to positively impact the lives of people with hearing and balance disorders and to have freedom and autonomy to practice in a way they choose. Some of the same factors that may seem to be challenges to the profession, corporate ownership or educational debt, also provide significant upsides. Corporate ownership and franchise options certainly may facilitate transitions into and out of practice ownership. In addition, even with substantial educational debt, audiologists, as a profession, are considered a good investment risk by lenders as they are ranked the lowest in loan failure rates among doctoring professions (Foltner, 2008).

With these factors in mind, the primarily purpose of this chapter is to address the critical transitions when an audiologist chooses to purchase or sell an established private practice. The transition process is not simply initiated one day and executed the next; it takes much planning time and energy to prepare for the purchase or sale of a practice. Although the concepts addressed in this chapter focus on transitions related to the independent practice of audiology, private practice is not the only setting in which these views are significant. The wise audiologist, even if wage-employed and not self-employed, should be aware of these factors.

It is obvious to state that the purchase or the sale of a practice requires considerable planning; this planning process is one of the most important steps in this transition. The purchase or sale of a practice requires a succession plan in order to facilitate the transition. Developing a succession plan focuses on preparing for the financial, professional, and emotional aspects of the sale. It is suggested that transition planning begin at least two years in advance of the transition; however, 3 to 5 years has been suggested as a more realistic timeframe in order to reach the goal of selling the practice in the manner which the buyer and seller desires: purchasing or selling the practice for a fair price and addressing a goal, whether practice ownership, retirement, or role change within the practice (Franks, 2006; Mabry & Ollapally, 2009; Nemes, 2006; Patsula, 2001). This lead time ensures that the audiologist owner will have the ability to address a number of issues, including the valuation of the practice as discussed in updating the business plan (Chapter 2), making necessary improvements in the physical structure (Chapter 5), planning for legal (Chapter 3) and fiscal responsibilities related to employees (Chapters 10 and 16), and the critical transition of patients (Chapter 11). Both the buyer and seller need to exercise significant care and due diligence in

this process. The process outlined in this chapter is designed to develop a smooth transition in the sales process.

Purchase and Sale of a Practice: Yin and Yang

Initially, it appears that the interests of an audiologist seeking to purchasing a practice and one trying to sell a practice would be polar opposites. After all, the goal for the buyer is to minimize the purchase price and the goal for the seller is to maximize the sale price. However, in reality, the roles of the buyer and seller are complimentary. As noted by Brady (2011), both the buyer and seller have similar goals. Both are interested in seeing the practice succeed; the buyer seeks to invest in a practice that will maximize profits while the seller wants to obtain the most value for their investment. Neither the buyer nor the seller wants to see the other fail in this shared relationship.

Optimizing both entry and exit strategies creates a win-win relationship for buyer and seller and ultimately, for the patient. This chapter "begins with the end in mind," as suggested by Covey (1999), focusing on aspects of the sale of the practice, which addresses both practice entry and exit strategies. It will become clear that the transition process of the buyer is intimately tied to the transition process of the seller.

When Is the Best Time to Sell a Practice?

The simple answer to the question of when is the best time to sell a practice is *when the seller does not have to sell!*

Timing of the sale of a practice is critical in terms of strategic positioning of the practice, both now and in the future (Mayer, 1998). Barlow, as cited in Nemes (2006), advises that audiology practices should be operated as if they will be sold in the near term, even if the owner has no intention of selling the practice, with all business decisions directed by the goal to develop a sustainable structure and measurable profits, in part to be attractive to a potential buyer. It is suggested that the time to plan an exit strategy for a practice is at the beginning and not the end of a career or practice (Kline, 2007a). In addition, funding a "buy out" vehicle at the outset of starting a practice assures long-term success in the sale of the practice (Mandell & O'Dell, 2008). This philosophy also helps to establish a process for successful transition in the case of unexpected illness or death of a practice owner.

Manning (2008) suggests that the principal objective of the seller is to obtain the best price for the practice with the most favorable terms in the shortest prior of time with the least stress. Planning is certainly a key to achieving that objective. Once the seller has made the commitment to develop a succession plan, there are several practical considerations that will maximize the value of the practice in preparation for sale. The value of the practice is ultimately based on two major factors: tangible assets and intangible assets, also known as goodwill (Franks, 2006). Both types of assets will contribute to a favorable appraisal and make the practice attractive to potential buyers. The practice owner should take an objective look at the physical appearance of the practice to ensure it is inviting and attractive. An unbiased party will be able to more effectively evaluate the condition of the physical space, particularly in a long-standing practice with a stable staff. In addition, the seller should be committed to increasing the productivity and profitability of the practice, as this reflects an upward trend in the practice and assurance that the buyer will purchase a vigorous practice (Franks, 2006).

Planning for the Ultimate Change: Entry and Exit Strategies

The purchase or sale of an audiology practice is clearly more difficult than buying or selling a home. Unlike the purchase or sale of a home, where valuation is often simply based on the floor and yard plan, the valuation of the practice encompasses both the physical space and other tangible and intangible assets that are potentially part of the purchase, including referral sources, equipment, employees, and patients. However, just as with home sales, the selling price can reflected diligent preparation and careful market research, as outlined in this chapter (Sullivan, 2006).

Although there is no standard for practice valuation, a professionally conducted appraisal is most likely to assure that the seller receives the maximum value for the practice and the buyer has sufficient information about the practice and its key features to understand why it is an attractive opportunity. The seller should be aware of models of valuation that may be considered in appraisal of the practice, along with the fact that the professional conducting the appraisal should be familiar with the profession of audiology. Professional appraisers may use several methods for calculating the value of assets (McDonald, 2005). A market approach compares the practice for sale to other similar practices that have recently been sold in the market. This method is difficult to apply in audiology due to the relatively small number of practices for sale in a given market at any period of time. A cost approach estimates the amount of money that would be required to duplicate the asset. This approach relies heavily on assumptions and is generally used as a secondary method in practice valuation. A book value approach, which is the sum total of cash, supplies, furniture, equipment, leasehold improvements, real estate, liabilities, and accounts receivable, is based on both fair market and depreciated costs. Although this method is not typically used for practice sales for an ongoing practice, it may be appropriate in situations where the practice must be closed, such as with illness or death. A modification of the book value approach takes into account the book value of the practice plus the value of "goodwill."

Another model of practice valuation in health care is the sum of tangible assets, accounts receivable, and intangible assets (Mabry & Ollapally, 2009). Tangible assets are relatively straightforward in valuation. The value of accounts receivable can be significant in a health care practice. The value of accounts receivable as part of the purchase price is obvious and often comprised of 5 to 6 months of service provided but not yet collected due to delays in reimbursement from third-party payers (Baum & Dowling, 2010; Mabry & Ollapally, 2009). The value of intangible assets to the practice presents conflicting views. Some believe that health care provides should not expect to be compensated for their professional reputation or

patient files (Baum & Dowling, 2010). Others suggest that despite the difficulty in assessing their value, intangible assets, and goodwill often comprise the greatest value of a health care practice (Mabry & Ollapally, 2009). Two types of goodwill may contribute to the overall value of the practice: practice goodwill and professional goodwill. Practice goodwill refers to the strengths of the business and is described as institutional goodwill, whereas professional goodwill refers to the practitioner's skills, knowledge, and reputation.

One model widely accepted in the health care industry is the composite valuation method, which compares common elements found in a practice: gross receipts, profitability, location, growth potential, collections, new patients, lease, equipment, staff, recall system in place, competition, patient base, transferability, practice production components (e.g., specialty services in the practice), and patient types—with an ideal practice to develop a percentile rating (Mattler, 2000). The model is heavily weighted toward practice income and patient base and the resulting percentile rating is then multiplied by factors addressing profitability and other market issues based on the appraiser's subjective judgment.

The seller may find that a potential buyer's potential lender requests modifications in valuation of the practice, particularly in a tight lending market. Although both buyers and sellers may view "goodwill" as one of the greatest assets of an existing practice, lending institutions may only be interested in providing a loan to cover the purchase of the tangible assets of the practice. In this case, the tangible assets may be appraised using a standard 3-tier format of purchase price, current market value

(CMV), and replacement cost (Silverman & Mohan, 2008).

The seller should develop a sales package, discussed later in this chapter, which presents a "turnkey" operation to the buyer. This "turnkey" operation will assure that the practice is ready to generate income from the first day of ownership, provide a salary to the owner and practice staff, and secure the capability to pay back the funding source. Even when a practice is a "turnkey" operation, there will be challenges for the new owner that go along with management of the practice. Some issues for the buyer may include:

- Inherited employees and office staff
- A patient database and referral base created and maintained in a method that may not reflect that of the buyer
- The "goodwill" (or "bad will") generated by audiologist owner or their staff
- The physical location of the practice: semipermanent and often difficult to change.
- The decorations, furnishing, and fixtures
- Clinical equipment inherited by the buyer.

In general, the above can either be benefits or liabilities to a turnkey operation. It is the responsibility of the seller to disclose information that provides insight into components of the practice purchase. Although a seller's responsibility is to provide the information and leave the clinic saleable, it is the buyer's responsibility to recognize that there are issues that need to be discussed and, where necessary, rectified.

The process of selling a practice requires due diligence on the part of both the buyer and seller. The audiologist selling the practice must prepare for the sale by working through a myriad of considerations to address potential concerns and ensure that the practice is in a saleable condition, which is discussed in detail later in this chapter. Although the sale of a practice can be a long process, taking from 6 to 9 months from initiation of discussion to transfer of the practice, a relatively quick and straightforward transition can occur if both parties are motivated and build a relationship of mutual trust (Baum & Dowling, 2010). Building trust between buyer and seller of a practice begins with the condition of the office and the financials. Buyers of practices do not want to purchase a clinic that is struggling, shabby, and requires substantial investment to make it profitable. At the first sign of recalcitrance, the buyer may wonder if the seller has something to hide. Reluctance on the part of the seller to provide information critical to the sale can erode trust that has been built between the parties and result in a less than smooth transition to a new owner. Additionally, it may cause the buyer and their practice appraiser, accountant, attorney, and the financial institution funding the purchase to be suspicious of hidden negative information. Failure to produce items of interest to the potential buyer and/or their representatives may result in delays due to the need to seek information for disclosure related to the sale. If a sale is to occur in good faith, it is necessary to ensure in advance that there will be full cooperation with the buyer and their representatives or there is no reason to progress to this stage of the sale. An audiologist purchasing a practice independently should be viewed as a colleague who will expect to make a living from conducting business in the practice and, after paying the purchase price of the practice, should have no surprises. Conversely, the seller should be assured that the potential buyer is negotiating in good faith, is serious regarding their inquiry into the practice, and will be able to secure funding to purchase the practice.

Preparing the Practice for Acquisition

General Considerations

Although there are situations and conditions where a sale can be obtained for a practice in "as is" condition, improvements made by the practice owner to prepare for a sale will make it more attractive. Drullinger (2006) indicates that there are specific items that the practice appraiser is looking for during the assessment process. Although some of these items lend themselves to preparation over a 3- to 5-year period, others are simply due diligence performance issues that must be presented when the sale is in progress. McAllister (2005) suggests that the first step in the assessment of the readiness of a practice for sale is for the seller to take an objective look at the practice. Although emotional clouding makes viewing the practice as others see it difficult, objectivity is absolutely necessary for the seller to obtain the best price. In preparation for the sale of the practice, many difficult questions must be addressed:

- What would an outsider think of this practice?
- How does it compare to other practices in the area?

- Has the neighborhood changed over the years?
- Is there a need to update the cosmetic aspects of the practice?
- Are the financials such that they will look attractive to a potential buyer?
- Is the practice management system updated?
- How are the equipment and computers in the practice?
- Are the employees ready for a sale?
- Will the practice accountant be available to assist in the sale?

These questions must be answered as they are what the buyer and their appraiser will consider basic information about the practice. The buyer may be considering the purchase of a number of practices; therefore, it is paramount for the seller to make their practice stand out among those being evaluated.

History of the Practice

As a component of the practice appraisal, the owner should prepare a history of the practice and put this information into a written document. This information should focus on the audiologist(s) in the practice, the length of time the practice has been in existence, current and previous locations, and special attributes, including specialized audiologic procedures performed (Mattler, 2000).

Leasehold and Physical Improvements

An initial consideration in the sale of the practice may revolve on an objective assessment of the community in which the practice is located. There may have been substantial changes in a neighborhood or a community over the time that the practice has been located there that may not be evident to the owner or employees due to the familiarity of the setting. In preparing for the sale of the practice, the audiologist should evaluate the neighborhood and become reacquainted with the advantages and disadvantages of the area as it has developed over time and with the demographics of the community (Mattler, 2000; McCall & Dunlop, 2004). Kline (2007b) suggests that understanding the demographics of the neighborhood is useful for the buyer to understand the potential growth or decline that might be anticipated in the area over the next decade. Although a decline may be predicted, this may not be a deal breaker for a potential buyer, depending on their vision and goals for the practice. For example, a mature neighborhood may provide easy access to an aging baby boomer market.

The building in which the practice is located also requires objective review. It is difficult to be objective about one's own practice, but this step is essential. Seeking consultation from someone outside of the practice that is willing to objectively assess the physical setting of the practice can help to provide a realistic assessment of the perception of the practice to help avoid surprises in the saleability of the practice. It is critical to demonstrate to a potential buyer that the practice has been progressive and has changed with over time, which may require updates of interior design, carpeting, and furniture. The potential buyer may have funds tied up in the purchase of the practice and, therefore, lack the financial resources for remodeling or relocation of the practice. The need for

major cosmetic modification may result in a potential buyer rejecting the purchase for a practice that requires less updating. One of the reasons to begin the sales process well in advance is to complete cosmetic overhauls and present the practice at its best; although a practice facelift may be expensive, it can help to attract interested buyers and/or enhance the practice price.

McCall and Dunlop (2004) suggest a number of considerations that should be attended to in evaluating the physical cosmetics of the practice:

- Exterior of the building in need of paint or modification in order to look more contemporary
- Sidewalks and approaches adequately lighted and in good repair
- Parking lot an appropriate number of well-marked parking spaces designated for the practice
- Carpet and tile cleanliness, up-to-date style and color
- Paint and woodwork up-to-date color, cleanliness, and touchup is recent
- Photographs and artwork current, not dated
- Attractive front desk area
- Display fixtures clean and up-to-date
- Adequate coat rack
- Adequate and attractive seating for patients in the waiting room
- Up-to-date magazines and product literature available to patients
- Clean restroom area, with appropriate decor and up-to-date features
- If an elevator in use in the building, it should be safe, clean, and operable
- Patient files and filing system clean and up to date; electronic medical records up-to-date

- General atmosphere of the sound room and counseling/fitting rooms
- Adequacy of the hearing aid laboratory
- Signage: positioning, style, and visibility
- Windows washed, signage/lettering readable and not deteriorated
- All ALDs and accessories stored/ displayed in an attractive manner that does not appear cluttered
- All light bulbs replaced and operating
- If available, storage should be clean and free of old equipment, cords, tables, and materials, as these items may be perceived as clutter to the buyer.

Attention to basic aspects of the facility are likely to yield significant benefit to the seller. Franks (2006) suggests that the seller should clean their office and desk prior to visits by potential buyers. McCall and Dunlop (2004) stress that it is critical that the overall atmosphere of the waiting room is pristine. A dated waiting room presents a shabby image that may justify a lower purchase price. An update of the waiting room may pay off in image presented to the patients, be consistent with the branding of the practice, and offer a contemporary image to a potential buyer.

Furthermore, both the seller and the buyer should know the current lease terms and monthly rent. The attorneys for the seller should critically review the specifics of the lease and the buyer, with specific options related to escalation and renewal capabilities for five years post-purchase/sale discussed. The buyer in the process of the sale should negotiate the new lease; however, the seller can be very

helpful in this process (DePaolo, 2008). If the audiologist selling the practice owns the facility, the terms for lease to the buyer should be carefully presented, with options for purchase of the real estate clearly addressed (Mattler, 2000).

Audiometric and Office Equipment

As discussed earlier in this chapter, the potential buyer of the practice is generally seeking a turnkey operation. An important component of a turnkey practice is audiometric and office equipment. A practice that utilizes an appropriate equipment depreciation schedule and funds equipment replacement as part of the business plan will have a clear advantage at the time of sale compared to the practice that has not addressed this critical aspect. An ongoing investment in equipment enhances the value of the practice both in capital and in "goodwill" as patients will perceive the practice as "state of the art," enhancing the practice reputation in the community. Audiologists using outdated equipment (e.g., electronystagmography rather than videonystagmography) may receiver a lower offer for their practice as a potential buyer will need to add equipment purchase or lease payments to the fixed expenses presented in the due diligence process. Since the addition of the new fixed expenses will add to the overhead of the practice, these expenses may reflect a change in the multiple selected for the practice by the buyer's appraiser and result in a price reduction to the seller.

Office equipment, such as computers, printers, office management software, and accounting programs must be replaced and/or updated in a systematic and organized way based on an infrastructure replacement cycle outlined in the business plan. This replacement cycle should be based on the usable life of the equipment and the schedule of depreciation. This cycle is less likely to be based on a fixed financial schedule but closely linked to business practices of the individual office (Ohm, 1999). Evidence of addressing software upgrades is critical in providing state of the art clinical care and assuring potential buyers that the office is well managed and up-to-date.

Files and file management needs to be an organized systematic method that allows for easy access to the records for each individual patient. Two options may be available, either a hard copy or an electronic medical record (EMR). Regardless of the filing system used, sample files should be available for the potential buyer to review. Some audiology offices have moved toward a "paperless" system, storing most or all information electronically. These systems require less physical space for storage, may be less costly, and provide for efficient access and retrieval of patient information. Although increasing in popularity, paperless systems are not yet the standard in audiology practices, thus not required to sell a practice. Having a paperless system is likely to garner the attention of potential buyers that are looking for a state-of-the-art practice and to facilitate care coordination. In addition, this system may be viewed as a necessary interface for some third party payers, particularly as part of current changes in the regulatory landscape (O'Malley, Grossman, Cohen, Kemper, & Pham, 2009). McAllister (2005) also describes this as a critical time to assure that the practice management system (PMS) is running effectively and efficiently and to objectively assess the potential need for a new PMS.

Staff Considerations

It is paramount that employees know that the practice is being sold. Employees that are satisfied and well trained can be a significant asset to the practice; conversely, issues with disgruntled or poorly performing employees can present an uncomfortable situation during the transition/sale (Franks, 2006; McDonald, 2005). Knowledge of a potential sale allows employees to plan for their future, whether seeking another position or assuring their role in the transition with a new practice owner. If a potential buyer is interested in a turnkey business, the audiologists, the receptionist/office manager, and billing personnel may be of particular interest to them. In order to facilitate this turnkey approach in relation to personnel, it is recommended that the audiologist selling the practice inform the employees of the impending sale, review the ethical/legal responsibilities with the employees, review retirement and healthcare plans and responsibilities to cover unused benefits (e.g., vacation or sick leave), and provide incentives for employees to stay during the transition period, if this is the desire of the new owner (American Medical Association, 1997).

The revenue generated by the business and productivity of each audiologist that contributes to that bottom line are important considerations in the purchase of a practice. Part of the practice valuation will be based on the productivity of the staff and which employees generate the revenue. If the majority of the revenue is generated by the audiologist who owns the practice, the owner is essential to the financial success of the practice. If the owner is leaving the practice, there is a risk of significant decrease in business if patients choose not to stay with the practice under the new ownership. Typically, if the audiologist selling the practice is the primary income producer, the valuation will be lower. However, if 50% or more of the revenue production has been transferred to a professional employee, the valuation is likely to be higher, particularly if the audiologist employee plans to stay with the practice after its sale. When a smaller percentage of revenue is generated by the audiologist owner, the chances of keeping existing patients within the practice upon the owner's departure are likely to be greater. If the owner of the practice is using the sale as an exit strategy for retirement or as a career change, the seller should plan the transition by slowly transferring patients to other audiologists in the practice (Bauer, 2004). This is typically done slowly so that the patients and staff in the practice gradually become accustomed to the original owner no longer being available to address issues or concerns. To a professional appraiser valuing a practice, this may be viewed as a solid indication that when the owner leaves the practice, business will be much the same and patients will remain loyal.

Normalizing Income and Expenses

Normalizing income and expenses is a critical step for the audiologist owner who may run legitimate personal expenditures through the practice. In this case, the seller adds back as income the amount of the expenses that are accrued by the practice owner, such as car lease expenses, travel expenses, and club membership and dues. Separating these major expenses accurately reflects the profitability of the practice and provides the buyer's financing source the actual income available to service the purchaser's salary and the debt created by the purchase (Lowes, 2006). These expenses should be separated prior to the appraisal so that their impact is obvious prior to the practice valuation.

Creating the Sales Package

Patsula (2001) indicates that once the practice components are in place, a sales package should be constructed. This gives the perspective buyer a concise orientation to the practice and organizes the discussion between the two parties as to the positives of the practice and the concerns of the buyer. This package provides essential information about the practice and serves as a checklist of discussion topics. The following items should be included in the practice sales package:

- History of the practice
- Description of how the practice operates
- Description of the physical facilities
- Discussion of the suppliers
- A review of marketing practices
- Description of the competition
- Review of personnel: including an organizational chart, job descriptions, and rates of pay and willingness of key employees to stay and work for the new owner
- Policy and procedure manuals
- Identification of all the owners
- Explanation of insurance coverage

- Discussion of any pending legal matters or contingent liabilities
- A compendium of 3 to 5 years of financial statements
- Accounts receivable, if part of the sale
- Inventory of equipment
- Hearing aid sales history
- A valuation report that states how the practice arrived at its asking price.

Basically, the sales package mirrors the practice's business plan, with the addition of real historical financial data offered by the seller. The practice owner must realize that they are selling their practice based on historic performance while the buyer is purchasing the practice on unknown future performance. The better the sales package tells the story of historic performance, the more likely the practice is to present a case for positive future performance.

Another portion of the sales package preparation is the anticipation of various discussion questions from the buyer, since thorough due diligence, the process of gathering information as it affects the purchase of the business, is essential for any buyer that plans to acquire a health-care entity (DePaolo, 2008; Doty & Campbell, 2000). Issues that concern the future viability of the practice may include:

- The age of the audiometric equipment and computers
- The anticipated transferability of patients to the new owner
- Patient relations and patient loyalty
- Practice reputation and image
- Competition threats and weaknesses
- Leasing costs for premises and equipment
- Location conditions

- Maintenance costs, heating, air conditioning, and other utility bills
- Parking availability
- Staff turnover.

The seller should be prepared to answer these and other specific questions key to any serious consideration of the practice purchase. The buyer may also request information about compliance plans and the billing audit to assure no undisclosed issues with billing or fraud and abuse problems exist (Doty & Campbell, 2000). The process of due diligence puts the seller in a vulnerable position by disclosing proprietary information to the buyer. The seller should ask potential buyers to sign a confidentiality agreement restricting the use of information provided for transactions related only to the purchase of the business (DePaolo, 2008).

Generating Interest in the Practice: Marketing to Potential Buyers

There are many reasons why a buyer will find one practice more attractive than others. It could be a significant financial opportunity, the location, the opportunity to learn and conduct specific procedures, the specifics in the sales package, or a myriad of other reasons. Development of a corporate profile, or a summary of the sales package, should be available to all potential buyers. Included in this profile should be brief descriptions of the practice, services offered, financials, assets, competitive factors, price, buy-in alternatives, along with a sales pitch that piques the potential buyer's interest to learn more (Manning, 2009). A practice broker, discussed later in this chapter, can generate interest or the audiologist owner marketing the practice on their own may generate it. For independent audiology practice sales, interest may be generated in a number of ways, including through print or Internet advertising, trade journals, and by word-of-mouth networking. Audiology is a relatively small profession; therefore, facilitating communication regarding the potential sale of a practice is fairly uncomplicated but does require a targeted approach in order to be effective. The size of the profession certainly facilities the ability to communicate about the sale; however, it should be noted that marketing of practice will eliminate any possibility of confidentiality regarding the sale. Print ads advertising the practice for sale may be placed in both trade journals, such as *The Hearing Journal* or *Hearing Review*, and communications from professional organizations, such as *Audiology Today*; however, these options have become less relevant with the advent of greater online and social media outlets. A number of Web sites provide information to those interested in buying or selling a practice, including *AudiologyOnline.com* and *AuDNet.com*. State audiology academies may provide a strong network to advertise the sale of a practice and to attract local buyers who may be particularly familiar with the reputation of the seller, thus understanding the goodwill aspects of the practice. Advertising on the state academy Web site and/or in E-newsletters is an effective approach for marketing the practice.

The marketing of the sale of a practice through word-of-mouth approaches requires taking advantage of networking opportunities in the profession of audiology. Manufacturer representatives and equipment distributors interface with a significant number of audiologists in a specific geographic area and may be able to reach a large number of audiolo-gists in a short period of time. Continuing education events and state, regional, and national conferences/conventions provide an opportunity to interact with audiologists and to market the practice. Networking with AuD programs may identify new and future audiologists who are seeking opportunities to enter a private practice.

Independent Versus Corporate Practice: Selling to a Corporate Entity

The corporate purchase of private practices is a trend that has affected medicine and other health care fields over the past several decades. This trend has recently become a consideration in private practice in audiology. In recent years, corporate entities in hearing care have been seeking to acquire independent audiology practices in order to expand their regional or national practice networks (Nemes, 2006). Affiliating with a corporate buyer may provide access to capital, expertise in billing and coding, specialized management services, and economies of scale not possible in an independent practice (Carlson, 1998). These potential advantages must be weighed against the practice mission, vision and values. Smriga (2011) suggests that the profession of audiology is viewed as a significant "customer" to corporate business, thus, collectively, audiology has the potential to influence corporate decisions. Conversely, there is a narrowing window for audiology to capitalize on the influence. As Smriga (2011) notes that "once control of a buying decision is lost, so is the economic influence it represents" (n.p.).

With that stated, the buyer and seller should use the same due diligence in exploring corporate purchase options as they would for purchase or sale of an independent audiology practice. This thorough approach will assist in providing a balanced perspective as to whether to remain independent and sell to an independent audiologist or to join or sell the practice to a corporate entity. Some corporate contacts are unsolicited and may be viewed as an opportunity to learn more about the market and as an opportunity to obtain additional viewpoints on the value of the practice, even if the seller has not considered a sale or affiliation with a corporate buyer. However, caution must be exercised to avoid potential pitfalls, which may include providing detailed financial information regarding the practice or accepting claims that other practices in the market have committed to an affiliation (Carlson, 1998). Corporate buyers may seek several approaches to obtaining independent private practices. They may seek a practice with reduced profitability in order to expand their network at minimal cost. Conversely, corporate buyers may seek independent practices that are well run in a desirable location, with diverse referral sources, and with a growing patient base (Nemes, 2006). Fell, as quoted in Nemes (2009), stated, for example, that HearUSA, a chain of hearing care centers that purchases practices, will continue to grow in its acquisition of practices, particularly since practice valuations are currently conservative, making it a positive acquisition environment.

A number of publicly held corporations are players in this corporate market and have been expanding market share in specific regions for much of the past decade. This makes them a significant force in the audiology market, thus viewed by some as competition to independent private practices. These corporate practices are often associated with a hearing instrument manufacturer which provides a significant distribution network for their products. Sonus, a national hearing care chain, is a division of Amplifon, has recently developed an audiology-based franchise model (Foltner, 2011). William Demant Holding Group, the parent company to Oticon and Sonic Innovations, among others owns the Avada corporate chain and has a significant investment in American Hearing Aid Associates (AHAA). GN ReSound owns the long established Beltone chain of franchises.

Discount stores such as Costco and Walmart actively offer hearing instruments as a product line in their stores. Although not actively purchasing independent practices, these stores have the potential to be formidable competition for hearing instrument sales in a given region, thus may impact the value of a practice in view of their proximity of one of these retailers.

For some audiologists, selling a practice to a corporate entity may result in a substantial economic windfall, among other benefits including increasing profitability of the practice of allowing the audiologist to change their role in the practice. However, it is critical to determine if the corporate group is truly interested in obtaining the independent practice or in merely investigating the practice to determine the competitive aspects of the independent practice in order to open an outlet close to the practice, without intent to purchase the practice. Conversely, talking with a representative of a corporate audiology entity may be a great opportunity to learn more about the marketplace and to help determine the value of a practice, information that may be useful in the long run. According to Carlson (1998), in order to avoid some potential pitfalls, it is important to consider the following:

- Avoid signing a "letter of intent" that restricts discussion with other corporate entities prior to the sale.
- Do not provide detailed financial data regarding the practice until the negotiations have advanced to the point where this is necessary, when the potential seller has determined that such an affiliation would be the right move for the practice.
- Do not take claims at face value that other practices in the market have committed to an affiliation with the corporate entity.

Another method of assessing the willingness of the corporation to enter as a partner in negotiation is to obtain a nonrefundable earnest commitment. This "earnest investment" would offset the time and effort involved in the due diligence process and, of course, apply the purchase price if the practice is actually purchased but would be forfeited if the practice is not purchased by the corporation.

The decision to affiliate with a retail/corporate practice or to remain in an independent practice setting is certainly influenced by financial considerations, but other factors may also play a role in the decision making. Corporate affiliation has impacted optometry over the past few decades and there are certainly potential parallels with the profession of audiology. In optometry, the number of retail chains resulted in direct competition with those in independent private practice, with young optometrists thought to be attracted to commercial/corporate optometry in order to earn an income without accruing the debt load

associated with starting or purchasing a private practice (Smriga, 2006). In contrast to other professions, such as optometry and medicine, the significant majority of dentists have maintained solo independent practices, which is thought to result in improved autonomy for the profession and earning ability for individual dentists (Mertz, 2002). Smriga (2011) points out that the corporate influence in audiology/hearing health care may also limit professional autonomy and potentially earning potential for audiologists. Audiologists who sell their practice to a corporate/commercial entity must be prepared to yield control of their practice and understand that the philosophy and corporate culture of the practice may change under the new ownership (Nemes, 2006). However, the ability to focus on patient care while receiving a salary and benefits package as an employee without the responsibilities of owning a practice may motivate an owner to consider a corporate audiology sale. Carlson (1998) advises a potential seller to recognize the risks in affiliating with a corporate organization and not to sell the practice based on the financial aspects only, as the affiliation should result in a partnership that the audiologist can live with, making their life easier, and their practice more competitive.

Using a Professional to Sell a Practice: Practice Brokers

Most audiologists have little knowledge or experience in negotiating the purchase or sale of a practice. Even with a strong business team, relying on the skill and knowledge of a practice broker can help to facilitate the sale of the practice. Using a real estate analogy, a practice broker would be similar to using a realtor to sell a home. McDonald (2005) suggests that the scenario of a practice owner selling their practice may have parallels to "for sale by owner" home sale: the home may be overpriced and the owner "in love with their own home," optimistic, and a "bit greedy." Specific knowledge in a number of key areas including practice valuation, marketing, real estate, negotiation, and advertising, may be of benefit in the sale of a practice. The buyer may have a team of professionals working on their behalf, including a practice appraiser. Adding a practice broker to the seller's team may provide considerable value and help both the buyer and the seller.

A practice broker can be viewed as a "matchmaker" between the buyer and seller. This independent broker may be able to address a number of complex tasks related to the sale of the practice. Reiboldt (2004) suggests that some of these activities may include:

■ Market analysis
■ Providing guidance in setting the sales price
■ Assisting with negotiations
■ Networking and advertising the practice
■ Providing direct mailing to potential buyers
■ Creating an Internet presence
■ Working with medical specialty lenders in order to maximize the amount of the loan to a potential buyer (which may assist the seller in obtaining a higher sales amount)
■ Screening calls and inquiries from potentially interested buyers;

procuring purchasers through recruiting and reference checks
■ "Showing" the practice.

Preparation for sale may include a consultation with a practice broker that can provide the proper presale advice to assist the audiologist in obtaining the most for their investment in the practice. Selling a practice can be a sensitive situation for the audiologist owner, due to the emotional and financial investment in the practice. A potential buyer will ask questions regarding how decisions have been made, why things are done in certain ways, and offer ideas about new services that may put the seller on the defensive. Beiting (2006) notes that a third party, such as a practice broker, can be helpful in reducing the emotion associated with the sale, being able to collate information for the seller, and negotiate a buy-sell agreement. The practice broker may also coordinate activities with attorneys, accountants, and lenders.

Although practice brokers can substantially reduce the burden of the sales process, they handle their business in a manner similar to that of a real estate broker. Similar to a real estate agent for a home, a practice broker is paid a commission for their services. Generally, these fees are about 10% of the purchase price of the practice (Reiboldt, 2004). Commission and other fees should be negotiated prior to the sale and both the buyer and seller's attorney should review the listing agreement.

Although practice brokers have historically been used in the purchase and sale of health care practices, a broker dedicated to the practice of audiology is a relatively unique. One current example is "My Practice" (http://www.mypractice

inc.com). Goals of this business include supporting independent practices in audiology, allowing the audiologist selling the practice be able to leave on their own terms, and providing the opportunity for the buyer to participate in a "learn to own" model where the practice owner can mentor the audiologist purchasing the practice. This particular broker model has targeted audiologists at the beginning of their careers, including students in AuD programs who may be offered the opportunity to include student loans into the purchase deal by buying an initial ownership stake in a practice (Nemes, 2009).

Sales Alternative: Employee Purchase of Practice

The audiologist interested in selling their practice may need to look no further for a potential buyer than in the staff of audiologists employed in the practice. This type of sale may include a number of options including out and out sale of the practice or selling portions of the business to employees using a number of approaches. The benefit to the audiologist owner may include infusion of cash into the business, reduced employee labor costs, or simply the ability to retire at a planned time. Grau (2007) states that an employee group is perfect option as they already know the patient base and mesh well with the business philosophy. In this sense, the employees become informed buyers, with considerable knowledge of the practice. Christensen (2003) suggests that one of the motivations for brining a new associate into a practice

is as a logical candidate to take over a practice. He adds that selling the practice to an employee/associate/partner is "the most painless way to exit from a practice."

Applegate (2002) notes that when the owner of a small business, such as an audiologist, wants to sell the practice to employees, there are several viable options to do so. Although the audiologist owner might be willing to negotiate a deal with an employee so that they may become a partner, audiology salaries are usually not conducive to obtaining the funds for a down payment on the practice without substantial collateral. Additionally, young practioners that have considerable debt related to their education may find that financing a practice, even with favorable terms, is a challenge. The audiologist owner may choose to fund the practice sale themselves, as it may be difficult for a young audiologist to borrow the full value of practice at a reasonable interest rate (Beitling, 2005).

Sale to employees often includes setting up options that may augment or replace some portion of salary or benefits in order to assist employees in being able to "own" the practice while providing a favorable situation for the owner. One such option is a "work-to-own" opportunity (Silverman & Mohon, 2008). Another option is employee stock ownership plans (ESOP), which provide for the owner to sell company "shares" of the practice to employees at a fair price. Employees that own shares in the practice may be more loyal and driven to perform, resulting in an increase in practice productivity. Selling stock in the practice may also provide a significant tax advantage in terms of capital gains, a topic that is addressed later in this chapter (Egerton & Egerton, 2005). A number of methods for establishing an ESOP are available and if an owner is interested in setting up this type of plan, consultation with an attorney and accountant are critical.

Retained Involvement

Some audiologists sell their practices and stay on to work in them for a specified period of time, often as a condition of sale. This option provides continuity of patient care and/or ongoing management the practice during the transition. Retained involvement is a common practice in sales to corporate entities as the corporate owner may need a practice manager for continuity and to provide patient care This allows for an effective transition for patients and staff alike and maximizes opportunities for success under new management.

Some audiologists may take advantage of a retained involvement approach known as "transitioning" in which the audiologist planning to sell a practice will look for another audiologist to join the practice that will purchase it and succeed the current audiologist at the time of their retirement (Wilson, 2005). If a favorable agreement can be reached, the senior audiologist will mentor the buyer for a period of time, often outlined in a legal document referred to as a "phase-out" agreement (Reiboldt, 2004). Although this transition period may take several years to plan and implement, it can be profitable for both the buyer and the seller.

There may be pros and cons to the audiologist being retained in the practice after sale. The audiologist, as a former owner, can be relieved of the pressures of management such as billing, insurance, and human resources, and can attend to patient care. This allows the audiologist to work as a salaried employee and have a greater degree of flexibility in their schedule. The audiologist retained as an employee in the practice must recognize that they will lose much of the autonomy and independence to which they are accustomed (Baum & Dowling, 2010). There may be a shift in the corporate culture of the practice: the new owners may change fundamentals such as marketing tactics or human resource options, and the audiologist retained in the practice must be able to accommodate this change if they are to stay on as a successful and productive employee. The new owner may take advantage of the knowledge and skills of the retained audiologists and include their input in decision making regarding the practice. However, the audiologist selling the practice and staying must be able to accept this potential loss of control.

The Successful Sale of the Practice: Tax Considerations

A goal in the sale of the practice is to maximize the profit to the seller. Attention to tax issues is critical in pursuit of this goal. The seller must seek appropriate counsel, including input from the attorney, financial advisor, and accountant. Burg (1995) suggests that the main tax goal in the sale of a practice should be to minimize the profit that is considered ordinary income and to assign the maximum profit possible to capital gains. Nearly everything that is owned and used for personal purposes, pleasure or investment is a capital asset. According to the IRS (2007), when a capital asset, such as an audiology practice, is sold, the difference between the selling price and the amount paid for the asset is a capital gain (or loss). There are number specific areas that the seller should consider in addressing tax aspects of the sale that may also impact the amount of capital gains.

One area of consideration is depreciation recapture. The owner of the audiology practice has had the tax benefit of depreciation of tangible business property, such as audiometers, computers, and office furniture over the life of the asset. The sale of these assets can qualify as capital gains only to the extent that the sale price exceeds the original cost of the asset, a rare situation (Bobryk, 1998). Generally, a buyer will not pay more for an asset than the original purchase price; therefore, the revenue from sale of these types of tangible business assets is taxed as ordinary income. An alternative approach that may result in benefits to both the seller and buyer is for the seller to lease equipment to the buyer (Burg, 1995). The seller will still be able to write off some of the depreciation, which offsets the revenue received from lease payment, while the buyer will benefit from having less working capital tied up in equipment.

Another consideration is leasehold improvements. Leasehold improvements are depreciated over a period of 31.5 or 39 years, depending on when the practice was purchased, and a longer period than for other types of tangible assets (Burg, 1995). The advantage for the seller is that the remaining leasehold write-off may be deducted in the sale year. If a $90,000 renovation was completed five years prior to the sale of the practice, it is possible that only $15,000 has been depreciated at the time of the sale. This would result in a $75,000 deduction for leasehold improvements at the time of sale.

Goodwill and the patient database are capital assets so the portion of the sale related to these are taxed as capital gains. Although this may provide benefit for the seller, the buyer may prefer to negotiate more of the sale be allocated to equipment or furnishings, as intangible assets are written off over 15 years but tangible assets can be written off two to three times as quickly (Burg, 1995). However, sale of these "hard assets" are taxed as ordinary income for the seller.

The tax and financial implications of the sale of an audiology practice are complex and require professional advice. An old adage is, "It's not what you earn, it's what you keep"; this suggests that the seller may benefit from accepting a slighter lower price if the sale can be structured to result in a more favorable tax treatment, as the long-term capital gains are currently taxed at a substantially lower rate than ordinary income. Trusted advisors in the sale of the practice will assure that the profit to the seller will be maximized in a legal and ethical manner.

Informing Patients That the Practice Has Been Sold

A critical task in the sale of a practice is informing patients about the impending transition. Practice management consultants encourage the audiologist selling the practice to contact patients by letter at least three months in advance of the sale or transition (Franks, 2006). The letter should inform active patients of the sale, the plan for the practice, and the assurance of continuity of care. If a colleague is to be taking over the practice, this audiologist should be introduced in the letter. If the audiologist owner will be remaining in the practice in a different role, this should also be addressed in the letter. Assuring patients that the practice infrastructure (e.g., location, staff, etc.) will remain constant will serve to ease the transition.

Exiting the practice can be an emotional time for the audiologist, their staff, and patients that have been loyal to the practice. Attention to the detail of communicating with staff will help to ease the transition, provide the patient with information that will ensure good will in the practice, and provide both the owner and patient the opportunity for closure. Some consultants also recommend that the audiologist buying the practice also contact patients via letter to introduce themselves and again ensure continuity of care.

Closing the Practice Without Selling

There may be situations in which an audiology practice will be closed without a sale. These situations, such as a health condition that precludes the owner from continuing to work, often occur suddenly. These again address the importance of having a succession plan in place. However, if this plan is not in place, the audiologist may have limited time in order to prepare the practice for closure. If addressed appropriately, the process for closure will require similar attention to detail as in the case of the

sale of the practice. Weiss (2004) suggests that walking away from a practice should be the last resort after serious attempts to sell the practice; however, in some situations, such as a rural practice with no buyers, there may be no other options. As noted later in this chapter, this type of "under duress" sale may provide a unique opportunity for both a motivated buyer and motivated seller, which may provide a better outcome than the inability to sell a practice. The audiologist will need to work closely with an accountant and attorney to insure that all patient, legal, and financial responsibilities are carefully considered prior to, during and after the closing of the practice.

Audiologists simply cannot abandon or abruptly withdraw from their patient responsibility. The continuity of audiological care is critical and attention to the disposition of patients to another audiology practice is absolutely necessary. It is also important that the audiologist(s) receiving these patients have a patient centric approach and assure new patients that their hearing instrument warranties and other commitments from the practice that is closing will be honored.

In order to ensure continuity of care for patients, the audiologist closing the practice should notify patients by letter, preferably at a minimum of three months prior to closure of the practice. This letter should include the following information:

- Practice closing date
- Name(s) of audiologists recommended and willing to accept new patients
- How copies of audiological records can be obtained or transferred to the new audiologist

- An authorization form for the patient to sign for release of records
- Where audiologic records will be stored after the practice is closed (Reiboldt, 2007; Weiss, 2004).

The audiologist should also plan on placing an announcement of practice closure in local newspapers a few weeks prior to the actual closing, a step that may be required in some states (Weiss, 2004).

In the case of the closure of the practice, special care should be given to the retention of patient records. An attorney should review a retention policy, with consideration to the statute of limitations for various potential lawsuits that may be faced by the audiologist or the practice (Reiboldt, 2007). A custodian for records must be established with previous patients being able to access records as necessary (Weiss, 2004). Records that are retained must be stored in a secure place and in a confidential manner. Options for storage, such as copying onto microfilm or scanning into read-only storage media, should be explored. Records that are no longer needed should be disposed of by utilizing a reputable record-shredding business.

In addition to notifying patients, closure of a practice requires communication with other entities and individuals, including:

- Liability/malpractice insurance company
- Medicare, Medicaid, and other third-party payers
- State licensing board
- Affiliated hospitals/referral sources
- Professional associations in which the audiologist holds memberships
- Insurers covering the practice, its employees, and facilities (Reiboldt, 2007; Weiss, 2004).

A location to receive practice mail and phone calls must be established. The assets of the practice will need to be sold, which can be done through a local equipment distributor or on a forum for selling used equipment, such as that at *Audiology-Online.com*. The final order of business is to address accounts receivable, as it may be possible to collect up to 90% of the outstanding AR (Weiss, 2004). It is recommended that a staff member be retained for a period of time to work on collections. Alternatively, a billing service may be more cost effective in the case of practice closure (Reiboldt, 2007).

When Is the Best Time to Purchase a Practice? Unique Considerations for the Buyer

In contrast to the answer to the question of when is the best time to sell a practice, the answer to this question is, *when the opportunity is right*. The buyer must strike a balance between being patience and flexibility in order to take advantage of that right opportunity. Obviously, the buyer has some significant choices to make, including purchasing an existing business or starting a practice "from scratch." Although there are pros and cons to each option, the opportunities for purchase of an established business may be significant. One of the best ways for the buyer to be ready to take advantage of potential opportunities is to have their financial house in order and maintain an exceptional credit score. Gerber (2009) recommends that in addition to a careful review of the purchase packet presented by the seller, a potential buyer should pay particular attention to several financial indicators of the practice and use these as benchmarks for decision-making. These indicators would include cost of goods sold (COGS), labor costs, and net income.

A seller assumes that a buyer will negotiate in good faith, which includes the ability to present options for financing the purchase of a practice. Although the current environment is stricter with lenders that it has been in the past, there are a number of options that a buyer may choose to pursue, in addition to those outlined earlier in the chapter. Potential buyers should investigate potential sources of funding including banks, credit unions, and the Small Business Administration (SBA). As noted earlier, audiologists, as a profession, are desirable candidates for funding, due to a very low loan failure rate and relatively high earning potential (Foltner, 2008). Manufacturer financing may available as a financing option, but this type of funding is likely to violate the federal anti-kickback statue and professional codes of ethics.

In addition to the financial aspects of purchase of a practice, a potential buyer should understand both the "brand" and core competencies of the practice and be sure that these are philosophically aligned with their view of audiology and their ability to make this practice their own. Kline (2007b) describes core competences as those profitable aspects of the practice that competitors have difficulty replicating and notes that a destroying a core competency of a practice is a "cardinal sin" that can contribute to failure of the practice under a new owner. She suggests that the buyer should leave the practice unchanged for the first 3 to 4 months under their ownership, with a commitment to leaving the core competencies of the practice unchanged.

The current economic environment may provide some unique opportunities for a potential buyer. An audiologist looking to sell a practice may find their business under a greater degree of scrutiny than in the past, limiting the pool of potential individual or corporate buyers. The current market may present great opportunities for an audiologist looking to buy a practice, as there may be fewer buyers competing for what is likely to be an increased number of practices for sale. Nemes (2009) suggests that the current demographic of baby boomer audiologist seeking to retire may result in a "landslide" of practices soon available for purchase. An increased number of practices for sale may result in great value opportunities for the buyer.

Young audiologists entering the profession may find some unique opportunities in the current practice environment beyond those presented by the current economic environment and supply and demand issues. Bringing young professionals into an established practice, a model used successfully in other doctoring professions such as optometry and dentistry, provides a viable practice transition model for audiology. Silverman and Mohon (2008) provide a model for targeting students enrolled in professional doctoral programs as potential buyers. Counter to conventional wisdom, they suggest that targeting potential buyers in their third year of a program may be an ideal time to establish opportunities. In this model, the transition from student to young professional provides the possibility for the audiologist to negotiate a lower starting salary with options to have equity ownership in the practice after the first 1 to 2 years. They point out that it is short-sighted for a young professional to focus on salary only, particularly if practice ownership is a career goal. This model allows young professionals to graduate into practice opportunities that provide a steady source of income with the ability to pay back student loans while pursuing buy in or "work to own" opportunities.

Much of this chapter has focused on the importance of preparation and planning for the sale of a practice; however, the reality is that some practice owners have not planned for inevitabilities. The sale of the practice happens under duress, in the case of death, sudden illness, divorce, or simply based on the owner's desire to "get away" (Kline, 2007a). This unfortunate situation creates an excellent opportunity for the potential buyer. In this case, it is critical for both the buyer and seller to understand that time is of the essence, as the value of the practice is based on access to patients, and if the practice is not functional due to lack of continuity of care, such as in the case of death of an audiologist in a solo-practice, the value of the practice can be destroyed quickly. A unique approach proposed in the chiropractic profession is having the doctor sign a no-cost contract with their professional program which states that if the doctor dies or becomes disabled, their family should immediately contact their professional program (Kline, 2007b). The school has one of its chiropractic partners take over the practice and brokers the sale with potential buyers, including advertising the availability of a practice for sale on their Web site. The goal is a quick sale, which allows continuity of the practice, and although may provide a bargain for a professional looking to purchase a prac-tice, also allows the family to receive a reasonable return on the investment. As the profession of audiology transitions to a greater number of audiologists working in independent practice settings, this type of model may certainly find its way into AuD programs across the country.

Summary and Conclusions

The transitions related to entering and exiting a practice are exciting and challenging. These transitions signify important milestones in the life of an audiologist: beginning a practice, entering into retirement, moving from employee to owner, or from owner to part-time employee or consultant. Developing a succession plan early in the practice is an effective way to assure that the transition will be seamless and maximize benefit to the buyer and seller. Updating business plans and attending to ongoing strategic positioning within the practice assures that the audiologist is prepared for all eventualities, including purchase or sale of the practice or a need to close. It cannot be stressed enough that the time to begin thinking about the sale is early in the life of the practice.

As noted by McDonald (2005), beginning with the end in mind suggests that an audiologist who opens a practice or purchases an existing practice will eventually want to sell it. Significant time should be spent in designing and developing a practice that will increase operational efficiencies and goodwill. McDonald (2005) suggests that "this investment of time and energy will result not only in a higher practice valuation but also in a more enjoyable (and profitable) professional life."

References

American Academy of Audiology. (2011). *2011 Compensation and benefits report.* Seattle, WA: Sector Intelligence, LLC.

American Hearing Aid Associates. (2005). *Corporate audiology in America.* Reno, NV: Author.

American Medical Association. (1997). *Closing your practice: Seven steps to a successful transition.* Chicago, IL: Author.

American Speech-Language-Hearing Association. (2010). *2010 Audiology survey report: Private practice.* Retrieved May 20, 2012, from http://www.asha.org

Applegate, J. (2002). *Twenty great ideas for your small business.* Princeton, NJ: Bloomberg Press.

Bauer, C. (2004). Plan for emotional changes, too: Here's how to make your transition out of practice a truly positive time. *Medical Economics, 81*(10), 60.

Baum, N. H., & Dowling, R. A. (2010). Thinking of selling your urology practice? Read this first. *Urology Times, 38*(13), 36–37.

Beiting, J. (2006). Part VI: Riding into the sunset: Many optometrists have discovered that if they can find a way to stay on the horse without having to manage the stable, "retirement" can be sweet indeed. *Review of Optometry, 143*(12), 27–31.

Bobryk, J. (1998). Tax traps in buying and selling a medical practice. *Physician's Management, 38*(1), 36–42.

Brady, G. Y. (2011). *Buying and selling an audiology practice: The basics.* Retrieved May 20, 2012, from http://www.audiologyonline.com/article_id=2351

Burg, B. (1995). Selling your practice? Avoid these tax traps. *Medical Economics, 72*(20), 68–73.

Carlson, R. P. (1998). When a physician practice management company comes calling. *Family Practice Management, 5*(6), 49–59.

Christensen, G. J. (2003). The best way to bring a dentist into your practice. *Journal of the American Dental Association, 134*(3), 367–369.

Covey, S. R. (1999). *Seven habits of highly effective people* (Rev. ed.). New York, NY: Simon and Shuster.

DePaolo, A. (2008). Buying of selling an audiology business. *ASHA Leader.*

Doty, L. W., & Campbell, A. T. (2000). Well-planned due diligence can protect buyers of healthcare entities. *Healthcare Financial Management, 54*(10), 56.

Drullinger, R. A. (2006). Practice valuation: The buying and selling of an audiology practice. *Seminars in Hearing, 27*(1), 57–76.

Eastern, J. S. (2006). Selling a medical practice. *Skin and Allergy News, 37*(11), 72.

Egerton, J. R., & Egerton, J. M. (2005). Selling our practice: A real roller-coaster ride. *Medical Economics, 82*(21), 73–76.

Engelmann, L., Berkey, D., Buck, T. P., Syfert, G., Tamres, M., & Williamson, S. (2008). Ensuring audiology's future in healthcare: Owning the profession through a culture of practice ownership. *Feedback (Suppl.), 19*(3), 1–12.

Foltner, K. (2008). Private practice: The BIG picture. *ADVANCE for Hearing Practice Management.* Retrieved May 20, 2012, from http://audiology.advanceseb.com/Editorial/Content/aspx?CC=114579

Foltner, K. (2011). Sonus creates first audiology-based franchise in hearing aid industry. Retrieved May 20, 2012, from http://wwwaudiologyonline.com/news/news_detail.asp?news_id=4650

Franks, D. (2006, November). Practice succession. *Southern California Physician,* pp. 1–3.

Gerber, G. (2009). When buying a practice, trust is not enough. *Optometry, 80*(12), 723–724.

Grau, D. (2007). Linked in. *Financial Planning, 37*(5), 89–91.

IRS. (2007). *Tax facts about capital gains and losses.* Internal Revenue Service. Retrieved May 27, 2007, from http://www.irs.gov/newsroom/article/0,,id=106799,00.html

Kline, C. M. (2007a). Buying and selling a practice—Keeping your edge. *Journal of the American Chiropractic Association, 44*(6), 2–5.

Kline, C. M. (2007b). Buying and selling a practice. Part II: Practice price and positive transitions. *Journal of the American Chiropractic Association, 44*(7), 2–6.

Lowes, R. (2006). How to value your practice: Whether you're selling to a hospital or getting a divorce, you need ropes. *Medical Economics, 83*(5), 66–70.

Mabry, C. D., & Ollapally, V. M. (2009) Selling a medical practice 101. *Bulletin of the American College of Surgeons, 94*(9), 6–9.

Mandell, D. B., & O'Dell, J. M. (2008). How to sell your medical practice for a million dollars. *Podiatry Management, 27*(3), 161–162.

Manning, L. (2008). How to sell your podiatry practice. *Podiatry Management 27*(6), 77–82.

Mattler, M. G. (2000). When and why should I have my practice appraised? *Journal of the American Dental Association, 131*(11), 1622–1624.

Mayer, T. (1998). Selling your medical practice: Calculate more than cash value in the bottom line. *Postgraduate Medicine, 104*(5), 25.

McAllister, D. (2005). Taking steps to prepare your practice for sale. *Coker Connection, 5*(9), 5–6.

McCall, K., & Dunlop, D. (2004). Marketing a practice. In B. Keagy & M. Thomas (Eds.), *Essentials of physician practice management* (pp. 394–409). San Francisco, CA: John Wiley & Sons.

McDonald, K. (2005). Practice builder: Understanding the factors that add to the value of a practice. *Podiatry Today, 18*(4), 20–25.

Mertz, E. (2002). *UCSF report finds dental practice patterns add to oral health disparity in the United States.* Press release, September 27. San Francisco, CA: Center for the Health Professions.

Nemes, J. (2006). Ready to sell? Experts offer advice on doing so successfully. *Hearing Journal, 59*(8), 19–26.

Nemes, J. (2009). Despite hard times, exit strategies exist for retirement-minded practice owners. *Hearing Journal, 62*(2), 19–23.

Ohm, N. (1999). How IT can move finance to change depreciation periods. *Gartner Group Archive Report.*

O'Malley, A. S., Grossman, J. M., Cohen, G. R., Kemper, N. M., & Pham, H. H. (2009). Are electronic medical records helpful for care coordination? Experiences of physician practices. *Journal of General Internal Medicine, 24*(2), 170–177.

Ousborne, A. L. (2007). Perception of the BIG picture. *Dental Economics, 97*(12), 49–50.

Patsula, P. (2001). *Selling your company. The Entrepreneur's Guidebook Series.* Patsula Media. Retrieved December 28, 2012, from http://www.smbtn.com/books/gb87.pdf

Reiboldt, M. (2004). *Buying, selling, and owning the medical practice* (2nd ed.). Chicago, IL: American Medical Association.

Reiboldt, M. (2007). *Financial management of the medical practice* (2nd ed.). Chicago, IL: American Medical Association.

Silverman, M. W., & Mohon, D. D. (2008). A case study in practice transition. *Optometry: Journal of the American Optometric Association, 79*(3), 149–153.

Smriga, D.J . (2006). For audiology, dentistry offers a good model for preserving independent private practice. *Hearing Journal, 59*(9), 36–42.

Smriga, D. J. (2011). Are we (still) asleep at the wheel? An update from seven years ago. Retrieved May 20, 2012, from http://www.audiologyonline.com/articles/pf_article_detail.asp?article_id=2387

Sullivan, J. D. (2006). Divesting strategies for medical practices. *Journal of Medical Practice Management: MPM, 22*(3), 159–161.

Weiss, G. G. (2004) How to close a practice: Whether you're turning your practice over to a colleague, selling it, or simply walking away, take the time to do it right. *Medical Economics, 81*(1), 69–73.

Wilson, K. (2005). Don't retire your practice; "transition" it. *Cosmetic Surgery Times, 8*(3), 46.

Index

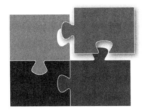

A

AAA (American Academy of Audiology)
  Code of Ethics, 391
  COE (Code of Ethics), 106
  Ethical Practice Guidelines on Financial
    Incentives for Hearing instruments
    position statement, 90–91
  Ethical Practices Committee (EPC), 106
  Practice Compliance Committee, 107
  scope of practice, 290
Accounting. *See* private practice accounting
    under Fiscal monitoring: cash flow
    analysis *main heading*
Advanced Beneficiary Notice form, 330
Advanced Bionics, 15
Affordable Care Act, 307
  and national debt, 10
AHAA (American Hearing Aid Associates),
    15, 16, 526
AKS (Anti-Kickback Statute), 90–91,
    110–112, 315–316
Americans with Disabilities Act, 85
Amplivox, 15
Audigy, 16
Authorization (sample) form, 333
Avada Network, 15, 526

B

Beltone, 526
Bernafon, 15, 16
Bill of rights example, patient,
    362–363
Bookkeeping. *See* private practice
    accounting *under* Fiscal
    monitoring: cash flow analysis
    main heading
Business planning, strategic. *See also*
    formal business plan *in this*
    section, audiology practice formal
    business plan format
  audiology practice formal business
    plan format. *See also* formal
    business plan *in this section*
  competitive analysis, 61–62
  executive summary, 57–58
  financial components, 63
  market assessment, 60–61
  mission statement, 58–59
  operational plan, 62–63
  overview, 57
  personnel, 62
  practice overview, 59–60
  summary, 63–64

Business planning, strategic *(continued)*
  audiology practice strategic conceptual
    planning
      analysis, internal/external, 52
      direction of strategy, 52–53
      formulation of strategy, 53
      overview, 51–52
  business ownership considerations,
    45–46
  business world entry considerations
    being one's own boss, 42–43
    earned benefits from manufacturers,
      44–45
    overview, 41–42
    practice rule setting, 44
    salary of self, 43–44
    and time off, 45
  formal business plan. *See also*
      audiology practice formal business
      plan format *in this section*
    advantages/utility, 55–56
    don'ts, 55
    do's, 54–55
    and market changes, 56–57
    preliminary considerations, 53–56
  overview, 39–41
  planning rationale
    overview, 47–49
    specific reasons, 49–51
  sidebars
    audiology business plan checklist,
      64–67
    computer-generated business plans,
      72
    executive summary questions, 58
    executive summary sample, 67–72
    ten principles essential to strategy
      development, 47–48
  strategy defined, 46–47

C

Career management
  communication, 432–433
  ethics, 440. *See also* Ethical
    considerations *main heading*
  fiscal responsibility, 438–439
  motivating others, 439–440

  negotiations, 433–434
  overview, 429–430, 440–441
  problem solving/analysis, 437–438
  promotional/public relations skills,
    434–435
  relationships, 430–432
  sales, 435–436
  skill sets, 430
Cash flow analysis. *See* Fiscal monitoring:
  cash flow analysis *main heading*
CMS (Centers for Medicare and Medicaid
  Services), 289, 290, 291
  billing, 290
  1500 claim form, 290, 306, 324
  hearing/balance assessment: Program
    Memorandum AB-02-080, 294
  HIPAA (Health Insurance Portability
    and Accountability Act), 320
  "incident to" billing, 299
  LCD (Local Coverage Determination),
    294
  MAC (Medicare Administrative
    Contractors), 294
  Medicare audits, 307
  Medicare compliance, 298
  NCD (National Coverage
    Determination), 294
  NPI (national provider identifier), 291,
    324
  pay for performance outcome measure,
    299–300
  RACs (Recovery Audit Contractors), 307
  and Stark law, 317, 318, 319
COE (Code of Ethics)
  and professional behavior, 99
Compensation strategies
  AAA (American Academy of
    Audiology), 452
  automobiles, 465
  benefits for employees, 82–83, 454–457
  country club dues, 465
  disability insurance, 464–465. *See
    also* Fiscal monitoring: cash flow
    analysis *main heading*
  insurance benefits
    disability/life, 459
    health, 458–459
  job satisfaction, 446–447

nature of compensation, 444–447
organizational commitment, 447
overview, 443–444, 465–466
philosophies of compensation
    entitlement-based programs, 449
    performance-based programs, 449
    skill-based compensation, 451–452
    straight salary, 449–450
    variable compensation model,
        450–451
the psychological contract, 445–446
retirement programs
    cash, 461
    deferred profit sharing, 461
    401(k) programs, 461–462
    overview, 460
stock options, 460
tangible base salary/salary range for
        employees computation, 452–454
types of compensation
    extrinsic (tangible), 448–449
    intrinsic (intangible), 447–448
vacations, holidays, personal time off,
        353–354, 459–460
Costco, 526
Counseling/employee considerations. *See
        also* Personnel management *main
        heading;* Policy and Procedures
        Manual *main heading*
    counseling attributes
        congruence with self, 390
        empathic understanding, 391–392
        forward through silence, 392–393
        timing, 393
        unconditional positive regard, 391
    overview, 390
    social styles
        assertion/responsiveness, 394
        descriptors, 395
        recognition of, 394–396
        supportive direction/collaboration,
            393–396
Counseling/patient considerations.
        See also Counseling/employee
        considerations *main heading;*
        Policy and Procedures *main
        heading*
    attributes of successful practitioners

empathic understanding, 391–392
    moving forward through silence,
        392–393
    overview, 390
    timing, 393
    unconditional positive regard,
        390–391
and bottom line, 396–401
hearing instrument repair counseling,
        480
hearing loss management attitudinal/
        behavioral change stages, 398
motivating toward action, 399–401
motivational engagement, 397–398
overview, 389–390
self-assessment measures, 397
CPT (Current Procedural Terminology)
        coding
    audiology diagnostic tests, 318
    and billing, 293
    "incident to," 298
    cochlear implant mapping/
        reprogramming, 318
    Editorial Panel, 291, 292
    evaluation and management codes
        (E & M), 303
    and HCPAC (Health Care Professionals
        Advisory Committee), 291
    hearing aids, 318
    and HIPAA (Health Insurance
        Portability and Accountability Act),
        291
    and MAC (Medicare Administrative
        Contractors) LCD (Local Coverage
        Determination), 294
    modifiers, 304–305
    overview, 291–292
    in Policies and Procedures Manual, 356
    and practice operational plan, 62
    and RUC (RVS [relative value scale]
        Update Committee of AMA)
        database, 291
    and Stark Law, 318
    on superbill, or encounter form, 301
    with technical and professional
        components, 299
    Transaction and Code Sets, 320
    utilization tracking, 291

D

Drucker, Paul (1909–2005), 46

E

Economics
  command economies, 3
  commoditization of amplification
      devices, 16–17, 132–135
  competitive landscape of the hearing
      industry
    amplification device
        commoditization, 16–17, 153
    buying groups, 17–18
    commoditization of amplification
        devices, 16–17
    distribution channels, 16
    horizontal integration:, 14
    horizontal integration: hearing
        industry, 15–16
    industry consolidation, 14–18
    overview, 14
    vertical integration: hearing industry,
        16
  competitive strategies, generic
    differentiation, 19–20
    focus, 20
    overall cost leadership, 19
  CPI (consumer price index)
    defined/calculated, 8
  currency values, 10
  cycles defined, 4
  deficit spending, 10
  deflation, 7
  depression defined, 4
  economic cycles defined, 3
  economic cycles/market economies,
      3–4
  economic indicators for audiologists,
      4–5
  Federal Reserve, 6, 7
  free markets, 3–4
  GDP (gross domestic product)
    calculation of, 5–6
    defined, 5
    versus GNP (gross national product),
        6

    as indicator, 5–6
    political manipulation, 6
    and productivity, 6
    and recession definition, 4
  GNP (gross national product), 6
    defined, 6
    versus GDP (gross domestic
        product), 6
  hybrid markets, 4
  inflation, 7, 8
  macroeconomics defined, 3
  market economies, 3–4
  market economy defined, 3
  microeconomics defined, 3
  Mind Tools, 36
  mixed economies, 3–4
  mixed economy defined, 3–4
  national debt
    and government spending
        reductions, 9–10
    overview, 8–9
    and tax raises, 9
  overview of current situation, 1–2
  Porter's five forces
    applicability to a practice, 29–36
    buyers' bargaining power, 23–24,
        31–32
    new market entrants' threats, 22–23,
        29–31
    overview, 20–21
    rivalry among incumbents, 27, 35–36
    suppliers' bargaining power, 24–26,
        32–34
    threat of substitutes, 26–27, 34–35
  power balance assessment/Porter's five
      forces
    buyers' bargaining power, 23–24,
        31–32
    new market entrants' threats, 22–23,
        29–31
    overview, 20–21
    rivalry among incumbents, 27, 35–36
    suppliers' bargaining power, 24–26,
        32–34
    threat of substitutes, 26–27, 34–35
  prime rate, 6–8
  realities of audiology private practice,
      2–3

recession defined, 4
sidebars
  business funding in a difficult
    economy: business defensive
    assets, 12
  business funding in a difficult
    economy: overview, 11
  business funding in a difficult
    economy: personal savings
    account, 12
  industry analysis typical steps, 18
  Porter's five forces, 28
  supply and demand, 3–4
EHR (electronic health records), 313–314
Electone, 16
Employee Handbook. *See* Policy and
  Procedures Manual
Employment options
  as employee, 77
  as independent contractor, 77–78
  as practice owner, 78
ENT (ear, nose, throat) physicians
  contractual relationships, 84
Ethical considerations
  AAA (American Academy of
    Audiology), Ethical Practices
    Committee (EPC), 106
  *Advisory Opinion: Hearing Aid
    Commissions* (AAA, Ethical
    Practices Committee), 114
  AKS (Anti-Kickback Statute), 110–112
    conflicts of interest (COI), 90–91
    safe harbor provision to protect
      employee payment, 111
  business ethics areas
    billing/coding, 106–107
    coding/billing, 106–107
  COE (Code of Ethics)
    overview, 98
  COE (Code of Ethics), state, sample,
    100–105
  conflicts of interest (COI)
    *Ethical Practice Guidelines on
      Financial Incentives from Hearing
      Instrument Manufacturers* (AAA
      & ADA), 110
    manufacturer relationships, 107–109
    overview, 107

dilemma solving, 114–115
documentation/record keeping,
  113–114
employee compensation, 114
Ethical Practices Committee (EPC),
  AAA (American Academy of
  Audiology), 106
marketing, 112–113
  safe harbor provision to protect
    employee payment, 113
  Stark law/Physician Self-Referral law,
    112–113
and marketing, 112–113
and Medicare/Medicaid, 106–107
overview, 97–98, 115
Physician Self-Referral law/Stark law,
  112–113
Practice Compliance Committee, AAA
  (American Academy of Audiology),
  106
professional behavior, 98
  and COE (Code of Ethics), 99
  standards, 98–99
professional organizations, 106
Stark law/Physician Self-Referral law,
  112–113
and Stark law/Physician Self-Referral
  law, 112–113
state licensure, 99–105
Ethical Practice Guidelines on Financial
  Incentives for Hearing instruments
  position statement, AAA (American
  Academy of Audiology), 90–91
Exit strategies, 93–94

F

Federal Trade Commission (FTC) and
  industrial consolidation, 14
Finance. *See under* Fiscal monitoring:
  cash flow analysis *main heading*
Fiscal monitoring: cash flow analysis
  accounting basics, 243, 245
  audiology private practice accounting
    cash and accrual methods, 246–247
    generally accepted accounting
      principles (GAAP), 247–249
    overview, 245–246

Fiscal monitoring: cash flow analysis
(continued)
  finance for audiologists
    borrowing money for the practice,
      276–278
    break-even analysis (BA): capital
      investment, 282–285
    budgeting: financial management,
      basic, 278–279
    capital investment, 282–285
    financial management, basic,
      278–285
    investing the profit, 275–276
    lease types, 279, 280–282
    lease *versus* purchase: financial
      management, basic, 279, 280, 281
    net present value (NPV): capital
      investment, 284–285
    overview, 275
    purchase *versus* lease: financial
      management, basic, 279, 280, 281
  financial accounting ratios
    activity ratios (AR), 265–269
    cross-sectional analysis: performance
      comparison, 260
    current ratio (CR)/quick ratios:
      liquidity ratios, 261–262
    debt, or leverage, ratios, 269, 270
    debt to assets (DA) ratio: debt, or
      leverage, ratios, 270, 271
    defensive interval measure (DIM):
      liquidity ratios, 263–264
    liquidity ratios, 261
    overview, 272–275
    performance comparison, 259–260
    practice monitoring with ratio
      calculation, 261
    profitability ratios, 270, 271
    profit margin on sales (PMOS):
      profitability ratios, 270, 271–272
    ratio calculation for practice
      monitoring, 261
    time series analysis, 260
    times interest earned (TIE) ratio:
      debt, or leverage, ratios, 270,
      271
    total assets turnover ratio (TAT):
      activity ratios (AR), 269

financial statements
  account balancing, 257–258
  assets: the balance sheet, 254–255
  the balance sheet, 253–255
  cash flow statement, 258–259
  the income statement, 255–257
  liabilities: the balance sheet, 255
overview, 286
private practice accounting
  bookkeeping types, 249–250
  double-entry bookkeeping:
    bookkeeping types, 249–250
  inventory control: bookkeeping
    types, 250
  payroll preparation: bookkeeping
    types, 252–253
  property tax accounting:
    bookkeeping types, 250
  receivables and payables:
    bookkeeping types, 250
sidebars
  bookkeeper key qualities, 251–252
  break-even analysis (BA), 283
  current ratio (CR)/quick ratio (acid
    test ratio) computation, 262
  debt to assets (DA) ratio: debt, or
    leverage, ratios, 271
  defensive interval measure (DIM)
    calculation, 263–264
  economic exchanges in an audiology
    practice overview, 244–245
  financial manager key qualities,
    251–252
  net present value (NPV) calculation,
    284–285
  profit margin on sales (PMOS), 272
  times interest earned (TIE) ratio:
    debt, or leverage, ratios, 271
  total assets turnover ratio (TAT), 269
Forms
  Advanced Beneficiary Notice, 330
  Authorization (sample), 333
FTC (Federal Trade Commission)
  and industrial consolidation, 14

G

GN ReSound, 15, 16, 526
Great Nordic, 15

H

Hansaton, 15
Hearing instrument manufacturer/
  supplier issues
  changing manufacturers, 486–488
  corporate (manufacturer)/private
    practice consolidation, 488–489
  costs/financial operations
    hearing instrument acquisition costs,
      477
    instrument repair benchmark
      establishment, 479–480
    manufacturer payment policies, 478
    range of instrument costs, 477
    rates of repairs, 479
    repair resolution/warranties,
      478–479
    warranties/repair resolution,
      478–479
  counseling patients about hearing
    instrument repairs, 480
  digital technology/patient satisfaction,
    471–472
  hearing instrument manufacturer and
    audiologist symbiosis, 471
  instrument acquisition costs
    monitoring, 488
  monitoring performance
    evidence-based decision making,
      485–486
    FDA standards, 484–485
    repair incidence, 485–486
  overview, 469–470
  patient advocacy, 489–490
  patient satisfaction/digital technology,
    471–472
  re-repairs by manufacturer/repair
    facility, 482
  return of repaired instruments by
    manufacturer/repair facility,
    481–482
  sidebars
    evaluating suppliers, 474
    importance of manufacturer field
      representatives, 481
    letter posing unresolved
      manufacturer problems, 487

technology
  assistive technologies/compatibility,
    473, 475
  connectivity ease, 475
  overview, 472–473
  user-friendly software, 475–477
want/need list for manufacturer
  services
  programming, 482–483
  re-repair warranty extensions, 483
  software upgrades, 483
worse-case repair scenario, 470–471
Hearing Planet, 15
HearPO, 16
HearUSA, 526
HEARx, 16
HIPAA (Health Insurance Portability
    and Accountability Act)/HITECH
    (Health Information Technology
    for Economic and Clinical Health
    Act). *See also* HITECH (Health
    Information Technology for
    Economic and Clinical Health Act)
    main heading
  abuse reporting disclosure exception,
    89
  and business associates, 88
  and CPT (Current Procedural
    Terminology) coding, 291. *See
    also* CPT (Current Procedural
    Terminology) coding *main
    heading*
  documentation/record keeping
    (HIPAA), 113–114
  enforcement/penalties, 89–90
  ICD-9 (International Classification
    of Diseases-9-CM codes), 291.
    See also ICD-9 (International
    Classification of Diseases-9-CM
    codes) *main heading for full
    listing*
  NPI (National Provider Identifier), 324
  NPP (Notice of Privacy Practices), 89
  permission to evaluate/treat, 88–89
  PHI (protected health information),
    88
  privacy officer, 89
  security, 87–88, 323

HITECH (Health Information Technology for Economic and Clinical Health Act), 324–325. *See also* HIPAA (Health Insurance Portability and Accountability Act)/HITECH (Health Information Technology for Economic and Clinical Health Act) *main heading*
  abuse reporting disclosure exception, 89
  and business associates, 88
  enforcement/penalties, 89–90
  NPP (Notice of Privacy Practices), 89
  permission to evaluate/treat, 88–89
  PHI (protected health information), 88
  privacy, 87–88
  privacy officer, 89
  security, 87–88
HMOs (health maintenance organizations), 300–301

I

ICD-9 (International Classification of Diseases-9-CM codes), 291
  hearing aids/supplies billing, 293
  ICD-10 codes introduction, 301–302
  supportive codes, 301
ICD-10 (International Classification of Diseases-10-CM codes), 301–302. *See* under ICD-9 (International Classification of Diseases-9-CM codes) *main heading*
Interacoustics, 15
International Classification of Diseases 9th Revision Clinical Modification (ICD-9-CM). *See* ICD-9 (International Classification of Diseases-9-CM codes) *main heading*
International Classification of Diseases 10th Revision Clinical Modification (ICD-10-CM). *See* ICD-10 *under* ICD-9 (International Classification of Diseases-9-CM codes) *main heading*
Interton, 16

L

Legal considerations, 80
  accountant selection, 77
  AKS (Anti-Kickback Statute), 90–91, 110–112
  arbitration, 86
  attorney selection, 75–77
  in audiology practice operation, 78–87
  banker selection, 77
  benefits/compensation, 82–83
  C corporations, 80
  certification, 93
  compensation/benefits, 82–83
  co-ownership, 81–82
  dispute resolution, 86–87
  employment law concerns, 93
  ENT (ear, nose, throat) physician contractual relationships, 84
  estate planning, 83
  exit strategies, 93–94
  expert testimony presentation, 84
  False Claims Act, 91–92, 106
  flexible health benefit plans, 83
  401(k), 82–83
  health insurance benefits, 82–83
  HIPAA (Health Insurance Portability and Accountability Act)/HITECH (Health Information Technology for Economic and Clinical Health Act). *See also* HIPAA (Health Insurance Portability and Accountability Act)/HITECH (Health Information Technology for Economic and Clinical Health Act) *main heading*
    abuse reporting disclosure exception, 89
    and business associates, 88
    enforcement/penalties, 89–90
    NPP (Notice of Privacy Practices), 89
    permission to evaluate/treat, 88–89
    PHI (protected health information), 88
    privacy officer, 89

HITECH (Health Information Technology for Economic and Clinical Health Act)/HIPAA (Health Insurance Portability and Accountability Act), 87–88. *See also* HITECH (Health Information Technology for Economic and Clinical Health Act)/HIPAA (Health Insurance Portability and Accountability Act) *main heading*
  abuse reporting disclosure exception, 89
  and business associates, 88
  enforcement/penalties, 89–90
  NPP (Notice of Privacy Practices), 89
  permission to evaluate/treat, 88–89
  PHI (protected health information), 88
  privacy officer, 89
insurance scope, 86
insurer/payor contractual relationships, 83–84
legal entity choice, 78–82
liabilities, nonprofessional, 78–79
licensure, state regulations, 92
LLC (limited liability company)/LLP (limited liability partnership) legal entities, 79, 81–82
mediation, 86
noncontributory-defined benefit plans, 82
nondiscrimination, 83
NPP (Notice of Privacy Practices), 89
office/facilities
  first refusal right, 85
  improvements, 85
  lease review, 84–85
  physical damage problems, 85
  renegotiation, 85–86
  "standard form" leases, 85
  subordination, nondisturbance, attornment agreement, 85
  zoning laws, 86
partnerships, limited, 80
partnerships, limited or general, 79, 80
patient relationships, 82–83
PHI (protected health information), 88
Physician Self-Referral law/Stark law, 91, 112–113
professional advisors to engage, 75–77
regulatory compliance, 87
retirement, 82–83, 93–95
retirement plans, 82–83
risk management, 86–87
sale of business, 93–94
S corporations, 79–80
SIMPLE IRAs, 82
Simplified Employee Pension Plans (SEPs), 82
sole proprietorship, 80, 81
Stark law/Physician Self-Referral law, 91, 112–113
state issues, 80–81
Licensure, state
  COE (Code of Ethics) sample, 100–105
  regulations, 92
Lyric, 15

M

Maico Audimeters, 15
Marketing effectiveness: developing/ growing the practice. *See also* Marketing fundamentals *main heading*
advertising defined, 162
effective message crafting, 173–174
evaluation
  content by title, 192
  data from Web site analytics, 189–190
  key words reports, 191–192
  phone tracking systems, 189
  referring Web sites, 191
  tracking marketing results, traditional, 188–189
  Web site analytics, 189–192
  Web site statistics terms, 190–191
execution, 173

Marketing effectiveness: developing/
growing the practice *(continued)*
  groundwork for effective plan
    business climate/competitive
      analysis, 169–170
    demographic/psychographic
      research, 167–169
    marketing strategy, budget, and
      goals, 170–173
    market research, 166–167
    psychographic/demographic
      research, 167–169
    USP (unique selling proposition),
      164–166
  marketing defined, 162
  media
    article marketing, 182–184
    billboards, 174
    blog feeds, 188
    blogger.com, 184
    blogging, 176–177
    blogging to attract visitors, 187–188
    bookmarking, social, 187
    direct mail, 174–175
    e-mail marketing, 181–182
    Facebook, 184
    guest blog posts, 188
    HubPages.com, 185
    links, online, 187
    networking, community, 175
    newspaper, 174
    nontraditional, 175–188
    online presence, 175–188
    outreach, community, 175
    pinging on Internet, 188
    PPC (pay-per-click), 176–177, 176–179
    press releases, Internet, 186–187
    radio, 174
    referral marketing, 175
    search engines, 176
    SEO (search engine optimization),
      179–181
    Squidoo.com, 185
    traditional, 174–175
    Twitter, 185–186
    video, Web site, 186
    Web sites, 175–176
    Web 2.0 Web sites, 184–187

    word-of-mouth Internet marketing,
      187–188
    WordPress.com, 185
    YouTube, 186
  online presence, 162–163
  overview, 161–162, 192–193
  sales defined, 162
  *Search Engine Optimization: An Hour
    a Day* (Grappone & Couzin), 179
  SWOT (strengths, weaknesses,
    opportunities, threats)
    analysis, 169–170. *See also*
    SWOT (strengths, weaknesses,
    opportunities, threats) analysis
    under Marketing fundamentals
    main heading
  3 E's of marketing/education, 163–164
Marketing fundamentals. *See also*
  Marketing effectiveness:
    developing/growing the practice
  advertising
    billboards, 149
    brochures/circulars, 149
    classified ads, 152
    coupons, 152
    demonstrations of products, 152
    direct mail by audiologists, 152–153
    direct mail sales of over-the-counter
      hearing instruments, 153
    direct-response radio and television,
      153–154
    educational seminars, 155
    exhibits/fairs, 154
    experiential advertising, 156–157
    Internet professional practice
      advertising, 156
    Internet sales of over-the-counter
      hearing instruments, 153
    magazine advertisements, 154
    newsletters, 154
    newspaper advertisements, 154–155
    personal letters, 155
    print articles/columns, 148–149
    radio advertisements, 155
    signage, 155
    speciality item printed practice
      information giveaways, 148
    telemarketing, 156

television, 156
Web sites, 150–152
yellow pages, 156
branding a practice
    categories of branding, 123–124
    decisions about, 124–125
    overview, 121–123
definition of professional marketing,
    120–121
expertise as added value, 132, 133
marketing specialists, 138
patient value promotion, 157–158
place of service provision, 134–135
plans. *See also* SWOT (strengths,
    weaknesses, opportunities,
    threats) analysis *under same main*
    heading
    competitive analysis, 146–147
    customer wants, needs, demands,
        129–130
    demographics, 128–129
    detailed marketing, 138–142
    Four Ps, 129, 130
    marketing map, 1-year, 139
    marketing mix, 129, 130
    organization, 142
    overview, 126, 128
    rationales for, 128
    and target market segmentation,
        128–129
and product
    branding by questioning consumers,
        135
    characteristics of product, 131
    commoditization, 16–17, 132–133
    manufacturer marketing
        partnerships, 132
    mix offered by practice, 131–133
    price setting/pricing mix, 133
    tangibility of product, 131
promotion
    advantages of practice location, 138
    advertising, 136
    ancillary products, 137
    of benefits, 138
    with current practice consumers,
        135–136
    for general public, 136

hints, 136–137
    with information, 138
    with marketing specialists, 138
    market offering, 136
    organizations, 138
    for patient referral from medical
        colleagues, 135
    publicity of special practice member,
        138
    with public relations, 136
    services, 137
    special event participation, 137–138
    types, 137–138
promotional mix: Kotler's 4 steps,
    157–158
rationale for marketing, 119–120
and rehabilitative treatment plans,
    132–133
research, 125–126. *See also* SWOT
    (strengths, weaknesses,
    opportunities, threats) analysis
    under same main heading
    competitive analysis, 146–147
    detailed, 138–142
    outline, 127
sidebar
    marketing analysis of the practice,
        professional, 143–144
    marketing map, 1-year, 139
sidebars
    database questionnaire, 144
    marketing questionnaire, 143–144
    research outline, 127
strategy development, 147–148
SWOT (strengths, weaknesses,
    opportunities, threats) analysis,
    169–170
    opportunities assessment, 145
    opportunities (example), 143
    overview, 142
    process of analysis, 145
    strengths assessment, 146
    strengths (example), 143
    threat assessment, 145
    threats (example), 143
    weaknesses assessment, 146
    weaknesses (example), 143
Web sites, 150–152

Medicare
  Advanced Beneficiary Notice, 296–297
  and AKS (Anti-Kickback Statute), 87
  billing for services not rendered, 106
  CERT (Comprehensive Error Rate
    Testing), 307
  compliance, 298
  fraud/abuse, 95, 307–308
  Medicare reimbursement formula, 290
  modifiers, 305–306
  nonparticipating status, 297–298
  other third-party payers, 300–301
  Part A, 295
  Part B, 295–296
  Part C, 296
  Part D, 296
  patient counseling of services covered,
    372
  Physician Self-Referral law/Stark law, 91
  positive reactions to budget cuts, 12–13
  practice employee mistakes, 99
  referrals, 91
  Stark law/Physician Self-Referral law,
    91
  teleaudiology services, 498
  threats to hearing industry, 23
Mind Tools, 36

O

Oticon, 15, 526

P

Patient bill of rights example, 362–363
Patient management
  angry/disgruntled patients, 375–379
  apathy costs, 359–360
  baby boomers, 379–382
  cognitive difficulty and staff, 371–372
  communication: verbal/nonverbal,
    363–365
  conflict resolution, 375–379
  and difficult patients/families, 372–379
  follow-up care, 382–386
  hearing loss issues and staff, 371
  loyalty and communication, 359
  loyalty benefits, 360
  loyalty development, 358–362

newsletters, 385–386
  noncompliance and extended care
    facilities (ECF), 374–375
  noncompliance patients/families,
    372–374
  and office staff, 366–372
  overview, 357–358, 386
  patient loyalty defined, 358–359
  personalization through involvement,
    382–383, 385
  and practice team, 370–372. *See also*
    receptionist *in this section*
  and receptionist, 367–370
  referrals from patients, 383, 385
  retrieving dissatisfied patients, 361–362
  satisfaction from verbal behaviors,
    365–366
  satisfaction levels, 361–362
  sidebars
    belligerent patient, 377–378
    brochure example, 383–384
  staff safety/conflict resolution, 375–379
  verbal behaviors and outcomes,
    364–365
  verbal behaviors to improve patient
    satisfaction, 365–366
  word-of-mouth dynamics, 360–361
Personnel management. *See also*
    Counseling/employee
    considerations *main heading;*
    Policy and Procedures Manual
    main heading
  adding audiologist to professional staff,
    426–427
  empowering associates, 423
  and leadership
    from employee to associate, 416–417
  orientation/training
    introducing to team members:
      on-boarding, 422
    on-boarding, 421–422
    overview, 420–421
    teaching the tasks: on-boarding, 422
  overview, 415–416, 427
  performance appraisal, 423–424
  recruiting
    interview, telephone, 419–420
    protocol, 418–419
    tendering an offer, 420

retention of employees, 424–425
sidebars
  recruiting protocol example, 419
  valuable character traits in potential
    candidates, 417
termination of employment, 425–426
Phonak, 15
Phonic Ear, 15
Policy and Procedures Manual. *See
  also* Counseling/employee
  considerations *main heading;*
  Personnel management *main
  heading*
Acknowledgment Form, Policy and
  Procedures Manual, 337
as all-encompassing compliance
  document, 338–339
legal considerations, 338
need for, 338
outline of manual, 340
overview, 335–336, 356
policies *versus* procedures, 336
proposed text overview, 339
sidebars
  Acknowledgment Form, Policy and
    Procedures Manual, 337
  outline of manual, 340
text, proposed/commentary
  Acknowledgment Forms, 343–344
  Administrative Staff Priorities, 345
  Billing and Collection Policy, 346
  Clinical Procedures, 356
  Confidentiality, 346–347
  Conflicts of Commitment/Conflicts of
    Interest, 347
  Consent Forms for Specific
    Procedures, 347
  Consent to Perform Cerumen
    Removal and/or Earmold
    Impression (example for all
    procedures), 347
  Disciplinary Actions, 348–349
  Drug/Alcohol Policy, 349–350
  Educational Allowances, 350
  E-mail Procedures, 352
  Emergency Medical Assistance
    Protocol, 350–351
  Equal Employment Opportunity
    (EEO) Policy, 350

Financial Agreement, 345–346
Hearing Instrument Lost Under
  Warranty Replacement, 351–352
Hearing Instrument Repairs, 352
Hearing Instrument Return Within
  Four Weeks Postfitting, 352
Inclement Weather, 355
Internet Procedures, general,
  352–353
Internet Usage, 352–353
Introduction, 341
Management Rights, 342–343
Operational Information of the
  Practice Access, 351
overview, 339
Paid Time Off (PTO), 353–354
Patient Satisfaction/Complaint
  Resolution, 347–348
Patients With Prior Collection
  Actions, 354
Performance Review, 351
Policies, 345–347
Position Descriptions, 354–355
Position Descriptions: Receptionist
  Description (example), 354–355
Practice Philosophy: A Mission of
  Commitment to Patients, 341–342
Professional Appearance/Dress
  Code, 351
Referring Patients to Other
  Practitioners, 355
Replacement of Lost Hearing
  Instrument Under Warranty,
  351–352
Tuition Assistance, 355
P&P Manual. *See* Policy and Procedures
  Manual
PPO (preferred provider organization),
  301
PQRS (Physician Quality Reporting
  System), 299–300
Practice entry and exit optimization
  closing practice without selling,
    532–533
  marketing to potential buyers, 523–524,
    524–525
  overview, 513–515, 535
  patient notification of practice sale,
    531–532

Practice entry and exit optimization
(continued)
  planning entry and exit strategies
    due diligence of seller and buyer,
      518–519
    planning sales disclosure
      information, 518
    sales package development, 518
    valuation, 516–518
  practice brokers, professional practice
    sellers, 527–529
  preparing practice for acquisition
    audiometric/office equipment,
      521–522
    files/file management organization,
      522
    improvements, 519
    income/expense normalization, 523
    physical location/needed building
      modification, 519–521
    practice history compilation, 519
    questions to address, 519
    staff considerations, 522–523
  purchase by employee(s)/ESOPs
    (employee stock ownership plans),
      529–530
  purchase timing, 533–535
  retained involvement (selling practice/
    staying to work in office), 530
  sales package creation, 523–524
  selling to a corporate entity, 525–527
  tax considerations of successful sale,
    530–531
  timing of practice sale, 513–516
Practice management, coding,
    reimbursement
  AKS (Anti-Kickback Statute), 315–316
  audits, 306–307
  billing practices, 292–293
  bundling *versus* unbundling/
    itemization, hearing aid fees, 304
  CERT (Comprehensive Error Rate
    Testing), Medicare, 307
  certification, 325
  Cerumen/Earmold Impression Waivers
    (samples), 331–332
  CMS (Centers for Medicare and
    Medicaid Services), 289, 290, 291,
    294. *See also* CMS (Centers for

    Medicare and Medicaid Services)
    main heading for complete listing
  collections, 306
  co-pays/co-insurances, 302–304
  CPT (Current Procedural Terminology)
    coding, 291–292. *See also* CPT
    (Current Procedural Terminology)
    coding *main heading;* CPT
    (Current Procedural Terminology)
    coding *main heading for full
    listing*
  CPT (Current Procedural Terminology)
    coding overview, 291, 292
  documentation, 311–312
    chart composition, 313
    chart composition/records retention,
      313
    EHR (electronic health records), 312,
      313–314
    overview, 311–312
    SOAP format, 311–312
  EHR (electronic health records), 312,
    313–314
  false claims, 319
  forms
    Advanced Beneficiary Notice, 330
    Authorization (sample), 333
  fraud/abuse, 307–308
  GPCI (geographic price cost index),
    290
  hearing aid fees bundling *versus*
    unbundling/itemization, 304
  HIPAA (Health Insurance Portability
    and Accountability Act)
    detailed, 319–323
    NPI (National Provider Identifier),
      324
    security, 323
  HITECH (Health Information
    Technology for Economic
    and Clinical Health Act). *See
    also* HIPAA (Health Insurance
    Portability and Accountability
    Act)/HITECH (Health Information
    Technology for Economic and
    Clinical Health Act) *main
    heading*
  HMOs (health maintenance
    organizations), 300–301

ICD-9 (International Classification of Diseases-9-CM codes), 291. *See also* ICD-9 (International Classification of Diseases-9-CM codes) *main heading for detailed listings*

ICD-10 (International Classification of Diseases-10-CM codes), 301–302

impaired practitioners, 326

informed consent, 326

insurance contract negotiations, 308–311

LCD (Local Coverage Determination), 294

liability, 325–326

MAC (Medicare Administrative Contractors), 294

Medicare
Advanced Beneficiary Notice, 296–297
compliance, 298
"incident to," 298–299
nonparticipating status, 297–298
opting out: not for audiologists, 298
overview, 293–295
Part A, 295
Part B, 295–296
Part C, 296
Part D, 296
participating provider status, 297

Medicare compliance, 298

Medicare modifiers, 305–306

Medicare reimbursement formula, 290

modifiers of CPT (Current Procedural Terminology) coding, 304–305

modifiers of Medicare, 305–306

MPFS (Medicare Physician Fee Schedule), 289, 294, 295

NCD (National Coverage Determination), 294

NPI (national provider identifier), 291

overview, 289–290

patients, dismissing, 327

patients, incompetent, 326–327

POS (point of service), 301

PPO (preferred provider organization), 301

PQRS (Physician Quality Reporting System), 299–300

RBRVS (Resource-Based Relative Value Scale), 289, 290

referrals to and from practice, 314

reports, 314

RVU (relative value unit), 290, 291

Stark laws, 317–319

state regulations/licensure, 325

Pricing strategy optimization
overview, 195–196, 240
price influences
avoidable business costs, 206–207
business costs, 203–213
competition pricing, 198–199
cost-plus business pricing, 207–213
cost-plus pricing, 198–199
customers as patients, 196–197
demand for products/services, 197–198
and expected profit, 213
fixed business costs, 204–205
fixed/incremental (variable) business costs/pricing, 206
incremental (variable) business costs, 205–206
price elasticity, 199–203
and product life cycle, 213
sunk business costs, 207
pricing fundamental concepts
bundling/unbundling, 223–226
communication of price methods, 229–232
discounting, 237–238
economic/differentiation value, 216–217
fencing (of segments), 221–222
hearing instruments' pricing tiers/segments, 219
metrics of pricing, 222–223
negotiation, 237–238
overview, 213–215
patient purchasing behaviors, 235–237
price level, 238–240
price structure, 221–226
price/value communication, 226–232
pricing objectives, 239–240
pricing policy, 232–238
purchase stages, 229
strategic pricing pyramid, 216
strategies, 231
value-based price segmentation, 217–221

Pricing strategy optimization *(continued)*
  7 principles of pricing, 240
  sidebars
    bundling/unbundling of prices, 224
    figuring cost-plus (markup) prices, 208–211
    five times cost rule-of-thumb pricing scheme, 208
    opportunity business cost of vestibular assessment, 204–205
    percentage of profit-over-cost scheme, 208–209
    product price elasticity, 202–203
    target-return pricing scheme, 209–211

R

Referral source management
  acquisition of referral sources, 403–404
  assessment of referral sources
    evidence-based assessment of referral source activity, 413–414
    overview, 412–413
  findings/recommendations
    communication to referrer
    format/content of report, 406–408
    interactions with difficult patients reporting, 409
    turnaround time of report, 405–406
  good words for referral sources, 404
  practice-to-practice marketing
    and client services, 411–412
    overview, 409–410
    practice image management, 410–411
  retention of referral sources, 404–405
Retirement, 82–83, 93–95
  cash, 461
  deferred profit sharing, 461
  401(k) programs, 461–462
  overview, 460
Rexton, 16

S

Safe harbors, 111, 116–117
Sale of business, 93–94

Search Engine Optimization: An Hour a Day (Grappone & Couzin), 179
Sennheiser, 15
Sidebars
  business planning, strategic
    audiology business plan checklist, 64–67
    executive summary questions, 58
    executive summary sample, 67–72
    ten principles essential to strategy development, 47–48
  economics
    business funding in a difficult economy: business defensive assets, 12
    business funding in a difficult economy: overview, 11
    business funding in a difficult economy: personal savings account, 12
    industry analysis typical steps, 18
    Porter's five forces, 28
  fiscal monitoring: cash flow analysis
    bookkeeper key qualities, 251–252
    break-even analysis (BA), 283
    current ratio (CR)/quick ratio (acid test ratio) computation, 262
    debt to assets (DA) ratio: debt, or leverage, ratios, 271
    defensive interval measure (DIM) calculation, 263–264
    economic exchanges in an audiology practice overview, 244–245
    financial manager key qualities, 251–252
    net present value (NPV) calculation, 284–285
    profit margin on sales (PMOS), 272
    times interest earned (TIE) ratio: debt, or leverage, ratios, 271
    total assets turnover ratio (TAT), 269
  hearing instrument manufacturer/supplier issues
    evaluating suppliers, 474
    importance of manufacturer field representatives, 481
    letter posing unresolved manufacturer problems, 487

marketing fundamentals
    database questionnaire, 144
    marketing analysis of the practice,
        professional, 143–144
    marketing map, 1-year, 139
    marketing questionnaire, 143–144
    research outline, 127
patient management
    belligerent patient, 377–378
    brochure example, 383–384
personnel management
    recruiting protocol example, 419
    valuable character traits in potential
        candidates, 417
Policy and Procedures Manual
    Acknowledgment Form, Policy and
        Procedures Manual, 337
    outline of manual, 340
pricing strategy optimization
    bundling/unbundling of prices, 224
    figuring cost-plus (markup) prices,
        208–211
    five times cost rule-of-thumb pricing
        scheme, 208
    opportunity business cost of
        vestibular assessment, 204–205
    percentage of profit-over-cost
        scheme, 208–209
    product price elasticity, 202–203
    target-return pricing scheme, 209–211
Siemens, 15–16
Software
    Business Plan Pro, 72
    Sales and Marketing Pro, 139
Sonic/Sonic Innovations, 15, 526
Sonova, 15, 153
Starkey, 16
Stark law/Physician Self-Referral law, 91,
    317–319
State regulations/licensure, 325

T

Teleaudiology services, 498

U

UHC (UnitedHealthcare), 16

Unitron, 15
University audiology clinic practice
        management
    challenges of university environment,
        495–496
    clinical educational activities issues
        AuD student roles, 502–503
        computer scheduling/billing,
            504–505
        human resource management
            opportunities, 503
        projects/assignments beyond clinical
            services, 503–504
        support for students, 504
    cost of services/reimbursement
        billing systems, 508
        contractual arrangements for unique
            services, 507
        financial responsibilities of, 505
        "free" service provision, 506
        nonprofit status, 505–506
        pricing, 506–507
        purchasing/accounts payable rules,
            508–509
        third-party payers, 507–508
    funding/support, 493
    marketing, 509–510
    overview, 491–493
    patient care considerations, 496–498
    patient-centered aspects, 510
    personnel
        administration of clinic, 498–500
        clinical faculty rank, 500–502
    physical facilities, 494–495
    referrals, 509
    service provision changes, 493–494

W

Walmart, 16, 526
WDH (William Demant Holding), 15, 16,
    526
Web sites
    AAA (American Academy of
        Audiology), 90
    salary reviews, 452
    ADA (Academy of Dispensing
        Audiologists), 90

Web sites *(continued)*
 billing codes, 294
 Blogger.com, 184
 Bureau of Labor Statistics, 95
 Business Plan Pro software, 72
 Center for Medicaid and Medicare
  Services (CMS) Fraud/Abuse, 95
 ClickPress.com, 186
 CMS ABN forms, 297
 CMS Fraud/Abuse, 95
 Ethical Practice Guideline for
  Relationships with Industry for
  Audiologist Providing Clinical
  Care (AAA), 110
 Ethical Practice Guidelines on
  Financial Incentives from Hearing
  Instrument Manufacturers (AAA
  & ADA), 110
 Facebook, 184

Health and Human Services (HHS)
  Information Privacy, 95
 hearing aid fees, itemization (AAA),
  304
 HearingPlanet, 139
 HIPAA (Health Insurance Portability
  and Accountability Act), 95
 HubPages.com, 185
 KnowThis marketing planning, 139
 LivePlan marketing planning, 139
 Medicare Fraud/Abuse, 95
 national debt clock, 8
 PressReleases.com, 186
 PRWeb, 186
 Squidoo.com, 185
 Twitter, 185–186
 Web 2.0 Web sites, 184–187
 WordPress.com, 185
 YouTube, 186